2003

The Jossey-Bass Health Series brings together the most current information and ideas in health care from the leaders in the field. Titles from the Jossey-Bass Health Series include these essential health care resources:

HEALTH ISSUES IN THE BLACK COMMUNITY

SECOND EDITION

Ronald L. Braithwaite
Sandra E. Taylor
Editors

Foreword by Rev. Jesse L. Jackson, Sr.

Jossey-Bass Publishers
San Francisco

Jossey-Bass books and products are available through most bookstores. To contact Jossey-Bass directly, call (888) 378-2537, fax to (800) 605-2665, or visit our website at www.josseybass.com.

Substantial discounts on bulk quantities of Jossey-Bass books are available to corporations, professional associations, and other organizations. For details and discount information, contact the special sales department at Jossey-Bass.

Printed in the United States of America.

Library of Congress Cataloging-in-Publication Data

Health issues in the black community / Ronald L. Braithwaite, Sandra E. Taylor, editors. — 2nd ed.
    p. cm. — (The Jossey-Bass health series)
  Includes bibliographical references and index.
  ISBN 0-7879-5236-2 (alk. paper)
    1. African Americans—Health and hygiene. [DNLM: 1. Blacks—United States.
  2. Health Status—United States. 3. Health Promotion—United States. 4. Social Problems—United States. WA 300 H433855 2001] I. Braithwaite, Ronald L., 1945–
II. Taylor, Sandra E., 1955– III. Title. IV. Series.
  RA448.5.N4 H395 2001
  362.1'089'96073—dc21

                                                          00-012798

SECOND EDITION
HB Printing   10 9 8 7 6 5 4 3 2 1

CONTENTS

To those who continue to work toward closing America's health gap

FOREWORD: ANOTHER CALL TO ACTION

In 1992, the first edition of *Health Issues in the Black Community* promulgated a "call to action" to address the health disparities documented in the 1985 *Report of the Secretary's Task Force on Black and Minority Health* from the U.S. Department of Health and Human Services. This report forecast 60,000 "excess deaths" for black and other minority citizens.

Sixteen years later, the health divide between the haves and the have-nots continues to grow, further marginalizing the well-being of African Americans. Ronald L. Braithwaite and Sandra E. Taylor and a host of contributing authors have offered challenges, strategies, and vision to examine the social, political, and economic factors that contribute to the leading causes of death in the black community. In doing so, they have issued another call to action.

Their vision lays the groundwork for this action. Without vision, the Bible says, the people perish. A grasshopper's vision is limited; its horizons are small. We must see ourselves as giants, with vision enough for an entire nation, not just part of it. The authors in this volume have offered their insights to help the nation grow.

The vision and courage of Martin Luther King Jr.—a black minister in the segregated South—made him a world leader. People sing "We Shall Overcome" in China, Poland, Indonesia, Africa, and Nicaragua. His words, his dream, incite passion across the globe. As we approach the new millennium, we must take stock of Dr. King's dream and honestly assess both the progress and the work that needs to be done.

Affirmative action has helped to put the majority in the room—women, blacks and browns, Asian Americans, Native Americans. We changed the room. We unlocked doors. We got a seat at the table. Equal treatment may not be completely achieved, but its value is beyond argument. We have lightened the burden of race. Examples of racism still abound, and discrimination has not been erased. But we can say with confidence and some pride, we have changed the room. We have lifted legal obstacles. That was the necessary first step. But it is not the last step.

Now that we've changed the room, it is time to change the house. Now we have to address the growing divide between upstairs and downstairs, between two nations—one affluent, one struggling; one with health insurance and the other without; one with access to quality health care and the other without; one locked in gated communities, one locked in dead-end neighborhoods. We must change the entire house, and to do so, we must recognize how it has been constructed.

Fourteen million American children—one in four—grow up in poverty, struggling for adequate food and shelter in the world's wealthiest nation. Welfare is down, but poverty is up. That is not right. Fifteen hundred Americans die every day from cancer. We possess the resources to boost research and end cancer as we know it; yet we fail to do so. That is not right.

Two million Americans are detained in our nation's jails and prisons—most of them are nonviolent substance abusing African American offenders. Rather than treat their disease of addiction, as part of their constitutional right to health care, we increase our budget to build more institutions, lining the walls of justice with catatonic men and women, incapable of breaking the chains of addiction and consequently discarded and spiritually deprived. That is not right.

Forty-seven million Americans without health insurance live just one serious illness away from financial ruin. This is not right. It's not right that African American suffer and die disproportionately because of higher rates of infant mortality, cancer, substance abuse, asthma, heart disease, diabetes, AIDS, and homicide. Blacks experience poorer nutrition, more untreated mental illness, more environmental exposure to toxins, and a lack of quality health care for elderly brothers and sisters.

These problems and challenges are immense and require the vision of giants, the creativity of geniuses, the energy of genies. We must see ourselves through a big door and not just through a tiny keyhole. We can no longer focus on one room and allow the larger house to fall. We must close the health disparity divide. We need a mandate for a national insurance policy that makes health care the right of everyone, not the privilege of the few.

The reaction to AIDS and other health epidemics has been too slow for too long. The stigma of AIDS, like any sexually transmitted disease, hampers efforts to educate people and treat the sick. "The first battle," as U.N. secretary general Kofi Annan has said, "to be won in the war against AIDS is the battle to smash the wall of silence and stigma surrounding it." America's leaders must do more. We must fight AIDS, both in the U.S. and in our motherland—Africa—the birthplace of our civilization. A continent rich with metals and precious stones. A continent full of rhyme and rhythm, a musical symphony describing in its harmony the gifts of human fulfillment.

As it is in Africa, AIDS is now the leading cause of death for African Americans between twenty-five and forty-four in the United States. Almost two-thirds (62 percent) of all women reported with AIDS are African American; 62 percent of all reported pediatric cases are African American children; 1 in 50 African American men and 1 in 160 African American women are estimated to be HIV infected. Like Africans, many African Americans do not know their HIV status; like Africans, many African Americans cannot access care and cannot afford adequate treatment. Like Africans, many African Americans are in poverty, and many of their communities lack the infrastructure needed to meet the needs of those infected and affected by AIDS. Simply speaking, as we begin to understand our commonalities, our differences will no longer be a continent away.

Presently, the United States is enjoying the longest economic expansion in its history. In this time of affluence, we have a duty to protect the next generation from premature illness and death. If we continue to allow people to die by the millions when we have the means to assist them, our failure to do the right thing will constitute a capital offense, a crime of malice.

Yet despite our resources and our ability to be good stewards, the media fixate on whether South African president Thabo Mbeki believes that HIV causes AIDS. The fact is that a Western orientation to treating AIDS in Africa may not necessarily be the best—or only—solution. We must ask critical questions. For example, what good are expensive drugs to a continent of destitute people? What good are complicated treatments to a continent without a health infrastructure? Why are the media spending so much time defending treatments that do not cure the disease, some of which are never delivered to the people with the disease? Why did it take so long for the drug companies to allow South Africa to approve generic drugs for treating AIDS? And what about the rest of the African continent?

There is more wealth in the world than ever before, more scientific knowledge about preventing and curing disease, yet many of the dreaded killers of our history—such as malaria and tuberculosis—are making a comeback while the modern plague of AIDS destroys Africa's hopes for a new century. As African Americans, we cannot stand by and let this plague roll on. This nation was built on the unpaid wages of slaves from the African continent. Our connections far outweigh our differences, and we must leverage our strength together.

We cannot separate Africa's attempt to address fundamental health challenges like AIDS from macroeconomic issues of poverty and crushing debt. Our legacy is to realize that despite our scientific efforts and interventions, poverty in and of itself threatens the social, economic, and political stability of all developed and undeveloped nations. And in order to stabilize HIV rates in sub-Saharan Africa, North America, Latin America, Western Europe, North Africa and the Middle East, Eastern Europe, and Central Asia, we must stabilize the growing rate of poverty. We cannot view these epidemics in isolation.

So many countries, constrained by limited national resources and significant debt repayment, are struggling just to provide basic education, clean drinking water, and primary health care. These are beyond the scope of any one of us, but they are not beyond the capacity of all of us together. When we come together and systematically address the callousness of poverty, we can then move beyond our errors of deliberate indifference.

So I invite you to leave the pages of this book with your mind made up. Let us decide to lift our sights. To revive our spirits. And to dedicate ourselves to contributing toward a new African and African American reality. We need to raise a moral challenge to this nation and this world. We can build a house with room for all.

What Shall We Tell Our Children in Fifty Years?

Tell them we always moved to a higher vision, to nonnegotiable ideals with faith in God. As long as we were morally centered and did not faint in the heat of battle, we prevailed. Tell them there are rivers and hills in front of us, but there are mountains and oceans behind us. Tell them we must choose the challenge of development over the rhetoric of despair. Tell them that we must resolve the contradiction between Wall Street and Harlem, decapitalized on the same island between the same two rivers in the same city. Tell them there was a health care gap and a life expectancy gap. Tell them that when Amidou Diallo is blown away by undisciplined police fire and Gideon Bush is blown away by overkill and there are attempts by the powers that be to offer justifications, the coalition of conscience had work to do. Yes, tell them that violence and institutional racism had implications for quality of life. Tell them, in the past tense let us hope, that violence was as American as apple pie. Tell them we had a major role in creating the dialogue that closed the health disparity gap.

Tell them the theme song of reflection in this century is that my mind reflects, my heart rejoices, how we got over. Hatred will lose; fear will be conquered. We have the courage to be. If we have the faith, God has the power. Let nothing separate us from the love of God or each other. Let nothing break our spirits. Let no one steal our joy. The road has been rocky, the hills have been steep. We made it. As a new century begins, as a new day dawns, we say with the writer, weeping endureth for a night, but joy cometh in the morning. It's morning time—it's hoping time—it's healing time. It has been a century of battles and scars and victories! We are winning every day.

Keep hope alive!

How Do We Build and Lead a Multiracial Coalition for Change?

We must focus not on that which divides us but on that which unites us. The ties that bind us together are strong and many: the need for comprehensive, affordable health care from birth to death; the need for investment in public education, from preschool to college; the need for good jobs, with good wages and benefits; the need to preserve a secure base for retirements; the need to make equal opportunity a reality not a promise; the need for a commitment to affordable housing and a decent environment; the need for a renewed emphasis on building strong families and strong communities, on valuing what we are rather than what we have.

Beyond color and culture, there lies the higher plateau of character. You inherit color and culture; you must earn character. Remain faithful. Remain optimistic. Remain enthusiastic. Remain young in outlook. Fight the good fight. Do justice. Leave no one behind. And always, keep hope alive!

When we fall behind, we suffer as a nation. We have fewer resources to devote to education and health care. We have fewer resources to care for the sick and needy. Diversity benefits us all. Inclusion is the key to growth. We do not need to create a whole host of new laws to close these gaps. We can start by enforcing and promoting those that are already on the books:

Leave no American behind. Keep hope alive!

About the Dash

We live life as if it is certain and death is uncertain. The fact is death is certain; life is uncertain. Upon your death and when your remains are taken to their final resting place, you will see in the City of the Dead on each tombstone a birth date and a date of death. But between those two numbers is a dash. You don't control or determine the birth date—where or when or to whom you are born. Nor the death date. But on that dash is where you must make your life's statement. Forces beyond our control determine the length of the dash.

I often feel that when an infant dies it is painful in part because the infant never knew the beauty or the challenges of life. When a very old person dies, there is reasonable anticipation, and you count the person's years and opportunities and accept it more readily. But when the dash is cut short, when the sun is eclipsed, we feel cheated. The length of the dash is uncertain. Jesus, thirty-three. Dr. King, thirty-nine. Princess Diana, thirty-six. Methuselah, nine hundred. He lived nine hundred years about nothing. There will be no schools or streets named after Methuselah. No one wants to wear his jersey or be identified with him. A long dash, but a journey devoid of substance.

You cannot determine the length of a dash, but you can determine the depth and the height. Jesus was born in a slum, yet he became King of Kings. The height of that dash is your achievements and the miles you covered.

Leave no American behind. Keep hope alive!

Washington, D.C.   Rev. Jesse L. Jackson, Sr.
April 2001   Founder and President
                                                                              Rainbow/PUSH Coalition

PREFACE

The first edition of *Health Issues in the Black Community* was released in 1992, evolving from our concerns about the many diseases and other health-related problems affecting the African American population. Almost ten years later, much like the widening digital divide in computer technology between the haves and the have-nots, the health status gap between disenfranchised and affluent citizens continues to widen. Hence the impetus for a second edition of *Health Issues in the Black Community* continues to be rooted in meeting the need for a readily accessible resource on an array of topics pertinent to African American health status and health disparities. Much like the first edition, this edition addresses contemporary health challenges confronting African Americans and discusses relevant strategies and policy implications for local, state, and federal governmental agencies as well as voluntary associations and community-based organizations.

Although this book is not intended to be an exhaustive treatment of all pertinent health problems affecting blacks, its twenty-six chapters provide information on some of the more salient health concerns that disproportionately affect this population as evidenced by the disparate morbidity and mortality indicators. Though the contributors present information from perspectives unique to their disciplines and professional experiences in research and practice, a common theme transcending the chapters is the need for demonstrative change if the black community is to achieve significantly improved health in the new millennium.

The purpose of this book is threefold: (1) to once again provide a forum for instigating debate and discussion on culturally relevant strategies and models for the prevention of disease and promotion of wellness in black communities; (2) to influence opinion leaders and provide a futuristic perspective on black health issues for students, academicians, public policymakers, and health administrators in the public health sciences and related disciplines; and (3) to document selected health conditions and advance viable strategies for ameliorating them. This volume's multidisciplinary perspective provides applicability across a wide range of areas. The disciplines of health education, public health, allied health, community health, nursing, nutrition, physical activity, psychology, medical sociology, medical anthropology, human services, social policy, social welfare, and ethics are all represented in the book. Many of the contributors are foremost experts in their fields.

Overview of the Contents

Part One, "Health Status Across the Life Span," sets the context by providing an overview of health issues pertinent to age and gender specific groups in the African American community. Chapter One introduces the breadth of African American health issues covered and outlines key demographic information. Chapter Two presents health status concerns for children and adolescents. Chapters Three and Four emphasize the health status of African American women and men, respectively. Chapter Five concludes this section with health concerns relevant to the black elderly. These chapters offer overviews of many diseases and conditions (for example, cancer, cardiovascular diseases, and diabetes) that are discussed in detail in the later chapters.

Part Two, "Social, Mental, and Environmental Challenges," addresses health-related dynamics in four areas. Chapter Six looks at the epidemiology of mental disorders over the fifteen-year period leading into the new millennium. Chapter Seven highlights the important and emerging role of the faith community in nurturing the basic health as well as the spiritual well-being of the population. Chapter Eight confronts the growing epidemic of intentional injuries in the black community. Chapter Nine discusses the culturally sensitive issue of organ and tissue donation and transplantation in the black community.

Part Three, "Chronic Diseases," reports on the status of several chronic disease areas that disproportionately affect African Americans. Chapter Ten covers the silent killer—hypertension—and heart disease and stroke. Chapter Eleven addresses cancer in the black community, and Chapter Twelve examines diabetes, commonly known as *sugar*. Chapter Thirteen covers sickle cell anemia and discusses new treatment breakthroughs. Chapter Fourteen addresses the re-emergence of tuberculosis, a new topic for *Health Issues in the Black Community*. The topic of Chapter Fifteen is also new in this edition, the prevalence of asthma in the black community.

Part Four, "Lifestyle Behaviors," draws attention to several self-defeating behaviors that negatively affect health status. In Chapter Sixteen, the devastating disease of HIV/AIDS and the behavioral modifications that can largely prevent it are discussed. Chapter Seventeen shows how tobacco is a major risk factor for numerous other diseases. Chapter Eighteen focuses on the use and abuse of illegal substances. The use and abuse of alcohol is discussed in Chapter Nineteen. Chapter Twenty addresses the importance of a balanced diet and good nutritional behaviors. Chapter Twenty-One captures the important role of physical activity as a health promoting behavior for African Americans.

Part Five, "Ethical, Political, and Ecological Issues," highlights several domains critical to improving the quality of life in African American communities. In Chapter Twenty-Two, environmental racism and justice issues are discussed. Chapter Twenty-Three revisits concepts of research ethics and African Americans' distrust of the medical establishment. Chapter Twenty-Four argues for a more responsive health policy. In Chapter Twenty-Five, the role of cultural relevancy in health promotion is examined, and Chapter Twenty-Six presents challenges for closing the gap and eliminating health disparities.

Again, a note is in order regarding the use of the terms *black* and *African American*. Both terms appear throughout this volume, in accordance with the preferences of the individual authors. The terms are used interchangeably in most chapters. Also, given the lack of consensus regarding the meaning of the terms *race* and *ethnicity*, the chapter authors tend to use them in combination, with the intent of covering all distinctions made by geographical regions of origin.

Finally, the chapters that make up this edition are not intended to be fully integrated. Rather, they are stand-alone contributions, consistent with our intention of offering a reference book or reader in the broad area of health issues for African Americans. It should also be noted that each chapter represents the views of its particular author or authors and in no way should be construed as representing a consensus of opinion among the contributors to this volume or the position of any affiliated organizations or agencies.

Acknowledgments

The second edition of *Health Issues in the Black Community* is the result of many dedicated persons' believing in a single mission of uplifting the health status of African Americans. We especially thank our contributing authors, who worked assiduously on the submission and revision of drafts. Recommendations from colleagues facilitated completion of this project and we remain grateful.

We are particularly indebted to Betty Stevens, who served as coordinating assistant for this effort. The research support of Alyssa Robillard, Miranda Lily, Sherene Brown, and Tara Ferebee-Harris was vital to the completion of this work. We also appreciate the technical support provided by Alexis Little, Shajuan Colbert, Lamonte Powell, Shalini Eddens, Robert Bailey, Kirsten Firla, and Keisha Cooper. The professional support of Torrance Stephens, and of Clair Sterk, chairperson of the Department of Behavioral Sciences and Health

Education in the Rollins School of Public Health of Emory University, has been invaluable in the completion of this work. We are also most appreciative to Lydia L. Watts, national director for HIV, Rainbow/PUSH Coalition, for her research contributions and assistance. Finally, we thank Jossey-Bass and its consummate professionalism for all aspects of support.

April 2001   Ronald L. Braithwaite
Atlanta, Georgia   Sandra E. Taylor

THE EDITORS

Ronald L. Braithwaite is a professor in the Department of Behavioral Sciences and Health Education at the Rollins School of Public Health of Emory University and is an adjunct professor in the Department of Community Health and Preventative Medicine at Morehouse School of Medicine, where he formerly directed a health promotion resource center. He received his B.A. (1967) and M.S. (1969) degrees from Southern Illinois University in sociology and rehabilitation counseling, respectively. He received his Ph.D. degree (1974) in educational psychology from Michigan State University. He has done postdoctoral studies at Howard University, Yale University, and the University of Michigan School of Public Health and Institute for Social Research.

Braithwaite has conducted evaluations of educational, health, and human service programs using several contemporary evaluation models. He has taught research design, statistics, program evaluation, testing and measurement, community organization, and minority health to nursing, medical, and public health students at the graduate level. Published widely in education and health journals, he is also coeditor of *Health Issues in the Black Community,* 1st edition (with S. E. Taylor, 1992), and *Prison and AIDS: A Public Health Challenge* (with Theodore M. Hammett and Robert M. Mayberry, 1996), and coauthor of *Building Health Coalitions in the Black Community* (with S. E. Taylor and J. N. Austin, 2000).

Braithwaite's work in community organization and development has gained national attention. He has also served as principal investigator for HIV/AIDS education and prevention programs in correctional settings funded by the Centers for Disease Control and Prevention, the federal Health Resources and Services Administration, and the Association of Schools of Public Health. He also serves as a senior justice fellow for the Center for the Study of Crime, Culture, and Communities at the Open Society Institute, and he has served as a consultant to numerous federal, state, and private organizations. His research involves both national and international HIV/AIDS intervention studies with juveniles and adults in correctional systems, substance abuse prevention, community coalition research, and mental health issues.

Sandra E. Taylor is a professor in the W.E.B. Du Bois Department of Sociology at Clark Atlanta University. Formerly, she headed the Department of Sociology and the Emory University School of Medicine's affiliate site of the Southeastern AIDS Training and Education Center (SEATEC) at Clark Atlanta University. She has held research appointments with the Nell Hodgson Woodruff School of Nursing and the Rollins School of Public Health of Emory University, where she currently serves as a visiting professor in the Department of Behavioral Sciences and Health Education. She received her B.A. degree (1977) in sociology from Norfolk State University, her M.A. degree (1978) in sociology from Atlanta University, and her Ph.D. degree (1983) in sociology from Washington University, and has done postdoctoral studies at the University of Michigan. She has studied abroad in the former East Germany and West Germany and in parts of West Africa.

Taylor's most recent publications are in the areas of health and illness with a specific focus on HIV/AIDS. Some of her recent research has been published in the *Journal of the National Medical Association,* the *Journal of Black Psychology, Patient Education and Counseling,* and the *Journal of Multicultural Counseling.* She is coeditor of *Health Issues in the Black Community,* 1st edition (with R. L. Braithwaite, 1992), and coauthor of *Building Health Coalitions in the Black Community* (with R. L. Braithwaite and J. N. Austin, 2000).

She has served as a consultant for various governmental and private sector initiatives and serves on the advisory boards of several health-related organizations. She also serves on the editorial or review boards for *Phylon, Race and Society,* and *Health Education and Behavior,* among other publications. Her current interests are the research and evaluation of community health programs and health promotion for inner-city youths and women.

THE CONTRIBUTORS

Hope E. Bannister manages a state-funded pregnancy prevention program located in Harlem, New York. Prior to that, she served as research coordinator at the Harlem Health Promotion Center, one of the prevention research centers funded by the Centers for Disease Control and Prevention. She received her B.A. degree (1993) in human biology from Brown University and her M.P.H. degree (1999) from Columbia University. She has authored several manuscripts on issues such as dating violence, violent crime, and emergency contraception as they affect adolescents.

Robert D. Bullard is Ware Professor of Sociology and director of the Environmental Justice Resource Center at Clark Atlanta University. His book *Dumping in Dixie: Race, Class, and Environmental Quality* (1994), is a standard text in the environmental justice field. A few of his related books are *Confronting Environmental Racism: Voices from the Grassroots* (1993), and *Unequal Protection: Environmental Justice and Communities of Color* (1996). He coedited *Just Transportation: Dismantling Race and Class Barriers to Mobility* (with G. S. Johnson, 1997). Bullard's latest book is *Sprawl City: Race, Politics, and Planning in Atlanta* (with G. S. Johnson, 2000). Bullard received his B.S. degree (1968) in government from Alabama A&M University, his M.A. degree (1972) in sociology from Atlanta University, and his Ph.D. degree (1976) in sociology from Iowa State.

Clive O. Callender is chairman of the Department of Surgery at Howard University Hospital and the first LaSalle D. Lefall Jr. Professor of Surgery at the Howard University College of Medicine. He is also the principal investigator for the national Minority Organ / Tissue Transplant Education Program (MOTTEP). He received his undergraduate degree from Hunter College, completed his M.D. degree (1963) at Meharry Medical College, surgical training at Freedmen's Hospital, transplant surgical training (kidney) at the University of Minnesota, and transplant surgical training (liver) at the University of Pittsburgh. Returning to Howard University Hospital in 1973, Callender helped develop the first minority-directed dialysis and transplant center and histocompatibility and immunogenetic laboratory in the United States.

Alwyn T. Cohall is associate professor of clinical public health and pediatrics at Columbia University's Mailman School of Public Health and the New York Presbyterian Hospital, where he is director of the Harlem Health Promotion Center, one of twenty-three prevention research centers funded by the Centers for Disease Control and Prevention. Additionally, Cohall is medical director of adolescent services at the Community Health Education Program of the Heilbrunn Center for Population and Family Health. He received his B.A. degree (1976) from Wesleyan University and his M.D. degree (1980) from the University of Medicine and Dentistry in New Jersey. Cohall has been instrumental in developing clinical care programs for youths in community centers, runaway and homeless shelters, and substance abuse residential treatment facilities. He has been a consulting physician at The Door and at Columbia University's Young Men's Clinic.

Giselle Corbie-Smith is assistant professor of social medicine and internal medicine at the University of North Carolina at Chapel Hill. She completed her M.D. degree (1991) at the Albert Einstein College of Medicine, trained as internal medicine intern, resident, and chief resident at the Yale University School of Medicine, and received her M.S. degree (2000) in clinical research at Emory University. Corbie-Smith's interest in minority health issues—especially access to care and the influence of culture, race, ethnicity, and social class on health—dates from early in her academic career. After she had completed her residency training, her interest in caring for underserved populations led her to take a faculty appointment at Grady Memorial Hospital, a public hospital that serves predominately poor, inner-city African American patients.

Thomas L. Creer is professor emeritus of psychology at Ohio University. Prior to assuming this position, he spent over a decade as coexecutive director of the National Asthma Center in Denver and director of the Behavioral Science Division at that center. Creer received a B.S. degree from Brigham Young University in 1956, an M.S. degree from Utah State University in 1961, and a Ph.D. degree from Florida State University in 1967. He has spent thirty-three years conducting research and writing widely published papers on chronic illness, particularly pediatric asthma. In recent years he has been interested in how patients can contribute to the control of their chronic illness by performing self-management skills. This research has been expanded from its original focus on asthma to include cystic fibrosis and renal transplantation.

M. Joycelyn Elders is professor emeritus of pediatrics in the Division of Endocrinology at the University of Arkansas Medical Sciences Center, Arkansas Children's Hospital. She received her M.D. degree in 1960 and her M.S. degree in 1964 from the University of Arkansas. Elders is author and coauthor of hundreds of professional publications in the areas of pediatrics, endocrinology, and public health. Elders is a former surgeon general of the United States (1993 to 1994) and an outspoken advocate for children's health. Prior to her stint in Washington, she was director of the Department of Health for Arkansas and served as president of Directors of Health of the United States.

Herman M. Ellis is associate professor and chair of the Department of Occupational and Preventive Medicine at Meharry Medical College and adjunct assistant professor in the Division of Environmental Sciences at the Columbia University School of Public Health. He received his B.S. degree (1971) from Manhattan College and his M.P.H. degree (1975) from the University of Michigan. He received his M.D. degree (1978) from Boston University School of Medicine. Presently, he is principal investigator on an HIV/AIDS grant from the Health Resources and Services Administration and Health Services Research Fellow of the Agency for Health Research and Quality. Ellis is vice chair of the American Association for World Health and a consultant to the National Conference of Black Mayors.

Angelina Esparza is community relations coordinator for the Center of Excellence for Research on Minority Health of the University of Texas M.D. Anderson Cancer Center. Esparza received her B.A. degree (1991) in psychology and anthropology from the University of Houston and was formerly employed with the Baylor College of Medicine Lipid Research Clinic. She has previously coauthored chapters on community outreach and health disparities. She is vice president of the Houston-based Hispanic Health Coalition, Inc., and a member of numerous boards and committees that promote equity in health for all populations.

Joyce Essien is a commissioned officer in the Public Health Service at the Centers for Disease Control and Prevention and the director of the Center for Public Health Practice at the Rollins School of Public Health, Emory University. She earned her B.S. degree (1969) and her M.D. degree (1971) from Wayne State University, and her M.B.A. degree (1988) from Georgia State University. Her career in medicine spans the fields of academic medicine, industry, and public health. She and her colleagues are engaged in interdisciplinary and applied research and capacity building to create systems of health that sustain improvements in population health. She has served on the boards of Exodus, Georgians for Children, and Agnes Scott College. She is a 1999 recipient of one of ten Women in Government Awards sponsored by *Good Housekeeping* magazine, the Council for Excellence in Government, the Rutgers Center for American Women and Politics, and the Ford Foundation for her work with Zap Asthma Consortium.

John M. Flack currently serves as professor and associate chairman for Clinical Research and Urban Health Outcomes of the Department of Internal Medicine, director of the Cardiovascular Epidemiology and Clinical Operations Program (CECA), and program director of the Academic Hospitalist Program (internal medicine hospital training and practice support program) in the Department of Internal Medicine at Wayne State University. He is also chief of medicine for the Detroit Medical Center Central Region Hospitals and vice president of the medical staff at Vector Hospital in Detroit. He received his B.S. degree (1978) in chemistry from Langston University and his M.D. degree (1982) from the University of Oklahoma Health Sciences Center, where he also completed an internal medicine residency and chief medical residency.

Robert L. Geller is associate professor of pediatrics at Emory University School of Medicine and also Chief of Pediatrics at Grady Health System in Atlanta. His clinical activities are focused on toxicological, asthma, and environmental issues, and he provides care for children in the Hughes Spalding Children's Hospital Pediatric Asthma Center. Geller received his M.D. degree (1979) from the Boston University School of Medicine.

Marcia Griffith, an employee of the Centers for Disease Control and Prevention, currently serves as program manager for ZAP Asthma Consortium, Inc., a position she has held since October 1997. She received her B.S. degree (1965) in health education from Brooklyn College, and an M.P.H. degree (1969) from Columbia University. Her areas of interest include maternal and child health and applied research. Griffith has worked extensively in program management and community development, especially in underserved communities.

Margruetta B. Hall is senior evaluator and owner of MBH Limited: Evaluation Research Services in Silver Spring, Maryland. She is principal program evaluation consultant to the national Minority Organ/Tissue Transplant Education Program (MOTTEP) at Howard University. Since 1989, she has served as principal researcher on several significant research projects focusing on organ donation and transplantation in the minority community. She received her B.S. (1967) and M.S. (1970) degrees in social psychology from Howard University, and her Ph.D. degree (1997) in evaluation research from the Union Institute Graduate School of Interdisciplinary Studies.

W. Rodney Hammond is director of the Division of Violence Prevention and Distinguished Science Fellow at the Centers for Disease Control and Prevention in Atlanta. He completed his Ph.D. degree (1974) in psychology at Florida State University and his postdoctoral study at Harvard University in Cambridge, Massachusetts. His professional and scientific efforts have focused on youth homicide and violence prevention as a public health concern. He developed Positive Adolescent Choices Training (PACT), a school-based prevention program distinguished by its successful outcome evaluations among at-risk youth. He is author and executive producer of the series *Dealing with Anger: A Violence Prevention Program for African American Youth,* which has been nationally recognized for its contribution to effective community programs and its application to persons at high risk.

Frederick D. Harper is professor of counseling in the School of Education at Howard University and managing editor of the *International Journal for the Advancement of Counseling.* He is also a former editor of the *Journal of Multicultural Counseling and Development.* He received a Ph.D. degree (1970) in counselor education from Florida State University and served as a research Fellow with the National Institute of Alcohol Abuse and Alcoholism. He has written a number of articles and books on alcohol and other drugs as they relate to African Americans, including *The Black Family and Substance Abuse* (1986) and *Alcoholism Treatment and Black Americans* (1979).

Sandra W. Headen is executive director of the National African American Tobacco Prevention Network and a community intervention consultant with the North Carolina Tobacco Prevention and Control Branch. She received her B.A. degree (1969) from Bennett College and her Ph.D. degree (1982) from Boston College. For twelve years, Headen was affiliated with the University of North Carolina at Chapel Hill as a faculty member in the Department of Health Behavior and Health Education and as a research associate in the Center for Health Promotion and Disease Prevention. Her work has focused on the health of youths and African Americans in the areas of diabetes and of tobacco and other substance abuse prevention, and on innovative approaches to smoking cessation for African American adults.

María A. Hernández-Valero is a National Cancer Institute postdoctoral fellow under the mentorship of Lovell A. Jones at the University of Texas M. D. Anderson Cancer Center, Center of Excellence for Research on Minority Health. She received her Ph.D. degree in 1996 from the University of Texas at Houston. She uses environmental and occupational epidemiology to assess the role of environmental and occupational exposures in the etiology of diseases, including cancer. Her research interest is cancer prevention among minority populations, and she currently conducts research among the underrepresented population of migrant farm workers.

M. Katherine Hutchinson is a postdoctoral fellow in the Center for Urban Health Research and the Center for Health Outcomes and Policy Research at the University of Pennsylvania School of Nursing. She received her B.S.N. degree (1979) from Michigan State University and her M.S. (1984) and Ph.D. (1994) degrees from the University of Delaware. Her research focuses on the influence of sexual partners and family structure and process variables on adolescents' and young adults' sexual risk behaviors and use of sexual protective strategies including condoms. She has presented and published numerous data-based papers on sexual communication between parents and teens and between young women and their sexual partners.

James S. Jackson is Daniel Katz Distinguished University Professor of Psychology, director of the Research Center for Group Dynamics and senior research scientist at the Institute for Social Research, professor of health behavior and health education in the School of Public Health, director of the Center for Afro-American and African Studies, and faculty associate at the Institute of Gerontology at the University of Michigan. He received his Ph.D. degree (1972) in social psychology from Wayne State University and has been a faculty member at the University of Michigan since 1971. In 1990, he helped establish and continues to direct the African American Mental Health Research Program, funded by the National Institute of Mental Health. His research interests and areas of publication include race and ethnic relations, health and mental health, adult development and aging, attitudes and attitude change, and African American politics.

Kimberly R. Jacob Arriola is a senior faculty associate in the Department of Behavioral Sciences and Health Education at the Rollins School of Public Health at Emory University. She completed her undergraduate work at Spelman College with a B.A. degree (1994) in psychology. She completed her M.A. (1996) and Ph.D. (1998) degrees in social psychology at Northeastern University in Boston. Her research interests are in the area of HIV/AIDS prevention among minority populations.

John B. Jemmott III received his Ph.D. degree (1982) in psychology from the Department of Psychology and Social Relations, Harvard University. From 1981 to 1999, he served as instructor, assistant professor, associate professor, and professor of psychology at Princeton University. He is currently Kenneth B. Clark Professor of Communication and director of the Center for Health Behavior and Communication at the Annenberg School for Communication of the University of Pennsylvania. Jemmott is a Fellow of the American Psychological Association and the Society for Behavioral Medicine. He has served on the Behavioral Medicine Study Section and the AIDS and Immunology Research Review Committee and is currently a member of the Office of AIDS Research Advisory Council of the National Institutes of Health (NIH). He has been the recipient of numerous NIH grants to conduct research designed to develop and test HIV risk-reduction interventions for inner-city African American populations.

Loretta Sweet Jemmott is associate professor and director of the Center for Urban Health Research at the University of Pennsylvania School of Nursing and holds a secondary appointment in the Graduate School of Education. Jemmott received her M.S.N. degree with a specialization in psychiatric mental health nursing in 1982, and her Ph.D. degree in education with a specialization in human sexuality education from the University of Pennsylvania in 1987. Since 1987, Jemmott's research has focused on designing and testing theory-based, culturally sensitive, and developmentally appropriate strategies to reduce HIV risk-associated sexual behaviors among African American and Latino populations. She has directed multiple HIV risk-reduction research projects and has published extensively in the areas of HIV/AIDS prevention and adolescent sexual behavior. Jemmott is a Fellow of the American Academy of Nursing and a member of the National Institute of Nursing Research Advisory Council and the Institute of Medicine.

Glenn S. Johnson received his Ph.D. in 1996 from the University of Tennessee. He is currently a research associate in the Environmental Justice Resource Center and assistant professor in the Department of Sociology at Clark Atlanta University. He coordinates several major research activities into fields including transportation, urban sprawl, smart growth, public involvement, facility siting, and toxics. He has worked on environmental policy issues for eight years and assisted Robert D. Bullard in the research for the book *Dumping in Dixie: Race, Class, and Environmental Quality* (1994). He is the coeditor of a book entitled *Just Transportation: Dismantling Race and Class Barriers to Mobility* (1997). His most recent book, coedited with Robert D. Bullard and Angel O. Torres, is entitled *Sprawl City: Race, Politics, and Planning in Atlanta* (2000).

Lovell A. Jones is professor in the Departments of Gynecologic Oncology and Biochemistry and Molecular Biology at the University of Texas M.D. Anderson Cancer Center and serves on the graduate faculty of the University of Texas Graduate School for Biomedical Sciences. Since 1988, he has served as director of the Experimental Gynecology/Endocrinology Center. In January 2000, he was named as the first director of the congressionally mandated Center of Excellence for Research on Minority Health. He received his Ph.D. degree (1977) in zoology with an emphasis in endocrinology and tumor biology from the University of California, Berkeley. Jones has published over one hundred scientific articles on topics ranging from hormonal carcinogenesis to health policy. He is the founding chair of the Biennial Symposium Series on Minorities, the Medically Underserved, and Cancer as well as the founding cochair of the Intercultural Cancer Council, the nation's largest multicultural health policy group focused on minorities, the medically underserved, and cancer.

Shiriki K. Kumanyika is professor of epidemiology and associate dean for health promotion and disease prevention at the University of Pennsylvania School of Medicine. She received her B.A. degree (1965) in psychology from Syracuse University, her M.S. degree (1969) in social work from Columbia University, her Ph.D. degree (1978) in human nutrition from Cornell University, and her M.P.H. degree (1984) from the Johns Hopkins University School of Hygiene and Public Health. Her research interests include the epidemiology and management of obesity and the role of obesity, sodium intake, and other dietary factors in chronic diseases, particularly in African American and older adult populations.

Robert S. Levine is professor of occupational and preventive medicine at Meharry Medical College. He received his B.A. degree (1963) from Columbia University and his M.D. degree (1968) from the Bowman Gray School of Medicine. He completed an internship in pediatrics at North Carolina Baptist Hospital and a residency in general preventive medicine at the University of Kentucky School of Medicine. He became a Fellow of the American College of Preventive Medicine in 1975. Since then, Levine has worked primarily in academic settings, first at the University of Miami School of Medicine and currently at Meharry Medical College.

Navdeep K. Mann is a third-year resident in the Department of Internal Medicine at Wayne State University. She attended medical school at Glancy Medical College in Amritsar, India, graduating with honors in 1997, and ranking among the top candidates in the entire country. She has conducted research in hypertension and renin-angiotensin-aldosterone systems and is currently doing research in immunology, focusing on the role of cathepsins and metastasis.

William J. McCarthy is adjunct associate professor of psychology at University of California-Los Angeles (UCLA) and associate researcher at the UCLA Cancer Center. He received his Ph.D. degree in 1980 from Yale University. His published research has included over fifty scientific papers on tobacco use cessation, correlates of tobacco use behavior, adopting low-fat diets, and decreasing cancer risk through a combination of increased physical activity and increased fruit and vegetable intake. He teaches graduate classes on health-related lifestyle change. He was the 1994 recipient of the Health Fitness Leader award of the Los Angeles County Board of Supervisors for his career of public service in promoting healthier lifestyle choices.

Chanda Nicole Mobley is a Dr.P.H. degree candidate in maternal and child health at the University of Alabama at Birmingham. She received her B.A. degree (1993) in psychology from San Diego State University, and her M.P.H. degree (1996) in behavioral sciences and health education from the Rollins School of Public Health at Emory University. She is a certified health education specialist and has worked extensively for several years in the areas of asthma health education and the development of asthma self-management skills, particularly in minority, underserved children and their families. She has also authored numerous articles and professional presentations on this subject.

Frederick G. Murphy is adjunct professor in the Department of Research at Oakwood College in Huntsville, Alabama, in the Department of Community Health and Preventive Medicine at Morehouse School of Medicine, and in the Department of Health Sciences at Georgia State University. His professional work is in the field of community organization and health promotion, and he is currently working on several community-based public health research projects as a public health consultant. Murphy holds both an M.S.P.H. degree (1977) and an M.P.I.A. degree (1977) from the Graduate School of International Affairs and an M.S.P.H. degree (1977) from the Graduate School of Public Health at the University of Pittsburgh.

Harold W. Neighbors is associate professor of health behavior and health education in the School of Public Health at the University of Michigan. He is also associate director for research training with the Center for Research on Ethnicity, Culture, and Health (CRECH) in the School of Public Health, where he is the principal investigator of the NIH-funded CRECH doctoral training program, Promoting Ethnic Diversity in Public Health Training. He also directs the school's Paul B. Cornely Postdoctoral Program and the CRECH Summer Public Health Scholars Program for Undergraduates. Neighbors has been an adjunct research scientist in the Program for Research on Black Americans in the Research Center for Group Dynamics at the Institute for Social Research since 1985. He received his Ph.D. degree (1982) in social and community psychology from the University of Michigan. His research interests and areas of publication include psychiatric epidemiology, with an emphasis on ethnic and cultural influences on the assessment (diagnosis and case finding) of mental disorder and the use of informal and professional services by African Americans.

Angela Odoms is a postdoctoral Fellow in the Community Health Scholars Program at the University of Michigan School of Public Health. She received a B.S. degree (1990) in foods and nutrition from the University of Illinois at Urbana-Champaign and M.S. (1994) and Ph.D. (1999) degrees in human and community nutrition from Cornell University. Her current research interests include examining social and cultural factors that influence dietary behaviors and chronic disease risk in African Americans, partnerships with faith communities in health promotion, and the use of the lay health adviser model in community-based research.

Deborah Prothrow-Stith serves as associate dean for faculty development as well as director and professor of the Division of Public Health Practice at the Harvard School of Public Health. She received her B.A. degree in 1975 from Spelman College and her M.D. degree in 1979 from Harvard Medical School. As a physician working in inner-city hospitals and neighborhood clinics, she recognizes violence as a significant public health issue. Appointed in 1987 as the first woman and youngest ever Commissioner of Public Health for the Commonwealth of Massachusetts, Prothrow-Stith expanded treatment programs for AIDS and drug rehabilitation. A chief spokesperson for a national movement to prevent violence, Prothrow-Stith developed and wrote the Violence Prevention Curriculum for Adolescents, the first such curriculum for schools and communities, and coauthored *Deadly Consequences* (with M. Weissman, 1991).

Sandra Crouse Quinn is an associate professor in the Department of Health Services Administration at the Graduate School of Public Health, University of Pittsburgh. Her research focuses on HIV prevention and policy, the history of public health activities in the African American community, and ethics. She received her Ph.D. degree (1993) in health education from the University of Maryland, College Park.

Preeti Ramappa is a research assistant at Wayne State University. She received her B.A. degree (1990) in natural sciences from the Marimallappa Junior College and her M.D. degree (1996) from J.S.S. Medical College. She served as a senior house officer at the coronary care unit in the department of internal medicine at J.S.S. Hospital in India.

Jaiwant K. Rangi is a first-year resident in the Department of Internal Medicine at Wayne State University, Detroit Medical Center. Rangi received her M.B.B.S. degree (1995) in medicine and surgery from Lady Harding Medical College in New Delhi, India. She worked as an internist with the Cardiovascular Epidemiology and Clinical Applications Program at Pal Hospital in Rajasthan before coming to the United States.

Ken Resnicow is a professor in the Department of Behavioral Sciences and Health Education at the Emory University Rollins School of Public Health. Prior to joining Emory, he was chief of child health and special populations research at the American Health Foundation in New York. His research interests include the design and evaluation of health promotion programs for special populations, particularly cardiovascular and cancer prevention interventions for African Americans; the relationship between ethnicity and health behaviors; substance use prevention and harm reduction; motivational interviewing for chronic disease prevention; and comprehensive school health programs. Resnicow is conducting several federally funded interventions to increase fruit and vegetable intake among African Americans recruited through black churches; an after-school substance use prevention program designed to test the effects of Afrocentric compared to traditional substance use prevention strategies; and a study to develop an obesity prevention program for overweight African American adolescent females.

Robert G. Robinson is associate director for program development of the Office on Smoking and Health, National Center for Chronic Disease Prevention and Health Promotion, Centers for Disease Control and Prevention (CDC). He has also served on editorial boards and in volunteer capacities for the American Cancer Society. Robinson holds a B.A. degree (1967) from the City University of New York, an M.S.W. degree (1969) from Adelphi University, and M.P.H. (1977) and Dr.P.H. (1983) degrees from the University of California at Berkeley. In his capacity at CDC, Robinson has developed national programs that target the needs of communities of color, women, blue-collar and agricultural workers, gays and lesbians, low-income individuals and families, and youths. In addition, he has developed policy and program initiatives for South America and sub-Saharan Africa. Robinson currently has a special focus on the problem of population disparities in public health. His work to further our understanding and knowledge of the underpinnings of race, community, and cultural competence is helping to advance models that may influence efforts to eliminate population differences and advance the nation further along the paths of equity and social justice.

Deborah Rohm Young is assistant professor of medicine in the Division of Internal Medicine of the Department of Medicine at the Johns Hopkins School of Medicine and a faculty member of the Welch Center for Prevention, Epidemiology, and Clinical Research. She holds a B.S. degree (1978) in kinesiology and an M.B.A. degree (1984) in business administration from UCLA, and a Ph.D. degree (1991) in health education from the University of Texas at Austin. She is an exercise epidemiologist with research experience and publications in physical activity assessment in community-based populations, evaluation of health benefits associated with physical activity, and determinants of and adherence to physical activity behavior. Her current research work involves conducting physical activity interventions in community settings, with a particular focus on African American populations.

Sherrill L. Sellers is an assistant professor in the School of Social Work at Florida State University and an adjunct faculty associate at the University of Michigan, Institute for Social Research. She holds M.A. degrees in social service from the University of Chicago (1992) and in sociology from the University of Michigan (1996), and received her Ph.D. degree from the joint social work and sociology program at the University of Michigan (2000). Her research interests include the life course, health consequences of social inequalities, and intergenerational relations. Her specialization is in gender, social mobility, and mental health.

Tony L. Strickland is associate dean for research in the College of Medicine, professor of psychiatry, and program director of the Memory Disorders and Cerebral Function Clinic at Charles R. Drew University of Medicine and Science. He is also associate professor of psychiatry-in-residence of the Neuropsychiatric Institute at the UCLA School of Medicine. He received his Ph.D. degree (1986) in clinical psychology (behavioral medicine) from the University of Georgia and completed his postdoctoral fellowship training in clinical neuropsychology at the Neuropsychiatric Institute of the UCLA School of Medicine. Strickland has extensive clinical and research experience in the areas of cerebral blood flow and neurobehavioral sequelae of substance abuse, ethnobiological variations in response to psychotropics, head trauma, and forensic neuropsychological evaluation.

Wendell C. Taylor is associate professor of behavioral sciences and the convener of the Behavioral Sciences Discipline at the University of Texas-Houston Health Science Center, School of Public Health, and Center for Health Promotion and Prevention Research. He is also adjunct associate professor in the College of Education Graduate Studies at the University of Houston and adjunct associate professor in the Department of Communications at Texas Southern University. He received his A.B. degree (1972) in psychology from Grinnell College, his M.S. degree (1974) in psychology from Eastern Washington University, his Ph.D. degree (1984) in social psychology from Arizona State University, and his M.P.H. degree (1989) from the University of Texas-Houston Health Science Center, School of Public Health. Taylor also completed a two-year postdoctoral fellowship in health promotion and health education at the Center for Health Promotion Research and Development, University of Texas. His research interests include health promotion in children and adolescents, physical activity and public health, cancer prevention, and health behaviors in underserved communities.

Stephen B. Thomas is director of the Center for Minority Health, the Philip Hallen Professor of Community Health and Social Justice in the Graduate School of Public Health, and professor in the School of Social Work at the University of Pittsburgh. Thomas received his B.S. degree (1980) from Ohio State University, his M.S. degree (1981) from Illinois State University, and his Ph.D. degree (1985) in community health from Southern Illinois University in Carbondale. Over the past fifteen years, he has applied his expertise in behavioral science and health education in the African American community, addressing several critical public health issues including HIV/AIDS, youth violence, substance abuse, and the need for more organ and tissue donations from African Americans.

Bailus Walker Jr. is professor of environmental and occupational medicine and of health policy and management at Howard University Medical Center. He is also director of the Joint Center for Political and Economic Studies. Walker holds an M.A. degree (1959) from the University of Michigan and a Ph.D. degree (1975) from the University of Minnesota. From 1994 to 1996, during the comprehensive health care reform debate in Congress, Walker was an American Public Health Association Health Policy Fellow in Congress, and later served as health policy advisor to Representative Louis Stokes of Ohio. In 1999, he was named chairman of the Black Caucus of Health Workers of the American Public Health Association. Walker is a Distinguished Fellow of the American College of Epidemiology.

Rueben C. Warren is associate administrator for Urban Affairs at the Agency for Toxic Substances and Disease Registry, U.S. Department of Health and Human Services, and adjunct professor at the Morehouse School of Medicine, at the Rollins School of Public Health at Emory University, and at Meharry Medical

College. Warren holds a B.A. degree (1968) from San Francisco State University, a D.D.S. degree (1972) from Meharry Medical College, and M.P.H. (1973) and Dr.P.H. (1975) degrees from the Harvard School of Public Health. He has published in the areas of public health, health education, and health services research. His current professional activities focus on public health issues in the areas of minority health, brownfields, and environmental justice.

Charles F. Whitten is currently Distinguished Professor of Pediatrics Emeritus and associate dean for Special Programs (part-time) for the Wayne State University School of Medicine. He received his A.B. degree (1942) in zoology from the University of Pennsylvania and his M.D. degree (1945) from Meharry Medical College. He has served as associate dean for curricular affairs and director of the Wayne State University Comprehensive Sickle Cell Center, sponsored by the National Institutes of Health, and he was one of two founders of the National Association for Sickle Cell Disease (now known as the Sickle Cell Disease Association of America) and served as its president and leader. He is also the founder and continuing president of the Sickle Cell Detection and Information Program of Detroit.

David R. Williams is professor of sociology, senior research scientist at the Institute for Social Research, and faculty associate in the African American Mental Health Research Center and the Center for Afro-American and African Studies at the University of Michigan. Previously, he was associate professor of sociology at Yale University and associate professor of public health in the Yale School of Medicine. He holds an M.P.H. degree (1981) from Loma Linda University and a Ph.D. degree (1986) from the University of Michigan. Williams currently serves on the editorial board of five scientific journals. He is interested in the determinants of socioeconomic and racial differences in mental and physical health. His research has examined the extent to which social and psychological factors—ranging from stress, racism, social support, and religious behavior to psychological resources and health behaviors—are linked to social status and may explain socioeconomic and racial variations in health.

Donella J. Wilson joined the American Cancer Society as scientific program director in January 1993. Prior to that, Wilson was an associate professor at Meharry Medical College for eight years. While at Meharry, she conducted research on sickle cell anemia and malaria and taught cell and molecular biology to graduate and medical students. She received a B.A. degree (1973) in biochemistry from Johnston College at Redlands University, California; an M.S. degree (1977) in immunogenetics from Texas Southern University; and a second M.S. degree (1979) and a Ph.D. degree (1981) in molecular biology from Purdue University. She completed postdoctoral studies at Harvard Medical School, M.I.T., and the Whitehead Institute.

Anne E. Streaty Wimberly is currently professor of Christian education at the Inter-denominational Theological Center (ITC). She received her B.S. degree (1957) in education from Ohio State University, an M.M.S. degree (1965) from Boston University, an M.T.S. degree (1993) from Garrett-Evangelical Theological Seminary, a graduate certificate (1979) in gerontology from Georgia State University, and a Ph.D. degree (1981) in educational leadership with a cognate in gerontology from Georgia State University. Wimberly is the author of *Soul Stories* (1994) and *Honoring African American Elders: A Ministry in the Soul Community* (1997).

Antronette K. Yancey is director of chronic disease prevention and health promotion for the Los Angeles County Department of Health Services and adjunct associate professor in the Department of Community Health Sciences at the UCLA School of Public Health. Yancey has directed numerous community health promotion projects targeting nutrition, physical activity, smoking, cancer screening behavior, and adolescent identity development. In addition to a number of scientific publications in the public health literature, she has written many lay articles and book chapters on self-image and physical activity and fitness. She completed her undergraduate work at Northwestern University in biochemistry and molecular biology (1979) and received her M.D. degree (1982) from Duke University School of Medicine and an M.P.H. degree (1991) from the UCLA School of Public Health.

HEALTH ISSUES IN
THE BLACK COMMUNITY

PART ONE

HEALTH STATUS
ACROSS THE LIFE SPAN

CHAPTER ONE

AFRICAN AMERICAN HEALTH

An Overview

Sandra E. Taylor, Ronald L. Braithwaite

This second edition of *Health Issues in the Black Community* echoes many of the points presented in the first edition. It continues to be not only a reference work on African American health but a call to action to address the ever-widening gap in health status between blacks and whites in the United States. Toward this end, selected health conditions and issues are presented, based on research and replete with practical solutions and recommendations. Many of the data and suggested strategies presented in 1992 remain virtually unchanged. Although a few improvements have occurred in the overall health status of African Americans, the scientific body of health data shows that blacks continue to lack parity (and are not even close to parity) with their white counterparts. As the United States celebrates its status as a global superpower in the new millennium, rigorous action must be directed to these health disparities if America is to be heralded as a genuine world leader.

The elimination of these disparities will require a composite of strategies including enhanced efforts at preventing disease, promoting overall health, and delivering appropriate care. The U.S. Department of Health and Human Services (DHHS) is focusing on six areas in which racial and ethnic minorities experience serious disparities in health access and outcomes: infant mortality, cancer screening and management, cardiovascular disease, diabetes, HIV/AIDS, and immunizations. This book devotes a chapter each to cancer, diabetes, hypertension, and HIV/AIDS, and all six areas are discussed to some extent throughout the book. The disparities in access and outcomes in these six areas apply to multiple racial and ethnic groups, including African Americans, Hispanics, Asian Americans and Pacific Islanders, and American Indians and Alaskan Natives. The attention of the DHHS to improvements in research as well as to action signals hope for all the racial and ethnic minority groups experiencing health disparities in the United States.

National Efforts Toward Closing the Gap

The national prevention initiative to improve the health of all Americans, Healthy People 2000 (U.S. Department of Health and Human Services [DHHS], 1991), and more recently Healthy People 2010 (DHHS, 2000a), is inextricably linked to President Bill Clinton's Initiative for One America, his Initiative on Race, and especially, his Initiative on Race and Health. This latter initiative is a much-needed step toward the action advocated by *Health Issues in the Black Community*. Along with DHHS, the U.S. surgeon general, David Satcher, and the assistant secretary for planning and evaluation, Margaret Hamburg, have taken on leadership roles in this noble effort. Given assurances of more rigorous research coupled with action strategies and the development of partnerships, African Americans and other groups sharing a disproportionate health burden can look to a brighter day. However, as discussed in many of the following chapters, making black America a healthier community is contingent upon everyone's sharing in the responsibility. Given the legacy of slavery and the subsequent institutionalized discrimination that still plagues African Americans, it is incumbent that a strategy such as the President's Initiative on Race and Health be actualized. A commitment to this and similar efforts can make a difference in the quest for "One America" (DHHS, 2000b; see also The White House, 2000).

It is well known that a number of factors affect a person's health status, including income, occupation, education, environment, and access to services. It has been further established that an additional factor, race, also has an impact (West, 1994). Both practitioners and research scientists argue that the disparity between black and white health is a function of the former's overrepresentation in lower socioeconomic groups. We do know, however, that when many of these variables, including income, are held constant, a difference between black and white health status still surfaces. Hence we arrive at an impetus for strongly following through on the President's Initiative on Race and Health. The evidence that race correlates with persistent health disparities among different populations in the United States rightly demands the attention of the policymakers and local, state, and national health and human service agency heads.

Selected Demographics

Before viewing some of the health conditions suffered by African Americans, it is helpful to put in context the numbers of this group, looking at how African Americans fare in comparison to nonblack groups. Table 1.1 depicts the black

TABLE 1.1. RESIDENT POPULATION ESTIMATES
OF THE UNITED STATES BY SEX AND RACE/ETHNICITY.

	Sept. 1, 2000	July 1, 1999	July 1, 1998	July 1, 1997	July 1, 1996	July 1, 1995
All races						
Population all ages	275,617	272,691	270,248	267,784	265,229	262,803
Median age (years)	35.8	35.5	35.2	34.9	34.7	34.3
Mean age (years)	36.5	36.4	36.2	36.1	35.9	35.8
Male population	134,402	133,277	132,030	130,783	129,504	128,294
Female population	140,510	139,414	138,218	137,001	135,724	134,510
Black						
Population	35,268	34,862	34,427	33,989	33,537	33,116
(Percentage of total)	(12.8)	(12.8)	(12.7)	(12.7)	(12.6)	(12.6)
Median age (years)	30.3	30.1	29.9	29.7	29.5	29.2
Mean age (years)	32.2	32.1	31.9	31.7	31.5	31.3
Male population	16,757	16,557	16,342	16,127	15,907	15,706
Female population	18,511	18,305	18,085	17,863	17,630	17,411

Note: Numbers in thousands. Estimates are consistent with 1990 population estimates base.

Source: U.S. Census Bureau, 2000, p. 1.

population and its growth from 1995 to 2000 as compared to all races (including whites; blacks; Hispanics; American Indians, Eskimos, and Aleuts; and Asian Americans and Pacific Islanders). These data depict a gradual positive growth in mean and median longevity for African Americans from July 1995 to June 2000; however, the black-white health disparity gap continues to persist.

In addition to answering the reader's questions about the general demographics of African Americans, these data provide a backdrop for the chapters on the health of black men and black women. The following data highlights, from DeBarros and Bennett (1997) of the U.S. Census Bureau, provide further insights into this population.

- In 1997, the black population was estimated at 34.2 million and represented 12.8 percent of the total population.
- In 1997, there were 8.5 million black families; of these, 3.7 million, or 46 percent, were married couple families.
- In 1997, nearly three-fourths (74 percent) of all black individuals twenty-five years old and over had at least a high school education; about 14 percent had at least a bachelor's degree.
- In 1996, black families had a real median income of $26,520.
- In 1996, the median earnings of black women and men working year-round and full time were $21,470 and $26,400, respectively, for a female-to-male earnings ratio of 0.81.

- In 1996, 2.1 million, or 26 percent, of black families had income below the poverty level.

Morbidity and Mortality

According to data from the National Center for Health Statistics, morbidity measures, the percentage of persons with activity limitations due to a chronic condition, have remained stable from 1990 to 1996, as has the percentage of persons reporting fair or poor health status. As family income decreases, the percentage of persons reporting fair or poor health or reporting activity limitations increases (National Center for Health Statistics [NCHS], 2000). Data for 1998 mortality rates continued to vary by race with age-adjusted death rates for the African American population exceeding those for the white population by 53 percent, a narrowing from about 55 percent in 1997 (a shift in the optimal direction). Between 1994 and 1997, the birthrate for unmarried women declined almost 11 percent for African American mothers, to 73.4 births per 1,000 unmarried black women aged fifteen to forty-four (another positive shift). However, among leading causes of death, the largest race differential was for homicide, which was nearly six times higher for African Americans than for the white population. The next highest race differential was for hypertension, with a rate nearly four times higher for African Americans than for white persons. Conversely, African Americans had lower rates for three leading causes of death—lung disease, suicide, and Alzheimer's disease (NCHS, 2000).

In the same NCHS report, life expectancy was reported to have increased to a record high of 76.7 years in 1998, up from 76.5 in 1997. A fifteen-year-old in 1998 could expect to live to be 77.5 years, a full year longer than a fifteen-year-old in 1993. The difference in life expectancy between the white and African American population was unchanged from 1997 to 1998, with the white population living six years longer than African Americans. The infant mortality rate remained unchanged in 1998, at 7.2 infant deaths per 1,000 live births. The rate for African American infants continued to be more than twice that of white infants (NCHS, 2000).

It has been established that low birthweight is associated with elevated risk of death and disability in infants. In 1997, the percentage of low birthweight infants (those weighing $< 2,500$ g at birth) increased to 7.5 percent overall, up from 7.0 percent in 1990. Since 1990, the low birthweight rate has increased for most racial and ethnic groups. However, among African Americans infants, low birthweight declined slightly, from 13.3 percent in 1990 to 13.0 percent in 1999 (another positive sign). Although there are certainly some small changes in the right direction, the age-adjusted death rates for African Americans in 1997 exceeded those for the white population by 77 percent for stroke, 47 percent for heart disease, 34 percent for cancer, and 655 percent for HIV infection. See

Table 1.2 for these and other differentials in age-adjusted death rates between African Americans and whites in the United States from 1950 to 1997 (Kramarow, Lentzner, Rooks, Weeks, & Saydah, 1999).

The contributing authors for each of the chapters have identified the health issues, barriers, and challenges to be faced in addressing the health disparity gaps experienced most profoundly by the African American population. Through their research efforts, including discussions of the most salient factors affecting each health issue, a composite picture of black health can be gleaned. From these authors, individually and collectively, a common theme emerges—the struggle for equity, access to quality healthcare, and an overall improved quality of life for all continues.

Call to the Nation

In Boston in November 2000, a "Call to the Nation" to eliminate racial and ethnic disparities in health was issued during its 128th annual meeting by the American Public Health Association (APHA), a national coalition of thirty-six federal, private, educational, health, congressional, senatorial, business, and professional organizations including the White House. The text of this call follows.

> The twentieth century witnessed unprecedented improvements in the health and longevity of millions of people in the United States. Stunning advances in medicine, public health, and the overall standard of living have led to many important health gains. Yet, despite decades of progress in these areas and significant achievements in civil rights protections, health disparities have persisted and, in many cases, have worsened. Racial and ethnic minorities— many of whom are economically disadvantaged—have not shared fully in this progress.
>
> Statistics amply demonstrate the disproportionately greater burden of disease, disability, and death experienced by racial and ethnic minorities in this country. As employers face a tight labor market and changing demographics in the labor force, this country's ability to effectively address health disparities also becomes critical to the continued health of the economy. Invisible in the numbers is the suffering of those who experience a disproportionate burden of health problems.
>
> Previous efforts to address the tragic legacy of these health inequities have not fully engaged the entire country. Given the broad roots of this problem, it is only with the combined efforts of all sectors and disciplines of society—the public and private sectors, business and labor, non-profit and community-based organizations, educational institutions, the faith community, and others—that we can hope to eliminate racial and ethnic health disparities. Major institutions, all levels of government, communities, and individuals—

TABLE 1.2. AGE-ADJUSTED DEATH RATES FOR SELECTED CAUSES OF DEATH BY SEX AND RACE/ETHNICITY, SELECTED YEARS 1950–1997.

Deaths per 100,000 Resident Population

Sex, Race, Hispanic Origin, and Cause of Death	1950[a]	1960	1970	1980	1985	1990	1994	1995	1996	1997
White										
All causes	800.4	727.0	679.6	559.4	524.9	492.8	479.8	476.9	466.8	456.5
Natural causes	—	—	—	497.7	471.9	442.0	431.4	428.5	419.2	409.7
Diseases of the heart	300.5	281.5	249.1	197.6	176.6	146.9	135.4	133.1	129.8	125.9
Ischemic heart disease	—	—	—	150.6	126.6	102.5	91.1	89.0	86.4	82.5
Cerebrovascular diseases	83.2	74.2	61.8	38.0	30.1	25.5	24.5	24.7	24.5	24.0
Malignant neoplasms	124.7	124.2	127.8	129.6	131.2	131.5	128.6	127.0	125.2	122.9
Respiratory system	13.0	19.1	28.0	35.6	38.4	40.6	39.7	39.3	38.9	38.4
Colorectal	—	17.9	16.9	15.4	14.7	13.3	12.5	12.3	11.8	11.6
Prostate[b]	13.1	12.4	12.3	13.2	13.4	15.3	14.6	14.0	13.5	12.6
Breast[c]	22.5	22.4	23.4	22.8	23.4	22.9	20.9	20.5	19.8	18.9
Chronic obstructive pulmonary diseases	4.3	8.2	13.4	16.3	19.2	20.1	21.6	21.3	21.5	21.7
Pneumonia and influenza	22.9	24.6	19.8	12.2	12.9	13.4	12.5	12.4	12.2	12.4
Chronic liver disease and cirrhosis	8.6	10.3	13.4	11.0	8.9	8.0	7.5	7.4	7.3	7.3
Diabetes mellitus	13.9	12.8	12.9	9.1	8.6	10.4	11.5	11.7	12.0	11.9
Human immunodeficiency virus infection	—	—	—	—	—	8.0	11.2	11.1	7.2	3.3
External causes	—	—	—	61.9	53.0	50.8	48.5	48.4	47.5	46.8
Unintentional injuries	55.7	47.6	51.0	41.5	34.2	31.8	29.5	29.9	29.9	29.6
Motor vehicle-related injuries	23.1	22.3	26.9	23.4	19.1	18.6	16.2	16.4	16.3	15.9
Suicide	11.6	11.1	12.4	12.1	12.3	12.2	11.9	11.9	11.6	11.3
Homicide and legal intervention	2.6	2.7	4.7	6.9	5.4	5.9	5.8	5.5	4.9	4.7

Black

All causes	1,236.7	1,073.3	1,044.0	842.5	793.6	789.2	772.1	765.7	738.3	705.3
Natural causes	—	—	—	740.2	713.5	701.3	686.5	685.8	662.3	632.7
Diseases of the heart	379.6	334.5	307.6	255.7	240.6	213.5	198.8	198.8	191.5	185.7
Ischemic heart disease	—	—	—	150.5	130.9	113.2	103.8	103.4	99.4	96.3
Cerebrovascular diseases	150.9	140.3	114.5	68.5	55.8	48.4	45.4	45.0	44.2	42.5
Malignant neoplasms	129.1	142.3	156.7	172.1	176.6	182.0	173.8	171.6	167.8	165.2
Respiratory system	10.4	20.3	33.5	46.5	50.3	54.0	50.6	49.9	48.9	47.9
Colorectal	—	15.2	16.6	16.9	17.9	17.9	17.2	17.3	16.8	16.8
Prostate[b]	16.9	22.2	25.4	29.1	31.2	35.3	35.3	34.0	33.8	31.4
Breast[c]	19.3	21.3	21.5	23.3	25.5	27.5	26.9	27.5	26.5	26.7
Chronic obstructive pulmonary diseases	—	—	—	12.5	15.3	16.9	17.7	17.6	17.8	17.4
Pneumonia and influenza	57.0	56.4	40.4	19.2	18.8	19.8	17.5	17.8	17.8	17.2
Chronic liver disease and cirrhosis	7.2	11.7	24.8	21.6	16.3	13.7	10.7	9.9	9.2	8.7
Diabetes mellitus	17.2	22.0	26.5	20.3	20.1	24.8	27.4	28.5	28.8	28.9
Human immunodeficiency virus infection	—	—	—	—	—	25.7	49.4	51.8	41.4	24.9
External causes	—	—	—	101.2	80.1	87.8	85.6	79.8	76.0	72.6
Unintentional injuries	70.9	66.4	74.4	51.2	42.3	39.7	38.1	37.4	36.7	36.1
Motor vehicle-related injuries	24.7	23.4	30.6	19.7	17.4	18.4	16.6	16.6	16.7	16.8
Suicide	4.2	4.7	6.1	6.4	6.4	7.0	7.1	6.9	6.6	6.3
Homicide and legal intervention	30.5	27.4	46.1	40.6	29.2	39.5	38.2	33.4	30.6	28.1

Note: Data are based on the National Vital Statistics System.

—Data not available.

[a] Includes deaths of persons who were not residents of the fifty states and the District of Columbia.

[b] Male only.

[c] Female only.

Source: Data for 1960 to 1993 from Grove & Hetzel, 1968; U.S. Public Health Service, 1997. Data for 1994 to 1997 from unpublished data: data computed by the Division of Health and Utilization Analysis from numerator data compiled by Division of Vital Statistics and denominator data from the U.S. Census Bureau (see Table 1.1) and unpublished Hispanic population estimates prepared by the Housing and Household Economic Statistics Division, U.S. Bureau of the Census.

both within and outside of the health care arena—must come together to amplify our knowledge, talent, and resources to reach this goal. Unless we focus our collective attention as a *nation* on racial and ethnic disparities in health, we can never hope to eliminate them.

Thus, at the beginning of a new millennium, we are issuing this Call to the Nation to Eliminate Racial and Ethnic Disparities in Health with the hope that organizations and individuals throughout the country will endorse and commit to achieving this historic goal. We are calling for the creation of a national coalition with an inclusive, diverse membership to lead this charge. And, we are calling upon this new national coalition to develop and implement a national strategy to eliminate racial and ethnic disparities in the United States.

As we experience the longest economic expansion in U.S. history, we believe the elimination of racial and ethnic disparities in health is a worthy, ground-breaking, and achievable goal for our prosperous and energetic nation. Now is the time to ensure that current and future generations of *all* Americans are healthier, happier, and more productive. With much enthusiasm, we urge others to join with us as we embark on this momentous undertaking [American Public Health Association, 2000].

Conclusion

At the federal level, moves are afoot to programmatically address the health disparity gap. In November 2000, President Clinton amended the Public Health Service Act in an effort to improve the health of ethnic minority groups. The short title for this act is the "Minority Health Disparities Research and Education Act of 2000." The amendment acknowledged the role that behavioral and social science research has on increasing the awareness and understanding of factors associated with health care utilization and access, patient attitudes toward health services, and risk and protective behaviors that affect health and illness. These factors have the potential to be modified to help close the health disparities gap among ethnic minority populations. Thus, the amendment established the National Center on Minority Health and Health Disparities within the National Institutes of Health.

Two major responsibilities of the National Center involve the development of centers of excellence for research education and training and the implementation of an extramural loan repayment program for minority health disparities research. The legislation requires that an evaluation be conducted and a report submitted by December 1, 2003, to Congress, the Secretary of Health and Human Services, and the director of the National Institutes of Health that provides (1) recommendations for the methodology that should be used to determine the extent of the resources of the National Institutes of Health that are to be dedicated to minority health disparities research and other health disparities research, including determining the amount of funds that are to be used to conduct and support such research; and (2) a determination of whether and to what extent, relative to fiscal year 1999, there has been an increase in the level of resources of the National Institutes of Health that are dedicated to minority health disparities research, including the amount of funds used to conduct and support such research. The report shall include provisions describing whether and to what extent there have been increases in the number and amount of awards to minority-serving institutions.

The amendment also requires a study and report by the National Academy of Sciences (NAS), wherein the NAS will conduct a comprehensive study of the data collection systems and practices of the Department of Health and Human Services, and any data collection or reporting systems required under any of the programs or activities of the department which relate to the collection of data on race or ethnicity, including other federal data collection systems (such as the Social Security Administration) with which the Department interacts to collect relevant data on race and ethnicity.

By November 2001, the NAS shall prepare and submit to the Committee on Health, Education, Labor, and Pensions of the Senate and the Committee on Commerce of the House of Representatives a report that (1) identifies the data needed to support efforts to evaluate the effects of socioeconomic status, race, and ethnicity on access to health care and other services and on disparity in health and other social outcomes and the data needed to enforce existing protections for equal access to health care; (2) examines the effectiveness of the systems and practices of the Department of Health and Human Services, including pilot and demonstration projects of the department, and the effectiveness of selected systems and practices of other federal, state, and tribal agencies as well as the private sector in collecting and analyzing such data; (3) contains recommendations for ensuring that the Department of Health and Human Services, in administering its entire array of programs and activities, collects or causes to be collected, reliable and complete information relating to race and ethnicity; and (4) includes projections about the costs associated with the implementation of the recommendations, and the possible effects of the cost on program operations. Other aspects of the act include provisions for (1) health professions education in health disparities, (2) grants for health professions education, (3) a national conference on health professions education and health disparities, and (4) an array of public awareness and information dissemination activities.

In summary, given that there is no silver bullet for addressing the complexity of issues, barriers, and challenges to the health disparity gap, a multilevel approach is advocated throughout the chapters of this book. The authors and the editors acknowledge and diligently reinforce the concept of partnerships inclusive of citizens; community-based organizations; health care providers; local, state, and federal sector participants; private, corporate, and foundation partners; and business, media, and faith-community involvement. A multidisciplinary approach that draws on the talent and expertise of diverse perspectives will be required to change behavioral, institutional, and cultural norms designed to improve the quality of life for disenfranchised populations.

References

American Public Health Association. (2000). *Call to the nation to eliminate racial and ethnic disparities in health.* (entire pamphlet). Washington, DC: Author.

DeBarros, K., & Bennett, C. (1997, June). Black population in the United States, March 1997 (update). *Current population reports: Population characteristics. (No. P20-498).* Washington, DC: U.S. Census Bureau.

Grove, R. D., & Hetzel, A. M. (1968). *Vital statistics rates in the U.S., 1940–1960. (No. 1677).* Washington, DC: U.S. Government Printing Office.

Kramarow, E., Lentzner, H., Rooks, R., Weeks, J., & Saydah, S. (1999). *Health and aging chartbook.* In National Center for Health Statistics, *Health, United States, 1999 with health and aging chartbook* (DHHS Publication No. PHS 99-1232). Washington, DC: U.S. Government Printing Office.

National Center for Health Statistics. (2000, July 24). *Gun deaths among children and teens drop sharply.* [News release and fact sheets]. Hyattsville, MD: Author.

U.S. Census Bureau. (2000, July 28). *Resident population estimates of the U.S. by sex, race, and Hispanic origin* [On-line]. Available: www.census.gov/population/estimates/nation/intfile3-1.txt

U.S. Department of Health and Human Services. (1991). *Healthy people 2000* (DHHS Publication No. PHS 91-50212). Hyattsville, MD: Author.

U.S. Department of Health and Human Services. (2000a). *Healthy people 2010: Understanding and improving health* (DHHS Publication No. 017–001–00543–6). Hyattsville, MD: Author.

U.S. Department of Health and Human Services. (2000b). *The initiative to eliminate racial and ethnic disparities in health* [On-line]. Available: www.raceandhealth.omhrc.gov

U.S. Public Health Service. (1997). *Vital statistics of the United States: Vol. 2. Mortality, Pt. A. (No. 97-1104).* Washington, DC: U.S. Government Printing Office.

West, C. (1994). *Race matters.* New York: Vintage Books.

The White House. (2000). *Building one America for the 21st century* [On-line]. Available: www.whitehouse.gov/Initiatives/OneAmerica/america.html

CHAPTER TWO

THE HEALTH STATUS OF CHILDREN AND ADOLESCENTS

Alwyn T. Cohall, Hope E. Bannister

What happens to a dream deferred?

Does it dry up

like a raisin in the sun?

Or fester like a sore—

and then run?

Does it stink like rotten meat?

Or crust and sugar over—

like a syrupy sweet?

Maybe it just sags

like a heavy load

Or does it just explode? [Hughes, 1951]

Langston Hughes penned these powerful words almost fifty years ago, describing the frequent evisceration of hopeful aspirations among African Americans. In a narrower context, the health status of African Americans can be viewed in a parallel fashion. Over the last century, dramatic reductions in mortality for many Americans have been achieved, chiefly through control of communicable diseases via improvements in public hygiene, aggressive immunization practices, and the development of antibiotics (Easterbrook, 1999). The average life expectancy has been extended from 49.2 years in 1900 to 1902 (National Center for Health Statistics, 1999) to 76.5 years in 1997 (Anderson, 1999), causing the late economist Julian Simon to declare the gift of greater life expectancy, "the most important achievement in human history" (Easterbrook, 1999, p. 25).

Unfortunately, African Americans have not shared equally in these impressive gains. At 71.1 years, their overall life expectancy is five years shorter than national averages. The disparity in average life expectancy is more pronounced for African American males compared to white males (9.3 years difference) than for African American females compared to white females (1.8 years difference).

In particular, African American children and adolescents are highly vulnerable and are disproportionately affected by both historical and contemporary health hazards. This chapter reviews the leading causes of mortality and morbidity for African American youths, examines potential causes for disparities in health outcome, and outlines strategies for remediation.

The data used in this chapter are obtained from a variety of sources, including divisions of the government (for example, the U.S. Census Bureau, National Center for Health Statistics, Healthcare Financing Administration, and Centers for Disease Control and Prevention) and not-for-profit organizations (for example, the Children's Defense Fund and the Alan Guttmacher Institute). Comparisons are made across race, age, and sex where possible. However, data are variably reported across these parameters, resulting in significant information gaps.

Many of the data are reported in aggregate, making it difficult to compare variables unless researchers have access to the entire data set on which to perform analyses. There is currently no single repository where comprehensive information about African American children and adolescents is kept.

Overview of Mortality Statistics

Over the last twenty-five years, the death rates for youths have fallen about 40.65 percent on average (Figure 2.1). In general, mortality rates are lower for females than for males, and for children aged five to fourteen as compared to children one to four or adolescents fifteen to twenty-four. Although many prominent health concerns noted in the early part of the century are less visible today, other health issues have emerged that endanger the well-being of the nation's children. For example, deaths resulting from injuries (unintentional and intentional) are three to ten times higher than the next leading cause of death in each child and youth age group (Figures 2.2, 2.3, and 2.4).

This is the kind of situation that prompted one public health official to remark, "What is the net gain if a child, through breast feeding or pasteurized milk, is prevented from dying of gastroenteritis, [but] pulls a stewpan of boiling water off the stove and is fatally scalded. What use to protect him from diphtheria to be killed by an automobile?" (Godfrey, 1937).

FIGURE 2.1. DEATH RATES BY AGE AND SEX, 1970–1997.

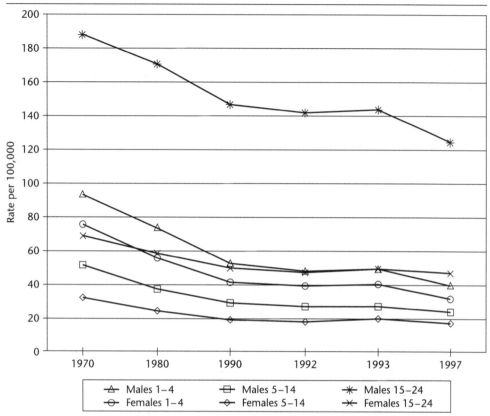

Source: U.S. Census Bureau, 1999; Hoyert, Kochanek, & Murphy, 1999, p. 6.

Infant Mortality Rates

Despite significant improvements, the United States ranks only twenty-third among all industrialized nations for infant mortality rates (IMR) (Guyer, MacDorman, Martin, Peters, & Strobino, 1998). Although the United States spends almost fifteen times more on overall health care expenditures than Canada does, the latter country's IMR (5.5 per 1,000) is lower than that of the United States (6.3 per 1,000) (Health Canada, Policy and Consultation Branch, 1997; U.S. Census Bureau, 1999).

Death rates for African American infants are two to three times higher than the national average. These higher rates are due primarily to the larger proportion of low birthweight (LBW) and very low birth weight (VLBW) infants born to African American mothers. VLBW infants (< 1,500 g) and LBW infants (1,500 g to 2,499 g) are responsible for three-quarters of the disparity in infant mortality rates (Iyasu, Becerra, Rowley, & Hogue, 1992). African American infants are

FIGURE 2.2. LEADING CAUSES OF MORTALITY
BY RACE/ETHNICITY, AGES 1–4, 1997.

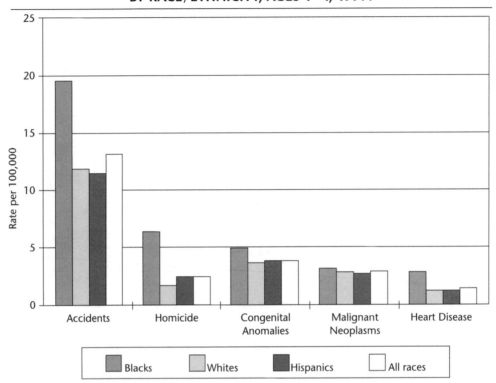

Source: Data adapted from Hoyert, Kochanek, & Murphy, 1999, pp. 29–37, 38–40.

four times more likely to be born with low birthweights and three times more likely to be born with very low birthweights (MacDorman & Atkinson, 1999; Poertner, 1998). Over a ten-year period from 1982 to 1992, the proportion of VLBW African American infants increased from 2.52 percent to 2.95 percent, whereas the proportion of VLBW white infants remained relatively constant (0.91 percent to 0.96 percent) (Centers for Disease Control and Prevention [CDC], 1994a).

Although LBW and VLBW infants make up the bulk of these premature deaths, it should also be noted that African American infants of normal weight and gestation have a 3 times greater risk of death from infections, a 2.5 greater risk of death from injuries, and a 2-fold greater risk of death from sudden infant death syndrome (SIDS). Infant mortality rates are higher for infants whose mothers are unmarried at either end of the age spectrum (nineteen or less and forty and over), who did not graduate from high school, who smoked cigarettes or used alcohol or drugs during the pregnancy, and who began prenatal care after the first

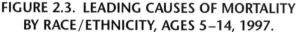

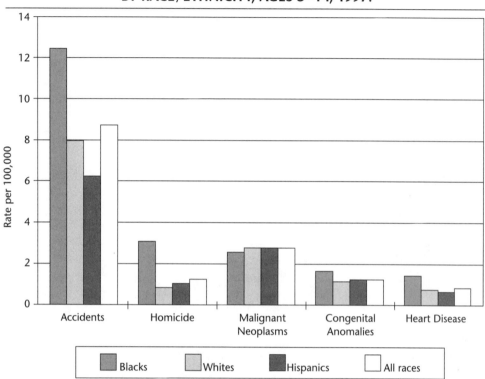

FIGURE 2.3. LEADING CAUSES OF MORTALITY BY RACE/ETHNICITY, AGES 5–14, 1997.

Source: Data adapted from Hoyert, Kochanek, & Murphy, 1999, pp. 29–37, 38–40.

trimester (MacDorman & Atkinson, 1999). Studies suggest that African American women (64 percent) were less likely than white women (81 percent) to enter into prenatal care during the first trimester. African American women (10 percent) were also more likely to enter into care during the third trimester or to receive no care than white women were (4 percent) (Rowley, 1995).

These racial disparities persist even among women who could be described as extremely low risk. This category includes women who are married, are aged twenty to thirty-four, completed high school, had adequate prenatal care, and had no evidence of substance use or medical problems during the pregnancy. Compared to white mothers, African American mothers were 2.64 times more likely to give birth to an infant who was small for gestational age (lighter than 2 standard deviations below the mean [less than 10th percentile] for normal new-borns of the infant's gestational age and sex) with a subsequent 1.61 greater risk for infant mortality. This suggests that additional explanations are required to explain differences in birth outcomes after controlling for epidemiological and

FIGURE 2.4. LEADING CAUSES OF MORTALITY
BY RACE/ETHNICITY, AGES 15–24, 1997.

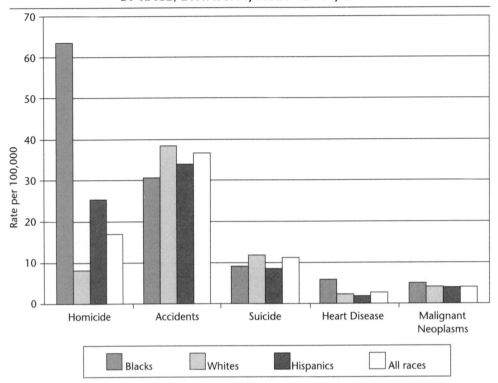

Source: Data adapted from Hoyert, Kochanek, & Murphy, 1999, pp. 29–37, 38–40.

socioeconomic risk factors (Alexander, Kogan, & Himes, 1999). Apparently the social advantages of income and education do not bestow the protection on African American women that they do on white women (Rowley, 1995).

Social determinants that may have an impact on pregnancy well-being and outcome include not only access to care but also the quality of the care and information that African American women receive. In some studies, African American women report receiving counseling about smoking, nutrition, and lifestyle issues less frequently than white women do during prenatal care visits. The withholding of this information may limit their opportunities for altering risk-taking patterns of behavior and could contribute to negative outcomes (Kogan, Kotelchuck, Alexander, & Johnson, 1994).

However, social factors do not tell the whole story. Biological factors such as low prepregnancy weight and anemia may have an impact on pregnancy outcomes not only for infants born today but for future generations as well. Studies of women exposed to extremes of poor nutrition show an increased risk of LBW infants spread out over subsequent generations (Marmot, Kogevinas, & Elston,

1987). African American mothers today may be paying for the hardship encountered by their grandparents and great-grandparents. Thus biological, social, racial, and genetic factors overlap and contribute to creating disparities in health care outcomes. The relative weight of these individual factors requires further elucidation.

Child and Adolescent Mortality Rates

Figures 2.2 through 2.4 summarize the five leading causes of death for children between the ages of one and twenty-four. Injuries are the leading cause of death in each age group. For most age ranges, African American children are more likely to die as a result of an accident than are white children. This holds true until the fifteen to nineteen age bracket when homicide becomes the leading cause of death for African American teenagers.

Injuries. African American children and adolescents (zero to nineteen years old) are more likely than white children to die from drowning, getting burned, suffocating, choking, getting cut, poisoning, and other injury mechanism (Baker, O'Neill, Ginsburg, & Li, 1992) (see also Table 2.1). Additionally, African American children and adolescents have a higher rate than their white counterparts of pedal cyclist and pedestrian deaths (in the motor vehicle traffic category) and unintentional, homicide, and undetermined deaths (in the firearm category).

TABLE 2.1. INJURY DEATH RATES BY CAUSE AND RACE/ETHNICITY, AGES 0–19, 1991–1992.

Injury Cause	African American (Rate per 100,000)	Non-Hispanic White (Rate per 100,000)	African American to White Rate Ratio
Motor vehicle traffic total			
Pedal cyclist	0.5	0.4	1.25
Pedestrian	2.4	1.4	1.71
Nontraffic			
Pedestrian	0.5	0.3	1.66
Firearm total	21.0	3.9	5.38
Unintentional	1.3	0.6	2.16
Homicide	17.8	1.0	17.8
Undetermined	0.3	0.1	3.0
Drowning	3.4	1.9	1.78
Fire/flame	4.0	1.3	3.07
Suffocation/hanging	1.7	1.4	1.21
Choking	0.8	0.3	2.66
Cutting/piercing	1.5	0.3	5.0
Poison: solid/liquid	0.6	0.5	1.2
Other	4.0	2.0	2.0

Source: Baker et al., 1996.

Violence. "Fate succumbs many a species: one alone jeopardises itself." Although W. H. Auden's words can generally describe the human race, they have particular resonance in describing the experience of African American children and youths. Many live in homes where domestic violence is present. It is estimated that annually one of every six U.S. couples experiences one or more episodes of domestic violence (Sorenson, 1996).

Pregnancy appears to be a high-risk period in which abuse may start or escalate. Estimates of prevalence of abuse during pregnancy ranges from 1 to 17 percent (Campbell, Poland, Waller, & Ager, 1992; Gazmararian et al., 1996). Outcomes of abuse during pregnancy include LBW infants (possibly secondary to the stress and associated cigarette smoking, substance abuse, poor dietary habits, and inadequate prenatal care) and miscarriage (Parker, McFarlance, & Socken, 1994; Stewart, 1993). When a live birth does occur, mothers and their children remain at-risk. Nineteen percent of women in one study were found to be abused postnatally compared to a baseline report of 10 percent during the prenatal period (Gielen, O'Campo, Faden, Kass, & Xue, 1994).

In addition, children may become targets of domestic violence. In 40 to 70 percent of households where domestic violence is present, child abuse also exists (McKibbon, Vos, & Newberger, 1989; Straus & Gelles, 1990). In 1997, child protective services estimated that almost one million children in the United States were victims of abuse and neglect (U.S. Department of Health and Human Services, 1999). African American children represented a disproportionate 29.5 percent of victims. Violence associated with child abuse may range from verbal abuse to physical abuse to sexual abuse.

Death is the most extreme outcome of abuse. In a review of homicides in children under the age of eleven in North Carolina, 85 percent of the 259 deaths recorded were due to child abuse. African American children were killed at three times the rate of white children. Fifty-nine percent of these deaths were incorrectly assigned to other causes. Similarly, on a national basis 62 percent of the homicides of children under eleven may have been incorrectly assigned, swelling the number of homicide deaths in this group from 2,973 to 9,467 (Herman-Giddens et al., 1999).

In 1997, 6,146 adolescents (aged fifteen to twenty-four) were victims of homicide. More than 57 percent of them were African American youths. African American males died from homicide at a rate that was 8.6 times that of white males. African American females are more than four times more likely to die as a result of homicide than white females are (Hoyert, Kochanek, & Murphy, 1999).

Overview of Morbidity Statistics

To get a more complete picture of the health status of African American children, an examination of morbidity patterns is also important. Major morbidities include the following:

Asthma

Approximately 2.7 million children and adolescents in this country have asthma (Gergen & Evans, 1988). In addition to being the leading chronic disease among youths, asthma is responsible for the majority of days lost from school (Fowler, Davenport, & Garg, 1992) and contributes significantly to the number of emergency room visits and hospitalizations. Data from the 1987 National Medical Expenditure Survey reveal that annually children with asthma obtain 3.1 times as many prescriptions, make 1.9 times as many ambulatory provider visits, have 2.2 times as many emergency room visits, and are hospitalized 3.5 times as often as children without asthma. On average, children with asthma incur about $1,129 in annual health care costs as compared to $468 for children without asthma (Lozano, Sullivan, Smith, & Weiss, 1999).

Minority children, particularly those who are poor and living in urban environments, are disproportionately affected by asthma. African Americans and Hispanics have five times more hospitalizations than whites and are four to five times more likely to die from asthma (Gergen & Weiss, 1990; Weiss, Gergen, & Crain, 1992).

Exposure to indoor allergens and pollutants such as dust mites, tobacco smoke, and cockroaches (Malveaux & Fletcher-Vincent, 1995) may contribute to the exacerbation of asthma. A study of 611 asthmatic children from eight cities found that 85 percent of them lived in homes with detectable cockroach antigen (Rosenstreich, Eggleston, & Kattan, 1997). Cockroach populations are highest in crowded urban areas (Sarpong, Wood, & Eggleston, 1996). African American race is an independent predictor of cockroach exposure and sensitization (Sarpong et al., 1996), suggesting either that African Americans are likely to have been exposed to a particularly potent cockroach antigen or that they have a specific genetic predisposition to sensitization that may initiate an immunological cascade resulting in asthma (Miller, 1999).

Although indoor allergens and pollutants are significant, the presence of external environmental toxins is also important to mention. Compared to non-urban children, children living in urban areas may be greatly exposed to higher levels of air pollution, in part fueled by the exhausts of cars, buses, trucks, and factories (Northridge et al., 1999).

Lead

National Health and Nutrition Examination Survey (NHANES) III data reveal that 4.4 percent (or 930,000) of the children in the United States between the ages of one and five have elevated lead levels ($> 10 \, \mu g/dl$). Children one to two years old have the highest rates of lead poisoning (5.9 percent). Poor children are eight times more likely than affluent children to have elevated lead levels. African American children are five times more likely than white children to have elevated lead levels. A primary reason for this disparity is the clustering of poor families, often African American, into substandard housing, where water damage and moisture often cause deterioration of the walls leading to peeling and cracking of paint. About 64 million homes still contain lead paint, and about 15 percent of homes have lead in pipes, faucets, or well pumps (Spake & Couzin, 1999). Younger children may ingest lead directly by drinking water contaminated by lead in the pipes or by eating paint chips or indirectly by playing with toys contaminated by lead dust particles (CDC, 1997).

Ingested lead from any source can affect the developing brain, leading to hyperactivity, attention-deficit disorder, and aggressive behaviors. It is estimated that 20 to 30 percent of children in special education have been affected by significant lead exposure. Children with elevated lead levels are six times more likely than others to have learning disabilities and seven times more likely to drop out of school (Spake & Couzin, 1999). Aggressive children may grow up to become bullying adolescents and to engage in antisocial activities such as vandalism, arson, and shoplifting.

Adolescent Sexuality

The 1997 Youth Risk Behavior Survey (YRBS) indicates an 11 percent decrease in the number of teenagers who are sexually active by the age of nineteen. Although African American teenagers are more likely than white teenagers to be sexually experienced, similar declines in sexual activity have also been noted among African American teenagers (from 81 percent to 73 percent).

Although there has been significant improvement overall in the use of contraception, much of that gain has been due to use of condoms. Use of condoms increased 23 percent overall from 1991 to 1997. The percentage of African American adolescents using condoms at last intercourse (64 percent) exceeded that of whites (56 percent) and Hispanics (48 percent) (CDC, 1998b).

It is important to note, however, that the rates of use of other contraceptive methods have fallen. The use of oral contraceptive pills (OCPs), for example, decreased by 4 percent between 1982 and 1995, with the largest decline noted among young African American women less than twenty-five years of age (Abma, Chandra, Mosher, Peterson, & Piccinino, 1997). The percentage of teenagers using OCPs fell by 15 percent (from 59 percent to 44 percent) between 1988 and 1995. Among young women aged twenty to twenty-four, the percentage dropped from 68 percent to 52 percent during the same time period. Over the same period, OCP use decreased by 60 percent among African American teenagers and decreased by 36 percent among young women aged twenty to twenty-four (CDC, 1998c).

Gonorrhea and chlamydia are two sexually transmitted diseases (STDs) that disproportionately affect African Americans. Although both can be easily treated with a short course of antibiotics, there are serious, long-term consequences for both males and females if these infections go undetected and untreated. Complications for females include pelvic inflammatory disease, ectopic pregnancy, and sterility, and males are at risk for orchitis and sterility. These potential dangers underscore the need for widespread screening for these diseases, particularly among adolescents of color, who suffer the highest rates of infection (Neinsten, 1996).

Although pregnancy rates have also decreased (CDC, 1998a), about one million teenagers become pregnant annually (Moore, 1996). Forty percent of adolescent females of color will become pregnant at least once before age nineteen, as compared to 21 percent of white females (Henshaw, 1997). Almost 90 percent of all teen pregnancies are unintended (Moore, 1996). In general, about 51 percent of teen pregnancies end in live births, 35 percent in induced abortions, and 14 percent in miscarriages or stillbirths (Moore, 1996).

Between 1992 and 1995, birthrates dropped for teens fifteen to nineteen, with the largest percentage decline (24 percent) noted among African American teens, compared to 17 percent for white teens (Ventura, Martin, Curtin, & Mathews, 1999). Rates have stayed constant for younger teens (Moore, 1996). The U.S. teen birthrate in 1997 (52.3 per 1,000) is still higher than the rate in 1980 (50 per 1,000) and is higher than in any other industrialized nation. Rates for African American adolescents (90.8 per 1,000), although lower than the rates for Hispanic adolescents (97.4 per 1,000), are about twice that of white adolescents (36 per 1,000) (Ventura et al., 1999).

Once a teen is pregnant, she is at increased risk for a subsequent pregnancy. Twenty-two percent of births to teens are not first births (Moore, Papillo, Williams, Jager, & Jones, 1999), although the live birthrate has declined by 16 percent since 1991 (Ventura et al., 1999).

Eighty-three percent of teens who give birth and 61 percent who have abortions are from poor and low-income families. One-third are products of teen pregnancies themselves. Between 50 and 60 percent of teens who become pregnant have a history of physical or sexual abuse (Alan Guttmacher Institute, 1994).

Mental Health and Substance Use

Various studies have implicated the extreme and often overwhelming levels of stress associated with living in poverty in the development of mental health problems among children and adolescents (Knitzer & Aber, 1995; McLoyd & Wilson, 1991). Posttraumatic stress disorder (PTSD) and depression are common. Exposure to violent acts is a significant contributor to PTSD. Although young men of color may be more exposed to violence, young women of color exhibit more symptoms of PTSD (Berton & Stabb, 1996).

The most extreme complication of depression is suicide. There has been a steady increase in completed suicides among African American adolescents over the last forty years. For example, rates per 100,000 among African American males ages fifteen to twenty-four have increased from 2.3 in 1960 (Holinger, Offer, Barter, & Bell, 1997) to 9.2 in 1997 (Hoyert, Kochanek, & Murphy, 1999; National Center for Injury Prevention, 1995).

Substance abuse is another maladaptive method for coping with stress, through self-medication. Pregnant teens, particularly those who have experienced physical or sexual abuse during the pregnancy and low levels of positive social support, are at high risk for depression and may cope with their stress by turning to alcohol or drugs (Curry, 1998). Depressed teen mothers are 3.3 times more likely than non-depressed peers to use drugs (Barnet, Duggan, Wilson, & Joffe, 1995). Risk for substance abuse may not necessarily decline following birth of the child. Forty-two percent of African American teen mothers screened positive for illicit drugs or admitted to drinking alcohol within four months of delivery.

Nevertheless, large-scale national studies of adolescent substance use behavior suggest that on average, African American youths are relatively less involved in substance use than their peers. The 1997 Youth Risk Behavior Survey indicated that both white and Hispanic youths were more likely to report current cigarette, alcohol, marijuana, and other illicit use than were African American youths (see Table 2.2) (Kann et al., 1998).

However, although African American youths historically have smoked fewer cigarettes than white youths, recent data indicate their increasing involvement, possibly as a result of creative advertising by the tobacco industry (CDC, 1998c). Additionally, although African American youths in general report lower levels of drug use, it should be kept in mind that many of the most popular surveys of youth drug use fail to address the prevalence of substance use among youths who have dropped out of school and who are at higher risk. Many of these disconnected youths are African American.

African American adolescents who fail to make strong connections academically or in the workplace may be lured into the underground economy of hustling and selling drugs and other illicit items (Williams & Kornblum, 1995). Adolescents who have been asked to traffic drugs, or who have seen others being asked, may become vulnerable to using drugs themselves (Li, Stanton, & Feigelman, 1999).

One teen strategy for filling the need to survive both economically and socially is to connect with a gang. Over the past fifteen years, there has been an explosive growth in gang involvement from about 2,000 gangs and 100,000 members in

TABLE 2.2. PERCENTAGE OF U.S. HIGH SCHOOL STUDENTS WHO HAVE USED ILLEGAL SUBSTANCES IN THEIR LIFETIMES, BY RACE/ETHNICITY, 1997.

Illegal Substance	African American (%)	Non-Hispanic White (%)	Hispanic (%)
Alcohol	73.0	81.3	83.1
Cigarettes	68.4	70.4	75.0
Marijuana	52.2	45.4	49.5
Cocaine	1.9	8.0	14.4
"Crack" or "freebase"	1.2	4.5	8.0
Injected drug use	1.0	1.8	2.2

Source: CDC, 1997, Table 16.

1980 to 1982 to 23,000 gangs and 650,000 members in 1995. In large part the underground economy supporting the sale and distribution of weapons and drugs has fueled this aggressive expansion of activities. It is common for gang members to both use and sell drugs. In one study of recently incarcerated gang members, positive urine toxicologies for marijuana ranged from 34 to 58 percent and for cocaine 4 to 12 percent (Sickmund, Snyder, & Poe-Yamagata, 1997).

Violence and Crime

Although African American youths make up 15 percent of the population, they represent 28 percent of all juvenile arrests. They are especially overrepresented in arrests for robbery (60 percent), murder (58 percent), forcible rape (45 percent), and aggravated assault (42 percent) (Sickmund et al., 1997). African American youths are also more likely to be disproportionately incarcerated in the juvenile justice and criminal justice systems. In 1995, there were over 108,700 juveniles held in detention, correctional, or shelter facilities. Sixty-four percent were held in public facilities and 36 percent in private facilities. Minority youths make up more than two-thirds of juveniles in custody in public facilities and about one-half of youths in private facilities (Sickmund et al., 1997). Although the incarcerated population is primarily male (86.5 percent), African American female adolescents represent the fastest growing category of young people in the juvenile justice system (Girls Inc., 1996; Sickmund & Snyder, 1999).

Use of marijuana or other illicit drugs, particularly in the absence of social support systems such as affiliations with academic and religious institutions, correlates with an increase likelihood of deviant behavior such as theft, vandalism, assault, and drug-related crimes (Brook, Gordon, Brook, & Brook, 1989).

HIV/AIDS

Despite making up only 14 percent of the population, African American children represent 62 percent of HIV/AIDS cases in the under-thirteen age group (U.S. Department of Health and Human Services, Division of STD Prevention, 1999).

Due to the advent of universal counseling and voluntary HIV testing during the prenatal period, more opportunities have arisen for earlier detection and administration of antiretroviral medications. Consequently, a dramatic decline in the number of U.S. infants born with HIV has been noted recently (Figure 2.5). Additionally, prompt recognition and management of HIV-infected infants has prolonged their survival. As a result, some infants born with HIV are now entering their adolescence.

Although the wave of perinatally infected children has crested and slowed, a new wave is emerging on the horizon. Adolescents make up a significant portion of the individuals who have recently acquired the virus primarily through sexual transmission. As of December 1998, there were 3,422 adolescents (ages thirteen to nineteen) reported with AIDS, 57 percent of whom were African American. In

FIGURE 2.5. PERINATALLY ACQUIRED AIDS
CASES BY QUARTER-YEAR OF DIAGNOSIS, 1985–1998.

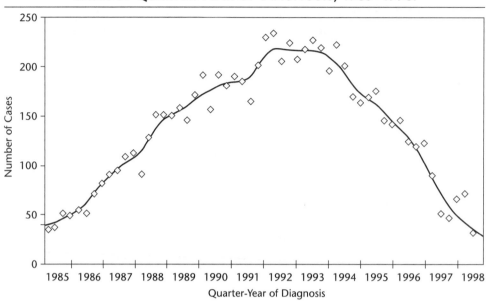

Note: Adjusted for reporting delays and redistribution of NIRs; data reported through March 1999.

Source: CDC, 2000, slide 3.

particular the percentage of young women infected by HIV is increasing. In 1998, of the 728 teenagers who tested positive for HIV, 62 percent were women, compared to 43 percent of those diagnosed with HIV in the twenty to twenty-four age group, and 29 percent in the over-twenty-four age group.

Chronic Disease

Furthermore, although the poor health status of African American youths alone is cause for concern, it should also be noted that many significant health problems of adults have antecedent risk factors that begin in childhood and become entrenched during adolescence. For example, cardiovascular disease and cancer are the leading causes of death for adults. These two diseases have in common many of the behavioral risk factors that contribute to their development. These behaviors include smoking, getting insufficient physical exercise, eating foods high in saturated fats, consuming too few fruits and vegetables, and episodically over-consuming alcohol. The YRBS indicates that 63 percent of youths have two or more risk factors; close to 8 percent report four or more risk factors. Risk of involvement in these risk factors for chronic disease is inversely related to socioeconomic status (Lowry, Kann, Collins, & Kolbe, 1996).

Additional reasons for concern are elicited from a review of data from NHANES III. This information showed that compared to white youths, African American children and young adults had higher body mass indices (BMIs) (a measure of body fatness), consumed a greater amount of calories from dietary fat, had higher blood pressure, and had higher levels of glycohemoglobin (which may indicate a preclinical stage of diabetes). Lower socioeconomic status (SES) was a significant predictor of BMI and glycosylated hemoglobin (Winkleby, Robinson, Sundquist, & Kraemer, 1999). The effect of SES on health will be further elaborated in the next section.

Contributing Factors

There are many contributing factors that may explain disparities in health status for African American youths.

Poverty

Much of the disparity in health status can be linked to poverty. Although our nation enjoys a strong, stable economy and income levels among the upper 20 percent of Americans have risen by 33 percent over the last twenty years, income levels of those families residing in the bottom 20 percent, after adjusting for inflation, have actually declined by 5 percent (Stevenson, 2000).

There are significant forces driving increasing numbers of families into poverty and limiting their options for escape. There has been a general decline in traditional manufacturing and blue-collar jobs, forcing many African Americans to seek employment in the relatively lower paying service industry and as unskilled labor, employment that rarely provides health benefits (Wilson, 1997). Additionally, although there has been an influx of new jobs as a result of the overall strength of the economy, these jobs may be located in suburbs surrounding the inner city, making access difficult for African Americans who rely primarily on public transportation. Furthermore, many of these new jobs (professional, managerial, and technical positions) require education at the postsecondary level or beyond, limiting the prospects for those African Americans who have dropped out of high school (Wilson, 1997).

As a result of decreased employment options for adults, the number of children living in poverty has increased by 70.7 percent between 1969 and 1997, to a total of 13.4 million in 1997. Close to 37 percent (36.8) of African American children are poor, compared to 15.4 percent of white children (U.S. Census Bureau, 1997).

The importance of connectedness between youths and family and between youths and social institutions has been underscored by findings from the National Longitudinal Adolescent Health Survey. Ninety thousand youths in grades 7 to 12 throughout the nation were surveyed; in-depth interviews were conducted at home with over 12,000 youths randomly selected from the larger pool. On the one hand, adolescents who perceived themselves as "connected" to home (experiencing feelings of warmth, love, and caring) and school (experiencing caring by teachers who have high expectations for student performance) were less likely to become involved in risk-taking behaviors (Resnick et al., 1997). On the other hand, youths who felt "disconnected" from family, school, and religious affiliations were more likely to become involved in a variety of risk-taking behaviors, such as substance use, premature sexual relations, and violence.

Similarly, the Search Institute reported in 1997 on a survey that was administered to over 100,000 teens across the United States to determine their exposure to risk or protective factors (Table 2.3). Only 8 percent of adolescents reported thirty-one or more assets, and 62 percent reported fewer than twenty assets. (Assets are factors that insulate adolescents from harm and help steer them toward health-promoting and life-affirming choices. Examples include external factors such as familial support and nurturance, supervised recreational or athletic outlets, strong schools, and religious affiliations, and internal factors such as empathy, self-control, hopefulness, motivation to succeed, healthy eating and recreation

TABLE 2.3. RISK AND PROTECTIVE FACTORS FOR ADOLESCENTS.

Individual Risk Factors	Individual Protective Factors
Impulsivity	Self-control
Anger/reactivity	Planning/decision-making skills
Aggressive behavior	Popularity/social skills/empathy
Life lacks meaning	Spiritual/religious/finds meaning
Disregard for others	Cares for others
Poor health behaviors	Healthy eating/exercise
Substance abuse	Restraint/integrates wellness into life
Sensation seeking	Tolerant of boredom
Language problems	Communication skills
Poor interpersonal boundaries	Ability to set boundaries
Affiliates with antisocial youth	Affiliates with prosocial youth
Disconnected from school	Motivated to achieve
Hopeless/"futureless"	Hopeful/optimistic
Negative view of self	Positive view of self

External Risk Factors	External Protective Factors
Poverty	
Parental crime	
Familial abuse/neglect	Familial support/nurturance
Familial substance abuse	Familial restraint/focus on wellness
Absence of supportive adults	Range of supportive adults
Poor access to health/ mental health care	Access to effective services
Poor schools	Strong schools/communities involved
Poor community resources	Strong resources/religious institutions
Neighborhood crime and violence	Neighborhood safety/closeness
Limited recreational outlets	Supervised recreational/athletic outlets

Source: Reprinted from Weist, Ginsburg, & Shafer, 1999, p. 173, by permission.

habits, and good communication skills.) Compared with those with more assets, the "bankrupt" youths reported more alcohol use (53 percent versus 3 percent), illicit drug use (42 percent versus 1 percent), sexual activity (33 percent versus 3 percent), violence (61 percent versus 6 percent), less success in school (53 percent versus 7 percent), and poorer health (88 percent versus 25 percent) (Search Institute, 1997).

Access to Care

Limited access to care closely rivals poverty as a key ingredient in contributing to disparities in health outcome. Poor children are less likely to have health insurance than are children of higher socioeconomic status. Between nine and ten million children under the age of eighteen (13 to 14 percent of all children) lack health insurance coverage. In addition to this already large number are those children who have experienced a period of time with no insurance. The 1991 National Maternal and Infant Health Survey (NMIHS) indicated that 23 percent of three-year-olds went at least one month in their lives without coverage; 60 percent of these were without insurance for more than six months or were never covered (Kogan et al., 1995). The increased number of uninsured children and youths is due to welfare reform practices that have resulted in a nationwide decline in Medicaid enrollment (from 17.2 million to 16.2 million). Compounding the problem of the uninsured child are those working parents who may not be offered benefit plans by their employers or who may not be able to afford the premiums.

Children without health insurance are less likely to visit the doctor for routine preventive health care services and more likely to have fewer physician visits overall. Consequently, they are not likely to receive early identification and treatment of health problems. Management of acute and chronic health problems is compromised by a lack of continuity of care. Less than 45 percent of children with no or inconsistent health coverage had a single site of health care. Nearly 20 percent had three or more sites (Kogan et al., 1995). Forty-one percent of children with asthma come from families with no health insurance (Lozano et al., 1999).

The 1994 National Ambulatory Medical Care Survey revealed that young people between the ages of eleven and twenty-one made relatively fewer visits to a doctor's office than other age groups. Teens represented 15 percent of the population, yet made only 9 percent of the visits (62 million visits). White teens made 79 percent of the visits (though representing 68 percent of the teen population); African Americans made 8 percent of these visits (though representing 16 percent of that population) (Ziv, Boulet, & Slap, 1999). White adolescents were more likely to have a private doctor or HMO (81 percent) than African American adolescents (59 percent) and were more likely to have the same source of care for both well and sick visits (Lieu, Newacheck, & McManus, 1993).

Adolescents are even more unlikely to be covered by insurance than younger children and to rely upon emergency rooms (ERs) for any health care. Lack of health insurance was more common among eleven- to twenty-one-year-olds (26 percent) than among young children (14 percent) or adults (23 percent). By age eighteen to twenty-one, 41 percent of male visits to the ER were uninsured as compared to 28 percent of female visits. African American teenagers accounted for a higher proportion of ER visits relative to their numbers in the overall population (Ziv, Boulet, & Slap, 1998).

Cultural Incompetence

Although poverty and limited access to care resources are undoubtedly key factors affecting the health status of African American children, they are by no means the only concerns that affect health care utilization. Assuming for a moment that income levels were standardized and that there were no impediments hindering access to care, would disparities in health outcomes be eliminated?

There is evidence to suggest that parents' use of physician services can be a strong predictor of their children's use of health care services (Hanson, 1998). So part of the answer for these differences in health utilization may be found in cultural differences in the perceived need for preventive health services and in the level of comfort with traditional versus natural remedies. Another potential explanation lies in the health service utilization histories of adult family members. For many parents of color, experiences with the health care system has been fraught with personal frustration and angst and rife with examples of differential treatment resulting from racism or a lack of cultural competency on the part of many health providers. Cultural competence and sensitivity require possessing a set of knowledge-based interpersonal skills that allows a provider to understand, appreciate, and work with individuals of cultures other than his or her own (Giger & Davidhizar, 1991). Lack of these skills may result in misdiagnosis, noncompliance, lack of cooperation, poor use of health services, and a general alienation of patients and families from the health care system (Nidorf & Morgan, 1987).

In addition to conflictual personal encounters, historical factors may also contribute to feelings of distrust. The legacy of the Tuskegee study wherein African American males infected with syphilis were denied treatment in order to monitor the natural progression of the disease's devastating effects on the human body (Gamble, 1997) has created an atmosphere in which many African American families fear and distrust the health care establishment.

The recent formal apology by President Clinton for the Tuskegee atrocities has done little to heal these wounds, particularly because there is abundant evidence that African Americans still receive unequal treatment for health conditions (Andrulis, 1998; Dominitz, Samsa, Landsman, & Provenzale, 1998; Makuc, Breen, & Freid, 1999; Oddone et al., 1998).

For these and other reasons, many families of color prefer seeking out health providers of race and ethnicity similar to their own; however, African Americans make up only 1.7 percent of the physician workforce, and that situation is unlikely to change in the near future as the percentage of underrepresented minorities entering medical school has declined by 11 percent from 1996 to 1997 (American Medical Association, 1998). Ensuring that all clinicians become culturally competent thus becomes even more important; however, medical schools and residency programs have been inconsistent in mandating curricula that would ensure that these skills are taught, practiced, and instituted.

Special Problems in Treating Teens

Cultural competency is not only an issue along ethnic and racial lines; it bears extra importance in treating adolescents. Many providers do not understand teens in general, and a lack of cultural competency may place African American teens at greater risk than other patients of being misunderstood. Several studies suggest that teens want to talk to their health care providers about a variety of concerns including acne, pubertal development, sex, contraception, STDs and HIV, substance abuse, depression, violence, and other sensitive topics (Malus, Lachance, Lamy, Macaulay, & Vanasse, 1987). However, in many instances, they leave the doctor's office with unanswered questioned and unsolved problems. Teenagers are reluctant to disclose sensitive personal matters without assurances of confidentiality and privacy (Klein, Wilson, McNulty, Kapphahn, & Collins, 1999). Clinicians provide these assurances infrequently. Many still interview teens with a parent present in the room. Additionally, due to increasing demands in the managed care setting for productivity, clinicians have less than fifteen minutes to spend assessing, examining, and treating patients. Counseling and education are often sacrificed (Marks & Fisher, 1987).

Furthermore, physicians report being inadequately trained for working with teenagers and often regard teens as their least favorite patients (Blum & Bearinger, 1990). Although these issues are generic for all teens, they are particularly problematic for minority adolescents who suffer a disproportionate share of health issues and are rarely engaged by the health care system for preventive health services. If and when they do appear in the system, they may need to contend with providers who not only are ill-prepared to handle their health concerns but may be rigid and judgmental. Even if afforded health insurance, minority teens who have been turned off by the health care system may be reluctant to reenter it for other than urgent or life-threatening concerns, once again perpetuating the cycle of crisis-oriented, health-seeking behavior.

Promising Initiatives

In reviewing the data presented, several recurrent themes emerge that must be addressed if we are to be successful in improving the health status of African American children and youths in the next millennium.

- *On a societal level,* poverty's impact puts families and children into situations of despair and potential despair that threaten destruction.
- *On a community level,* inadequate housing, schools, and programs offer limited insulation and protection against the harshness of the environment and instead often reinforce and intensify adversity.

- *On a family level,* the sum total of current and historical assaults on African Americans creates maladaptive and health destroying patterns of behavior among adults that too often ensnare children and youths.
- *On an individual level,* children and adolescents often grow up with limited resources and few options for avoiding risk-taking behaviors or for getting assistance in eliminating problematic behaviors once initiated.

Although it is far too easy to paint a bleak picture, it is perhaps more beneficial to begin looking at opportunities for success. Although many children and youths grow up in less than ideal circumstances, many are still able to overcome the odds and become productive citizens. For adolescents to achieve self-directed behavior change, they need to be provided not only with reasons to alter their high-risk behavior but also with the means, resources, and social supports to do so (Durant, Cadenhead, Pendergrast, Slavens, & Linder, 1994). Additionally, rather than focusing primarily on a blaming-the-victim construct that attempts to explain health disparities narrowly as a result of a higher prevalence of risky health behaviors among the disadvantaged (Lantz & House, 1998), we should begin to take a more holistic approach that examines and modifies the social context of African American children and adolescents (Roberts, 1999).

Focus on Building Social Capital

Social capital refers to familial and community-level resources that support and nurture. Runyan et al. (1998) developed a social capital index rating score based on the presence or absence of family and community resources. They assessed 667 children aged two to five living with high-risk families in five cities. Using various psychological and developmental measures, they determined that about 13 percent were doing "well" as determined by their scores on these tests. However, the presence of any social capital indicator increased the odds of doing well by 29 percent; adding two indicators increased the odds by 66 percent (Runyan et al., 1998).

Therefore, identifying promising strategies to build and sustain social capital in high-risk communities should be considered. Such an approach, if successful, may be extremely beneficial in restoring a sense of balance to families threatened by external and internal chaos. An example of this approach is the Free to Grow initiative sponsored by the Robert Wood Johnson Foundation (RWJ) in conjunction with the Head Start Bureau. Currently operational in five cities, with plans for additional expansion with support from RWJ and federal agencies, Free to Grow uses various approaches to identify and obtain treatment services for families affected by substance abuse; to mobilize community residents to work with law enforcement officials to reduce drug trafficking and sale of alcohol to minors; and to train parents to advocate for improvement of the physical, social, and cultural environments of local schools.

Focus on Improving Access to Care

Three avenues are especially important to explore in improving access to care: increasing insurance coverage, developing better models of care, and training health care professionals to be more culturally aware and sensitive.

Insurance Coverage. Undoubtedly, Medicaid has served an important role in improving access to care for indigent populations and in reducing health care differentials between the poor and the privately insured (Rowland, Salganicoff, & Keenan, 1999). However, with the increasing emphasis on welfare reform and the uncoupling of Medicaid (health benefits) from welfare (AFDC [Aid to Families with Dependent Children], now TANF [Temporary Aid to Needy Families]), it becomes critical to ensure that babies (and children) are not being thrown out with the bath water. Better education needs to be provided to parents and guardians to inform them that their children may still be eligible for health benefits despite the family's loss of welfare (Klerman, 1999).

Medicaid managed care has the potential to improve coordination of care for those families eligible for Medicaid. Medicaid managed care enrollees in New York report better access to care and higher levels of satisfaction compared to conventional Medicaid beneficiaries (Sisk et al., 1996). However, satisfaction is far from uniform across the country. In a study comparing the effect of Medicaid expansion on utilization of health care services in three states (Florida, Michigan, and Maine), two of the three (Michigan and Maine) still reported high rates of unmet needs and increased use of the emergency room. Improvements in Florida were attributed to expanded hours of clinic availability (including evening hours), steering of patients with nonurgent complaints away from the ER into these evening clinics, and assessment of a copay if the ER was utilized for nonurgent services. Additionally, Florida placed increased emphasis on preventive care and on educating parents about the importance of having a "medical home." Higher levels of patient satisfaction and lower levels of family disenrollment from the plan were noted compared to programs in the other two states. However, although both the demonstration and control groups in Florida (13.8 percent and 7.4 percent of the Medicaid managed care and Medicaid-eligible population) and Michigan (11.9 percent and 33.0 percent) had significant percentages of African Americans in their study, Maine had none in its demonstration group and only 0.3 percent in its control group (Rosenbach, Irvin, & Coulam, 1999).

Innovative Models of Care. Although ensuring insurance coverage is an important part of promoting access to care, innovative models for reaching out to families and youths are also needed. For example, in terms of reaching children and youths, school-based health clinics are creative attempts to employ resources efficiently. School-based clinics are satellite primary health care clinics usually affiliated with an area hospital or community health center but sited at an elementary, intermediate, or high school. Most of them offer a varied array of primary health care services. A major advantage of these clinics is that they eliminate traditional access barriers such as transportation and hours of operation because they function at the school site and in conjunction with the school day. Asthmatic children who suffer an attack during the school day can be treated in the clinic with appropriate medications and returned to class. In contrast, in schools without clinics parents may need to leave work to bring their child to a doctor's office or to the emergency room for evaluation and treatment. In addition to reducing the need for ER services, clinic staff are often involved in educational and monitoring activities, which may reduce the need for acute care visits of any type.

Although these clinics represent an innovative model for working with in-school youths, other subpopulations of young people exist that are perhaps even more at risk, due to their marginalization from mainstream activities and their involvement in the juvenile justice system. The Health Link Project, sponsored by the Hunter College Center on AIDS, Drugs and Community Health, works with incarcerated minority adolescents and young adults to help prepare them for successful reintroduction into their community of origin. In addition to providing them with health education and with risk-reduction skills while they are in jail, the program facilitates their transition back to the community by connecting them with health services; drug treatment; and housing, entitlement, and employment services upon their discharge (Roberts, 1999).

Training of Health Care Professionals. Just as important as making health care accessible to children is the quality of the health care service delivery. Several medical schools and residency programs are involved in efforts to ensure cultural sensitivity among physicians. The Association of American Medical Colleges conducted a survey in the fall of 1997 to determine the extent to which cultural competency is taught. Although 86 percent of medical schools offer their students at least one opportunity to participate in learning about multicultural medicine, only 71 percent have made such education part of a required course (Association of American Medical Colleges, 1998).

In an attempt to counteract the negative perceptions health providers have about teenagers, the Young Men's Clinic, sponsored by the Community Health Education Program at Columbia University's Mailman School of Public Health, offers first-year medical students a six-month elective designed to teach them the nuances of working with adolescents in a primary care clinic (Armstrong et al., 1999). Students consistently rate this elective as one of the most positive experiences of their medical school career.

Focus on Improving Screening, Management, Referral, and Coordination of Care

Better screening, management, referral, and coordination of care would be of great value in improving the health of African American children and youths. With respect to reducing childhood injuries, for example, there are several promising interventions. As noted by Scholer (1999), several maternal and child characteristics are frequently associated with an increased risk of fatal injuries: maternal age, maternal education, presence of other children in the home, and low birthweight of index child. Recognition of these risk factors by health care staff and intensive, focused intervention may result in reduced pathology.

Olds and colleagues (1997) conducted a longitudinal randomized study with four hundred pregnant women to test the efficacy of frequent home visits by nurses on the life course of high-risk mothers and infants. The results indicated that home visitation influenced better health outcomes such as decreased substance abuse and decreased child abuse and neglect. Those children in the home had fewer arrests, fewer sexual partners, and smoked less.

Focus on Reducing Environmental Hazards

For older children and adolescents, external and environmental factors contribute significantly to the injuries they sustain. Collaborations between communities, medical centers, and governmental agencies can drastically decrease unintentional injuries. The Harlem Hospital Injury Prevention Program, for example, has coordinated a series of interventions that have put window bars on apartment windows; increased the use of infant car seats in private vehicles and in taxis; increased the use of bicycle helmets; created Safer Streets, a program designed to teach elementary school children about traffic safety; renovated and remodeled playgrounds to provide children with play alternatives safer than playing in the street; and developed adult-supervised recreational activities (a bicycle riding program; baseball, basketball, and soccer leagues; and artistic programs in art and dance). These various initiatives have provided a safer environment for young people. Because of programs such as this and others like it, the number of unintentional injuries caused by assault and firearms among children and youths in the Harlem community decreased by 50 percent between 1989 and 1992 (Durkin, Kuhn, Davidson, Laraque, & Barlow, 1996).

Although reducing external hazards is important, there is increasing evidence that the internal environment of a child's home can be equally toxic. Reducing exposure to lead is of paramount importance. Although the price tag for extensive lead abatement in the millions of dwellings containing lead paint could conceivably run into billions of dollars, more conservative approaches may be reasonably cost efficient and effective in improving public health. Community residents can be taught to identify specific signs of deterioration, such as moisture damage, in buildings. At-risk buildings can be screened inexpensively for the presence of lead by sending samples of paint or dust or water to environmental laboratories. Correcting sources of water leakage, repairing damaged walls, and replacing old plumbing are logical physical interventions (Ryan, Levy, & Walker, 1999).

Limiting exposure to environmental irritants can be an important component of a comprehensive program emphasizing prevention as well as early and sustained intervention. Lowering the cockroach burden in urban dwellings may reduce a significant trigger for asthma among African American children (Gergen, Mortimer, & Eggleston, 1999; Sarpong et al., 1996).

Focus on Improving Life Options

Rutter (1987) encourages youth advocates to focus on creating protective services for youths that will alter the course of their life trajectories from risk taking to adaptation. Strategies include (1) reducing the impact of risks, (2) reducing the likelihood of negative chain reactions from risk exposure, (3) promoting self-esteem and self-efficacy, and (4) creating options and opportunities.

As noted previously, teen pregnancy has the potential to be a disruptive force in the lives of many young people. Although a substantial number of youths engage in sexual relations on a regular basis, contraceptive use remains inconsistent. In terms of reducing both the risk impact and the likelihood of negative chain reactions, one underused strategy for decreasing unintended pregnancies is emergency contraception (EC). The most popular type of emergency contraception consists of a concentrated dose of oral contraceptive pills dispensed in two portions within seventy-two hours of unprotected intercourse. Emergency contraception is approximately 75 percent effective in preventing an unintended pregnancy and has been safely used by thousands of women all over the world. However, minority adolescents, despite being at high risk for unintended pregnancies, are generally unaware of this modality (Cohall, Dickerson, Cohall, & Vaughan, 1998). Current efforts are under way, supported by the Open Society Institute and other foundations, to increase minority teens' awareness of EC and facilitate its appropriate use (Simkin, Radosh, Cohall, Cohall, & Bannister, 1999). Emergency contraception often serves as the initial introduction to the health care system for many young women of color and, if negotiated successfully, may ease the way for their consistent health care utilization. Clinical evidence suggests that many young women who use EC do so successfully, use it only once, and eventually transition to more reliable forms of birth control (Cohall, Bannister, Cohall, & Vaughan, 2000).

One example of promoting youths' self-esteem and self-efficacy and opening up opportunities is the comprehensive pregnancy-prevention model developed by Michael Carrera and colleagues that provides at-risk youths, predominately minority, with an array of services that develop and support life skills and critical decision making. In addition to receiving tutoring and assistance in improving academic skills, youths are exposed to adult role models from similar racial or ethnic backgrounds who have successfully overcome environmental obstacles to achieve prominent careers in medicine, law, business, and architecture. Efforts to bolster self-esteem include participation in entrepreneurial activities, performing arts, and sports. Additionally, youths (and their parents) are provided with a structured course on sexuality. Teens are given support in sexual decision making; health professionals are available to provide medical, psychosocial, and reproductive health services. As an additional incentive, youths in the program are guaranteed admission to local colleges if they graduate from high school. Evaluation of the program shows that participants tend to have better educational outcomes and lower pregnancy rates compared to both local and national samples of minority youths (Carrera, 1995).

Conclusion

Although there have been improvements in the overall health status of African American children over the years, significant disparities with the health status of white children are found in several health indicators. Poverty and its attendant stressors—lack of access to health resources; cultural insensitivity of health providers; and personal, familial, and historical distrust of the health care delivery system—are key factors that create imposing barriers to effective health promotion and health service utilization. Although there is some good news (Table 2.4), the overall health status of African American children and adolescents is far from satisfactory.

It is important that we develop a standard method by which data are reported. There should also be a single repository for health statistics on African American children. This would not only allow easier access to information but would also facilitate the collection of data to better inform program development and policy. Only with such data resources can more valid assessments about the health status of African American children and adolescents be made.

Our nation has lived through the shame of the Tuskegee travesty. Its legacy of imperious disregard for human life is a dark stain that cannot be erased by apologies or appeals. It should not be forgotten, or repeated. Yet the wide disparities in health status between African American children and youths and their white peers suggest that in fact there are mini-Tuskegees occurring all over this country today. Failure to act aggressively to counter the pathogens of poverty, lack of health insurance, and cultural insensitivity is no less a disgrace than withholding treatment for syphilis. Although the cure for health disparities is not as simple as a shot of penicillin, there are concrete, tangible efforts that can be made today to sustain the flickering flames of our next generation of dream-makers and allow their hopes and goals to be sustained and realized.

TABLE 2.4. GOOD NEWS ABOUT THE HEALTH OF AFRICAN AMERICAN CHILDREN AND ADOLESCENTS.

Compared to White Children, African-American Children and Adolescents
Are less likely to drink alcohol
Are less likely to smoke cigarettes
Are less likely to use cocaine, crack, or freebase
Are less likely to use injected drugs
Are less likely to die from malignant neoplasms (ages 5–14)
Are less likely to die as a result of accidents (ages 15–24)
Use condoms at a higher rate

References

Abma, J., Chandra, A., Mosher, W., Peterson, L., & Piccinino, L. (1997). Fertility, family planning and women's health: New data from the 1995 National Survey of Family Growth. *Vital Health Statistics, 23*(19), 1–114.

Alan Guttmacher Institute. (1994). *Sex and America's teenagers.* New York: Author.

Alexander, G., Kogan, M., & Himes, J. (1999). Racial differences in birthweight for gestational age and infant mortality in extremely-low-risk U.S. populations. *Paediatric and Perinatal Epidemiology, 13,* 205–217.

American Medical Association. (1998). *Minority physicians data source: Total physicians by race/ethnicity.* www.ama-assn.org/ama/pub/print/article/168-187.html.

Anderson, R. (1999). United States, life tables, 1997. *National Vital Statistics Reports* (Vol. 47, No. 28). Hyattsville, MD: National Center for Health Statistics.

Andrulis, D. (1998). Access to care is the centerpiece in the elimination of socioeconomic disparities in health. *Annals of Internal Medicine, 129,* 412–416.

Armstrong, B., Cohall, A., Vaughan, R., Scott, M., Tiezzi, L., & McCarthy, J. (1999). Involving men in reproductive health: The Young Men's Clinic. *American Journal of Public Health, 89,* 902–905.

Association of American Medical Colleges. (1998). Teaching and learning of cultural competence in medical school. *Contemporary Issues in Medical Education, 1,* 1–2.

Baker, S., Fingerhut, C., Higgins, L., Chen, L., & Braver, E. (1996). Injury to children and teenagers: State-by-state mortality facts. Baltimore, MD: Johns Hopkins Center for Injury Research and Policy.

Baker, S., O'Neill, B., Ginsburg, M., & Li, G. (1992). *The injury fact book* (2nd ed.). New York: Oxford University Press.

Barnet, B., Duggan, A., Wilson, M., & Joffe, A. (1995). Association between postpartum substance use and depressive symptoms, stress and social support in adolescent mothers. *Pediatrics, 96,* 659–666.

Berton, M., & Stabb, S. (1996). Exposure to violence and posttraumatic stress disorder in urban adolescents. *Adolescence, 31,* 489–498.

Blum, R., & Bearinger, L. (1990). Knowledge and attitudes of health professionals toward adolescent healthcare. *Journal of Adolescent Health, 11,* 289–294.

Brook, J., Gordon, A., Brook, A., & Brook, D. (1989). The consequences of marijuana use on intrapersonal and interpersonal functioning in black and white adolescents. *Genetic, Social and General Psychology Monographs, 115,* 349–369.

Campbell, J., Poland, M., Waller, J., & Ager, J. (1992). Correlates of battering during pregnancy. *Research in Nursing and Health, 15,* 219–226.

Carrera, M. (1995). Preventing adolescent pregnancy: In hot pursuit. *Siecus Reports, 23,* 16–19.

Centers for Disease Control and Prevention. (1994a). Differences in infant mortality between blacks and whites: United States, 1980–1991. *Morbidity and Mortality Weekly Report, 43,* 288–289.

Centers for Disease Control and Prevention. (1994b). *Pregnancy, STDS and related risk behaviors among U.S. adolescents.* Atlanta, GA: Author.

Centers for Disease Control and Prevention. (1997). Update: Blood lead levels: United States, 1991–1994. *Morbidity and Mortality Weekly Report, 46,* 141–146.

Centers for Disease Control and Prevention. (1998a). State-specific pregnancy rates among adolescents: United States, 1992–1995. *Morbidity and Mortality Weekly Report, 47,* 497–504.

Centers for Disease Control and Prevention. (1998b). Trends in sexual risk behaviors among high school students: United States, 1991–1997. *Morbidity and Mortality Weekly Report, 47,* 749–752.

Centers for Disease Control and Prevention. (1998c). *Tobacco use among U.S. racial/ethnic minority groups: A report of the surgeon general.* Atlanta, GA: Author.

Centers for Disease Control and Prevention. (2000). *Pediatric HIV/AIDS surveillance.* L262, slide series through 1999. Atlanta, GA: Author.

Cohall, A., Bannister, H., Cohall, R., & Vaughan, R. (2000). *EC and adolescent girls: What happens after the morning after?* Manuscript in preparation.

Cohall, A., Dickerson, D., Cohall, R., & Vaughan, R. (1998). Inner-city adolescents' awareness of emergency contraception. *Journal of the American Medical Women's Association, 53,* 258–261.

Curry, M. (1998). The interrelationships between abuse, substance abuse and psychosocial stress during pregnancy. *Journal of Obstetric Gynecology and Neonatal Nursing, 27,* 692–699.

Dominitz, J., Samsa, G., Landsman, O., & Provenzale, D. (1998). Race, treatment, and survival among colorectal carcinoma patients in an equal-access medical system. *Cancer, 82,* 2312–2320.

Durant, R., Cadenhead, C., Pendergrast, R., Slavens, G., & Linder, C. (1994). Factors associated with the use of violence among urban black adolescents. *American Journal of Public Health, 84,* 612–617.

Durkin, M., Kuhn, L., Davidson, L., Laraque, D., & Barlow, B. (1996). Epidemiology and prevention of severe assault and gun injuries to children in an urban community. *Journal of Trauma-Injury Infection and Critical Care, 41,* 667–673.

Easterbrook, G. (1999, October 11). Reproductivity. *New Republic, 221*(15), 22–26.

Fowler, M., Davenport, M., & Garg, R. (1992). School functioning of U.S. children with asthma. *Pediatrics, 90,* 939–944.

Gamble, V. (1997). Under the shadow of Tuskegee: African Americans and healthcare. *American Journal of Public Health, 87,* 1773–1778.

Gazmararian, J., Lazorick, S., Spitz, A., Ballard, T., Saltzman, L., & Marks, J. (1996). Prevalence of violence against pregnant women. *Journal of the American Medical Association, 275,* 1915–1920.

Gergen, J., & Evans, R. (1988). National survey of prevalence of asthma among children in the U.S., 1976–1980. *Pediatrics, 81,* 1–7.

Gergen, P., Mortimer, K., & Eggleston, P. (1999). Results of the National Cooperative Inner-City Asthma Study (NCICAS) environmental intervention to reduce cockroach allergen exposure in inner-city homes. *Journal of Allergy and Clinical Immunology, 103,* 501–506.

Gergen, P., & Weiss, K. (1990). Changing patterns of asthma hospitalization among children, 1979 to 1987. *Journal of the American Medical Association, 264,* 1688–1692.

Gielen, A., O'Campo, P., Faden, R., Kass, N., & Xue, X. (1994). Interpersonal conflict and physical violence during the child-bearing years. *Social Science and Medicine, 39,* 781–787.

Giger, J., & Davidhizar, R. (eds.). (1991). *Transcultural nursing: Assessment and intervention.* St. Louis: Mosby.

Girls Inc. (1996). *Prevention and parity: Girls in juvenile justice.* New York: Author.

Godfrey, E. (1937). The role of the health department in the prevention of accidents. *American Journal of Public Health, 27,* 152–155.

Guyer, B., MacDorman, M., Martin, J., Peters, K., & Strobino, D. (1998). Annual summary of vital statistics, 1997. *Pediatrics, 102,* 1333–1349.

Hanson, K. (1998). Is insurance for children enough? The link between parents' and children's healthcare use revisited. *Inquiry, 35*(3), 294–302.

Health Canada. Policy and Consultation Branch. (1997). *National Health Expenditures in Canada.* Toronto: Author.

Henshaw, S. (1997). Teenage abortion and pregnancy statistics by state, 1992. *Family Planning Perspectives, 29,* 115–122.

Herman-Giddens, M., Brown, G., Verbiest, S., Carlson, P., Hooten, E., Howell, E., & Butts, J. (1999). Underascertainment of child abuse mortality in the United States. *Journal of the American Medical Association, 282,* 463–467.

Holinger, P., Offer, D., Barter, J., & Bell, C. (1997). *Suicide and homicide among adolescents*. New York: Guilford Press.

Hoyert, D. L., Kochanek, K. D., & Murphy, S. L. (1999, June 30). Deaths: Final data for 1997. *National Vital Statistics Reports* (Vol. 47, No. 19). Hyattsville, MD: National Center for Health Statistics, 1–95.

Hughes, L. (1951). Dream deferred. *Montage of a dream deferred*. New York: Holt.

Iyasu, S., Becerra, J., Rowley, D., & Hogue, C. (1992). The impact of the very low birth weight on the black-white infant mortality gap. *American Journal of Preventive Medicine, 8,* 271–277.

Kann, L., Kinchen, S., Williams, B., Ross, J., Lowry, R., Hill, C., Grunbaum, J., Blumson, P., Collins, J., & Kolbe, L. (1998). Youth risk behavior surveillance: United States, 1997. *Morbidity and Mortality Weekly Report, 47*(SS-3), 1–89.

Klein, J., Wilson, K., McNulty, M., Kapphahn, C., & Collins, K. (1999). Access to medical care for adolescents: Results from the 1997 Commonwealth Fund Survey of the Health of Adolescent Girls. *Journal of Adolescent Health, 25,* 120–130.

Klerman, L. (1999). How legislation and health systems can promote adolescent health. *Adolescent Medicine: State of the Art Reviews, 10,* 23–40.

Knitzer, J., & Aber, J. (1995). Young children in poverty: Facing the facts. *American Journal of Orthopsychiatry, 65,* 174–176.

Kogan, M., Alexander, G., Teitelbaum, M., Jack, B., Kotelchuck, M., & Pappas, G. (1995). The effects of gaps in health insurance on continuity of a regular source of care among preschool-aged children in the U.S. *Journal of the American Medical Association, 274,* 1429–1435.

Kogan, M., Kotelchuck, M., Alexander, G., & Johnson, W. (1994). Racial disparities in reported prenatal care advice from health providers. *American Journal of Public Health, 84,* 82–88.

Lantz, P., & House, J. (1998). Socioeconomic factors and determinants of mortality: Results from a nationally representative prospective study of U.S. adults. *Journal of the American Medical Association, 279,* 1703–1708.

Li, X., Stanton, B., & Feigelman, S. (1999). Exposure to drug trafficking among urban, low-income African American children and adolescents. *Archives of Pediatrics and Adolescent Medicine, 153,* 161–168.

Lieu, T., Newacheck, P., & McManus, M. (1993). Race, ethnicity and access to ambulatory care among U.S. adolescents. *American Journal of Public Health, 83,* 960–965.

Lowry, R., Kann, L., Collins, J., & Kolbe, L. (1996). The effect of socioeconomic status on chronic disease risk behaviors among U.S. adolescents. *Journal of the American Medical Association, 276,* 792–797.

Lozano, P., Sullivan, S., Smith, D., & Weiss, K. (1999). The economic burden of asthma in U.S. children: Estimates from the National Medical Expenditure Survey. *Journal of Allergy and Clinical Immunology, 104,* 957–963.

MacDorman, M., & Atkinson, J. (1999). Infant mortality statistics from the 1997 period linked birth/infant death data set. *National Vital Statistics Reports* (Vol. 47, No. 23). Hyattsville, MD, National Center for Health Statistics.

Makuc, D., Breen, N., & Freid, V. (1999). Low income, race, and the use of mammography. *Health Services Research, 34,* 229–239.

Malus, M., Lachance, P., Lamy, L., Macaulay, A., & Vanasse, M. (1987). Priorities in adolescent healthcare: The teenager's viewpoint. *Journal of Family Practice, 25,* 159–162.

Malveaux, F., & Fletcher-Vincent, S. (1995). Environmental risk factors of childhood asthma in urban centers. *Environmental Health Perspectives, 103,* 59–62.

Marks, A., & Fisher, M. (1987). Health assessment and screening during adolescence. *Pediatrics (Suppl.),* 135–155.

Marmot, M., G., Kogevinas, M., & Elston, M. A. (1987). Social/economic status and disease. *Annual Review of Public Health, 8,* 111–135.

McKibbon, L., Vos, E. D., & Newberger, E. (1989). Victimization of mothers of abused children: A controlled study. *Pediatrics, 84,* 531–535.

McLoyd, V., & Wilson, L. (1991). *The strain of living poor: Parenting, social support, and child mental health.* New York: Cambridge University Press.

Miller, R. (1999). Breathing freely: The need for asthma research on gene-environment interactions. *American Journal of Public Health, 89,* 819–822.

Moore, K. A. (1996). *Teen fertility in the U.S.: Facts at a glance.* Washington, DC: Planned Parenthood Federation of America.

Moore, K. A., Papillo, A., Williams, S., Jager, J., & Jones, F. (1999). *Facts at a glance.* Washington, DC: Child Trends.

National Center for Health Statistics. (1999). *United States, decennial life tables for 1989–1991: Some trends and comparisons of the United States life table data, 1900–1991.* Hyattsville, MD: Author.

National Center for Injury Prevention. (1995). [Unpublished data.] Atlanta, GA: Centers for Disease Control and Prevention.

Neinsten, L. (1996). Sexually transmitted diseases. In L. Neinstein (ed.), *Adolescent healthcare: A practical guide* (pp. 853–908). Baltimore: Williams and Wilkins.

Nidorf, J., & Morgan, M. (1987). Cross-cultural issues in adolescent medicine. *Primary Care, 14,* 69–82.

Northridge, M., Yankura, J., Kinney, P., Santella, R., Shepard, P., Riojas, Y., Aggarwal, M., Strickland, P., & Crew, T. E. (1999). Diesel exhaust exposure among adolescents in Harlem: A community-driven study. *American Journal of Public Health, 89,* 998–1002.

Oddone, E., Horner, R., Diers, T., Lipscomb, J., McIntyre, L., Cauffman, C., Whittle, J., Passman, L., Kroupa, L., Heaney, R., & Matchar, D. (1998). Understanding racial variation in the use of carotid endarterectomy: The role of aversion to surgery. *Journal of the National Medical Association, 90,* 25–33.

Olds, D. L., Eckenrode, J., Henderson, C. R., Kitzman, H., Powers, J., Cole, R., Sidora, K., Morris, P., Pettit, L. M., & Luckey, D. (1997). Long-term effects of home visitation on maternal life course and child abuse and neglect. *Journal of the American Medical Association, 278,* 637–643.

Parker, B., McFarlance, J., & Socken, K. (1994). Abuse during pregnancy: Effects of maternal complications and birth weight in adult and teenage women. *Obstetric Gynecology, 84,* 323–328.

Poertner, G. (1998). Birthweight distribution and survival differences by infant race. *Abstract book of the Association for Health Services Research, 15,* 67.

Resnick, M., Bearman, P., Blum, R., Bauman, K., Harris, K., Jones, J., Tabor, J., Beuhring, T., Sieving, R., Shew, M., Ireland, M., Bearinger, L., & Udry, J. (1997). Protecting adolescents from harm: Findings from the National Longitudinal Study on Adolescent Health. *Journal of the American Medical Association, 278,* 823–832.

Roberts, L. (1999). Creating a new framework for promoting the health of African American Female Adolescents: Beyond Risk-Taking. *Journal of the American Medical Women's Association, 54,* 126–128.

Rosenbach, M., Irvin, C., & Coulam, R. (1999). Access for low-income children: Is health insurance enough? *Pediatrics, 103,* 1167–1174.

Rosenstreich, D., Eggleston, P., & Kattan, M. (1997). The role of cockroach allergen in causing morbidity among inner-city children with asthma. *New England Journal of Medicine, 336,* 1356–1363.

Rowland, D., Salganicoff, A., & Keenan, P. (1999). The key to the door: Medicaid's role in improving healthcare for women and children. *Annual Review of Public Health, 20,* 403–426.

Rowley, D. (1995). Framing the debate: Can prenatal care help to reduce the black-white disparity in infant mortality? *Journal of the American Medical Women's Association, 50,* 187–193.

Runyan, D. K., Hunter, W. M., Socolar, R. S., Amaya-Jackson, L., English, D., Landsverk, J., Dubowitz, H., Browne, D. H., Bangdiwala, S. I., and Mathew, R. M. (1998). Children who prosper in unfavorable environments: The relationship to social capital. *Pediatrics, 101,* 12–18.

Rutter, M. (1987). Psychosocial resilience and protective mechanisms. *American Journal of Orthopsychiatry, 57,* 316–331.

Ryan, D., Levy, B., & Walker, B. (1999). Protecting children from lead poisoning and building healthy communities. *American Journal of Public Health, 89,* 822–824.

Sarpong, S., Wood, R., & Eggleston, P. (1996). Short term effects of extermination and cleaning on cockroach allergen Bla g 2 in settled dust. *Annals of Allergy, Asthma, and Immunology, 76,* 257–260.

Scholer, S. (1999). Sociodemographic factors identify U.S. infants at high risk of injury mortality. *Pediatrics, 103,* 1183–1188.

Search Institute. (1997). *The asset approach: Giving kids what they need to succeed.* Minneapolis, MN: Author.

Sickmund, M., & Snyder, H. (1999). *Juvenile offenders and victims: 1999 national report.* Washington, DC: Office of Juvenile Justice and Delinquency Prevention.

Sickmund, M., Snyder, H., & Poe-Yamagata, E. (1997). *Juvenile offenders and victims: 1997 update on violence.* Washington, DC: Office of Juvenile Justice and Delinquency Prevention.

Simkin, L., Radosh, A., Cohall, A., Cohall, R., & Bannister, H. (1999). *Preparing health practitioners to prescribe ECP to adolescents: Training and practice issues.* Paper presented at the annual meeting of the American Public Health Association, Chicago.

Sisk, J., Gorman, S., Glied, S., Reisinger, A., DuMouchel, W., & Hynes, M. (1996). Evaluation of Medicaid managed care: Satisfaction, access, and use. *Journal of the American Medical Association, 276,* 50–55.

Sorenson, S. (1996). Violence and injury in marital arguments: Risk patterns and gender differences. *American Journal of Public Health, 86,* 35–40.

Spake, A., & Couzin, J. (1999). In the air that they breathe: Lead poisoning remains a major health hazard for American children. *U.S. News and World Report, 127,* 54.

Stevenson, R. (2000, January 23). In a time of plenty, the poor are still poor. *New York Times,* Sec. 4, p. 3.

Stewart, D. (1993). Physical abuse during pregnancy. *Canadian Medical Association Journal, 149,* 1257–1263.

Straus, M., & Gelles, R. (1990). *Physical violence in American families: Risk factors and adaptations to family violence in 8,145 families.* New Brunswick, NJ: Transaction.

U.S. Census Bureau. (1997). *Statistical Abstract of the United States: 1997.* Washington, DC: Author

U.S. Census Bureau. (1998). *Poverty in the United States: 1997* (Current Population Reports Series P60–201). Washington, DC: Author.

U.S. Census Bureau. (1999). *Statistical Abstract of the United States: 1999.* Washington, DC: Author.

U.S. Department of Health and Human Services. (1999). *Child maltreatment, 1997: Reports from the states to the National Child Abuse and Neglect Data System.* Washington, DC: U.S. Government Printing Office.

U.S. Department of Health and Human Services. Division of STD Prevention. (1999). *Sexually transmitted disease surveillance, 1998.* Atlanta, GA: Centers for Disease Control and Prevention.

Ventura, S., Martin, J., Curtin, S., & Mathews, T. (1999). Births: Final data for 1997. *National Vital Statistics Reports* (Vol. 47, No. 18). Hyattsville, MD: National Center for Health Statistics.

Weiss, K., Gergen, P., & Crain, E. (1992). Inner-city asthma: The epidemiology of an emerging U.S. public health concern. *Chest, 101* (Suppl. 6), 362S–367S.

Weist, M. D., Ginsburg, G., & Shafer, M. (1999). Progress in adolescent mental health. *Adolescent Medicine: State of the Art Reviews, 10,* 165–174.

Williams, T., & Kornblum, W. (1995). *Growing up poor.* San Francisco: New Lexington Press.

Wilson, W. (1997). *When work disappears: The world of the new urban poor.* New York: Knopf.

Winkleby, M., Robinson, T., Sundquist, J., & Kraemer, H. (1999). Ethnic variation in cardiovascular disease risk factors among children and young adults. *Journal of the American Medical Association, 281,* 1006–1013.

Ziv, A., Boulet, J., & Slap, G. (1998). Emergency department utilization by adolescents in the United States. *Pediatrics, 101,* 987–994.

Ziv, A., Boulet, J., & Slap, G. (1999). Utilization of physician offices by adolescents in the United States. *Pediatrics, 104,* 35–42.

CHAPTER THREE

THE HEALTH STATUS OF BLACK WOMEN

Sandra E. Taylor

All the women are white, all the blacks are men, but some of us are brave.

BLACK WOMEN'S STUDIES (HULL, SCOTT, & SMITH, 1982).

African American women have historically been at the bottom of the totem pole relative to a number of status factors including income and occupation. In health this trend of low priority tends to continue. Statistics on various health conditions underscore the abysmal status of black women's health vis-à-vis the health of their white counterparts. For example, black women aged forty-five to sixty-four are ten times more likely than white women of the same age to die of diseases of the heart and are five times more likely to die of diabetes (National Center for Health Statistics [NCHS], 1999). Treatment decisions can compound the situation as evidenced in research showing that physicians are less likely to refer women and blacks than white men for catheterization. Findings from this research suggest that the race and sex of a patient independently influence how physicians manage chest pain (Schulman et al., 1999). Other illnesses, chronic diseases, and mortality rates experienced by black women indicate a similar dilemma. This chapter discusses some of these conditions in an overview of black women's health by examining selected publications including governmental data. It provides information on the current health status of African American women through a review and synthesis of these various sources.

The state of black health is in decline as evidenced by several indicators, as discussed in a number of chapters in this book. One glaring indicator is the declining state of black women's health. Black women in the United States suffer a disproportionate risk of ill health in part just because they are black women. The privileges that come with being born white and male extend into one of the most cherished and desired of all attributes, health. Black women in America are disproportionately faced with many conditions that are preventable, or at least controllable. This is evident in various diseases including cancer, diabetes, and cardiovascular, or heart disease. Especially poignant is the fact that black women are particularly vulnerable to the leading cause of death for black males aged eighteen to forty-four and women aged twenty-four to thirty-six. A majority of the women who have AIDS-related illness or are HIV positive are black. Furthermore, black women with AIDS do not live as long or die as well as their white or male counterparts.

Of the various preventable health conditions and diseases discussed in this chapter, none rivals the magnitude of the HIV/AIDS epidemic for black women. Black women are woefully overrepresented as a proportion of reported HIV/AIDS cases compared to white women. HIV/AIDS is thirteen times more common among African American women than among Caucasian women. The Centers for Disease Control and Prevention (CDC) report that through June 1999, among all women, African American women represented 57 percent of total reported AIDS cases. The numbers are even higher for HIV infections as reported from the thirty-three states with confidential HIV infection reporting—of this total (HIV infection among women), black women accounted for 68 percent (CDC, 1999a).

HIV/AIDS, like some other conditions, affects black women more dramatically partially due to failure to diagnose it correctly in its early stages in these women. Additionally, it is harder to maintain health or reverse the situation when a condition is diagnosed in its latter stages. These reasons are often discussed in the context of other related factors when examining black-white differences in health.

Many theories have been argued and various hypotheses tested to explain the disproportionate number of blacks facing health problems. In the sociological literature these theories include the (1) genetic hypothesis, (2) physical exertion hypothesis, (3) associated disorder hypothesis, (4) psychological stress hypothesis, (5) diet hypothesis, and (6) medical care hypothesis (Cockerham, 1998). Throughout the literature, irrespective of discipline, studies abound on these and other hypotheses. Researchers are beginning to pay attention to issues of multiculturalism and the need for the inclusion of black women and other women of color in their sample populations. Despite this awareness, however, the result still tends to be a sample inclusive of black men and a preponderance of white women, if and when the latter are at all represented. In contrast, far fewer studies are available that include black women or that examine factors specifically related to black women's health. The sparseness of the empirical literature on black women's health appears to be directly related to their health status.

Much of the scientific literature that does exist on black women's health has been criticized for examining it outside the contexts important to black women. One emerging argument is that black women's social and psychological contexts are often ignored by medical practitioners and researchers in their health analyses. Landrine and Klonoff (1997) argue that even though the health of black women tends to be neglected altogether in psychological research, where it is addressed (for example, in medical and public health journals), cultural and social context variables are methodologically inadequate. These authors discuss the growing contention that the health of black women must be understood in the particular cultural context in which these women find themselves. For example, understanding this cultural context is a particular bone of contention for Burkett (2000).

Burkett (2000) analyzed the content of articles published from 1989 to 1998 in three major medical journals: the *Journal of the American Medical Association*, the *American Journal of Public Health*, and the *New England Journal of Medicine*. Her findings suggest that explanations for illness and mortality are limited to black women's individual behaviors and that few address the context in which these behaviors occur. Her research has important implications for the improved health status of black women in that the content of the articles analyzed can serve to inform healthcare providers and the medical community about this particular population. This in turn can positively affect health care providers' capacity to adequately address the specific needs of their black women patients.

That psychosocial factors affect black women's health status has also been argued by Lawson, Rodgers-Rose, and Rajaram (1999). They conclude that research on black women should conceptualize their health as a complex interaction of psychosocial risks that have a profound effect on that health. Examining the relationship between psychosocial factors and health status, the study illuminates an array of relationships. For example, the study shows that black women in the lower economic groups are more likely to be treated for allergies and pelvic inflammatory disease in comparison to their middle- and upper-income counterparts. The study also found that women who had experienced comparatively more incidents of racism received more medical treatments for yeast infections, pregnancy-related problems, allergies, and pelvic inflammatory disease. Additionally, these data showed that the women who had histories of physical, psychological, and early sexual abuse were more likely to be treated for depression, allergies, yeast infections, and hypertension compared to those women with no such histories.

Even in the new millennium, black women are still too often stereotyped in medical and health care settings. These stereotypes, along with prevailing myths, act to hamper any elevation in health status. Taylor (1999) discusses how negative images and labels function together to become oppressive mechanisms for black women. By discussing images of black women in terms of (1) the mammy, (2) the matriarch, (3) the welfare mother, (4) the Jezebel, and (5) the black lady overachiever, the author illuminates how very little things have changed in the struggle for a color-blind and gender-neutral society. She analyzes the processes that sustain "whiteness" and racism in nursing practice, research, and academics. Health care disciplines and professions have failed to adequately address this problem. In fact, it has been argued that some health care disciplines actively perpetuate sexist and racist attitudes and practices. Eliason (1999), in her discussion of health disparities between African American and European American women, contends that the nursing profession has been a partner in perpetuating the racism of health care and society. Although her focus is on nursing research and practice, this argument can be appropriately applied to other disciplines. The health care literature is replete with accounts of how the medical profession has historically responded in disparaging ways to blacks and women. As other health and health-related disciplines build the literature on black women and their neglect, it appears that the field of medicine is likely to share its onerous distinction with these other disciplines.

The long history of excluding black women from empirical research points to the low status afforded this group. Klonoff, Landrine, and Lang (1997) discuss this void, focusing on the particular case of black women's absence in health psychology and behavioral medicine research. According to these authors, psychology stands conspicuously apart from other health disciplines in the exclusion of black women from studies. They argue that although the major health disciplines have failed in their consideration of black women for empirical analysis, no discipline has fared worst than psychology. Others have also pondered the absence of black women. Vivian Pinn, associate director of the Office of Research on Women's Health at the U.S. National Institutes of Health, raises the question directly in her article "Where Are African American Women?" (1996). The lack of information about the overall health of black women and the attitudes that lead to this void in the literature portend a bleak picture when data are analyzed.

In a recent CDC study, maternal mortality figures show that black women are three to six times more likely than white women to die from complications of pregnancy. Furthermore, this disparity did not improve from 1987 through 1996 (CDC, 1999b). The total maternal mortality ratio (MMR) for black women increased slightly over the two five-year periods, from 18.8 to 20.3, whereas it decreased for white women, from 5.5 to 5.0. The national MMR was 7.7 for both the five-year period between 1987 and 1991 and the five-year period from 1992 through 1996. Hence there was no improvement over time despite a national health objective to reduce the MMR to 3.3 per 100,000 live births by the year 2000. The study also points out that black women have a higher risk than white women of dying from every pregnancy-related cause of death reported, including the three leading causes (hemorrhage, pregnancy-induced hypertension, and embolism).

It seems unfathomable that as we enter the millennium and the age of the mapping of the human genome that any woman in the United States should die due to pregnancy or childbirth complications. The irony of this travesty is that American women are experiencing health hazards that faced women one hundred years ago. The data on maternal mortality are so appalling that they prompted congressional attention. Appropriately, women in the U.S. Congress introduced the Safe Motherhood Monitoring and Prevention Research Act of 1999. The bill's intent is, among other things, to provide funding for monitoring systems at the local, state, and national level so we can better understand the burden of maternal complications and mortality and decrease ethnic and racial disparities. This congressional act and similar decisions are necessary if any appreciable progress is to be made in the improvement of health for black women. Advocacy for this particular group on an array of levels is key in gaining parity across health indices.

Strategic Efforts for the Promotion of Black Women's Health

A number of health promotion initiatives have recently emerged to address morbidity and mortality disparities among black women. Many of these have come in the form of coalition or partnerships that include the governmental, business, and religious sectors. Whether public or private, the most successful partnerships have tended to involve strong community organization (Braithwaite, Taylor, & Austin, 2000).

The Food and Drug Administration (FDA) of the U.S. Department of Health and Human Services (DHHS) created the Office of Women's Health (OWH) in 1994. Among other purposes, the office was created to provide scientific and policy input on women's health issues, many of which have particular relevancy for low-income women and women of color. These OWH initiatives have led to various health promotion campaigns through partnerships with grassroots organizations, other federal agencies, state and local governments, and private industry.

The Health Resources and Services Administration (HRSA) has recently created the Office of Women's Health to improve health services for women and girls, especially women of color and medically underserved groups. HRSA has historically played a significant role in education and training efforts for increasing access to primary and preventive health care for vulnerable groups. Its Office of Women's Health extends this mission through initiatives in prenatal care, immunizations, physical examinations, and other preventive health care programs. The office also promotes access to health care for homeless women and children and residents of public housing. A number of additional efforts particularly consequential for black women include support services to women living with HIV/AIDS (through programs under the Ryan White CARE Act) and nurse-managed clinics focusing on domestic violence prevention and interventions.

The National Institutes of Health (NIH) and the CDC collaborated in 1995 to sponsor several university-based prevention research studies whose findings might translate into community interventions. To the extent that a major focus was on community approaches to more healthful behaviors, black women were largely represented. This effort, part of the Women's Health Initiative (WHI) of NIH, sought to enhance knowledge of several conditions that affect black women disproportionately, including cancer, hypertension, and heart disease.

Other research and applied initiatives that are more expressly designed for health promotion and disease prevention among black women include local and state government efforts. Unfortunately, however, these efforts are not always representative of the systematically developed programs necessary for a sustained change in the status of black women's health. Moreover, only a few states sponsor any initiative specifically targeted to black women's health. As discussed later in this chapter, a recent telephone survey to key contacts in all fifty states confirms the need for more health promotion initiatives.

Perhaps no single organization has done as much as the National Black Women's Health Project (NBWHP) in organizing around issues relating to the overall health and welfare of African American women. This organization, founded by Bylle Avery in 1981, is viewed as the key voice on black women's health issues. Its mission is to improve the health of African American women by providing wellness education and services, self-empowering strategies, health information, and advocacy. The current president and CEO, Julia Scott, advocates (as do other key activists in NBWHP) for a change in research priorities in addition to changes in the other, more common situations that make good health problematic for black women.

Through statewide initiatives, NBWHP has affected the lives of countless black women. One state-based model of particular note is the California Black Women's Health Project (CBWHP), established in 1994 as a health promotion and wellness empowerment model to address community-specific needs. This program has received many accolades from formal organizations and agencies and from the women who directly participate. Like many health initiatives involving coalitions or partnerships, this effort is best conceptualized as a process model that can inspire community change (Brown, Jemmott, Mitchell, & Walton, 1998).

The NBWHP sponsors various forums from the publication of books and other timely health articles to immunization programs and health screenings. If it did not exist, it would most certainly need to be created. Still, it alone cannot correct even a fraction of the problems that need addressing to improve black women's health. We now turn to some of these health problems.

Heart Disease, Hypertension, and Stroke

Black women experienced a heart disease mortality rate of 553 per 100,000 during 1991 to 1995, compared to a rate of 388 per 100,000 for white women during this same time period (CDC, 1999c). Gerhard et al. (1998) contend that differences in coronary risk factors may place the black women in their study at increased risk compared to the white women studied. The black women studied (aged eighteen to forty-five) had a higher body mass index and higher systolic and diastolic blood pressures. They also had a two- to threefold greater rate of coronary heart disease than their premenopausal white counterparts.

Although it is established that heart disease kills more people in the United States, including black women, than any other killer, there are few studies of risk factors for coronary heart disease in African American women. One recent study (Rosenberg, Palmer, Rao, & Adams-Campbell, 1999) shows that high body mass index was associated with coronary heart disease in the absence of control for hypertension, diabetes mellitus, and elevated cholesterol, but it was not associated when they were controlled. This suggests that obesity may influence risk as a result of its effects on blood pressure, glucose tolerance, and cholesterol levels. The data further suggest that important risk factors for coronary heart disease are similar in black women and white women (Rosenberg, Palmer, Rao, & Adams-Campbell, 1999).

Hypertension, or high blood pressure, is related to both heart disease and stroke. Black women have recently experienced lowered rates of stroke with the improvement of hypertension treatments. Still, hypertension is more prevalent among blacks than whites, due in part to social and environmental factors. Krieger (1990) found that the stress of racial discrimination is directly related to hypertension among black women. Other studies show the positive relationship between stress management and lowered incidents of morbidity and mortality due to heart disease, hypertension, and stroke.

Cancer

Breast cancer is the leading cause of cancer deaths among black women; lung cancer (mostly attributable to tobacco use) is the major cause of cancer deaths among all women. Although white women are more likely to develop breast cancer, black women are more likely to die of this disease. The five-year survival rate for black women with breast cancer is 43 percent; the rate for white women is 90 percent.

Moormeier (1996) reviewed articles and clinical studies from 1966 to 1995 on breast cancer in black women and concluded what we have known for some time—that the discrepancy in survival rates between black and white women exists because breast tumors in black women are consistently diagnosed at a more advanced stage of disease, because tumor biology in black women is different from that in white women, and because of confounding comorbid conditions and socioeconomic factors. This article also confirms statistics that show the incidence of breast cancer is lower in black women than in white women and discusses differences in reproductive factors as a plausible explanation. Although deaths due to breast cancer are decreasing among white women but not among black women, recent prevention and intervention strategies signal hope for reducing this burden for the African American female population.

Mortality differences between black and white women are also apparent for women with cervical cancer. The death rate from cervical cancer is more than twice as high for black women as it is for white women. Race has been found to be an independent predictor of cervical cancer survival; even when accounting for factors such as age, stage of disease, and treatment patterns, race remains a predictor (Howell, Chen, & Concato, 1999).

Diabetes

Nearly 6 percent of black men and 8 percent of black women have diabetes. More than two million blacks are estimated to have this disease. As discussed in Chapter Twelve, diabetes disproportionately affects African Americans. Rates for African Americans are 2.5 times higher than rates for whites. Among black women, diabetes has reached epidemic proportions, with one in four black women fifty-five and older having diabetes. Much of the literature on black women and diabetes points to the importance of screening and early detection of diabetes among high-risk women and the need for improved quality of care and for patient education services appropriate to the needs of these women (McNabb, Quinn, & Tobian, 1997).

Diabetes is the leading cause of new cases of blindness, end-stage renal disease, lower extremity amputation, and premature death. More than 3.5 million women in the United States have been diagnosed, and an equal number have diabetes but are unaware of the fact (CDC, 1999c).

Although diabetes is no longer considered a serious risk during pregnancy, women with diabetes should closely monitor their blood glucose before and during pregnancy. A temporary form of diabetes that develops during pregnancy, gestational diabetes, is 80 percent more common in African American women than in white women. Gestational diabetes typically dissipates after pregnancy; however, women with gestational diabetes are at an increased risk for developing type II diabetes.

Lupus

Lupus is three times more common in black women than in white women. It is a disease of the immune system that can affect the joints, skin, kidneys, lungs, heart, and brain. Although the cause of lupus is unknown, the autoimmune disease is neither contagious nor necessarily hereditary. Systemic lupus erythematosus (SLE), which affects different parts of the body, is the most serious form of the disease. Discoid, or cutaneous, lupus mainly affects the skin. Affected persons may have a red rash or a color change of the skin on the face, scalp, or other parts of the body. A third type, drug-induced lupus, is triggered by prescription medications. The most common drugs that can lead to drug-induced lupus are procainamide, used for heart problems; hydralazine, used to treat hypertension; and Dilantin, used for seizures. Unlike SLE, this form of lupus is usually found in older men and women of all races. Studies on lupus are inconclusive as to how the disease affects the immune system, why black women are especially vulnerable, and the extent to which it runs in families. However, research funded by NIH as well as private sponsors shows a promising outlook for lupus patients (Sullivan, 1996).

Reproductive Health

We have seen how maternal morbidity has affected black women. Other reproductive health areas in which all women have special health care needs include
fertility, contraception, menstruation, and menopause. Many health issues in
these areas, especially in fertility and contraception, are affected in part by lifestyle choices. For example, smoking can affect fertility and the unborn child. Similarly, overeating and a high-fat diet can adversely affect a woman's pregnancy.

Teen Pregnancy

Teen mothers are more likely to live in poverty and to interrupt their education
than are older mothers. Also, the overall quality of a young mother's life is greatly
compromised in comparison to the lives of young women who wait until they are
older to become pregnant. Yet, even though conventional wisdom suggests that
teenage pregnancy is undesirable for all these reasons, it has also been argued that
because health risks for black women increase after the teen years, these years
may be the best years for black women to bear children, given their health trajectories over the life cycle. Hence Geronimus (1994) argues that policy concerns
have been misdirected, focusing on the age of black motherhood rather than on
the economic and social conditions under which it occurs and to which it is forced
to adapt.

Given this argument, health risks are more associated with discrimination
and the social policies that do not support the procreation of black families than
with the biological consequences of giving birth during the teen years. Nevertheless, young black women bear a disproportionate burden of poor health outcomes
compared to young white women (as evidenced in rates of HIV infection, poor
nutrition, victimization and exposure to traumatic violence, incarceration, and
mortality). So it would appear that these women are also vulnerable to health
risks during pregnancy. Therefore risk behavior should be examined along with
gender, race, and socioeconomic status in assessing health outcomes, especially in
the case of black female adolescents who live in inner cities (Roberts, 1999).

Fibroids and "Female Problems"

Uterine leiomyoma or fibroid tumors (fibroids) are the most common pelvic tumors occurring in women (affecting up to 40 percent of all women) and are more
often found in black women than in white women. Fibroids are noncancerous
growths found in or attached to the uterus; they consist of fibrous smooth muscle
cells that grow from the muscular womb lining. Generally, they do not cause
problems and can remain undetected. However, they can be associated with

menstrual abnormalities and pelvic pressure or pain and may be associated with infertility, spontaneous abortion, and premature delivery.

Hysterectomy, the surgical removal of the uterus, is the most commonly performed nonobstetric surgical procedure in the United States (NCHS, 1999). Approximately one-third of all women will have undergone this procedure by their sixtieth birthday. (Cesarean section is the most common of all surgical procedures.) In addition to being performed for the treatment of fibroid tumors, many hysterectomies are performed in attempts to cure endometriosis, which can cause women to suffer from pain during intercourse, pelvic pains, dysmenorrhea, and infertility. Endometriosis affects women from all racial and ethnic groups. According to CDC data from 1980 through 1993, annual rates of hysterectomies did not differ significantly by race (Lepine et al., 1997). Over 50 percent of hysterectomies are performed due to either fibroid tumors or endometriosis (Lepine, et al., 1997). Uterine prolapse or cancer is the other condition most often associated with hysterectomy.

Certain other health conditions uniquely faced by women, including menopause, are becoming increasingly controversial with respect to treatment. For example, estrogen replacement therapy (use of an artificially produced form of the hormone to raise estrogen levels) is increasingly viewed by medical authorities as a choice patients can make. This is in part an outgrowth of resistance to *medicalization,* the process in which medicine comes to control areas of life that were previously considered nonmedical (Zola, 1972). Until the time comes when the medical establishment acknowledges and acts on gender biases, women must be actively engaged in decisions about their ultimate treatments (Scully, 1994). Knowing as much as possible about a condition and its treatment is especially consequential for disenfranchised women, many of whom are African American.

Intimate Violence

Approximately two million women are assaulted by their partners each year. On average each year from 1992 to 1996, approximately 8 in 1,000 women aged twelve or older experienced a violent victimization perpetrated by their partner (this figure contrasted with 1 in 1,000 men aged twelve or older) (Greenfield et al., 1998). Battering causes more physical injuries to women than car accidents and muggings. Approximately one-third of all violence is caused by someone close to the victim (for example, husband, fiancé, or boyfriend); hence the term *intimate violence.* Research indicates that as many as 30 percent of women treated in emergency departments have injuries or symptoms related to physical abuse (NCHS, 1999).

Black women are at greater risk for abuse than are white women and remain in abusive relationships longer than white women. On average each year from 1992 to 1996, approximately 12 per 1,000 black women experienced intimate violence, compared with about 8 per 1,000 for white women (rates not adjusted for socioeconomic status which may account for the higher rates in black women) (Greenfield et al., 1998). A sample of 323 women (91.6 percent black) revealed that 25 percent of those surveyed had been beaten by a spouse (Lawson et al., 1999). In addition, 75 percent of those studied reported psychological abuse. This sample consisted of middle-class black women. Thus, if we accept the data showing that low-income women are at greater risk than their middle-class counterparts, these figures become even more astounding. In either case, these abuses play a role in contributing to the poor health status of black women.

Psychological or emotional abuse has received less attention than has physical abuse in both the published literature and in public awareness campaigns. Russo et al. (1997) found that although lower-income women were more likely to experience partner violence, this did not hold for their having had experienced abuse during childhood. The study found that childhood physical and sexual abuse and partner violence were intercorrelated.

Both abuse history and partner violence were related to greater risk for depressive symptoms, lower life satisfaction, and lower perceived health care quality. Sexually abused women had more difficulties in interpersonal relationships, including lower perceived health care quality, even with self-esteem and depressive symptoms held constant (Russo, Denious, Keita, & Koss, 1997). Psychological consequences for women of intimate violence can include depression, suicidal thoughts and attempts, lowered self-esteem, alcohol and other drug abuse, and posttraumatic stress disorder, among other conditions (NIH, 1998).

Mental Health Issues

African American women cope with a plethora of problems, some of which emanate from a racist and sexist society. There is no hard evidence that explains why some of these women surmount stressors while others develop lapses in mental health functioning. However, research does show the positive impact of social supports, whether religious or familial or from some other source. Still, black women are experiencing increasing challenges to optimal mental health. Depression is a particular problem that is on the increase for this group. Early diagnosis and treatment are essential for preventing depression from becoming chronic. Improvements in education and training programs and in the development of culturally competent mental health services delivery systems are recommended to address the needs of black women. Additionally, changes in research paradigms are necessary if these women are to enjoy a heightened quality of life.

Lifestyles and Health Behaviors

A substantial proportion of mortality in the United States can be attributed to three major behaviors: using tobacco, eating an unhealthy diet, and being sedentary or physically inactive. A disproportionate number of black women consume foods that are low in fiber and high in fat. A disproportionate number of black women also maintain a sedentary lifestyle not conducive to good health. However, black women do not use tobacco, alcohol, and drugs more than their white counterparts. For example, CDC data show smoking to be less common among African American women compared to white women (21 percent and 24 percent, respectively). Regardless of the behavioral choice, studies show the benefits from lifestyle enhancements and augmented health behaviors. Using data from the South Carolina mortality files and the Behavioral Risk Factor Surveillance System, Macera et al. (1996) suggest that physical inactivity and poor dietary habits (excess caloric intake, low fruit and vegetable consumption) would be good choices for interventions not only because they affect mortality, but also because they exert interim effects on morbidity.

Obesity

Obesity is more common among black women than whites as is high serum cholesterol, a factor often found in conjunction with obesity. Even among college-educated black women, this holds. Factors that contribute to obesity include diet (high fat content), stress (which leads to overeating for consolation purposes), and attitudes (a body weight that is often considered fat or despicable by whites may often be considered desirable, attractive, or *phat* by blacks). Black women are less likely to be concerned about picking up a pound and less likely to diet. However, obesity is a risk factor for several diseases including cardiovascular disease, diabetes, and hypertension. A recent study by Rosenberg, Palmer, Adams-Campbell, and Rao (1999) assessed the relationship of body mass index to prevalent hypertension among both African American women who had completed college and less educated black women. Using data from the Black Women's Health Study (which examined 64,530 black women aged twenty-one to sixty-nine who responded to mailed health questionnaires in 1995), the authors found a high prevalence of obesity and hypertension and a strong association of obesity with hypertension among highly educated African American women.

Using data from this same study, Adams-Campbell, Rosenberg, Washburn, Kim, and Palmer (2000) found this to hold and also that strenuous physical activity increased with education. Higher levels of walking for exercise and moderate and strenuous activity were associated with higher levels of participation in strenuous exercise in high school. At the same time, the authors conclude what we have known for some time—that physical activity levels are not very high for black women. To reverse this problem, they suggest that educational efforts to increase levels of physical activity start at an early age. In 1988 to 1991, 34 percent of all women aged twenty to seventy-four were overweight. Over one-half of African American women over twenty years of age are overweight (NCHS, 1999).

Barriers to physical activity have been identified as competing responsibilities, lack of motivation, fatigue, no person with whom to exercise, and lack of child care, among other reasons (Nies, Vollman, & Cook, 1999).

Women Who Are Especially Vulnerable: Special Populations

Black women who are incarcerated or homeless have even greater needs than other black women. Both groups' health is at particular risk.

Women in Prisons

Because of the disproportionate number of black women in prisons, the penal system can be seen as yet another health hazard for African American women. Incarcerated persons often complain about their medical conditions going untreated and the lack of adequate health care in these institutions. Across the country, legal counsel has been sought in numerous cases to argue on behalf of prisoners whose health has been severely endangered. Pregnant women and women who give birth while incarcerated report on experiences of incredible neglect and undue suffering. Those with chronic conditions and other diseases report on the unavailability of prescriptions or on not being given medications on schedule. The result of incarceration is too often a weaker individual both mentally and physically.

Women inmates have been found to have higher rates of antisocial and borderline personality disorders compared to women in community epidemiological studies (Jordan, Schlenger, Fairbank, & Caddell, 1996). The authors of that study concluded that the high rates of psychiatric and psychological disorders associated with exposure to traumatic events suggest that incarcerated women have a need for treatment for mental health problems.

For black women prisoners, like black men prisoners, HIV/AIDS is a particular risk. Although the vast majority of inmate AIDS deaths and current AIDS cases continue to occur among men, HIV seroprevalence is very often higher among female than male inmates. Data from one study show aggregate AIDS incidence rates in state and federal systems to be 464 cases per 100,000 among men and 705 cases among women (Braithwaite, Hammett, & Mayberry, 1996). This same study shows that in responding city and county jail systems, the rates were 342 cases per 100,000 among men and 201 cases among women. To the extent that incarceration rates are rising faster among women than men, and given that women in both prisons and jails are more likely to be drug users than are male inmates, women prisoners are increasingly at risk for HIV/AIDS.

Homeless Women

Although racial and ethnic research has not reported data separately for homeless men and women, statistics do show that a majority of the homeless population are people of color, primarily African Americans, and that this population includes a growing number of women and children. In a sample of St. Louis homeless (three hundred women and six hundred men), North and Smith (1994) found that the homelessness of white individuals was internally related whereas the homeless African Americans was externally related: that is, white homelessness was more often related to substance abuse in men and non-substance abuse psychiatric illness in women; African American homelessness was more often related to socioeconomic problems arising from lower incomes for men and reliance on a failing welfare system for women and their dependent families.

In addition to their obvious problems (such as lack of food, clothing, and shelter), homeless persons also face such problems as a higher rate of mental illness compared to the general population and a higher incidence of life-threatening conditions, including HIV infection. Because these problems represent conditions that affect society as well as the individual, implications for public health are present. More developed modes of treatment for mental disorders and of HIV prevention and treatment should be integrated into comprehensive health and medical programs serving homeless populations.

Conclusion

It would be a mistake of course to lump all black women together as if they constituted a monolithic group. And there are differences in socioeconomic characteristics and geography among black women that are important in understanding their specific health conditions and risk factors for disease. Nevertheless, it is clear that the health needs of black women in general have been grossly ignored and that black women face the problem of being overlooked and understudied largely because of their African ancestry. However, given community and national partnerships and the voices of black women themselves, there is reason to believe that the current bleak picture does not have to constitute a stagnant situation. A number of published resources discuss health promotion, wellness, and empowerment strategies useful to black women (Aldridge & Rodgers-Rose, 1993; Boston Women's Health Book Collective, 1998; Villarosa, 1994; White, 1994).

History has shown how black women have been active in the black health reform movement and have played a pivotal role in linking government and private sector health initiatives with those to be served. In a review of Susan Smith's acclaimed work (1995), Elders (1996) discusses this link in the context of black women's recognition of their plight and their struggle for change. An awareness and sense of empowerment have and continue to be important factors in this change.

Policy Issues

It is vital that the dominant white medical and research communities develop an enhanced understanding of the needs, beliefs, and values of black women. The health care professions' lack of knowledge and insights about black women continues to exacerbate an already critical problem. From exclusion from clinical trials to all-too-common medical delayed diagnosis or misdiagnosis, improvements have been negligible. In the instance of clinical trials the dominant medical research community has argued that it has faced difficulties recruiting black women to participate in studies. It is popular to argue that black women may be reluctant to participate in clinical trials because of the shadow cast by the Tuskegee syphilis experiment and other incidents of medical abuse. Gamble (1997) contends not only that the Tuskegee abomination accounts for the virtual absence of black women in studies but also that the battle against racism in medicine is far from over. Moreover, Gamble argues that the battle against racism must be an integral part of the campaigns and ongoing strategies to improve the health of black women. However, even though the infamous Tuskegee syphilis experiment is often used as a rationale for low recruitment or lack of recruitment of black women into both therapeutic and nontherapeutic clinical trials, some black women do not agree with this claim. According to Freedman (1998), in interviews with middle-class, professional, and semiprofessional black women, these women say they would be more likely to participate given trials that are relevant to their primary medical concerns.

Recommendations

Many studies on the health of black women point out the need for more health care exams, planning, and community-based interventions that emphasize empowering black women to take control of their particular health issues. This has been debated in the context of public health and the role of government in improving morbidity and mortality rates.

It is time for a national review on leading causes of morbidity. States should implement review mechanisms to help identify and investigate specific conditions (as many states have recently done to learn more about maternal mortality). In order to gauge how states were faring in the development and implementation of programs for black women's health, the author of this chapter and the author of Chapter Four (on black men's health) conducted a telephone survey. Findings from this survey indicate that only a miniscule number of states have ongoing programs or have interventions currently in practice (see Table 4.1 in Chapter Four). Included among the initiatives are HIV/AIDS, cancer awareness, and mental health programs. Of these programs, a majority were largely supported by federal funds. For example, the Health Care Financing Administration (HCFA) offers mammogram screening and other interventions geared toward older and Hispanic women in selected major cities throughout the country, including Atlanta, Chicago, Cleveland, Los Angeles, Philadelphia, San Antonio, and Washington, D.C.

Studies that will advance our knowledge of ways to improve the health status of black women are sorely needed, as is research on the health status of all women of color. Whether the differences in mortality and morbidity among women in America are due to culture, environment, or genetic predisposition, white women enjoy a significantly higher health status than do women of color (Adams, 1995). Leveling these differences is a goal from which all in our society can benefit.

As it is for the other health issues discussed in this volume, improved prevention is undoubtedly the single most important factor for improving black women's health. This holds whether we reflect on the conditions discussed in this chapter or on additional conditions, such as asthma, arthritis, disabilities, and sexually transmitted diseases (all of which affect black women disproportionately). The need for a greater emphasis on prevention in the research and medical treatment of black women is a requirement that will be met through the orchestrated efforts of all parties genuinely concerned about the growing disparities in black women's health.

Lastly, a recommendation related to economics is in order. Because most black women work outside the home, employers should have strategies in place for incorporating health promotion and disease prevention programs into the workplace. The labor market is a strategic environment for disseminating health messages. Attention to these and other recommendations is important if black women in American society are to attain greater parity in health outcomes.

References

Adams, D. L. (Ed.). (1995). *Health issues for women of color: A cultural diversity perspective.* Thousand Oaks, CA: Sage.

Adams-Campbell, L. L., Rosenberg, L., Washburn, R. A., Kim, K. S., & Palmer, J. (2000). Descriptive epidemiology of physical activity in African American women, *Preventive Medicine, 30,* 43–50.

Aldridge, D., & Rodgers-Rose, L. (1993). *River of tears: The politics of black women's health.* Newark, NJ: Traces.

Boston Women's Health Book Collective. (1998). *Our bodies, ourselves for the new century.* New York: Simon & Schuster.

Braithwaite, R. L., Hammett, T. M., & Mayberry, R. M. (1996). *Prison and AIDS: A public health challenge.* San Francisco: Jossey-Bass.

Braithwaite, R. L., Taylor, S. E., & Austin, J. N. (2000). *Building health coalitions in the black community.* Thousand Oaks, CA: Sage.

Brown, K. A., Jemmott, F. E., Mitchell, H. J., & Walton, M. L. (1998). The well: A neighborhood-based health promotion model for black women. *Health and Social Work, 23,* 146–152.

Burkett, T. (2000, April). *Black women's health: A content analysis of the Journal of the American Medical Association, the American Journal of Public Health, and the New England Journal of Medicine, 1989–1998.* Paper presented at the Southern Sociological Society Association meeting, New Orleans.

Centers for Disease Control and Prevention. (1999a). *HIV/AIDS Surveillance Report, 11*(1).

Centers for Disease Control and Prevention. (1999b). State-specific maternal mortality among black and white women: United States, 1987–1996. *Morbidity and Mortality Weekly Report, 48,* 492–495.

Centers for Disease Control and Prevention. (1999c). *Women and heart disease: An atlas of racial and ethnic disparities in mortality.* Atlanta, GA: Author.

Cockerham, W. C. (1998). *Medical sociology.* Upper Saddle River, NJ: Prentice Hall.

Elders, M. J. (1996). Sick and tired of being sick and tired [Review of the book *Black women's activism in America*]. *Lancet, 347,* 454–455.

Eliason, M. J. (1999). Nursing's role in racism and African American women's health. *Health-care for Women International, 20,* 209–219.

Freedman, T. G. (1998). Why don't they come to Pike Street and ask us? Black American women's health concerns. *Social Science and Medicine, 47,* 941–947.

Gamble, V. N. (1997). The Tuskegee Syphilis Study and women's health. *Journal of the American Medical Women's Association, 52*(4), 195–196.

Gerhard, G. T., Sexton, G., Malinow, M. R., Wander, R. C., Connor, S. L., Pappu, A. S., & Connor, W. E. (1998). Premenopausal black women have more risk factors for coronary heart disease than white women. *American Journal of Cardiology, 82,* 1040–1045.

Geronimus, A. (1994). The weathering hypothesis and the health of African American women and infants: Implications for reproductive strategies and policy analysis. In G. Sen & R. C. Snow (Eds.), *Power and decision: The social control of reproduction* (pp. 77–100). Cambridge, MA: Harvard University Press.

Greenfield, L., Rand, M. R., Craven, D., Klaus, P. A., Perkins, C. A., Ringel, C., Warchol, G., Matson, C., & Fox, J. A. (Eds.). (1998, March). Violence by inmates: Analysis of data on crimes by current or former spouses, boyfriends, and girlfriends. *Bureau of Justice Statistics Factbook.* (NCJ-167236. Washington, DC: U.S. Department of Justice.

Howell, E. A., Chen, Y. T., & Concato, J. (1999). Differences in cervical cancer mortality among black and white women. *Obstetrics and Gynecology, 94,* 509–515.

Hull, G. T., Scott, P. B., & Smith, B. (Eds.). (1982). *All the women are white, all the blacks are men, but some of us are brave: Black women's studies.* New York: Feminist Press at the City University of New York.

Jordan, B. K., Schlenger, W. E., Fairbank, J. A., & Caddell, J. M. (1996). Prevalence of psychiatric disorders among incarcerated women. II. Convicted felons entering prison. *Archives of General Psychiatry, 53,* 513–519.

Klonoff, E. A., Landrine, H., & Lang, D. L. (1997). Introduction: The state of research on black women in health psychology and behavioral medicine. *Women's Health, 3,* 165–181.

Krieger, N. (1990). Racial and gender discrimination: Risk factors for high blood pressure? *Social Science and Medicine, 30,* 1273–1281.

Landrine, H., & Klonoff, E. A. (1997). Conclusions: The future of research on black women's health. *Women's Health, 3,* 367–381.

Lawson, E. J., Rodgers-Rose, L., & Rajaram, S. (1999). The psychosocial context of black women's health. *Healthcare for Women International, 20,* 279–289.

Lepine, L. A., Hillis, S. D., Marchbanks, P. A., Koonin, L. M., Morrow, B., Kieke, B. A., & Wilcox, L. S. (1997, August 8). Hysterectomy surveillance—United States, 1980–1993. *Morbidity and Mortality Weekly Reports, CDC Surveillance Summaries, 46*(SS-4), 1–14.

Macera, C. A., Lane, M. J., Mustafa, T., Giles, W. H., Blanton, C. J., Croft, J. B., & Wheeler, F. C. (1996). Trends in mortality and health behaviors: Status of white and African American women. *Journal of the South Carolina Medical Association, 92*(10), 421–425.

McNabb, W., Quinn, M., & Tobian, J. (1997). Diabetes in African American women: The silent epidemic. *Women's Health, 3*(3-4), 275–300.

Moormeier, J. (1996). Breast cancer in black women. *Annals of Internal Medicine, 124,* 897–905.

National Center for Health Statistics. (1999). *Health, United States, 1999 with health and aging chartbook* (DHHS Publication No. PHS 99-1232). Hyattsville, MD: Author.

National Institutes of Health (NIH). (1998). *Women of color health data book.* (NIH publication no. 98-4247). Rockville, MD: Office of Research on Women's Health.

Nies, M. A., Vollman, M., & Cook, T. (1999). African American women's experiences with physical activity in their daily lives. *Public Health Nursing 16,* 23–31.

North, C. S., & Smith, E. M. (1994). Comparison of white and nonwhite homeless men and women. *Social Work, 39,* 639–647.

Pinn, V. W. (1996). Status of women's health research: Where are African American women? *Journal of the National Black Nurses Association, 8,* 8–19.

Roberts, L. (1999). Creating a new framework for promoting the health of African American female adolescents: Beyond risk taking. *Journal of the American Medical Women's Association, 54,* 126–128.

Rosenberg, L., Palmer, J. R., Adams-Campbell, L. L., & Rao, R. S. (1999). Obesity and hypertension among college-educated black women in the United States. *Journal of Human Hypertension, 14,* 237–241.

Rosenberg, L., Palmer, J. R., Rao, R. S., & Adams-Campbell, L. L. (1999). Risk factors for coronary heart disease in African American women. *American Journal of Epidemiology, 150,* 904–909.

Russo, N. F., Denious, J. E., Keita, G. P., & Koss, M. P. (1997). Intimate violence and black women's health. *Women's Health, 3,* 315–348.

Schulman, K. A., Berlin, J. A., Harless, W., Kerner, J. F., Sistrunk, S., Gersh, B. J., Dube, R., Taleghani, C. K., Burke, J. E., Williams, S., Eisenberg, J. M., & Escarce, J. J. (1999). The effect of race and sex on physicians' recommendations for cardiac catheterization. *New England Journal of Medicine, 340*(8), 618–626.

Scully, D. (1994). *Men who control women's health.* New York: Teachers College Press.

Smith, S. L. (1995). *Black women's health activism in America, 1890–1950.* Philadelphia: University of Pennsylvania Press.

Sullivan, E. G. (1996). Lupus: The silent killer. In Catherine Fisher Collins (Ed.), *African-American women's health and social issues* (pp. 25–35). Westport, CT: Auburn House.

Taylor, J. Y. (1999). Colonizing images and diagnostic labels: Oppressive mechanisms for African American women's health. *Advances in Nursing Science, 21,* 32–45.

Villarosa, L. (Ed.). (1994). *Body and soul: The black women's guide to physical health and emotional well-being.* New York: Harper Perennial.

White, E. C. (Ed.). (1994). *Black women's health book: Speaking for ourselves.* Seattle, WA: Seal.

Zola, I. K. (1972). Medicine as an institution of social control. *Sociological Review, 20,* 487–504.

CHAPTER FOUR

THE HEALTH STATUS OF BLACK MEN

Ronald L. Braithwaite

During the 1970s, African American men were labeled an "endangered species." Thirty years later, African American men face a multitude of health, sociopolitical, and psychological issues, and thus they continue to be an "endangered species." Several factors account for their increasing scarcity and absence from family life. The number and percentage of black men in prison is higher than it is for any other racial or ethnic subgroup (Braithwaite, Hammett, & Mayberry, 1996). Although African American men make up approximately 6 to 7 percent of the total U.S. population, they represent more than 60 percent of the two million persons under correctional supervision. African Americans are imprisoned at seven times the rate of whites. Thirty-three percent of black men between the ages of twenty and twenty-nine are either in jail, on probation, or on parole (Whitehead, 2000). These findings exacerbate and amplify the reality behind the endangered species hypothesis.

Black men experience a shorter life expectancy (67.6 years) than does any other racial or ethnic minority subgroup (74.5, 74.8, and 80.0 years for white men, black women, and white women, respectively) (Murphy, 2000). African American men in every age group up to age sixty-five and over experience higher mortality rates than any other racial or ethnic subgroup. Their death rate for heart disease is one and one-half times greater than that of African American women and two times greater than that of Caucasian males (Courtenay, 2000). Furthermore, accidents and homicide contribute disproportionately to the decline of black men. According to the National Center for Health Statistics (NCHS) (Murphy, 2000), accidents were the leading cause of death for black males aged five to fourteen years and twenty-five to forty-four years and the second most common cause of death for black males aged fifteen to twenty-four. Homicide was the leading cause of death for black males aged fifteen to twenty-four and second for those five to fourteen years old. HIV/AIDS is yet another contributing factor in the decimation of black men. For black males aged twenty-five to forty-four, AIDS was the second leading cause of death in 1999.

This chapter draws attention to health issues pertinent to African American men with emphasis on their nonutilization and underutilization of the American health care system. The leading causes of mortality in this population are discussed, and examples of statewide approaches to closing the black-white disparity gap in health status are identified.

Health Care Utilization Among African American Men

One construct that has emerged over the last thirty years to explain the disconnection of African American men from the American health care system is stoicism. Stoicism has its roots in ancient philosophy, and philosophers such as Zeno and Chrysippus were contributors to this school of thought (Rist, 1969). Although stoicism is a broad philosophy with several tenets (Timothy, 1973), its idea of indifference to pleasure or pain is the reason that it can be important in considering individuals' attitude toward health care. In particular, indifference to pain or discomfort may be an important factor contributing to failure to seek health care as well as delays in seeking health care.

Wagstaff and Rowledge (1995) examined the relationship between stoicism and negative attitudes toward the poor in both men and women. Men were shown to be more stoic. Study participants identified as stoic displayed less emotional reaction to stories with emotional content. Morse and Penrod (1999) discuss concepts associated with illness and injury including "enduring" and "suffering." Enduring was defined as "an emotionless state that focuses on the present" (p. 146). In the face of illness or injury, African American men may often not acknowledge their physical weakness, choosing instead to focus on more immediate needs and concerns. They display an emotionless posture and take an instrumental approach to solving problems with everyday living.

Moynihan (1998) discusses a theory of masculinity as it relates to health care and research, and advances the idea that men's stoic attitudes toward health care contribute to both physical and mental health conditions. It may well be the case that African American men learn pathological levels of stoic tolerance of discomfort that often prevent appropriate behavioral responses to pain, illness, and stress. This presents yet another barrier to achieving optimal health in African American men. As such a barrier, stoicism among African American men is a plausible explanation for the disparity gap in health between African American men and other subgroups in the U.S. population.

There is considerable disparity in health care utilization rates between higher and lower socioeconomic groups, between women and men, and between African Americans and Caucasians (Kaiser Family Foundation, 1999). These disparities are often attributed to differences in both income and insurance access (Agency for Healthcare Research and Quality, 2000). African American men, in particular, experience greater morbidity and mortality than other racial or ethnic subgroups because of their underutilization of the health care system. One theory posits that African American men have learned to deal with pain differently than others do and in accordance with their roles and subcultures. This theory suggests that African American men become indifferent to pain or discomfort and do not seek out health care services until absolutely necessary, and then most often in emergency room settings. Unfortunately, these stoic attitudes place them at higher risk for adverse health conditions and for late diagnosis of health conditions.

Although impassiveness toward pain and discomfort was a conscious choice for followers of stoic thought, this is likely not the case for African American men. Several factors may contribute to their stoic attitudes toward health, including a lack of adequate health insurance, traditional attitudes about male gender roles, fear of a poor prognosis, and distrust of the medical community. Each of these topics is discussed in the following pages.

Inadequate Health Insurance

Approximately forty-four million Americans are without health insurance coverage. The uninsured are primarily children and people under the age of sixty-five. Young adults aged eighteen to thirty-nine years accounted for the highest rates of uninsurance from 1989 to 1996, with 22 percent without coverage in 1994 (Carrasquillo, Himmelstein, Woolhandler, & Bor, 1999). Although most Americans who have health insurance obtain it through their employment, many lack coverage either because they cannot afford to pay for it or because it is not offered through their employment. For example, between 1988 and 1994, employment-based health insurance covered four million fewer people than in previous years (Schroeder, 1996). Consequently, low-income earning employees and their families are predominantly uninsured. Americans who earn less than 200 percent of the federal poverty level (or $27,300 for a family of three) are likely to be uninsured (Kaiser Family Foundation, 2000). Thus employment is not indicative of adequate access to affordable health coverage. In 1998, three of five men living on $16,000 or less were uninsured (Sandman, Simantov, & An, 2000). In 1996 the rates of uninsurance are higher for males as compared to females (17.1 percent versus 14.2 percent), and the percentage of increase in uninsurance was higher for males than females (Carrasquillo et al., 1999).

Although a lack of health care coverage affects millions of Americans, ethnic and racial minorities are at a greater risk of being uninsured. A lack of health insurance is more common among African American men than among white men. According to the Men's Health Network (2000a), "Poor black men are 6–7 times as likely to be uninsured as their white counterparts" (p. 1). Even when compared to their female counterparts, African American men are less like to have any form of health insurance coverage (see Figure 4.1).

FIGURE 4.1. PERCENTAGE UNINSURED
BY RACE/ETHNICITY AND SEX, 1996.

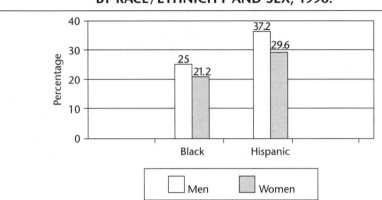

Source: Kass, Weinick, and Monheit, 1996, p. 4.

Traditional Attitudes About Male Roles

Men have traditionally been socialized that they should not cry, that they should be cavalier about certain things that affect them, that it is weak to show pain, and that it is cowardly to run from danger. They have also been encouraged to detach themselves psychologically from feelings of fatigue or discomfort that might prevent them from completing their tasks. Ignoring these feelings may lead to a short-term increase in performance but at the long-term expense of increasing risk of injury and illness. Nowhere is this more evident than in the way men and women seek health care. Across all income levels, African American men are twice as likely as women to have had no physician contacts in the past year (Men's Health Network, 2000a). Women consistently report their symptoms to doctors more than men do (Kronke & Spitzer, 1998). Such traditional attitudes about the male roles in society manifest with greater morbidity and mortality in African American men.

Fear of Poor Prognosis

Males tend to be hesitant to acknowledge fear in any capacity. Their stoic attitudes toward health and health care utilization may be a result of fear of a poor prognosis. When males experience pain and discomfort, many elect not to seek health care professionals because they do not want to hear "bad news." This may be a reason African American men suffer the consequences of prostate cancer more often than white men. Early detection increases the chances of survival in this and other diseases, but fear may serve to incapacitate men when it comes to seeking and utilizing health care services and thus serve as a barrier to early detection and treatment of chronic health conditions.

Distrust of the Medical Community

African Americans are distrustful of the U.S. health care system because of historical evidence of racial discrimination (Thomas & Quinn, 1991; Dula, 1994). Misguided medical research such as the Tuskegee syphilis trials may have contributed to the atmosphere of distrust in the health care system among African Americans and the economically disadvantaged (Thomas & Quinn, 1991). Fear of becoming a medical guinea pig may override any health concerns for many who remember the consequences of medical research gone wrong. Conspiracy theories about potential genocide of African American people circulate throughout the community regularly enough to perpetuate fear and distrust of the medical community. This is another reason why contact with the health care system can be limited or nonexistent. This distrust has severely compromised the health and well-being of African American men who could benefit from regular preventive health care.

The Tuskegee medical experiment on poor, uneducated African American males is often cited as the singular reason for African American distrust of the medical community. However, such an interpretation neglects the pervasive distrust that predates the Tuskegee study. African Americans' fears date back to the antebellum period, when slaves and free blacks were often used in experiments. In one experiment, slave women were used to develop a surgical procedure to repair vesicovaginal fistulas. These women underwent up to thirty painful operations, often without anesthesia (Dula, 1994). In another experiment, a slave underwent a series of experiments to test remedies for heatstroke. The slave was forced to sit naked on a stool that was placed on a platform in a pit that was heated to a high temperature. Over a period of three weeks, the slave was placed in the pit five or six times and given different medications to determine which medication best enabled him to withstand the heat (Dula, 1994).

African Americans' distrust of the medical establishment continues as a twentieth century phenomenon because of more recent events as well. For example, in the 1970s, misinformation about sickle cell screenings led to job and housing discrimination against African Americans, increased costs for life and health insurance, and social stigmatization resulting in low self-esteem (Dula, 1994). Experiments that are disproportionately focused on the black population such as the sterilization abuses in the 1960s, the current search for a gene that controls violent behavior, and certain biomedical research on the AIDS virus have contributed to the ongoing mistrust in the African American community.

According to Cornelius Baker, former executive director of the National Association of People with AIDS, fear coupled with their collective memory about exploitation by the medical community has led blacks not to comply with taking indicated medications (Stryker, 1997). For example, a case manager who works for an agency that provides services for people with AIDS in New York City refuses to take HIV medication because the Tuskegee study taught her, she says, "not to jump at the first thing they come out with" (Richardson, 1997, p. A6).

Life Expectancy

America's ethnic minority populations have historically experienced poorer health outcomes than have whites. Moreover, men in America die nearly seven years younger than women and have higher death rates for all of the fifteen leading causes of death (Courtenay, 2000). African American males age sixty-five and over experience higher mortality rates for all causes of death than any other racial subgroup. Based on the 1998 mortality rates, females are expected to outlive males by 5.7 years, and the white population is expected to outlive the black population by 6.0 years. Data from the NCHS (Murphy, 2000) on life expectancy at birth by race and sex in the United States show that white females continue to have the highest life expectancy at birth (80.0 years), followed by black females (74.8 years), white males (74.5 years), and black males (67.6 years) (see Figure 4.2). This variance in life expectancy among the races is attributed largely to environmental and situational factors that are life threatening (Lober, 1997).

In a recent article by Jonathon Leach (1998) on men's health issues, males are described as the "weaker gender." This labeling is based on the epidemiological evidence that women suffer more bouts with illnesses on the whole but men tend to experience higher incidents of morbidity and mortality. Men tend to be more vulnerable to heart disease than women due to the cardio-protective effect of estrogen in women. Premature death in African American men, in general, is linked to lifestyle habits such as smoking, alcohol use, substance abuse, unhealthy diet, and self-defeating and deleterious risk-taking behaviors (Leach, 1998; Lober, 1997).

Contemporary scientists have focused a great deal on women's health issues while neglecting attention to men's health issues. Men's issues have been relegated to the male genital organs and the prostate, with mentions for comparative purposes in the literature on women's health (Leach, 1998). The next few pages highlight the leading causes of death of African American males.

Cardiovascular Disease

Cardiovascular disease or heart disease is the leading cause of death in the United States. Approximately twice as many men as women die from heart disease (119.3 as compared with 60.4) (Men's Health Network, 1999). The heart disease rate for African American men is one and one-half times greater than the rate for African American women and over two times greater than the rate for Caucasian males (Men's Health Consulting, 2000).

The term *cardiovascular disease* (CVD) encompasses a number of diseases caused by deficits in the circulatory system. These diseases include stroke and coronary heart disease. Risk factors for CVD include smoking, high cholesterol, hypertension, excessive alcohol intake, obesity, diabetes, lack of exercise, and a sedentary lifestyle. Hypertension is considered by some to be the single most

**FIGURE 4.2. LIFE EXPECTANCY AT BIRTH
BY RACE/ETHNICITY AND SEX, 1990–1998.**

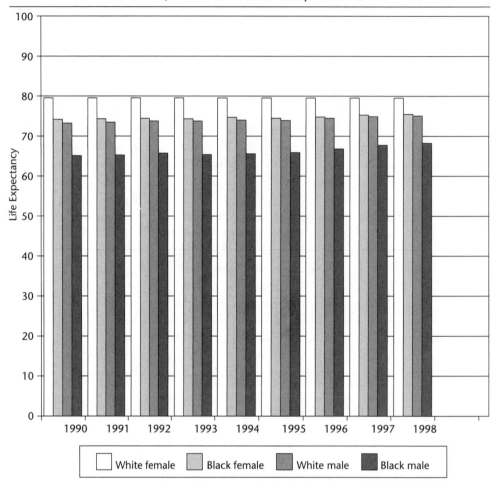

Source: Murphy, 2000, p. 22.

important risk factor for CVD, particularly in African Americans. Nearly twice
as many African American males as females have high blood pressure, and one
and one-half times more males have hypertension. When contrasted with Caucasians, African Americans are twice as likely to have moderately high blood
pressure and three times as likely to have severe hypertension (Men's Health Consulting, 2000). Obesity can contribute to heart disease by elevating blood pressure. It can also contribute by inducing type 2 diabetes, which is a risk factor for
heart disease (American Heart Association, 2000; World Health Organization,
1999; Feldman & Fulwood, 1999). Studies have found that men with a body mass
index ranging from 25 to 29 have a 70 percent increased risk of coronary heart
disease and men with a body mass index of 29 to 33 have a threefold higher risk
of coronary heart disease (World Health Organization, 1999).

Over the last two decades a decline in the CVD mortality rate has become evident. This decline is attributed to the improvement in medical technology and a reduction in the risk factors that cause CVD (Feldman & Fulwood, 1999). Although African Americans have participated in this decrease in the CVD mortality rate, they still have a higher ratio of stroke and coronary heart disease as compared to non-Hispanic whites. Socioeconomic status along with obesity, hypertension, diet, and smoking are believed to be chiefly responsible. In general African Americans tend to have a larger body mass index than non-Hispanic whites. What is considered a traditional *soul food* diet may contain multiple high-fat and high-cholesterol foods that contribute to the risk factors for CVD. Twenty-three percent of the African American population lives in poverty and lacks adequate transportation. This coupled with limited high-quality community food chain resources can make obtaining proper nutrition difficult (Feldman & Fulwood, 1999; American Heart Association, 2000).

Cancer

Cancer is the second leading cause of death for men in general. For college-age African American men, it is the fourth leading cause of death. Fifty percent more men than women die of cancer. The excess deaths are concentrated in three kinds of cancer: lung, colorectal, and prostate (Men's Health Network, 2000). Overall, African Americans have a higher incidence of cancer and a higher cancer mortality rate than any other racial or ethnic group does. Multiple factors contribute to this occurrence including a lack of knowledge about cancer symptoms, the detection of cancer in the later stages of disease development, a lack of access to cancer treatment services and state-of-the-art medical technology, a fatalistic view that cancer equals death, an overreliance on religious faith as a means of healing, a mistrust of the medical system, and lifestyle factors.

In the United States, lung cancer is the most common type of cancer in men, with prostate cancer being the second and colon or rectum cancer the third most common types (American Cancer Society, 1996; Feldman & Fulwood, 1999). Lung cancer is the leading cause of cancer deaths among African American males. Over twice as many African American males as females die from lung cancer (Men's Health Network, 2000). Before the age of sixty, African American men are four times more likely to develop lung, colon or rectum, and prostate cancer than are all other races combined. The mortality rate for prostate cancer among African American men is the highest in the world for that disease (Weinrich, Reynolds, Tingen, & Starr, 2000).

Prostate cancer is one of the most common causes of cancer mortality despite being one of the most treatable forms of cancer. It is the second leading cause of cancer death among African American males. African American men have seven times the incidence of prostate cancer that non-Hispanic white men do. The reasons for the disparity are not completely known but may be related to a higher level of biologically available testosterone and other genetic and environmental factors in African American men. Prostate cancer is an androgen-dependent tumor; the presence of testosterone promotes this cancer's growth (Ross, Shinizu, Paganini-Hill, Honda, & Henderson, 1987).

Studies of African American men's knowledge about prostate cancer have indicated a lack of association between prostate cancer and its symptoms (such as blood in the urine, pain while urinating, and difficulty urinating). Additionally, a majority of study subjects were unaware of their high risk for prostate cancer development or at what age to begin screening for prostate cancer. Many study participants held the fatalistic view that once they developed prostate cancer, they were going to die (Feldman & Fulwood, 1999; Mandelblatt, Yarboff, & Kerner, 1999). In studies performed to identify the barriers to prostate screening, cost, lack of knowledge, and avoidance ("putting it off") were identified as the major barriers for men in general. For African American men, lack of transportation has been identified as an additional barrier (Weinrich et al., 2000).

Accidental Injuries

Accidental injuries are among the top five causes of mortality in African American males of all ages. Accidental injuries include those occurring in motor vehicle accidents, occupational accidents, and accidents in the home. Injuries from accidents are the second leading cause of death for African American men of college age (Hoyert, Kochanek, & Murphy, 1999; Men's Health Consulting, 2000).

More than 95 percent of the employees in the top ten most hazardous jobs are men. Of persons killed in occupational accidents in 1999, over 90 percent were men (Men's Health Network, 1999). Although non-Hispanic white men in general are more likely to be injured in the workplace, African American men are more likely to die of injuries incurred in the workplace. Traditionally, "dirty" and dangerous jobs were referred to as *Negro work* and reserved for African American laborers. This led to high exposure to industrial hazards and increased incidence of occupational disease among African American workers (Loomis & Richardson, 1998).

Currently there is a disparity in the labor force structure. Non-Hispanic whites are more likely to be employed in managerial, sales, or administrative positions, which have lower occupational fatality rates. African Americans are more likely to have jobs that are more physical or that require exposure to chemical and environmental hazards (Wagener & Winn, 1991; Loomis & Richardson, 1998). Similarly, a 1997 retrospective study at the University of North Carolina at Chapel Hill examined the employment patterns of African American workers and non-Hispanic white workers in North Carolina and the rate of unintentional fatal occupational injuries occurring between 1977 and 1991. Results showed that even when disparities in the labor force structure are removed, the occupational mortality rates for African American men are still higher than those for non-Hispanic white men. This suggests that factors in addition to these disparities are contributing to the greater occupational mortality in African American men. These other factors are likely to involve unequal access to the labor market, unequal distribution of hazardous assignments within a job, and discrimination (Loomis & Richardson, 1998).

Interpersonal Violence

Interpersonal violence is a public health issue that affects both morbidity and mortality. The term *interpersonal violence* encompasses a group of acts involving the willful infliction of pain or death. These acts include homicide, domestic violence, rape, assault, and suicide (Cubbin, Pickle, & Fingerhut, 2000; Trowers, 1998–1999). Eighty percent of the victims of interpersonal violence know the perpetrator. Although women are more likely to be victims of rape and domestic violence and to attempt suicide, men are more likely to be victims of violent deaths and to make successful suicide attempts. Interpersonal violence often occurs in association with the use of alcohol and illegal drugs by both the victims and the perpetrators (Centerwall, 1995; Cubbin, Pickle, & Fingerhut, 2000).

African Americans are overrepresented as both the perpetrators and victims of interpersonal violence, with the exception of suicide. Homicide ranks thirteenth in the United States as a leading cause of death. For African American men of all ages, however, homicide ranks fifth, and it remains second for youths, ages fifteen to twenty-four. Over his lifetime an African American male runs a one in twenty-nine chance of becoming a murder victim (Livingston, 1994; Hoop & Herring, 1996; Cubbin, Pickle, & Fingerhut, 2000; Hoyert, Kochanek, & Murphy, 1999).

African Americans in general are less likely to commit suicide than are members of non-Hispanic white populations. However, young African American males (ages fifteen to twenty-four) have a relatively high rate of suicide. In other racial groups the rate of suicide tends to be higher in the older age groups. The high rate of suicide among young African American males is believed to be caused by psychosocial stressors. These stressors include economic, political, and social disadvantages (Livingston, 1994).

Two of the central issues in the study of violence are why individuals vary in their propensity to commit violence and why populations vary in their rates of violence. The theory of social disorganization (that is, the "inability of a community structure to realize the common values of its residents and maintain effective social controls") is one explanation that has been offered (Cubbin, Pickle, & Fingerhut, 2000, p. 2; also see Centerwall, 1995). It is believed that social disorganization leads to an increase in crime. Other theories have focused on socioeconomic deprivation, advancing the idea that a lack of legitimate economic opportunities will lead to frustration, which may in turn lead to the commission of crime (Cubbin, Pickle, & Fingerhut, 2000).

HIV/AIDS

When acquired immune deficiency syndrome (AIDS) first surfaced in the early 1980s, it was considered a disease of white, middle- and upper-class, urban gay men. It was believed to be caused by a promiscuous homosexual lifestyle and was called the gay-related immune disease (GRID). Today the face of AIDS has changed as the disease has become an epidemic primarily among poor, urban racial and ethnic minorities, particularly African Americans and Hispanics (Lober, 1997; Ward & Duchin, 1998). African Americans are 12.6 percent of the total U.S. population but represent 28 percent of all HIV/AIDS cases in the United States, a disproportionately high number. Among African American males the prevalence of HIV is 186.3 per 100,000; for non-Hispanic white males the prevalence of HIV is 32.5 per 100,000. Of the AIDS cases reported in the United States in 1998, 45 percent were among African Americans and 33 percent were among non-Hispanic whites (Hoyert, Kochanek, & Murphy, 1999; Feldman & Fulwood, 1999; Kaiser Family Foundation, 1998).

According to the NCHS (Hoyert, Kochanek, & Murphy, 1999), the primary mode of HIV transmission among African American males is the exchange of body fluids in connection with the use of intravenous drugs. In 1998, 37 percent of the new HIV cases in African American males reported intravenous drug use as the primary mode of transmission, followed by anal intercourse at 27 percent. Comparatively, the primary mode of HIV transmission among non-Hispanic white males is unprotected anal intercourse. Male-to-male sexual transmission was involved in 69 percent of all new HIV cases for non-Hispanic white males. In 1998, non-Hispanic white males had a lower percentage than African American males did of new HIV cases attributable to intravenous drug use (11 percent) (Hoyert, Kochanek, & Murphy, 1999; Kaiser Family Foundation, 1998).

Diabetes

Diabetes mellitus is a major public health problem in the African American community. It is the seventh leading cause of death for African American males of all ages. Most of the current articles written about diabetes highlight the disparity between racial groups rather than between genders. However, according to the National Institute of Diabetes and Digestive and Kidney Diseases (1999), women twenty years old and older have a higher prevalence of diabetes than men in the same age group (8.1 million and 7.5 million, respectively). The prevalence of diabetes in African Americans is 70 percent higher than in whites. Approximately 2.3 million African Americans have diabetes. African Americans are 1.7 times more likely to develop type 2 diabetes as whites (American Diabetes Association, 2000; National Institute of Diabetes and Digestive and Kidney Diseases, 1999).

In the African American population in particular, the high prevalence of type 2 diabetes is caused by a combination of environmental and genetic factors. Some African Americans have inherited a gene that provided their ancestors with a means for surviving harsh climates and periods of famine. Today in Western industrialized societies, there are few cycles of feast and famine, and the presence of this gene can make weight control difficult and increase the risk of developing diabetes (Black Healthcare, 2000). The Western diet is an environmental risk factor for the development of diabetes. The high carbohydrate intake characteristic of the Western diet contributes to hyperglycemia (American Heart Association, 2000).

Looking Toward the Future: Developing Men's Health Care Initiatives

In order to assess how states are faring in implementing programs that address African American men's health, the chapter author conducted telephone interviews with key contacts in each state health department during 2000. These contacts were asked if there was a statewide initiative addressing men's and women's health in general and specifically African American men's and women's health. If no statewide initiative was in place, the contacts were then asked if there was any categorical state funding that targets specific health issues pertinent to men's and women's health. The interviews were fifteen to thirty minutes in length. Information was collected on statewide health care initiatives for men in general and women in general and for African American men specifically and for African American women specifically. Information was also obtained on the type of program available for these men and women (see Table 4.1).

The results of the survey are summarized in Table 4.1. The results for women's health are discussed in Chapter Three. The results for men's health indicate

TABLE 4.1. SURVEY OF STATE HEALTH DEPARTMENTS ON MEN'S AND WOMEN'S HEALTH INITIATIVES.

States	Men's Health	African American Men's Health	Women's Health	African American Women's Health	Comments
Alabama	–	–	+	–	Initiatives on local level
Alaska	*	*	*	*	
Arizona	–	–	+	–	
Arkansas	+	+	+	+	
California	+	+	+	+	
Colorado	–	+	+	+	
Connecticut	*	*	*	*	
Delaware	–	+	+	+	
Florida	–	+	+	+	
Georgia	+	+	+	+	
Hawaii	–	–	+	–	
Idaho	*	*	*	*	
Illinois	*	*	*	*	
Indiana	–	PP	+	PP	Initiatives on local level
Iowa	–	PP	+	PP	Minority Health Advisory Task Force developing policies on African Americans

(*Continued on page 74*)

TABLE 4.1. (*continued*)

States	Men's Health	African American Men's Health	Women's Health	African American Women's Health	Comments
Kansas	−	+	+	+	
Kentucky	−	−	+	−	
Louisiana	*	*	*	*	
Maine	−	−	+	−	Initiatives on local level
Maryland	*	*	*	*	
Massachusetts	*	*	*	*	
Michigan	+	+	+	+	
Minnesota	*	*	*	*	
Mississippi	*	*	*	*	
Missouri	−	+	+	+	Initiatives on local level
Montana	−	−	+	−	Low African American population
Nebraska	+	+	+	+	
Nevada	+	+	+	+	
New Hampshire	+	+	PP	PP	Effective September 1, 2000
New Jersey	+	+	+	+	
New Mexico	−	+	PP	PP	Effective within the next year
New York	+	+	+	+	
North Carolina	+	+	+	+	
North Dakota	+	+	−	−	Low African American population
Ohio	+	+	+	+	
Oklahoma	+	+	+	+	
Oregon	+	+	+	+	
Pennsylvania	+	+	+	+	
Rhode Island	+	+	+	+	
South Carolina	+	+	+	+	
South Dakota	+	+	−	−	Low African American population
Tennessee	+	+	+	+	
Texas	+	+	+	+	
Utah	+	+	+	+	
Vermont	+	+	+	+	
Virginia	+	+	+	+	
Washington	+	+	+	+	
West Virginia	+	+	+	+	
Wisconsin	+	+	+	+	
Wyoming	+	+	+	+	
Washington, D.C.	*	*	*	*	

+ Statewide initiative

− No statewide initiative

PP Policy pending

* Missing data

that few states have statewide initiatives that specifically target African American men's health. Instead, the states administer categorical funding that targets specific health issues, such as HIV/AIDS in the African American community.

Michigan is one of the states that has recognized the need to address men's health specifically. In response to the increasing rate of premature deaths among African American males, Michigan sponsored the African American Male Initiative as a way for the community to combat the causes of these deaths (Michigan Department of Community Health, 2000). In March 1995, the Department of Public Health in Michigan organized a sixty-five-member statewide task force to address the major health problems that disproportionately affect African American males. In July 1997, in response to the work of the task force, the Michigan Department of Community Health (MDCH) created the African American Male Initiative, which seeks to

- Advocate for and promote responsive, consumer-oriented health care providers and services
- Advocate for and support development of activities to bring about healthier lifestyles
- Support research and policies that can lead to improved health status.
- Educate individuals and families to take charge of their health [Michigan Department of Community Health, 2000, p. 3]

One of the MDCH goals is to assist local communities in developing community-based coalitions to address the health needs of African Americans on the local level. The MDCH promotes this concept by using a model developed in Washtenaw County, Michigan. Calhoun County was the first county to successfully adopt the concept, developing the African American Health Issues Forum (Michigan Department of Community Health, 2000).

Similarly, Georgia has recognized that there is a health crisis affecting men's health and well-being in the state. In response, the state has created the Commission on Men's Health. The bill instituting the commission was introduced on January 25, 2000, passed by the state senate on February 16, and signed by Governor Barnes on March 10, 2000. The duties of the commission (Georgia Commission on Men's Health, 2000) are to

- Develop strategic, public policy recommendations and programs, including community outreach and public-private partnerships that are designed to educate Georgia's men on the benefits of regular physician checkups, early detection and preventive screening tools, and healthy lifestyles practices
- Focus on improving health outcomes of men in specific disease areas including, but not necessarily limited to, prostate and testicular cancer, cardiovascular disease (including high blood pressure, stroke, and heart attacks), depression and suicide, and diabetes

- Monitor state and federal policy and legislation that may affect areas of men's health
- Recommend assistance, services, and policy changes that will further the goals of the commission
- Submit a report of its findings and recommendations under its charter to the governor, the president of the senate, and the speaker of the house of representatives not later than October 1 of each year [Childers et al., 2000, p. 6]

Recently, Senator Strom Thurmond of South Carolina introduced a bill on the floor of the U.S. Senate (S. 2925) to create an Office of Men's Health (OMH) within the U.S. Department of Health and Human Services. The OMH will co-ordinate and promote the status of men's health in the United States.

In addition to statewide initiatives, some nonprofit organizations have committed themselves to increasing public awareness around issues relating to men's health. The Men's Health Network, for example, was created to address the continuing silent crisis in the health and well-being of men. The goals of the network (Men's Health Network, 2000b) are to

- Save men's lives by reducing the premature mortality of men and boys
- Foster health care education and services that implement positive lifestyle decisions for men of all ages and their families
- Increase the physical and mental health of men so that they can live fuller and happier lives
- Significantly reduce the cycles of violence and addiction that disproportionately afflict so many men

Conclusion

As African American males engage the new millennium, they do so with challenges and obstacles to their physical and psychological well-being. This subpopulation has and continues to suffer from societal forces that relegate them to places among the lowest rungs on the ladder of upward mobility. Forces that promote overt and covert discrimination in employment, housing, and access to health care resources marginalize their health status and reinforce the endangered species hypothesis. The increasing scarcity of African American men and the imbalance in their ratio to African American women severely threaten the vitality of the African American family.

A Policy Issue

Although this chapter primarily addresses health disparities between African American males and other subpopulations in America, failure to link African American males' plight to the unparalleled struggles they have historically faced and still face would result in an incomplete and inaccurate description. The disparity in health status experienced by African American males comes as no surprise when one considers the structural and institutional barriers they continue to confront in their quest to achieve parity and equal footing in a land of slippery slopes and uneven playing fields. No longer can the victims be blamed for the shortcomings of institutions. Emphasizing personal behavioral change among African American males without emphasizing institutional policy change is blaming the victim. The insensitive and antiquated policies and practices of governmental agencies that continue to disregard the health and human service needs of African American males feed the demise of the African American family. When we consider the participation of African American males in health promotion and wellness-oriented programs, we must be aware that the line between system responsibility and individual responsibility is thin. Indeed, there are responsibilities on both sides that can serve to enhance the health status of black men.

Much of the confusion attending the victim-blaming debate has to do with the assumption of a direct relationship between attributions of cause for problems and attributions of responsibility for correcting them. These two processes are not always distinguished from each other (Caplan & Nelson, 1973). Many assume that if individuals are held personally responsible for changing their lifestyles, then they must be blamed for adverse health outcomes. Emanating from this assumption is the further mistaken assumption that health promotion programs that emphasize personal responsibility and individual change are victim blaming programs. However, encouraging African American males to participate in health education programs says nothing about attributing blame. Rather, it asks African American males to participate in creating a solution. A greater emphasis on personal responsibility does not have to and should not replace system blame and social change perspectives. The real issue is how to better incorporate individual behavior change and personal responsibility into the health promotion paradigm in a way that is sensitive to both the historical and situational circumstances of African American males.

Green (1987) criticizes academicians for pitting health education strategies against social change strategies as if we could actually have the latter without the former. His point is relevant to health promotion among African American males—social change and health promotion can and should go together. Similarly, Green and Kreuter (1990) argue that the community is the perfect intersection for health promotion, allowing escape from the simplistic dichotomous debate that pits victim blame against system blame as if the two must be viewed as polar opposites.

Recommendations

Given the concept of shared responsibility for closing the health disparity gap, several recommendations are offered to advance this nation to a higher level of actualization and implementation:

1. Convening African American males into small groups to discuss health issues pertinent to them is a needed step and beginning method for getting them to open up and talk about their issues. Leadership for convening such groups can and should be provided by churches, community-based organizations, health departments, and voluntary associations. The American Cancer Society has begun such an effort through its Men-to-Men program designed to attract African American males through prostate cancer support groups.

2. A national campaign is needed to confront the many faces of despair and the faces of hope among African American males. Galvanizing this population is important, as evidenced several years ago by the Million Man March, an example of African American males' interest in and need for coming together at a national and local level to atone and develop strategies for confronting issues in a proactive manner. Reverend Jesse L. Jackson's impetus and leadership role in drawing attention to the HIV/AIDS epidemic in the African American community is another example.

3. Increasing substantially are the numbers of African American males who participate in local community health-oriented coalitions. Such engagement can enhance their involvement with organized entities concerned about health promotion and disease prevention initiatives (see Braithwaite, Taylor, & Austin, 2000, for methodological strategies for coalition development).

4. Schools of public health must take a more aggressive role and responsibility for training contemporary health educators in community development with ethnic minorities and with a focus on being responsive to the needs of African American males. This will require that these institutions modify their curricula to become more culturally relevant and inclusive of the needs of special populations.

5. State health departments need to follow the lead of Georgia, Michigan, and South Carolina by adopting legislative policies that direct resources and programs to address the health concerns of males and particularly those of African American males.

References

Agency for Healthcare Research and Quality. (2000). *Addressing racial and ethnic disparities in healthcare* (AHRQ Publication No. 00-PO41). Rockville, MD: Author.

American Cancer Society. (1996). *Cancer and African Americans* [On-line]. Available: www.2cancer.org/siteSearch/aframer.htm

American Diabetes Association. (2000). *Diabetes in African Americans* [On-line]. Available: www.diabetes.org/africanamerican/diabetesin.asp

American Heart Association. (2000). *African Americans and cardiovascular diseases* [On-line]. Available: www.americanheart.org/statistics/biostats/bioafr.htm

Black Healthcare. (2000). *Diabetes in African Americans* [On-line]. Available: www.blackhealth care.com/BHC/Diabetes/Description/asp.htm

Braithwaite, R. L., Hammett, T. M., & Mayberry, R. M. (1996). *Prisons and AIDS: A public health challenge.* San Francisco: Jossey-Bass.

Braithwaite, R. L., Taylor, S. E., & Austin, J. N. (2000). *Building health coalitions in the black community*. Thousand Oaks, CA: Sage.

Caplan, N., & Nelson, S. (1973). On being useful: The nature and consequences of psychological research on social problems. *American Psychologist, 28,* 199–211.

Carrasquillo, O., Himmelstein, D., Woolhandler, S., & Bor, D. (1999). Going bare: Trends in health insurance coverage, 1989 through 1996. *American Journal of Public Health, 89,* 36–42.

Centerwall, B. (1995). Race, socioeconomic status, and domestic homicide. *Journal of the American Medical Association, 273,* 1755–1758.

Childers, E. M., McClinton, J., Epps, C. V., Smith, L. R., Smyre, C., & Manning, J. H. (2000). *HB-1235 Commission on Men's Health*. Available: www2.state.ga.us/legis/1999_00/leg/fulltext/hb1235.htm

Courtenay, W. H. (2000). Constructions of masculinity and their influences on men's well-being: A theory of gender and health. *Social Science and Medicine, 50,* 1385–1401.

Cubbin, C., Pickle, L. W., & Fingerhut, L. (2000). Social context and geographic patterns of homicide among U.S. black and white males. *American Journal of Public Health, 90,* 579–587.

Dula, A. (1994). African American suspicion of the healthcare system is justified: What do we do about it? *Cambridge Quarterly of Healthcare Ethics, 3,* 347–357.

Feldman, R., & Fulwood, R. (1999). The three leading causes of death in African Americans: Barriers to reducing the excess disparity and to improving health behaviors. *Journal of Healthcare for the Poor and Underserved, 10,* 45–71.

Georgia Commission on Men's Health. (2000). HB 1235.

Green, L. W. (1987). [Letter to the editor]. *Health Education Quarterly, 14,* 3–5.

Green, L. W., & Kreuter, M. W. (1990). Health promotion as a public health strategy for the 1990s. *Annual Review of Public Health, 11,* 319–334.

Hoop, J. W., & Herring, P. (1996). Promoting health among black American populations: An overview. In R. M. Huff & M. V. Kline (Eds.), *Promoting health in multicultural populations: A handbook for practitioners* (pp. 201–221). Thousand Oaks, CA: Sage.

Hoyert, D. L., Kochanek, K. D., & Murphy, S. L. (1999). Deaths: Final data for 1997. *National Vital Statistics Reports* (Vol. 47, No. 19) [On-line]. Available: www.cdc.gov/nchs/releases/99facts/99sheets/97mortal.htm

Kaiser Family Foundation. (1998). *The untold story: AIDS and black Americans: A briefing on the crisis of AIDS among African Americans* [On-line]. Available: www.kff.org/content/archives/1372/afr_amerre.html

Kaiser Family Foundation. (1999). *Key facts: Race, ethnicity and medical care*. Menlo Park, CA: Author.

Kaiser Family Foundation. (2000). *The uninsured and their access to healthcare* [On-line]. Available: www.kff.org/content/archive/1407

Kass, B. L., Weinick, R. M., & Monheit, A. C. (1996). *Racial and Ethnic Differences in Health 1996. MEPS Chartbook No. 2*. Available: www.meps.ahrq.gov/papers/chartbk2/cashlf4.htm

Kronke, K., & Spitzer, R. L. (1998). Gender differences in the reporting of physical and somatoform symptoms. *Psychosomatic Medicine, 60,* 150–155.

Leach, J. (1998). Key issues in men's health. *Practitioner, 242,* 616–618, 620.

Livingston, I. L. (1994). *Handbook of black American health: The mosaic of conditions, issues, policies, and prospects*. Westport, CT: Greenwood Press.

Lober, J. (1997). *Gender and the social construction of illness*. Philadelphia: Saunders.

Loomis, D., & Richardson, D. (1998). Race and risk of fatal injury at work. *American Journal of Public Health, 88,* 40–44.

Mandelblatt, J. S., Yarboff, K. R., & Kerner, J. F. (1999). Equitable access to cancer services: A review of barriers to quality care. *Cancer, 86,* 2378–2390.

Men's Health Consulting. (2000). *African American men's health* [On-line]. Available: www.menshealth.org/code/afroamer.html

Men's Health Network. (1999). *The silent health crisis.* Washington, DC: Men's Health Network Policy Department.

Men's Health Network. (2000a). *The crisis in minority men's health.* Washington, DC: Men's Health Network Policy Department.

Men's Health Network. (2000b). *Goals.* [On-line]. Available: www.menshealthnetwork.org/new-goals.html

Michigan Department of Community Health. (2000). *Making the survival of the African American male a priority in Michigan* [On-line]. Available: www.mdch.state.mi.us/aami/right.htm

Morse, J. M., & Penrod, J. (1999). Linking concepts of enduring, uncertainty, suffering, and hope. *Image: Journal of Nursing Scholarship, 31,* 145–150.

Moynihan, C. (1998). Theories in healthcare and research: Theories of masculinity. *British Medical Journal, 317,* 1072–1075.

Murphy, S. L. (2000). Deaths: Final data for 1998. *National Vital Statistics Reports* (Vol. 48, No. 11) [On-line]. Available: www.cdc.gov/nchs/releases/00news/finaldeath98.htm

National Institute of Diabetes and Digestive and Kidney Diseases. (1999). *Diabetes statistics* [On-line]. Available: www.niddk.nih.gov/health/diabetes/pubs/dmstats/dmstats.htm

Richardson, L. (1997, April 21). An old experiment's legacy: Distrust of AIDS treatment. *New York Times,* p. A6.

Rist, J. M. (1969). *Stoic philosophy.* New York: Cambridge University Press.

Ross, R. K., Shinizu, H., Paganini-Hill, A., Honda, G., & Henderson, B. E. (1987). Case-control studies of prostate cancer in blacks and in Southern California. *Journal of the National Cancer Institute, 78,* 869–874.

Sandman, D., Simantov, E., & An, C. (2000). *Out of touch: American men and the healthcare system* [On-line]. Available: www.cmwf.org/programs/women/sandman_men'ssurvey 2000_374.asp

Schroeder, S. A. (1996). The medically uninsured: Will they always be with us? *New England Journal of Medicine, 334,* 1130–1133.

Stryker, J. (1997, April 13). Tuskegee's long arm still touches a nerve. *New York Times,* p. A6.

Thomas, S. B., & Quinn, S. C. (1991). The Tuskegee Syphilis Study, 1932–1972: Implications for HIV education and AIDS risk education programs in the black community. *American Journal of Public Health, 81,* 1498–1505.

Timothy, H. B. (1973). *The tenets of stoicism, assembled and systematized: From the works of L. Annaeus Seneca.* Amsterdam: Hakkert.

Trowers, R. (1998–1999). *Interpersonal violence: Perspectives from an emergency physician* [On-line]. Available: www.blackhealthnet.com/articles.asp

Wagener, D. K., & Winn, D. W. (1991). Injuries in working populations: Black-white differences. *American Journal of Public Health, 81,* 1408–1413.

Wagstaff, G., & Rowledge, A. (1995). Stoicism: Its relation to gender, attitudes toward poverty, and reactions to emotive material. *Journal of Social Psychology, 135,* 181–184.

Ward, J. W., & Duchin, J. S. (1998). The epidemiology of HIV and AIDS in the United States. *AIDS Clinical Review,* 1–45.

Weinrich, S. P., Reynolds, W. A., Tingen, M. S., & Starr, C. R. (2000). Barriers to prostate cancer screening. *Cancer Nursing, 23,* 117–121.

Whitehead, T. L. (2000). The "epidemic" and "cultural legends" of black male incarceration: The socialization of African American children to a life of incarceration. In J. P. May & K. R. Pitts (Eds.), *Building violence: How America's rush to incarcerate creates more violence* (pp. 82–89). Thousand Oaks, CA: Sage.

World Health Organization. (1999). *Cardiovascular diseases* [On-line]. Available: www.chef.whoint:9654/?WHOhg+WHOhg.html

CHAPTER FIVE

HEALTH AND THE ELDERLY

James S. Jackson, Sherrill L. Sellers

The development of better national health policies—policies that are responsive to life-course considerations and realities of family life in the United States—is essential if we are to improve the health of the African American population, especially older blacks. Recent research on aging and discriminated-against minorities has focused on three major themes—heterogeneity, vulnerabilities due to societal maltreatment, and family strengths (see for example, Berkman & Mullen, 1997; LaVeist, 2000; Miles, 1999). These themes are especially relevant for aging African Americans and their families (Tucker, 2000). Projections indicate that the number of African American elders will rise dramatically over the next thirty years (Angel & Hogan, 1994). Their past history, including racial inequality, socioeconomic disparities, and individual and group coping resources, will influence their morbidity, family and community relationships, and mortality.

A life-course framework is needed to explore how sociohistorical context influences and interacts with individual and group resources to both impede and facilitate the quality of life and health of successive cohorts of African Americans over the group life course and in the nature of their individual human development and aging experiences (Baltes, 1987; Burton, Dilworth-Anderson, & Bengtson, 1991; Smith & Kington, 1997a). For example, relationships between socioecologic factors, such as high crime rates, family dysfunction, high noise levels and social isolation, and negative health factors (such as hypertension) can affect all members of the African American family and community, thus possibly initiating poorer health among younger as well as older African Americans (Berkman & Mullen, 1997; Smith & Kington, 1997a). A life-course perspective illuminates the fact that current and aging cohorts of blacks have been exposed to the conditions that will influence profoundly their social, psychological, and health statuses as they reach older ages in the years and decades to come (Baltes, 1987; Barresi, 1987; Jackson & Sellers, 1996).

This life-course perspective provides the overarching framework for this chapter. After a brief review of the health of older black Americans, we address three areas—period and cohort influences (heterogeneity), socioeconomic disparities (social maltreatment), and race-relevant risk and coping mechanisms (risk and resources). In discussing these issues we draw heavily from previous work on the African American life course (Jackson & Sellers, 1996) and especially from a chapter in Robert Kastenbaum's *Encyclopedia of Adult Development* (Jackson, 1993).

For the most part, African Americans have been portrayed in the scientific literature in a simplistic and undifferentiated manner. An underlying assumption of prior research has been that there is extensive homogeneity in values, motives, social and psychological statuses, and behaviors among black Americans (Jackson, 1991; Jaynes & Williams, 1989). It is true that categorical treatment based upon race produces extensive group uniformity in attitudes and behaviors. It is equally true, however, that a rich heterogeneity exists among blacks in these same status, attitudinal, and behavioral dimensions (Jackson, 2000; Jackson, 1991). Older African Americans span the same spectrum of social and economic circumstances, psychological statuses, and social beliefs as do the millions of other older Americans of different ethnic and cultural backgrounds (Jackson, 1991, 1993; Stanford, 1990).

Recent studies show that older African Americans are a diverse and heterogeneous population possessing a wide array of group and personal resources (Farley, 2000; Jackson, 1993; Stanford, 1990). Older black Americans are one of the fastest growing segments of the population, and along with elders of other ethnic minority populations in three decades will constitute a fifth of the over-sixty-five-year-old group (Siegel, 1999). The changing age and ethnic structure of America will have important influences on the health and functioning of these older blacks (Gibson, 1986; Jackson, 2000; Richardson, 1996; Siegel, 1999). A large proportion of the future older black Americans of this coming century have already been born. A continuing gender imbalance, segregated geographic distribution, and disproportionate numbers in poverty, among other factors, will have profound influences upon family structure, health status, and the well-being of black elders in the twenty-first century (Miles, 1999; Siegel, 1999).

The Role of Racial Categorization

Throughout this chapter, we will use the terms "black" and "African American" interchangeably. Both refer to Americans who share a common ancestral descent from people historically indigenous to sub-saharan Africa. Ethnic and racial categories derive their interpretations from (1) the sociohistorical and current circumstances that different groups with well-defined physical characteristics face, and (2) the own- and other-group attitudes and behaviors toward members who belong to these categories (Dressler & Bindon, 2000; Jackson, 2000; Jackson & Sellers, 1996). While some genetic and biological factors may vary with the categorization of peoples of African descent (for example, sickle cell anemia, hypertension, lupus), we believe that the more fundamental nature of being African American derives from both self- and other-definitions and continuing discrimination and maltreatment (Dressler & Bindon, 2000; Jackson & Sellers, 1996; Neel, 1997).

It is not yet clear how race group categorization fits in models of health, human development, and aging (Wilkinson & King, 1987; Williams & Jackson, 2000). However, it is particularly important to integrate into models of health and aging the conditions under which race, ethnicity, sociocultural, and socioeconomic factors may serve as important resources in the coping processes and adaptation of Americans of African descent to their environmentally-disadvantaged circumstances (Dressler, 1985, 1991; Wilkinson & King, 1987). For example, Cooper (1984; 1991) suggests that the biologic concept of race has no scientific meaning and the social definitions of race and ethnicity should be viewed solely as clues for searching out environmental causes of observed differences between groups (Neel, 1997). Other work in illness behavior and behavioral medicine notes the independent role of cultural and lifestyle differences among racial groups in accounting for behavioral and health outcomes (Cooper, 1984, 1991; Dressler, 1985, 1991; Dressler & Bindon, 2000; Driedger & Chappell, 1988; Richardson, 1996). Treating race and ethnicity as one of many sociocultural factors, rather than as distinct predisposing cultural and social environment indicators (Jackson, Antonucci, & Gibson, 1990a), has precluded the types of research and analyses that examine the contributory role of sociocultural factors to health behaviors within racial and ethnic groups (James, 1984; Myers, 1984). Researchers such as James (1984, 1985) and Myers (1984), among others (for example, J. J. Jackson, 1988), have even questioned the appropriateness and validity of socioeconomic status and other sociocultural measures (occupation, coping resources, lifestyle factors) when making comparisons across race and ethnic groups (Markides, Liang, & Jackson, 1990).

Human development, aging, and the life course are the central concerns in an approach to understanding ostensible health race effects. Ethnic and racial groups have divergent life experiences because of sociostructural, socioeconomic, and cultural reasons (Dressler & Bindon, 2000; Driedger & Chappell, 1988). These different experiences will have significant influences, both positive and negative, on individual, family, and group well-being and health at all stages of the life course, ultimately influencing the adjustment to major life transitions (such as loss of spouse, retirement, and disability) in older ages. In this approach we conceptually place race as first and foremost a summary construct that "stands-in" for a host of other social, psychological, and possibly biological variables (Wilkinson & King, 1987).

Health of Older Blacks

Compared to Americans of European descent, at every point of their life span, African Americans have greater morbidity and mortality (Braithwaite & Taylor, 1992; Jackson, 1991; Jackson & Sellers, 1996; LaVeist, 2000). Among African Americans, as with most racial-ethnic groups in the United States, cancer and cardiovascular disease are the two leading causes of death (LaVeist, 2000). However, because of hypertension, which afflicts one out of every three African Americans, blacks have a 60 percent greater risk of death and disability from stroke and coronary disease than whites. In particular, the rate of cardiovascular disease is 80 percent higher than the rate for white women (National Center for Health Statistics, 1996). Similarly, cancer incidence rates for blacks are 6 to 10 percent higher than for whites.

Mortality statistics are equally troubling. The infant mortality rate for blacks is twenty deaths per 1,000, twice the rate that occurs among whites (LaVeist, 2000). The average life expectancy for whites is approximately 76.8 years, compared with 70.3 years for blacks (LaVeist, 2000), with an almost eight-year difference between white men (73.8) and black men (66.1). Hypertension is particularly deadly. Black women are twice as likely as white women to die of hypertensive cardiovascular disease (National Center for Health Statistics, 1996). Overall cancer mortality rates for African Americans are 20 to 40 percent higher than the general population, according to the National Cancer Institute.

To summarize these statistics, African Americans, especially older blacks, are at disproportionate risk for negative health outcomes when compared with European Americans (Smith & Kington, 1997b). A number of factors may contribute to this disparity, ranging from biological dispositions (Baquet & Ringen, 1987) to dietary habits (Hargreaves, Baquet, & Gamshadzahi, 1989), to a failure to receive adequate health care (Williams & Rucker, 2000). The specific mechanisms, however, that produce these differential outcomes are less clear (LaVeist, 2000; Williams, 1999). Given the complex sociohistorical context of African Americans, it may be less useful in determining exact mechanisms to compare between racial and ethnic group outcomes than within groups. For example, black-white comparisons may be less illuminating than the examination of various intra-group social and cultural factors as possible sources of risk and resilience for African American men, women, and children (Dressler & Bindon, 2000; Jackson, 1991; Jackson & Sellers, 1996).

Significant improvements in the life situations of blacks (Farley, 1987, 2000), particularly in health, have occurred over the last forty years (Jackson, 1981; Jackson, 1993; Jackson, 2000). Within the fast-growing elderly segment of the American population, African Americans are one of the fastest growing subpopulations (Jackson, 1988; Gibson & Jackson, 1991; Angel & Hogan, 1994; Miles, 1999). On the other hand, recent literature (see for example, Farley, 2000; Gibson, 1986; Jaynes & Williams, 1989) documents the negative life events and structural barriers, particularly for poor blacks, that still exist. These problems include the difficulties of single-parent households, high infant morbidity and mortality, childhood diseases, poor nutrition, lack of preventive health care, deteriorating neighborhoods, poverty, adolescent violence, un- and under-employment, teen pregnancy, drug and alcohol abuse, and broken marriages. While the exact causal relationships are not known (Williams, 1990; Williams, 1999; Williams & Collins, 1995), it is clear that these are predisposing factors for high morbidity and mortality across the entire life span (for example, Berkman & Mullen, 1997; Dressler, 1991; Haan & Kaplan, 1985; Hamburg, Elliott, & Parron, 1982).

Period and Cohort Influences on the Health of Aging Blacks

It is important to develop a life-course framework within which the nature of the economic, social, and health status of black Americans can be explained and understood in the context of historical and current structural disadvantage and blocked mobility opportunities (Jackson, 1991; Jackson, Antonucci, & Gibson, 1990a, 1990b). This framework contextualizes individual and group experiences by birth cohort, period events, and individual aging processes. Riley and her colleagues (Riley, 1994a; Riley, 1994b; Riley & Loscocco, 1994; M. W. Riley & J. W. Riley, 1994; J. W. Riley & M. W. Riley, 1994) have for a number of years proposed that cohort succession and structural lag (in other words, "changes in social structures that provide role opportunities and norms that do not keep pace with the twentieth-century metamorphoses in people lives") (J. W. Riley & M. W. Riley, 1994, p. 17), must be considered in models of aging, health, and human development. Their main argument has been that as people age they encounter changing role opportunities and circumstances in society. At the intersections of lives and structures, the influence is reciprocal, such that lives influence structures and structures influence lives. This interplay between individual lives and role opportunities for individuals can never be synchronized. Thus, structural lags will continue.

Researchers have begun to explore the nature of African American reactions to their unequal status in the United States (Brown, Sellers & Gomez, under review; Neighbors & Sellers, under review). Specifically, this research has addressed the question of how structural disadvantages in the environment are translated at different points in the individual and group life courses into physical- and mental-health outcomes. This work has focused on such things as self-esteem, personal efficacy, close personal and social relationships, neighborhood, church and family integration, political participation, group solidarity, and physical and mental health (Brown, Sellers, & Gomez, under review; Gibson & Jackson 1991; Jackson, Antonucci, & Gibson, 1990b).

The main theoretical focus was to explore the intersection of age, period, and cohort-related phenomena as they influence the African American family and individual experience. These studies focus on how the age cohort into which blacks are born; the social, political, and economic events that occur to blacks born together; and the individual aging process at different points in a person's life course influence the adaptation and quality of life of individuals, families, and larger groups of African Americans. For example, blacks born before the 1940s faced very different environmental constraints and have experienced a very different set of life tasks, events, opportunities, and disappointments than those born in the 1970s (Baker, 1987; Smith & Kington, 1997a). In addition to significant changes in the legal structure, health care advances and delivery, family changes, urban migration, and macroeconomic influences all differed dramatically across birth cohorts, as they will for future cohorts of blacks (Richardson, 1996). For example, blacks born since the struggles of the Civil Rights Movement (CRM) have a very different set of expectations of what life should offer than those who came of age before this point. While there is overlap across the generations within families, and across birth cohorts, the fact is that the CRM and its corollary events changed irrevocably the level of aspirations and expectations of African Americans, especially those who came of age during and following this period (Sellers, 2000). After the CRM, a substantial number of blacks were able to improve their social status through occupational achievement, educational advancement, and home ownership in better neighborhoods. In the past thirty years, relative to whites, blacks have experienced substantial occupational upward mobility (Levy, 1998).

Paradoxically, the CRM was conducive to upward mobility but constrained by persistent racial prejudices. Thus, the group that came of age after the CRM has been caught in a historical bind. On one hand, the expectation was for continued upward social mobility; on the other, it became clear that the full promise of the CRM was not to be realized. Further, a changing economy not only dampened prospects for upward mobility but also threatened past gains (Hochschild, 1995).

In essence, the post-CRM birth cohort constitutes a "disappointment" generation (Jackson, 1993). Not only have their legitimate aspirations not been fulfilled, the nature of racial oppression has changed dramatically from the pre-CRM period. The struggle for equal opportunity is a very different and more difficult one than the struggle for equal rights under the law (Jackson, 2000). How this may affect the "disappointment" generation as they age is unknown. It may be that the adaptive mechanisms of fatalism, worldview, or religious orientation may not be as effective for a more cynical, while no less deprived, group of African Americans as they grow older. On the other hand, somewhat greater access to health care (through Medicare, Medicaid, and so on) may eventually offset some of the negative consequences of continued structural barriers to individual and group mobility and achievement.

In a more pessimistic vein, it may be that African Americans middle-aged at the time of the CRM have benefitted the most from what now appear to be the "radical" changes that occurred during the mid-1960s and 1970s. New cohorts of middle-aged and elderly blacks may exist in an environment of fewer tangible goods and services as well as a more pessimistic and worsening social and psychological atmosphere.

While several authors have indicated the necessity of considering life-course models—history, cohort, and period effects in the nature of black status (see for example, Barresi, 1987; Manton & Soldo, 1985)—few have actually collected the type of data or conducted the analyses that would shed any light on these processes. For example, in reviewing the material on health, mortality, morbidity, and risk factors, it appears that the examination of black health status has been conducted in a relative vacuum. This has been as much the fault of a lack of good conceptual models of black health status as it has been the lack of quality trend data on sizable numbers of representative samples of black Americans.

It is clear though that older blacks arrive in adulthood and older ages with extensive histories of disease, ill health, and varied individual adaptive reactions to their poor health (Smith & Kington, 1997b). The available cohort data for cause-specific mortality and morbidity across the life course over the last few decades indicates that there are accumulated deficits that perhaps place black middle-aged and older people at greater risk than comparable chronologically aged whites (Jackson, 1991). Similarly, the fact that blacks actually outlive their white counterparts in the very older ages suggests possible selection factors at work that may result in hardier older blacks (Gibson & Jackson, 1987, 1991; Manton & Stollard, 1997). These selection factors may act on successive cohorts of blacks in a "sandwich-like" manner, leaving alternate cohorts of middle-aged and older blacks of relative wellness and good functional ability.

The cohort experiences of blacks undoubtedly play a major role in the nature of their health experiences over the life course in terms of the quality of health care from birth, exposure to risk factors, and the presence of exogenous environmental factors. Another contributing factor is the stressor role of prejudice and discrimination across the life course, even though it may differ in form and intensity as a function of birth cohort, period, and age (Baker, 1987; Cooper, Steinhauer, Miller, David, and Schatzkin, 1981; Dressler, 1991; Williams & Williams-Morris, 2000).

Socioeconomic Status and the Health of Blacks over the Life Course

The role of socioeconomic status (SES) has been touted as a major risk factor and implicated in the effects of other risk factors in mortality and morbidity (Williams, 1999; Haan & Kaplan, 1985; Smith & Kington, 1997a; 1997b). Impressive evidence exists that SES plays a major role in a wide variety of diseases, such that increasing SES is associated with better health and lowered morbidity (Adler & Ostrove, 1999). This effect has been shown at both the individual and ecological levels on blood pressure, general mortality, cancer, cardiovascular heart diseases (CHD), and cerebrovascular disease, diabetes, and obesity (James, 1985). What has not been shown is how SES status from conception, birth, or early in the life course affects these health outcomes in adulthood and older ages (Smith & Kington, 1997b; Williams, 1999). Perhaps, over the full life course, advantaged blacks would be considerably more similar to their white counterparts than less-advantaged blacks to theirs (Jackson, 1993); but current middle-to-high-SES blacks would be at an intermediate position, and the full-life-course-disadvantaged blacks would continue to show worse health status conditions than their comparable low-SES white counterparts (Smith & Kington, 1997a).

This nonsymmetrical effect of SES on health has been suggested by a few researchers (such as Haan & Kaplan, 1985). For example, James (1985) speculated on the role of SES in CHD using a similar argument. Thus, an emerging theme in some of the empirical literature is that similarity in income and education may serve to equate upper-income race groups but have fewer effects on certain health outcomes among lower-income groups (see for example, Kessler & Neighbors, 1986). The causes of these observed effects are not known and may be due to several factors (Williams, 1999). For example, income and other socioeconomic control variables may serve to underequate different race groups at lower-income levels and overequate at upper-income levels. In a racially divided society in which blacks have had to struggle to be successful (Jaynes & Williams, 1989), perhaps harder than whites in comparable income (or education and occupation) positions, blacks at these upper levels may in fact have more of the underlying factors that are correlated with education, income, or occupation levels than comparable whites, thus countering the effects of discrimination. Therefore, blacks at these upper socioeconomic positions may show health outcomes equal or superior to comparable-level whites.

Lower socioeconomic-status blacks, however, are not as well off as comparable low-income whites, perhaps due to discrimination and lack of resources (Williams & Rucker, 2000; Williams & Williams-Morris, 2000). It is probable that whites at these levels would still maintain a decided advantage over blacks; thus blacks would show decidedly poorer health outcomes. It may also be true that different health outcomes may show differential effects of the interaction between race and SES. It may be that SES is less effective in reducing health outcome differentials between blacks and whites in which stress plays a major etiological role (McEwen & Seeman, 1999). On the other hand, health outcomes in which social and economic resources may play a major role (for example, infectious diseases, HIV/AIDS) may show marked differences between blacks and whites (LaVeist, 2000).

We suggest that controls for socioeconomic status should be progressively more effective in newer aged cohorts. Current older blacks, of both upper and lower socioeconomic status, have had longer to suffer the difficulties associated with racial group membership. The older blacks from upper socioeconomic status groups will show continued health deficits and older blacks in lower socioeconomic positions will show continued poorer health outcomes. These differences should be much less prominent in younger age groups. Thus, these younger groups may show no appreciable differences when socioeconomic controls are applied at either upper- or lower-status levels. Geronimous (1991) has proposed a related notion (weathering theory) to account for why younger teen mothers among African Americans may have better birthing and postpartum health experiences than relatively older teen mothers. In addition, the weathering perspective may explain the differences in findings (Haan & Kaplan, 1985; Williams, 1999) in studies on socioeconomic status and health (Kaplan, 1999). The use of younger age cohorts may have been more likely to show a clear effect of socioeconomic status to eliminate health status differentials while, for the reasons outlined above, the use of older age groups may have been much less effective. (Anderson & Shumaker, 1989; Taylor & Seeman, 1999). The impact of aging and socioeconomic status on the health of black Americans requires additional research (Adler & Ostrove, 1999).

Race-Relevant Risks and Coping Mechanisms and the Health of Aging Blacks

Contemporary cohorts of blacks being born today are at considerable risk. Studies indicate that black Americans are most likely to spend the majority of their childhoods in low-income, single-female-headed households. Poverty in turn places black Americans at risk for inadequate diets, fewer educational opportunities, greater exposure to crime, and limited opportunities for occupational advancement (Massey & Denton, 1993; Wilson, 1996). Job prospects will be poor in young adulthood, and a large proportion of blacks will die or suffer chronic disease prior to reaching middle adulthood. Only a comparative few will have the advantage of intergenerational economic transfers from parental sources (Oliver & Shapiro, 1995). Even for those born into contemporary middle-class homes (since this is an often fragile situation for most blacks), providing a tangible legacy for children, even college funding, is problematic (Oliver & Shapiro, 1995). Dental visits, preventive health maintenance, well-baby checks, poor hearing and vision checks, and the like will go undone. Other "luxuries" of life are difficult to afford (Jackson, 1993). Recent data (Williams & Collins, 1995) suggests that blacks at every family income level have lower wealth than comparable whites. At the lowest-income quintile, whites have ten thousand dollars in wealth while comparable black families have one dollar. In every new generation of African Americans, wealth is thus re-created and consumed. This results in structural disadvantage that increases risk for poor health over the life course.

There are also psychological and social psychological costs of life among black Americans—lack of perceived control, discouragement and discrimination that sap energy, and thwarted aspirations and expectations of a successful life

(Neighbors & Sellers, under review; Williams & Williams-Morris, 2000). When the barriers to educational and occupational mobility and the high probability of exposure to environmental risk factors (Berkman & Mullen, 1997) are considered, the early health morbidity, disability, and excess mortality of older black Americans become understandable (LaVeist, 2000; Miles, 1999; Williams & Rucker, 2000).

Older age among blacks does not have to be a time of inevitable poor health (Jackson, 1993; Manton & Stollard, 1997; Rowe, 1985; Smith & Kington, 1997b). Changes in lifestyle, environmental risk reduction, and medical interventions can have positive influences on the quantity and quality of life among middle-aged and older black adults (Williams & Rucker, 2000). Survey data (for example, Gibson & Jackson, 1987, 1991; Manton & Stollard, 1997) show that many older blacks are free from functional disability and limitations of activity due to chronic illness and disease. In fact, blacks and whites after the age of sixty-five, within sex groups, differ very little in years of expected remaining life (Elo & Preston, 1997; LaVeist, 2000; Smith & Kington, 1997b). Health care has improved significantly for middle-aged and older black adults, and consecutive cohorts are better educated and better able to take advantage of available opportunities. Yet, without extensive environmental intervention, it is highly likely that a significant proportion of older black adults of the mid-twenty-first century, born in the mid- to late-twentieth century, are at severe risk for impoverished conditions, and poor social, physical, and psychological health in older age. This poor prognosis is predicated less on biological dimensions of racial differences (Neel, 1997) than on the physical, social, psychological, and environmental risk factors correlated with racial and ethnic group membership in the United States (Berkman & Mullen, 1997; Dressler & Bindon, 2000; Williams & Jackson, 2000).

In the face of severe structural, social, and psychological constraints, one wonders how older black Americans do as well as they do. Studies that address the coping skills, capacity, and adaptability of Americans of African descent at different points in the life course are particularly important (Jackson, 1991). It is possible that the most important race effects, if they do occur, are probably in the form of interactions with other ethnic, structural, or cultural factors (for example, religion, socioeconomic status, and world views) (Jackson, Antonucci, & Gibson, 1990a; Jackson, 2000; Markides, Liang, & Jackson, 1990).

Blacks may utilize, over the individual life course, different mechanisms than whites to maintain levels of productivity, physical and mental health, and effective functioning (Williams & Williams-Morris, 2000). One race-relevant adaptive mechanism may be the use of a fatalistic psychological orientation. In the face of significant and severe structural barriers, a cognitive orientation to life that stresses the existence of systematic, systemic blockages to upward mobility may be very important among blacks in understanding why hard work and prodigious individual efforts do not lead to positive outcomes (Neighbors, Jackson, Broman, & Thompson, 1996; Neighbors & Sellers, under review). A fatalistic view may be even more important at the upper end of the individual life course as both blacks and whites have to come to grips with the failures and missed opportunities of their lives. A coping orientation that employs reasonably accurate assessment of environmental constraints can lead to external attributions of failure and can protect blacks from some of the life disappointments (Williams & Williams-Morris, 2000). This coping strategy may be particularly effective for understanding failure due to racism and discrimination.

Another possible protective mechanism may be the sense of collectivity or group identity and consciousness that places the good of the group on an equal or greater priority status than the good of the self. Thus, even though individual mobility and achievement may not be great, concerns about the group may serve as a very important filter for interpreting one's own contributions. Religious orientation seems to serve a similar role for blacks, perhaps part of a group "world view" that provides a charitable and spiritual organizing and guiding set of values for life (Levin, Chatters, & Taylor, 1995).

Summary and Conclusions

The African American life course, perhaps more so than in the majority population, highlights the continuities and discontinuities of a life-span perspective on health. From birth to death, African Americans are at greater risk for debilitating social, psychological, and physical conditions that negatively influence the quality of individual and family life and, in many instances, result in "premature" death: greater fetal death rates, greater homicide statistics in adolescence and mid-life, and greater risk of death from chronic health conditions early in old age (Miles, 1999; Smith & Kington, 1997b). However, all blacks are not born into such circumstances. Though people argue over its relative proportions (Vanneman & Cannon, 1987), there exists a black middle-class, and some blacks in the United States can look forward to relatively comfortable styles of living over their life courses (Farley, 2000). This heterogeneity is intertwined with categorical group membership and experience of racial discrimination.

Even with economic and social resources, the pernicious nature of racial discrimination and other structural barriers can negatively influence the aspirations and expectations of youth and young adults—aspirations and expectations that the majority assume as a given right of citizenship (Jackson, 2000). The often-portrayed success stories of African Americans in sports, the arts, and entertainment worlds are exceptions to the working-class, near-poverty, and poverty existence of a large proportion of blacks (Jackson, 2000), especially older blacks (Siegel, 1999). Numerous writers have theorized about how responding to the stress of blocked opportunities can affect the well-being of black Americans, and a few studies have found associations between aspirations, achievements, and health (Neighbors & Sellers, under review). These studies hint at potential cohort differences that have yet to be explored.

A life-course perspective suggests the need to consider human development, historical context, and structural position as factors that influence the health of present and future cohorts of black elders. Different birth cohorts, historical and current environmental events, and individual differences in developmental and aging processes interact with one another to affect physical and mental health. Racial group membership plays an important part in the health of these elders; cultural resources provide important coping and adaptive mechanisms in alleviating the distinct socioeconomic and psychological disadvantages of categorical racial membership (Jackson, 1993; Stanford, 1990; Williams & Williams-Morris, 2000). The unique social history and the nature of their group and individual developmental experiences all serve to place new elderly cohorts of African Americans at disproportionate risk for poor physical and mental health (LaVeist, 2000). This can be seen in population statistics, such as continuing disproportionate rates of mortality, disintegrating neighborhoods, numbers of women and children in poverty, joblessness, and unemployment (Jackson, 2000). Individual efforts are not enough to improve the health of black elders. We argue that without significant intervention, the health future of older black Americans is clear and it is dismal (Richardson, 1996). The majority of future black American elders in the twenty-first century have already been born and are at various stages of their individual and family life courses (Siegel, 1999; Smith & Kington, 1997a, 1997b). Unfortunately, we can predict what the most likely life experiences will be for a sizeable proportion of these coming elderly African Americans (Jackson, 2000). Fortunately, we have time to change factors related to the health of future cohorts of African American middle-aged and elderly. Whether the nation is willing to invest the resources to reverse these all-too-predictable negative health outcomes in older-age black Americans is not clear (Jackson, 1993, 2000; Jackson & Sellers, 1996; Williams & Rucker, 2000).

References

Adler, N. E., & Ostrove, J. M. (1999). Socioeconomic status and health: What we know and what we don't. In N. E. Adler, M. Marmot, B. S. McEwen, & J. Stewart (Eds.). *Socioeconomic status and health in industrial nations: Social, psychological, and biological pathways* (pp. 3–15). New York: The New York Academy of Sciences.

Anderson, N. B., & Shumaker, S. A. (1989). Race, reactivity, and blood pressure regulation. *Health Psychology, 8,* 483–486.

Angel, J. & Hogan, D. (1994). The demography of minority aging populations. In *Minority elders: Five Goals toward building a public policy base* (pp. 9–21). Washington, DC: The Gerontological Society of America.

Baker, F. M. (1987). The Afro-American life cycle: Success, failure, and mental health. *Journal of the National Medical Association, 7,* 625–633.

Baltes, P. B. (1987). Theoretical propositions of life-span developmental psychology: On the dynamics between growth and decline. *Developmental Psychology, 23,* 621–626.

Baquet, C., & Ringen, K. (1987). Health policy: Gaps in access, delivery, and utilization of the Pap smear in the United States. *Milbank Quarterly, 65*(2), 322–347.

Barresi, C. M. (1987). Ethnic aging and the life course. In D. E. Gelfand & C. M. Barresi (Eds.). *Ethnic dimensions of aging.* New York: Springer.

Berkman, L. F., & Mullen, J. M. (1997). How health behaviors and the social environment contribute to health differences between black and white older Americans. In L. G. Martin & B. J. Soldo (Eds.). *Racial and ethnic differences in the health of older Americans* (pp. 163–182). Washington, DC: National Academy Press.

Braithwaite, R. L., & Taylor, S. E. (Eds.). (1992). *Health issues in the black community.* San Francisco: Jossey-Bass.

Brown, T., Sellers, S. L., and Gomez, J. (under review). Internalization of stereotypes and the self-esteem of black Americans.

Burton, L. M., Dilworth-Anderson, P., & Bengtson, V. L. (1991). Creating culturally relevant ways of thinking about diversity. *Generations, 15,* 67–72.

Cooper, R. (1984). A note on the biological concept of race and its application in epidemiological research. *American Heart Journal, 108,* 715–723.

Cooper, R. (1991). Celebrate diversity—or should we? *Ethnicity and Disease, 1,* 3–7.

Cooper, R. S., Steinhauer, M., Miller, W., David, R., & Schatzkin, A. (1981). Racism, society and disease: An exploration of the social and biological mechanisms of differential mortality. *International Journal of Health Services, 11*(3), 389–414.

Dressler, W. (1985). Extended family relationships, social support, and mental health in a southern black community. *Journal of Health and Social Behavior, 26,* 39–48.

Dressler, W. (1991). Social class, skin color, and arterial blood pressure in two societies. *Ethnicity & Disease, 1,* 60–77.

Dressler, W., & Bindon, J. R. (2000). The health consequences of cultural consonance: Cultural dimensions of lifestyle, social support, and arterial blood pressure in an African American community. *American Anthropologist, 102*(2), 244–260.

Driedger, L., & Chappell, N. (1988). *Aging and ethnicity: Toward an interface.* Toronto, CA: Butterworth.

Elo, I. T., & Preston, S. H. (1997). Racial and ethnic differences in mortality at older ages. In L. G. Martin & B. J. Soldo (Eds.). *Racial and ethnic differences in the health of older Americans* (pp. 10–42). Washington, DC: National Academy Press.

Farley, R. (1987). Who are black Americans? The quality of life for black Americans twenty years after the civil rights revolution. *The Milbank Quarterly (Supplement 1), 65,* 9–34.

Farley, R. (2000). Demographic, economic, and social trends in a multicultural America. In J. S. Jackson (Ed.), *New Directions: African Americans in a diversifying nation* (pp. 11–44). Washington, DC: National Policy Association.

Geronimous, A. T. (1991). Teenage childbearing and social and reproductive disadvantage: The evolution of complex questions and the demise of simple answers. *Family Relations, 40,* 463–471.

Gibson, R. C. (1986). Blacks in an aging society. *Daedalus, 115,* 349–372.

Gibson, R. C., & Jackson, J. S. (1987). Health, physical functioning, and informal supports of the black elderly. *Milbank Quarterly (Supplement I), 65,* 1–34.

Gibson, R. C., & Jackson, J. S. (1991). The black oldest old: Health, functioning, and informal support. In R. M. Suzman, D. P. Willis, & K. G. Manton (Eds.), *The oldest old* (pp. 506–515). New York: Oxford University Press.

Haan, M. N., & Kaplan, G. A. (1985). *The contribution of socioeconomic position to minority health.* In *Volume II: Crosscutting issues in minority health. Report of the Secretary's Task Force on Black and Minority Health.* Washington, DC: U.S. Department of Health and Human Services.

Hamburg, D. A., Elliott, G. R., & Parron, D. L. (1982). *Health and behavior: Frontiers of research in the biobehavioral sciences.* Washington, DC: National Academy Press.

Hargreaves, M. K., Baquet, C., & Gamshadzahi, A. (1989). Diet, nutritional status, and cancer risk in American blacks. *Nutrition and Cancer, 12* (1), 1–28.

Hochschild, J. (1995). *Facing up to the American dream.* Princeton, NJ: Princeton University Press.

Jackson, J. J. (1981). Urban black Americans. In A. Harwood (Ed.), *Ethnicity and medical care.* Cambridge, MA: Harvard University Press.

Jackson, J. J. (1988). Social determinants of the health and aging black populations in the United States. In J. S. Jackson (Ed.), *The black American elderly: Research on physical and psychosocial health.* New York: Springer.

Jackson, J. S. (Ed.). (1988). *The black American elderly: Research on physical and psychosocial health.* New York: Springer.

Jackson, J. S. (Ed.). (1991). *Life in black America.* Newbury Park, CA: Sage Publications.

Jackson, J. S. (1993). Racial influences on adult development and aging. In R. Kastenbaum (Ed.), *The encyclopedia of adult development* (pp. 18–26). Phoenix, AZ: Oryx Press.

Jackson, J. S. (Ed.). (2000). *New Directions: African Americans in a diversifying nation.* Washington, DC: National Policy Association.

Jackson, J. S., Antonucci, T. C., & Gibson, R. C. (1990a). Cultural, racial, and ethnic minority influences on aging. In J. E. Birren & K. W. Schaie (Eds.). *Handbook of the psychology of aging* (3rd Edition) (pp. 103–123). New York: Academic Press.

Jackson, J. S., Antonucci, T. C., & Gibson, R. C. (1990b). Social relations, productive activities, and coping with stress in late life. In M.A.P. Stephens, J. H. Crowther, S. E. Hobfoll, & D. L. Tennenbaum (Eds.), *Stress and coping in later life families.* Washington, DC: Hemisphere Publishers.

Jackson, J. S., & Sellers, S. (1996). African American health over the life course: A multidimensional framework. In P. M. Kato and T. Mann (Eds.), *Handbook of diversity issues in health psychology* (pp. 301–317). New York: Plenum Press.

James, S. A. (1984). Coronary heart disease in black Americans: Suggestions for research on psychosocial factors. *American Heart Journal, 108,* 833–838.

James, S. A. (1985). Coronary heart disease in black Americans: Suggestions for future research on psychosocial factors. In A. M. Ostfield (Ed.), *Measuring psychosocial variables in epidemiologic studies of cardiovascular disease.* (NIH Publication No. 85–2270). Washington, DC: Public Health Service, U.S. Department of Health and Human Services.

Jaynes, G. D., & Williams, R. M., Jr. (Eds.). (1989). *A common destiny: Blacks and American society.* Washington, DC: National Academy Press.

Kaplan, G. A. (1999). What is the role of the social environment in understanding inequalities in health? In N. E. Adler, M. Marmot, B. S. McEwen, & J. Stewart (Eds.), *Socioeconomic status and health in industrial nations: Social, psychological, and biological pathways* (pp. 116–119). New York: The New York Academy of Sciences.

Kessler, R., & Neighbors, H. (1986). A new perspective on the relationships among race, social class and psychological distress. *Journal of Health and Social Behavior, 27,* 107–115.

LaVeist, T. A. (2000). African Americans and health policy: Strategies for a multiethnic society. In J. S. Jackson (Ed.), *New Directions: African Americans in a diversifying nation* (pp. 144–161). Washington, DC: National Policy Association: Washington.

Levin, S., Chatters, L., & Taylor, R. (1995). Religious effects on health status and life satisfaction among black Americans. *Journal of Gerontology: Social Sciences* 508: S154-S163.

Levy, F. (1998). *The new dollars and dreams.* New York: Russell Sage Foundation.

Manton, K. G., & Soldo, B. J. (1985). Dynamics of health changes in the oldest old: New perspectives and evidence. *Milbank Quarterly, 63,* 206–285.

Manton, K. G., & Stollard, E. (1997). Health and disability differences among racial and ethnic groups. In L. G. Martin & B. J. Soldo (Eds.), *Racial and ethnic differences in the health of older Americans* (pp. 43–104). Washington, DC: National Academy Press.

Markides, K. S., Liang, J., & Jackson, J. S. (1990). Race, ethnicity, and aging: Conceptual and methodological issues. In L. K. George & R. H. Binstock (Eds.), *Handbook of aging and the social sciences* (3rd Edition), (pp. 112–129). New York: Academic Press.

Massey, D., & Denton, N. (1993). *American apartheid: Segregation and the making of the underclass.* Cambridge: Harvard University Press.

McEwen, B. S., & Seeman, T. (1999). Protecting and damaging effects of mediators of stress: Elaborating and testing the concepts of allostasis and allostatic load. In N. E. Adler, M. Marmot, B. S. McEwen, & J. Stewart (Eds.), *Socioeconomic status and health in industrial nations: Social, psychological, and biological pathways* (pp. 30–47). New York: The New York Academy of Sciences.

Miles, T. P. (Ed.) (1999). *Full-color aging: Facts, goals, and recommendations for America's diverse elders.* Washington, DC: Gerontological Society of America.

Myers, H. F. (1984). Summary of workshop III: Working group on socioeconomic and sociocultural influences. *American Heart Journal, 108,* 706–710.

National Center for Health Statistics (1996). Health, United States, 1995. Hyattsville, MD: Public Health Service.

Neel, J. V. (1997). Are genetic factors involved in racial and ethnic differences in late-life health? In L. G. Martin & B. J. Soldo (Eds.), *Racial and ethnic differences in the health of older Americans* (pp. 210–232). Washington, DC: National Academy Press.

Neighbors, H., Jackson, J., Broman, C., and Thompson, E. (1996). "The mental health of African Americans: The role of self and system blame." *Ethnicity & Disease. 6:* 167–175.

Neighbors, H., & Sellers, S. (under review). Effects of goal-striving stress on the mental health of black Americans.

Oliver, M., & Shapiro, T. (1995). *Black wealth / white wealth.* New York: Routledge.

Richardson, J. (1996). *Aging and health: African American elders.* (2nd Edition). (Stanford Geriatric Education Center Working Paper Series, Number 4: Ethnogeriatric Reviews). Stanford, CA: Stanford Geriatric Education Center, Division of Family & Community Medicine, Stanford University.

Riley, M. W. (1994a). Changing lives and changing social structures: Common concerns of social science and public health. *American Journal of Public Health, 84,* 1214–1217.

Riley, M. W. (1994b). Aging and society: Past, present, and future. *The Gerontologist, 34,* 436–446.

Riley, M. W., & Loscocco, K. A. (1994). The changing structure of work opportunities: Toward an age-integrated society. In R. P. Abeles, H. C. Gift, & M. C. Orey (Eds.), *Aging and the quality of life.* New York: Springer.

Riley, M. W., & Riley, J. W. Jr. (1994). Age integration and the lives of older people. *The Gerontologist, 34,* 110–115.

Riley, J. W. Jr., & Riley, M. W. (1994, June). Beyond productive aging: Changing lives and social structure. *Aging International,* 15–19.

Rowe, J. W. (1985). Health care of the elderly. *New England Journal of Medicine, 312,* 827–835.

Sellers, S. L. (2000). Dreams delivered, dreams deferred: Mental and physical health consequences of social mobility. Ph.D. dissertation, University of Michigan, Ann Arbor.

Siegel, J. S. (1999). Demographic introduction to racial/Hispanic elderly populations. In T. P. Miles (Ed.). *Full-color aging: Facts, goals, and recommendations for America's diverse elders* (pp. 1–20). Washington, DC: Gerontological Society of America.

Smith, J. P., & Kington, R. (1997a). Demographic and economic correlates of health in old age. *Demography, 34* (1), 159–170.

Smith, J. P., & Kington, R. (1997b). Race, socioeconomic status, and health in late life. In L. G. Martin & B. J. Soldo (Eds.), *Racial and ethnic differences in the health of older Americans* (pp. 105–162). Washington, DC: National Academy Press.

Stanford, E. P. (1990). Diverse black aged. In Z. Harel, E. A. McKinney, & M. Williams (Eds.), *Black aged: Understanding diversity and service needs.* Newbury Park, CA: Sage Publications.

Taylor, S. E., & Seeman, T. (1999). Psychological resources and the SES-health relationship. In N. E. Adler, M. Marmot, B. S. McEwen, & J. Stewart (Eds.), *Socioeconomic status and health in industrial nations: Social, psychological, and biological pathways* (pp. 210-226). New York: The New York Academy of Sciences.

Tucker, M. B. (2000). Considerations in the development of family policy for African Americans. In J. S. Jackson (Ed.), *New directions: African Americans in a diversifying nation.* (pp. 162–206). Washington, DC: National Policy Association.

Vanneman, R., and Cannon, L. (1987). *The American perception of class.* Philadelphia: Temple University Press.

Wilkinson, D. T., & King, G. (1987). Conceptual and methodological issues in the use of race as a variable: Policy implications. *The Milbank Quarterly, 65* (Supplement 1), 56–71.

Williams, D. R. (1990). Socioeconomic differentials in health: A review and redirection. *Social Psychology Quarterly, 53,* 81–99.

Williams, D. R. (1999). Race, socioeconomic status, and health: The added effects of racism and discrimination. In N. E. Adler, M. Marmot, B. S. McEwen, & J. Stewart (Eds.), *Socioeconomic status and health in industrial nations: Social, psychological, and biological pathways* (pp. 173–189). New York: The New York Academy of Sciences.

Williams, D. R., & Collins, C. (1995) U.S. Socioeconomic and racial differences in health: Patterns and explanations. *Annual Review of Sociology. 21*: 349–386.

Williams, D. R., & Jackson, J. S. (2000). Race/ethnicity and the 2000 census: Recommendations for African American and other black populations in the United States. *American Journal of Public Health, 90*(11), 1728–1730.

Williams, D. R., & Rucker, T. D. (2000). Understanding and addressing racial disparities in health care. *Health Care Financing Review, 21* (4), 75–90.

Williams, D. R., & Williams-Morris, R. (2000). Racism and mental health: The African American experience. *Ethnicity & Health, 5*(3/4), 243–268.

Wilson, W. (1996). *When work disappears: The world of the new urban poor.* New York: Random House.

PART TWO

SOCIAL, MENTAL,
AND ENVIRONMENTAL
CHALLENGES

CHAPTER SIX

THE EPIDEMIOLOGY
OF MENTAL DISORDER

1985 to 2000

Harold W. Neighbors, David R. Williams

In 1985, the landmark report of the Task Force on Black and Minority Health (the Heckler Report) was instrumental in stimulating a tremendous amount of research and writing on racial health disparities (U.S. Department of Health and Human Services [DHHS], Task Force on Black and Minority Health, 1985). Due to its heavy emphasis on mortality, however, the report was conspicuous in how little it had to say about racial differences in mental health. As a result, it did not stimulate much public health research on serious mental disorders. Although the period between 1985 and 2000 has yielded much information on physical health problems, it has not drawn enough attention to the mental health challenges that African Americans face. Thus the picture of African American mental health that has been drawn on the basis of epidemiological studies conducted over the last fifteen years is interesting but incomplete.

The issue of black-white differences in the epidemiology of mental illness has a long and varied history (Cannon & Locke, 1977; Dohrenwend & Dohrenwend, 1969; Fischer, 1969; Kramer, Rosen, & Willis, 1973; Pasamanick, 1963; Thomas & Sillen, 1972). For much of that history, the epidemiological research focused on methodologically limited anecdotal accounts and nonrepresentative treatment rate studies (Fischer, 1969; Jaco, 1960; Kramer et al., 1973; Schermerhorn, 1956). During the 1980s, more rigorous community surveys of psychological distress often found significantly higher symptom rates among blacks compared to whites, although these differences were eliminated when socioeconomic status was controlled (Neighbors, 1984; Vega & Rumbaut, 1991). By the late 1980s, publications from the Epidemiologic Catchment Area (ECA) program of the National Institute of Mental Health (NIMH) provided, for the first time, information on discrete mental disorders, free from much of the clinical ambiguity associated with symptom checklists and unencumbered by the selection bias of treatment rate studies. Although epidemiologists continue to study racial differences in psychological distress, a large part of what we now know about the prevalence of mental disorder among African Americans comes from community surveys of specific diagnostic categories (Brown, Ahmed, Gary, & Milburn, 1995; Robins & Regier, 1991; Somervell, Leaf, Weissman, Blazer, & Bruce, 1989; Williams, Takeuchi, & Adair, 1992a, 1992b).

The purpose of this chapter is to review the empirical findings on black-white differences from community epidemiological surveys of well-being, psychological distress, and serious mental disorder. Within-race demographic comparisons (gender, age, socioeconomic status, and marital status) are summarized for particular disorders (for example, mood and anxiety disorders) in order to illustrate some of the more interesting descriptive statistics in need of further investigation. Clinical issues related to treatment are not addressed—with the exception of diagnosis, which we argue is directly relevant to improving epidemiological case finding.

The Public Mental Health Perspective

Perhaps more than any other health construct, the concept of mental health encompasses a tremendously wide variety of topics, issues, and meanings (Fellin, 1996; Mechanic, 1999; Taylor, 1992). As a result, no chapter on mental health can cover all factors that have been placed in this broad area. Therefore the emphasis here is on public health approaches resting on a sound psychiatric epidemiological foundation. The goal of this nation's public mental health efforts should be to direct resources toward developing tools for clearly identifying African Americans who are experiencing disability due to psychological pain and toward developing interventions designed to raise these individuals to a relatively symptom-free level of functioning. This is not to imply that there is no benefit in encouraging African Americans to strive for self-development and self-actualization (Franklin & Jackson, 1990, p. 300; Jahoda, 1958; Peterson, 1999, p. 116). In fact it is clear that the vast majority of African Americans are seriously engaged in the process of self-betterment and the struggle for upward social mobility. Rather, this chapter will address the mental health implications of such striving efforts, and what can be done to reduce the psychiatric morbidity that results from race-based blocked opportunities. We must focus our energies on increasing the overall mental health of African American communities by reducing stress and increasing resiliency among those blacks suffering the incapacitating effects of life in the United States.

Effective public health interventions are based on accurate, comprehensive epidemiology. The conceptualization of epidemiology presented here includes more than the counting of mental disorder. It addresses the full spectrum of the epidemiological paradigm, including the development of theories concerning risk and protective factors, the utilization of services, and preventive intervention. When it comes to research on African Americans, however, the psychiatric epidemiological picture remains largely descriptive. Although theory-based risk factor research is accumulating, this review shows that we still do not have enough information on how various biological, psychological, and social factors increase or decrease vulnerability to mental disorder among African Americans.

Important Research Questions

This chapter draws attention to a set of interesting and important research questions. The goal is to stimulate a new generation of research investigators to accept the challenge of clarifying the results presented here. Many argue that the stress associated with racial status and exposure to discrimination should increase the vulnerability of African Americans to mental disorder (Cannon & Locke, 1977; Fischer, 1969; Kramer et al., 1973). As a result, the *minority status* hypothesis predicts higher rates of mental disorders for blacks than for whites at *all* levels of socioeconomic status (Halpern, 1993; Kessler & Neighbors, 1986; Mirowsky & Ross, 1980; Parker & Jones, 1999). Yet the epidemiological data are not consistent with this hypothesis. Blacks have comparable or lower rates of mental disorder than whites do (Kessler, McGonagle, et al., 1994; Robins & Regier, 1991). Despite this general trend, there are significant racial differences for a few mental disorders. For example, rates of anxiety disorders, particularly phobias, are significantly higher for blacks than for whites; whereas rates of depression are lower for blacks. Some have speculated that cultural factors explain the findings for both depression and phobia (Brown, Eaton, & Sussman, 1990; Magee, Eaton, Wittchen, McGonagle, & Kessler, 1996; Warheit, Holzer, & Arey, 1975). Yet the empirical evidence demonstrating that protective processes operate differently for blacks than for whites remains unsatisfactory.

Cultural factors also come into play in the assessment of psychopathology. Because so much of what we now know about race and mental disorder is based on findings from the ECA program (Robins & Regier, 1991; data collected from July 1980 to August 1984) and the National Comorbidity Survey (NCS) (Kessler, McGonagle, et al., 1994), the data on race are largely a function of a methodological approach characterized by highly structured questionnaires that employ the same diagnostic criteria used by clinicians, that is, the criteria of the *Diagnostic and Statistical Manual of Mental Disorders (DSM)*. Yet it is frequently argued that racial groups often differ in their presentation and expression of mental disorder. This presents a particularly important challenge for psychiatric epidemiology because the rigid implementation of *DSM* criteria via highly structured survey instruments does not allow assessments of psychopathology to be adjusted on the basis of such cultural differences (Neighbors, Trierweiler, et al., 1999; Rogler, 1999; Vega & Rumbaut, 1991, p. 359; Wakefield, 1999, pp. 30–39, 50–54).

Studies of help-seeking show that like members of other population groups, many African Americans who could be helped by specialty mental health services do not access the professional help they need. On the one hand we need interventions designed to overcome both the psychological and structural barriers African Americans face in seeking professional help. This means effective mental health education programs designed to facilitate the recognition of mental disorders and to overcome the stigma associated with admitting to emotional difficulty. On the other hand it is not at all clear that increasing access to mental health services for African Americans will result in quality care (Neighbors et al., 1992). Some literature indicates that African Americans are at increased risk for being misunderstood, misdiagnosed, and mistreated (Adebimpe, 1981; Bell & Mehta, 1980, 1981; Neighbors, Jackson, Campbell, & Williams, 1989; Strakowski, McElroy, Keck, & West, 1996; Whaley, 1997). For example, rates of treated mental disorder have consistently shown that blacks have a higher rate of schizophrenia and a lower rate of mood disorder than whites. However, although these data have been interpreted as evidence of widespread misdiagnosis among African Americans, they are consistent with black-white differences in the community prevalence of these two disorders. It is possible that the treatment rates for depression and schizophrenia are a function of racial differences in the true prevalence of mental illness and of the fact that depressed African Americans are less likely to enter treatment than depressed whites.

Finally, public health researchers are increasingly being called on to clarify exactly what they mean by the concept of race and whether it differs from the related construct of ethnicity. Issues related to conceptualizations of race and ethnicity have important implications for sampling, recruiting study participants, classifying respondents for data analysis, and devising explanatory frameworks for the nature of racial differences in mental disorder. Clearly, race matters for mental health, although there are differing opinions as to how and why. Although for some this means doing a better job of measuring the impact of discrimination, for others it is a matter of understanding the relative importance of biology, genetics, and the environment (Farone & Tsaung, 1995; Lawson, 1990, 1996; Lin, Poland, & Silver, 1993; Lin, Poland, & Wallaski, 1993).

A Closer Look at the Epidemiological Evidence

The epidemiological data in five areas of concern—well-being and distress, depression, anxiety disorder, phobia, and suicide—will provide an initial picture of the mental health status of African Americans.

Well-Being and Distress

African Americans are disadvantaged compared to whites on most subjective indicators of the quality of life. Blacks report lower levels of life satisfaction, happiness, and marital happiness, and higher levels of anomia and mistrust than whites. There has been no change in the black disadvantage on these quality-of-life indicators between 1972 and 1996 (Hughes & Thomas, 1998). In addition, these racial disparities in the quality of life cannot be explained by socioeconomic status. However, blacks have comparable or better mental health than whites on other indicators. For example, there are no black-white differences in self-esteem (Jackson & Lassiter, in press; Porter & Washington, 1979, 1993). Similarly, elevated rates of psychological distress among African Americans as compared to whites are not consistently found. Although some studies find that blacks have higher rates of distress compared to whites, other studies find the opposite, and some studies find no racial differences at all (Dohrenwend & Dohrenwend, 1969; Neighbors, 1984; Vega & Rumbaut, 1991; Williams & Harris-Reid, 1999). Moreover, blacks have comparable or lower rates of mental disorder than whites. The ECA study found very few differences between blacks and whites in the rates of both current and lifetime psychiatric disorders. The absence of a racial difference in drug use history and the prevalence of alcohol and drug dependence is especially noteworthy given popular perceptions of elevated rates of drug use in the black community. The more recent National Comorbidity Survey found that blacks do not have higher rates of mental disorder than whites for any of the major classes of disorders. Instead, lower rates of disorders for blacks when compared to whites are especially pronounced for mood disorders and the substance abuse disorders (alcohol and drug abuse). Anxiety disorders, especially phobias, however, stand out as one area where blacks had considerably higher rates than whites.

Taken together, national epidemiological estimates from both the ECA and the NCS show that the prevalence of serious mental illness in African Americans is equivalent or below that of whites. Focusing on overall rates of any disorder is not, however, particularly useful because it obscures important subgroup differences for specific disorders. The manner in which rates of disorder vary once demographic categories such as age, sex, marital status, and socioeconomic status are taken into account has not been inspected adequately. Unfortunately, the NCS remains a relatively untapped data resource. A comprehensive investigation of NCS data for black-white differences in *DSM* disorders has yet to be published. Therefore some of the best information in this area still comes from the ECA study.

Depression

The ECA found that overall, blacks and whites did not differ in the lifetime prevalence of major depression (Robins & Regier, 1991; Robins, Helzer, Croughan, & Ratcliff, 1981; Somervell et al., 1989), but factoring in the effect of age, gender, and socioeconomic status reveals some interesting patterns (see Table 6.1, columns 1 to 4). The most dramatic racial difference in depression occurred among men aged thirty to forty-four, where white men display a higher lifetime prevalence rate than black men (7.2 percent compared to 2.6 percent). A similar but much less dramatic racial difference was found for the one-year and

TABLE 6.1. THE RELATIONSHIP OF AGE AND RACE TO MOOD, GENERALIZED ANXIETY, AND PHOBIA (ONE-YEAR AND LIFETIME PREVALENCE) FOR MEN AND WOMEN.

Men

	Any Mood Disorder				Generalized Anxiety Disorder				Any Phobic Disorder			
	One-Year		Lifetime		One-Year[a]		One-Year[b]		One-Year		Lifetime	
	Black	White	Black	White	Black	White	Black	White	Black	White	Black	White
18–29	2.9	2.8	5.3	6.3	8.80	3.10	7.38	2.88	11.46	5.84	16.18	10.65
30–44	1.4	2.9	2.6	7.2	2.28	2.06	1.68	1.11	10.48	5.82	14.29	10.27
45–64	1.1	1.8	1.9	3.7	6.76	1.35	6.71	0.91	12.71	6.23	20.26	9.93
65+	0.2	0.6	1.9	1.5	0.90	1.50	1.02	0.83	12.04	4.20	15.30	7.18

Women

	Any Mood Disorder				Generalized Anxiety Disorder				Any Phobic Disorder			
	One-Year		Lifetime		One-Year[a]		One-Year[b]		One-Year		Lifetime	
	Black	White	Black	White	Black	White	Black	White	Black	White	Black	White
18–29	7.6	5.8	11.1	10.9	10.55	5.42	8.24	3.14	22.99	12.24	27.23	14.84
30–44	5.1	8.3	10.5	16.1	6.89	4.69	3.97	3.03	18.04	16.35	24.60	22.33
45–64	2.8	3.6	6.0	9.5	3.44	5.35	1.68	4.24	21.03	10.49	30.63	15.56
65+	1.8	1.4	3.4	3.4	2.76	2.82	2.71	2.28	14.80	8.45	24.17	13.01

Note: "One year" means that there was some sign of the disorder within one year before the interview.

[a]GAD with no exclusions for other *DSM* disorder.

[b]GAD excluding people with panic or major depression.

Source: Robins & Regier, 1991 (data abstracted from the NIMH Epidemiologic Catchment Area study, p. 60, p. 165, and pp. 187–188).

lifetime prevalence of depression for women in the same age group (16.1 percent for white women over a lifetime compared to 10.5 percent for black women). Blacks also had lower one-year and lifetime rates for both men and women aged forty-five to sixty-four. The most dramatic difference for this age group was seen in lifetime rates for black women (9.5 percent compared to 6 percent for white women). There were no appreciable racial differences in depression among elderly (sixty-five-plus) men or women.

Black women show higher rates of depression than black men at all age groups for both one-year and lifetime prevalence. For both black men and women, the highest rates of depression occur in the eighteen to twenty-nine age range, and both one-year and lifetime rates decline with age (Weissman, Bruce, Leaf, Florio, & Holzer, 1991, p. 60). In a detailed analysis of race and depression, Somervell et al. (1989) found no black-white differences in the six-month prevalence of depression. Taking age into account, however, a high rate of depression was revealed among black women aged eighteen to twenty-four. This is consistent with ECA findings. Black women aged eighteen to twenty-four in both the New Haven and Baltimore ECA sites had a higher lifetime prevalence of depression than white women; a higher six-month prevalence of depression for black women was seen at all five ECA sites. Williams, Takeuchi, and Adair (1992b) focused more closely on socioeconomic status, race, and psychiatric disorder. They found that, unlike the pattern for whites, the six-month prevalence of depression among blacks was not related to socioeconomic status. Neither was there a relationship between socioeconomic status and lifetime depression among black men, although there was a significant positive relationship between lifetime depression and education. Black men with some college were more likely to be depressed than less educated black men. Lifetime depression was not related to socioeconomic status among black women. Brown, Ahmed, Gary, and Milburn (1995) conducted a regional study of major depression in a community sample of African Americans. The one-year prevalence of depression was higher for men than for women but the difference was not significant. The highest rates of depression were among those aged eighteen to twenty-nine (the youngest examined). Depression was not related to income or to education.

Williams, Takeuchi, and Adair (1992a) used the ECA data to examine racial differences in mental disorder when marital status was also considered. Married blacks and whites had lower rates of psychiatric disorders than the previously married (separated, divorced, and widowed) did. Widowed black women, for example, had levels of major depression that were three times higher than those of their married counterparts. Never-married black men and women and white men had rates of depression comparable to married respondents' rates. The absence of an elevated risk of psychiatric illness for never-married black women is especially instructive because of concerns about the psychological consequences of being a female head of household, given the rise of such households in the black community. An examination of which sex benefits more in mental health terms from marriage found that among the separated and divorced, black men had a higher rate of depression than black women. Gender differences were also evident among the never married and widowed. For never-married blacks, men had higher rates of depression than women; whereas among the widowed, as mentioned, black women were at higher risk of major depression.

Generalized Anxiety Disorder

Warheit, Bell, Schwab, and Buhl's study (1986) of northern Florida, using a twelve-item symptom checklist, found significantly higher anxiety scores for blacks than for whites. Blazer, Hughes, George, Swartz, and Boyer (1991) concluded that despite wide variation in the definitions used in epidemiological studies conducted between 1970 and 1986, generalized anxiety disorder (GAD) was more common in blacks than in whites. In general, these early findings were confirmed by the ECA (see Table 6.1, columns 5 to 8). Blacks had higher one-year prevalence rates of generalized anxiety than whites. The ECA used three different definitions of

GAD. Blacks who had GAD without depression or panic had significantly higher rates than whites. Among blacks and whites with GAD with or without other *DSM* diagnoses (that is, with no exclusions for other diagnoses), the overall difference was quite noticeable (6.09 percent for blacks versus 3.47 percent for whites). Among men less than thirty years of age and men forty-five to sixty-four, blacks had higher rates than whites for all three measures of GAD; there were no racial differences among the elderly or among the thirty to forty-four age group. Black women aged eighteen to twenty-nine and thirty to forty-four exceeded white women for all three GAD measures. The differences were most pronounced for GAD with no exclusions for other disorders. Interestingly, white women aged forty-five to sixty-four had slightly *higher* rates of GAD than black women of that age did. No racial differences in GAD were found among the elderly. For black men, GAD was highest in the youngest age group across all three measures. Among black men, the GAD rates drop for those aged thirty to forty-four and then rise again among those aged forty-five to sixty-four, to rates almost comparable to those less than thirty years of age. The lowest rates of GAD among black men were for those aged sixty-five and above. For black women the GAD rates were also highest among those less than thirty years of age. Unlike black men, however, black women consistently exhibited less GAD with age. Similar to black men, black women incurred the lowest rates of GAD at age sixty-five and older.

Phobia

Black-white comparisons for phobia, also an anxiety disorder, are even more interesting than those for GAD. Historically, blacks have consistently exhibited higher rates of phobia than whites. As far back as the mid-1970s, Warheit et al. (1975) reported significantly higher rates of phobic symptomatology for African Americans than for whites, even with controls for socioeconomic status. Similarly, the ECA study reported that blacks had higher rates of phobia for one-month, one-year, and lifetime prevalence (Table 6.1, columns 9 to 12). In fact, 23.4 percent of blacks in the ECA study met lifetime criteria for phobic disorder. Controlling for sex did not change this pattern. In terms of phobia subtypes, blacks exceeded whites for agoraphobia and simple phobia but not for social phobia. Controlling for sex yields this same pattern for men, but black women exceeded white women for social phobia as well as for agoraphobia and simple phobia. Twenty-four percent of black women met lifetime prevalence criteria for simple phobia. Controlling for both sex and age, black men exceeded white men in both the one-year and lifetime prevalence of phobia at all age groups. There was no relationship of phobia to age for black men; the rates were high for all ages, but highest in the forty-five to sixty-four age group. For one-year and lifetime phobia, black women exceeded white women at all ages, although black and white women aged thirty to forty-four were very similar. There were no noticeable trends for phobia by age for black women. Finally, blacks also had higher rates of any phobic disorder (one-year prevalence) than whites when data were controlled for education (Robins & Regier, 1991).

Brown et al. (1990) performed a multivariate analysis of racial differences in phobia using data from the ECA study. This analysis showed that African Americans were 1.52 times more likely than whites to report recent phobia. In a very comprehensive analysis of respondents in wave 2 of the Durham ECA site, Hybels et al. (1997) found significantly higher phobia rates for blacks when controlling for social network structure, social interaction, social support, religiosity, self-confidence, physical health, and comorbidity as well as for the typical list of demographic characteristics (age, gender, socioeconomic status, marital status, urbanicity). Even with all of these controls, a multivariate logistical analysis showed that Durham blacks were 1.97 times more likely than whites to meet criteria for phobia. The initial findings from the NCS also revealed that the prevalence of phobias was significantly higher among African Americans and that blacks were twice as likely as whites to meet criteria for one-month agoraphobia (Magee et al., 1996). Blacks were also 33 percent more likely than whites to meet criteria for simple phobia. Closer inspection of the NCS data revealed that black women had a higher current rate of agoraphobia and simple phobia than white women did. White males, however, had rates of simple and social phobia that were two and three times higher than the rates for black men (Magee, 1993).

Suicide

In general, suicide rates have been and remain much lower for blacks than whites, a pattern that is remarkably consistent with the general finding of no black-white differences in mental disorder. Racial differences in suicide have been termed a "cultural paradox," given that African Americans have experienced discrimination, decreased economic opportunity, and low social status (Gibbs, 1997). A closer inspection of the suicide data, however, reveals some troubling trends. In fact, suicide is now the third leading cause of death for African American youths fifteen to twenty-four years old. Suicide among elderly African Americans, over seventy-five years old, increased more than 50 percent from 1980 to 1992 (Davis, 1979; Kachur, Potter, James, & Powell, 1995). Interestingly, suicide among black girls ten to nineteen years old decreased over this period. Paradoxically, although more black men than women complete suicide, African American females are more likely to attempt suicide, and their rate of attempts is virtually equal to that of white women (Cannetto & Lester, 1995; Kachur et al., 1995; Lester, 1998; Molock, Kimbrough, Lacy, & McClure, 1994; Summerville, Kaslow, & Doepke, 1996).

Within the black population, women are much more protected from completing suicide than are black men (Cose, 1995). Little is known, however, about why these protective factors do not prevent women from *attempting* suicide and why these factors protect women but not men (Baker, 1988; Early, 1992; Gibbs, 1997; Singh, Kochanek, & MacDorman, 1996; Smith & Carter, 1986). It could be, on the one hand, that there are no gender differences in the underlying processes, and that the outcome difference may be due entirely to the differential lethality of the methods chosen. Certainly, men tend to use more effective suicide strategies than women. The difference may, on the other hand, have something to do with the concept of black male masculinity. Majors and Billson (1993) discuss the mental health implications of the construct *cool pose,* a cluster of behaviors designed to deliver a message of strength and control. Majors and Billson speculate that the cool pose may in fact mask feelings of self-doubt and insecurity. It may then increase the risk of suicide because its use as a coping strategy results in losing touch with one's feelings. Although interesting explanations for the observed patterns abound, few have been tested empirically. For example, some have speculated that because blacks report being more religious than whites, religiosity operates to protect African Americans from suicide (Neeleman, Wessely, & Lewis, 1998). Some research suggests that social support from family and friends protects African American women against suicide and that low social status (particularly for single mothers) may actually *increase* involvement in suicide-protective support systems (Nisbet, 1996). The protective effects of religiosity or family support have not been linked empirically to suicidal ideation, nor has the *differential* impact of such factors been tested across races.

One of the more popular explanations for the black male suicide increase has to do with the stress of upward social mobility and the provocative hypothesis that academic and economic achievement and success are detrimental to black mental health (Centers for Disease Control and Prevention, 1998). It has been argued that upwardly mobile African Americans are exposed to stressful events (for example, racial slurs, social isolation) associated with moving into new, more racially integrated social environments. Assimilation into the middle class might also draw African Americans away from the traditional social institutions that have operated as protective factors. As blacks move up economically and into more racially integrated settings, they may lose access to some culturally based protective factors such as family and religious support. This line of thinking is provocative because conventional wisdom would suggest that economic success leads to improvements in mental health. But as the depression and anxiety data show, middle and upper socioeconomic status blacks are just as depressed and anxious as low socioeconomic status blacks. It is possible that the impact of upward social mobility varies as a function of differences in the ways black men and women are socialized. We do not know enough to determine whether successful upward mobility is the culprit that explains the increasing rates of suicide among young African American males or whether it is the persistently poor who have lost hope who are committing suicide in ever higher numbers. Furthermore, we do not understand why such stresses do not affect black women in a similar manner. These mobility-related hypotheses about the mental health effects of assimilation remain largely untested. In summary, despite some very troubling trends and suicide's importance as an "ultimate outcome" of risk for depression, epidemiological research on race and suicide remains much too descriptive. More studies are needed before we can better understand the impact of specific risk and protective factors on race and suicide.

The African American Experience: Risk and Protection

African Americans must continually confront issues of acculturation and identity, discrimination, goal-striving stress, and the stress of imposed and sometimes internalized inferiority. Learning how they do so and with what results is important to improving black mental health.

Acculturation and Identity

The concept of acculturation offers a promising direction for broadening psychiatric epidemiological research on race beyond its preoccupation with describing demographic differences. The relationship between acculturation and mental health has been applied much more to Hispanics and Asians than to American Indians and African Americans (Banks, 1996; Landrine & Klonoff, 1996a; Snowden & Hines, 1999; Williams-Flournoy & Anderson, 1996). There is, however, some overlap between research on African American identity and acculturation models. Black identity and acculturation research overlap most with respect to the concept of psychological acculturation (Marger, 1997), where the focus is on the individual's changes in self-concept and the extent to which individuals feel that they belong to a mainstream, largely white society as opposed to their own particular racial group. Models of black identity development and acculturation are concerned both with the mental health implications of separation (segregation), assimilation, and feelings of marginalization and with the ability to successfully integrate aspects of multiple cultures (to be multicultural) (Berry, Poortinga, Segall, & Dasen, 1992). Some African Americans are able to become multicultural with relatively little cost to mental health and self-concept; others find it much more difficult and stressful.

Black racial group identity and other forms of psychological acculturation are partly a function of how members of other racial groups (for example, whites) respond to the acculturation strategies adopted by African Americans. The manner in which highly visible phenotypic characteristics (for example, skin color) are used to facilitate or limit access to societal resources has important implications for factors such as social status, social mobility, power, control, and social support. The African American identity literature is dominated by social and clinical psychology and, as such, is certainly relevant to mental health. The issues of identity and acculturation have not, however, been adequately explored with respect to the epidemiology of mental disorders. Psychiatric epidemiology has much to learn by linking more directly with the body of knowledge about these matters. Rogler, Cortes, and Malgady's review (1991) demonstrates that the acculturation and mental health literature is still fraught with conceptual ambiguities, measurement problems, and conflicting results. Nevertheless, acculturation remains an increasingly promising but underexplored explanatory framework for racial differences in mental disorder.

Discrimination

A growing body of research is examining the mental health consequences of exposure to discrimination. In a national probability sample of blacks, whites, Hispanics, and Asians, Williams (2000) found that reports of discrimination due to race or cultural background were positively related to psychological distress. In the first wave of the National Survey of Black Americans (NSBA), Williams and Chung (in press) documented that perceptions of racial discrimination were related to higher levels of psychological distress and lower levels of life satisfaction and happiness as well as to poorer physical health. Prospective analyses of the NSBA data revealed that discrimination was inversely associated with life satisfaction but unrelated to happiness and psychological distress (Jackson et al., 1996). Several recent studies have provided more comprehensive assessments of discrimination than the single-item global measures used in most early studies of discrimination and mental health. Landrine and Klonoff (1996b) developed an eighteen-item scale of racist events, and found that this measure of discrimination was positively related to psychological distress. Thompson (1996) found that a multiple-item measure of exposure to discrimination was predictive of higher levels of psychological distress in a probability sample of African Americans in St. Louis, Missouri. Ren, Amick, and Williams (1999) found that experiences of discrimination were positively related to self-report measures of physical and mental health in a nationally representative sample.

Williams and colleagues (Forman, Williams, & Jackson, 1997; Williams, Yu, Jackson, & Anderson, 1997) developed a scale to capture minor but recurrent experiences of discrimination. This measure of chronic, everyday discrimination assesses the frequency of experiences such as being treated with less courtesy, being shown less respect, and receiving poorer service than others in restaurants or stores. Two recent studies found that blacks report markedly higher levels of both minor and major experiences of discrimination (Kessler, Mickelson, & Williams, 1999; Williams et al., 1997). Such discriminatory events adversely affected self-rated health, chronic physical conditions, psychological distress, and life satisfaction in the metropolitan Detroit study (Williams et al., 1997). Importantly, these associations between discrimination and health were independent of other measures of stress. Perceptions of discrimination were related to psychological distress, major depression, and generalized anxiety in the national study (Kessler et al., 1999).

Goal-Striving Stress

Climbing the ladder of success is a central feature of the American dream. As integral members of U.S. society, black Americans fully endorse the core value of achievement and the idea that hard work and persistence can ensure socioeconomic success (Clark, 1965; Gurin, Gurin, Lao, & Beattie, 1969; Hyman, 1953; James, 1994). As the findings on discrimination show, the mental health of

African Americans has a lot to do with how blacks deal with expectations for success and aspirations for achievement in the face of race-based obstacles. This is the delicate psychological balancing act faced by African Americans living in the United States. The manner in which each black person resolves the counteracting forces of the upward pull of his or her dream and the downward pressure of discrimination is the key to whether or not he or she will make a successful adaptation to life in the United States (Edwards & Polite, 1992). The desire for a better life coupled with the fact of blocked opportunities can be frustrating, disappointing, and worse, psychologically damaging (Dressler, 1988; Neighbors, Jackson, Broman, & Thompson, 1996). Yet few psychiatric epidemiological investigations have empirically examined the relationship between aspirations, achievements, and the stress of blocked opportunities.

The concept of goal-striving stress is a useful but underutilized way to capture the social psychological effects of race-based discrimination. Parker and Kleiner (1966) were the first to apply the concept of goal-striving to a psychiatric epidemiological investigation of black Americans. Goal-striving stress is the psychological discrepancy between aspiration and achievement, weighted by the subjective probability of success and the disappointment experienced if those aspirations are not achieved. Parker and Kleiner found that low socioeconomic status blacks displayed *low* goal-striving stress and high psychological distress; the opposite was true for high socioeconomic status blacks. Further analyses of the data showed that social mobility modified the relationships among socioeconomic status, goal-striving, and mental health. Upwardly mobile, high socioeconomic status blacks had high goal-striving stress and high rates of distress, which Parker and Kleiner interpreted as failure to reduce striving even after achieving success. Downwardly mobile, poor African Americans had high goal-striving stress scores and high symptoms, which Parker and Kleiner saw as a failure to reduce aspirations associated with past status. Stable, persistently poor blacks had low goal-striving stress and low symptoms. For this group, Parker and Kleiner speculated that the reduction of active goal-striving was psychologically adaptive. It is time we linked such concepts as goal-striving (and related constructs like John Henryism) to the epidemiology of mental disorder (Neighbors & Lumpkin, 1990, pp. 63–64). Recently, analyses from the National Survey of Black Americans found that high goal-striving stress lowers happiness, life satisfaction, and self-esteem and increases psychological distress as well as clinical depression for African Americans regardless of age, sex, income, or education (Neighbors & Sellers, 2000; Sellers, 2000).

The Stress of Inferiority

Another significant psychological effect of racism and discrimination is its attack on the ego identity of its victims. By this we do not mean self-hatred. Rather, we refer to the erosion of self-confidence that can result when others voice skepticism about the cognitive and behavioral abilities of African Americans (Wilson, 1999).

Negative images of blacks are pervasive in American culture. Although focusing on academic achievement (a stereotype threat), the research of Claude Steele (Steele, 1992, 1999) clearly shows the pervasive impact of negative stereotypes on self-concept and test performance. These beliefs about biological or cultural black inferiority can attack the self-worth of some African Americans. The term *internalized racism* describes their acceptance of the negative societal beliefs and stereotypes about their group. It has been suggested that in a color-conscious, racially stratified society, one adaptive response of populations defined as inferior is to accept the dominant society's ideology of their inferiority (McCarthy & Yancey, 1971; Pettigrew, 1964). For some African Americans the normative cultural characterization of the superiority of whiteness and the devaluation of blackness, combined with the economic marginality of blacks, can lead to self-perceptions of worthlessness and powerlessness.

Several lines of evidence suggest that the internalization of cultural stereotypes by stigmatized groups can create expectations, anxieties, and reactions that can adversely affect social and psychological functioning. Fischer et al.'s review of research from several countries (1996) indicates that groups that are socially regarded as inferior have poorer academic performance than their more highly regarded peers (this has been found for Koreans versus Japanese in Japan, Scots versus the English in the United Kingdom, and Eastern European–origin Jews versus Western European–origin Jews in Israel). Research in the United States revealed that under experimental conditions, when a stigma of inferiority is activated, performance on an examination is adversely affected. African Americans who were told in advance that blacks perform more poorly on exams than whites, women who were told that women perform more poorly than men, and white men who were told that whites usually do worse than Asians, all had lower scores on an examination than control groups who were not confronted with a stigma of inferiority (Fischer et al., 1996; Steele, 1992, 1999). Similarly, studies of mental patients revealed that the expectation of negative stigmatization adversely affected social networks, job performance, and self-esteem (Link, 1987; Link, Streuning, Cullen, Shrout, & Dohrenwend, 1989).

Jerome Taylor and his colleagues at the University of Pittsburgh have empirically examined the mental health consequences of internalized racism. In a study of 289 African American women, Taylor and Jackson (1990) found a positive association between internalized racism (believing in the innate inferiority of blacks and feeling uncomfortable around other blacks) and psychological distress (see also Taylor, Henderson, & Jackson, 1991; Taylor & Jackson, 1991). These associations remained significant after adjustment for stress, social support, religious orientation, socioeconomic status, marital status, and physical health. Other studies with Taylor's instrument (the nationalization scale) have produced similar results (Tomes, Brown, Semenya, & Simpson, 1990). Support for the adverse health consequences of internalized racism also comes from analyses of the NSBA (Williams & Chung, in press). In this study, blacks were asked the extent to which they regarded seven negative stereotypes and seven positive stereotypes as true of most black people. The endorsement of negative stereotypes was positively related to psychological distress. The rejection of positive stereotypes as true was inversely related to happiness and life satisfaction. These associations were significant after controlling for sociodemographic factors (age, education, and gender) and discrimination.

Much is yet to be learned about the determinants and consequences of internalized racism. Hughes and Demo (1989) found an inverse association between internalized racism (measured in terms of the endorsement of stereotypes) and self-esteem among blacks, but we do not currently understand the causal dynamics underlying this association. Research is needed to explicate the ways in which racial group self-esteem and personal self-esteem relate to each other and combine to affect health. The research so far provides intriguing leads but as yet has not been subjected to rigorous examination within the context of black mental health.

The Classification of Psychopathology

The ability and means to make accurate diagnoses within the context of African American culture, a recognition of racial influences on epidemiological case-finding, and an understanding of the meaning of race and ethnicity all affect the provision of effective mental health care for African Americans.

Diagnosis

Psychiatric diagnosis is centrally important to quality mental health care because it predicts and informs treatment. However, psychiatric diagnosis is especially difficult because the diagnosis of mental disorder depends disproportionately on symptoms and behaviors observed and reported by the patient and on complicated inferences made by clinicians. Diagnosis within the context of race is fraught with difficulties and serious problems that we are only beginning to address in depth.

Historically, there have been two perspectives on the manner in which race influences diagnosis (Neighbors, Jackson, Campbell, & Williams, 1989). The first perspective assumes that blacks and whites exhibit symptomatology in essentially the same manner and that diagnostic criteria are equally applicable to both blacks and whites. Diagnostic errors then are the result of stereotypes that clinicians have about black people. The second perspective assumes that blacks and whites display psychopathology in different ways but that diagnosticians incorrectly assume racial similarity in symptom presentation. Diagnostic errors then result from the fact that clinicians are unaware of or insensitive to cultural differences in the way the same disorder can be manifested in blacks and whites.

These conflicting perspectives raise critical questions that need to be answered before we can determine the appropriateness of applying diagnostic models and instruments developed on whites to blacks.

Numerous studies of patient samples have shown that whites are more likely than blacks to be diagnosed with a mood disorder and that African Americans are more likely than whites to be diagnosed with schizophrenia (Neighbors, Jackson, Campbell, & Williams, 1989; Snowden & Cheung, 1990). There has been much discussion, however, about how to interpret the meaning of these relationships. Many scholars argue that these statistics are indicative of widespread misdiagnosis among African Americans. Although the misdiagnosis hypothesis is varied and complex, the fundamental premise is that clinicians have not been sensitive enough to black-white differences in the expression of symptoms of emotional distress. Specifically, researchers suggest that unfamiliarity with the cultural aspects of African American behavior and language leads to misinterpretation and misdiagnosis of African American patients (Jones & Gray, 1986; Lawson, 1986). Although much has been written about the misdiagnosis of African American psychiatric inpatients, a careful review of the empirical literature reveals that the data are neither clear nor definitive (Adebimpe, 1981; Good, 1993; Neighbors, Trierweiler, 1999; Whaley, 1997). Thus, although treatment statistics suggest that schizophrenia is overdiagnosed in African Americans, more in-depth explorations are needed of black-white differences in presenting symptoms and their impact of these differences on the diagnostic process.

Studies comparing two diagnoses for each patient, one clinical and the other arrived at by researchers using semistructured instruments and adhering strictly to *DSM* criteria, often find that black patients with a clinical diagnosis of schizophrenia are more often than white patients given a research diagnosis of depression. This finding raises two important issues. First, it underlines the importance of exploring diagnostic divergence under varying interview conditions as a useful technique for exploring racial influences on diagnosis. If two reasonable diagnostic processes disagree, we must be willing to assume that one of those diagnostic techniques is *more* accurate or valid. More important, pinpointing the precise location of the diagnostic divergence—for example, more disagreement when distinguishing bipolar disorder from schizoaffective disorder among blacks than among whites—should document more precisely where race poses a particularly difficult diagnostic challenge for clinicians. Second, it highlights the importance of arriving at a set of clinical procedures that skillfully implement diagnostic taxonomies like *DSM-IV,* procedures that can interpret responses to carefully crafted questions in the context of racial culture.

Interestingly, despite the indictment of clinical judgment as the culprit in racial bias in diagnosis, the mental health field has taken the position that for clinicians to become competent diagnosticians, they must acknowledge differences among patients that are due explicitly to racial group membership. The challenge is for clinicians to learn how to take cultural context into account in an appropriate manner. As a result the importance of using *clinical judgment* in the application of *DSM* criteria must not be underemphasized. Indeed, it is absolutely crucial that sociocultural contextual information be taken into account in making diagnostic judgments of psychologically painful symptoms, troubling thoughts, and disturbing behaviors. In essence the field is searching for a reasonable and effective way to *control* the manner in which cultural context is brought into play in clinically important processes such as diagnosis (Grier & Cobbs, 1968, pp. 177–179). The best solution is to rely on procedures that inquire about the entire range of diagnostic categories, using criteria in conjunction with interviewing techniques that allow enough *flexibility* to effectively incorporate knowledge and understanding of the patient's culture. These diagnostic issues have important implications for psychiatric epidemiology.

Racial Influences on Epidemiological Case-Finding

There are many ways that culture may affect the epidemiology of mental disorder, but the one most relevant to this review is the assumption that symptom expression varies as a function of racial group membership (Kleinman, 1996). The notion of racial differences in the patterning of symptomatology creates important challenges for psychiatric epidemiological case-finding, which relies heavily on mimicking the clinical diagnostic process. The *DSM,* by making criteria explicit and specific, has implied that it can reduce diagnostic bias (for example, misdiagnosis) by guiding clinicians to treat *all* patients in the same manner, regardless of race. The *DSM* also set the stage for the large psychiatric epidemiological community studies on which the present review is based (Rogler, 1999, p. 426). The problem with the approach is that it contradicts a fundamental assumption underlying cultural psychiatry. Persons of different racial groups often differ from one another and, as a result, should *not* be treated the same (Aponte, Rivers, & Wohl, 1995; Dana, 1993; Gaw, 1982; Kleinman & Good, 1985; Lefley & Pedersen, 1986; Marsella & Pedersen, 1981; Mezzich, Kleinman, Fabrega, & Parron, 1996; Rogler, 1999). To make an "accurate" diagnosis, case-finding procedures *must* have the ability to distinguish symptoms of pathology from normative cultural experiences that are not indicative of mental disorder (American Psychiatric Association, 1994; Frances, 1998). This raises an interesting dilemma for psychiatric epidemiology as it is currently practiced, using questionnaire instruments like the Diagnostic Interview Schedule (DIS) and the Composite International Diagnostic Interview (CIDI) administered by nonclinical survey interviewers. Because diagnostic instruments like these are highly structured, it is difficult to take cultural context into account.

Psychiatric epidemiology has been relying on instruments like the DIS and the CIDI for so long that the innovative case-finding technology they represent is often taken for granted. But we cannot afford to forget just how radical it is that our best prevalence estimates are arrived at by nonclinical survey interviewers and computer algorithms based on *DSM-III, DSM-III-R,* and *DSM-IV* criteria. We cannot ignore the fact that the methodological foundation on which all of our mental health statistics is based is an ambitious, pragmatic approximation of the clinical interview. The original ECA studies included a clinical reappraisal as an evaluation of how well the DIS operated. Those studies showed that for some disorders there was low agreement between the DIS and clinical diagnoses (Anthony et al., 1985; Eaton, 2000; Helzer et al., 1985; Hendricks & Bayton, 1983; Kessler & Zhao, 1999). This should not be surprising given that epidemiological investigations and clinical reappraisals are such different diagnostic procedures. Clearly these differences in diagnostic outcomes are due to the role that clinical judgment plays in determining the presence or absence of psychopathological symptoms. On one hand, nonclinical survey interviewers employed in large epidemiological studies like the ECA and the NCS have to accept all responses *at face value.* They are not allowed to cross-examine respondents to probe beyond the standard questions that make up the DIS and CIDI questionnaires. Nor are they allowed to make a sociocultural interpretation of the meaning of the responses provided. On the other hand, as a function of their clinical expertise, clinicians have the flexibility to decide whether there is something about a response that needs clarification. Thus clinicians, unlike survey interviewers, can continue probing until they are satisfied that the response is or is not indicative of the presence of psychopathology.

Perhaps the inability of highly structured instruments to compensate for cultural influences when assessing psychopathology is a key to understanding some of the paradoxical findings presented here. For example, earlier we suggested that the lack of black-white differences in depression could be explained on the basis of the counterbalancing effects of risk and protective factors. Yet it is equally plausible that the case-finding methods employed in psychiatric epidemiology are underdiagnosing depression among African Americans. A number of writers have noted the curious finding that many black respondents with very high depressive symptom checklist scores *do not* meet diagnostic criteria for major depression (Sue, Chun, & Gee, 1995; Vega & Rumbaut, 1991; Williams & Harris-Reid, 1999). Similarly, many authors suggest that African Americans with mood disorders present in such varied and different ways that the identification of major depression is especially difficult (Adebimpe, Hedlund, Cho, & Wood, 1982; Brown, Schulberg, & Madonia, 1996; Fabrega, Mezzich, & Ulrich, 1988; Fabrega, Mulsant, Rifai, & Al, 1994; Jones & Gray, 1986; Lawson, 1986; Leo, Narayan, Sherry, Micchalek, & Pollock, 1997; Strakowski et al., 1996). Another possibility is that depressive symptoms and a major depressive episode are not the same phenomenon. Checklists likely capture a mental state more akin to demoralization, which is qualitatively different from clinical disorder (Dohrenwend, Shrout, Egri, & Mendelsohn, 1980; Seiler, 1973). Although more research is needed to substantiate this possibility, the implications for psychiatric epidemiology are immensely important because the screening item that qualifies respondents for detailed follow-up questions in the depression module of the DIS requires a positive response to "feeling sad" (dysphoria) for two weeks or more. If clinical judgment continues to be eliminated from psychiatric epidemiological case-finding, the only alternative for obtaining more accurate diagnoses is to make culturally based modifications to the diagnostic instruments. It is currently difficult to find concrete examples of ways investigators have modified diagnostic instruments for use with African Americans in community epidemiological surveys.

The Meaning of Race and Ethnicity

This chapter has reviewed empirical studies, most of which did not make much distinction among ethnic groups from different countries of origin. We have employed the term *race* to refer to a socially constructed category of limited biological and genetic significance. As such, the term race overlaps with the concept of ethnicity (Landrine & Klonoff, 1996b). We opted in this chapter to employ the term race as a convenient descriptor to refer to a research variable most often operationally defined by self-identification by the respondent. Such self-definitions of race have been shown to be associated with important mental health outcomes. Certainly, there is considerable ethnic variation in both the so-called black and white groups, but the vast majority of psychiatric epidemiological investigations do not attend to this within-group ethnic variation. Most of the studies reviewed here asked respondents to self-identify within the traditional U.S. racial categories (African American, Caucasian, Hispanic, and so forth) and not to differentiate themselves in terms of their specific ethnic group memberships (Haitian, Nigerian, Jamaican, Irish, Italian, and so forth). Thus the two groups described as black and white should be viewed as aggregations of various ethnic groups. Although there are important commonalities among blacks in the United States, there is also considerable heterogeneity in the black population. Green (1978), for example, has argued that there are nine distinctive "cultural-ecological areas" for the black population that vary in history, economics, and a broad range of social characteristics. These cultural-ecological areas are (1) Tidewater-Piedmont (eastern Maryland, Virginia, and North Carolina); (2) coastal Southeast (South Carolina and eastern Georgia); (3) black belt (central and western Georgia, Alabama, Mississippi, parts of Tennessee, Kentucky, Arkansas, Missouri, Louisiana, and Texas); (4) French tradition (Louisiana, eastern coastal Texas, and southwestern Mississippi); (5) areas of Indian influence (Oklahoma and parts of Arkansas and Kansas); (6) Southwestern areas (west Texas, New Mexico, Arizona, and California); (7) old Eastern colonial areas (New Jersey, Pennsylvania, New York, Massachusetts); (8) Midwestern and far Western areas (Illinois west to Washington State); and (9) post-1920 metropolitan North and West ghetto areas (major inner cities in such cities as New York, Detroit, Chicago, and San Francisco). Health researchers have not explored the usefulness of this typology for predicting variations in African American health.

Immigrants from the Caribbean area and the African mainland are important ethnic subgroups in the black population. These immigrant groups are also characterized by considerable heterogeneity. For example, the black population from the Caribbean basin countries is a diverse group including

Spanish-speaking persons from Cuba, the Dominican Republic, and Panama; French-speaking persons from Haiti and the other French-speaking Caribbean territories; Dutch-speaking individuals from Aruba and the Netherlands Antilles; and English-speaking persons from the former British colonies in the Caribbean Sea and the mainland territories of Belize and Guyana. The 1990 census estimated that there were almost one million Americans of English-speaking West Indian ancestry and an additional three hundred thousand of Haitian ancestry. However, some research suggests that persons of West Indian or other Caribbean descent are at least 10 percent of the black population in the United States (Hill, 1983). In addition, the 1990 census indicated that there were almost half a million persons of sub-Saharan African ancestry in the United States. Although these ethnic subpopulations are relatively small within the entire black population, they constitute a substantial proportion of that population in some areas. For example, it is estimated that at least 25 percent of New York City's black population consists of foreign-born West Indians (Vickerman, 1999). Variations in the mental health status of blacks by ethnicity have not been systematically addressed in the literature. One recent national study found that blacks of Caribbean descent had higher levels of both stress and psychological distress than native-born blacks (Williams, 2000). However, the sample size of Caribbean-origin blacks was relatively small, and these findings await further replication.

Conclusion

Numerous questions are raised by this review, and there is much opportunity offered by the many research directions that have been suggested. Clearly the epidemiology of mental disorder between and within racial and ethnic groups is a field ripe for investigation. There is especially a need to link theories and findings from the social sciences with epidemiology and public health. Although psychology and sociology have been concerned with the study of race and ethnicity for quite some time, they have not focused as much on risk for serious mental disorder. Similarly, the psychiatric epidemiology of race has focused too much on the demographic correlates of disorders and not enough on the psychological and sociological processes that influence racial differences in the prevalence of illness.

The relationship between socioeconomic status and depression among African Americans deserves more attention. The typical inverse relationship between these two variables was not uniformly observed in the ECA, and the patterns that emerged suggest that education for blacks does not translate into mental health protection in the same way that it does for whites (Robins & Regier, 1991; Williams et al., 1992b). Another area in need of further investigation emerged from the fact that younger African Americans appear to be particularly vulnerable to mental health problems. Depression is much higher among young adults, particularly young black women (Somervell et al., 1989). The same is true for generalized anxiety and phobia. Furthermore, suicide is increasing at an alarming rate among young black men. How do we explain this increased risk among younger blacks? Could it be that the desire to "make it" in this country coupled with the uncertainty about exactly how to guarantee a positive return on the personal investment is in itself an anxiety-provoking proposition (Bowman, 1992; Dressler, 1991)?

This speculation underlines the importance of understanding the meaning of anxiety in the lives of African Americans. We have presented evidence that phobia and generalized anxiety may be more prevalent among blacks than whites. Although depression reflects disappointment about the past, anxiety is characterized by feelings of apprehension and worry about the future, precisely the kind of uncertainty that we suspect most African Americans must cope with in the course of their day-to-day struggles for upward social mobility. The majority of African Americans must confront these issues in integrated settings such as work and school, where race is consistently salient. The inevitability that differences in skin color will be highlighted places a pervasive racialized context around attempts to understand both successes and failures. The attributional uncertainty that many blacks feel as they weigh the relative importance of personal capabilities and institutional racism can weigh heavily on their "nerves." Although this heightened vigilance concerning race can be seen as an added stress that all African Americans must carry, it can also be viewed as a psychological protection that keeps the negative effects of prejudice and discrimination from damaging the psyche. Because so many African Americans feel that they cannot afford to let their guard down, they keep their racial defenses up. This degree of caution practically guarantees a certain level of social distrust, particularly of whites. Such feelings of distrust are experienced on a continuum (Whaley, 1998). Maintaining a healthy level of distrust (Grier & Cobbs, 1968) without allowing it to develop into a more painful, maladaptive sense of paranoia is a complicated and delicate balancing act. It is no coincidence that the vocabulary of mental health in the black community is dominated by the language of "nerves" and "worry" (Neighbors, 1996). Realistically, African Americans should be worried and somewhat nervous about what the future may bring. Even when blacks have been successful, racial problems remain that must be dealt with (Cose, 1995). It is possible that the necessity of maintaining a perspective of cultural mistrust that derives from the potential for racial victimization and exploitation may increase risk for anxiety disorders among African Americans. More research is necessary before we can state definitively that these processes are operative.

In general, the epidemiological findings reported here fail to show a higher prevalence of morbidity for blacks as compared to whites. This seems paradoxical; we easily assume that blacks should routinely evidence higher levels of mental disorder as a result of greater stress exposure (Halpern, 1993; Mirowsky & Ross, 1980; Somervell et al., 1989). Supporting this easy assumption are at least two underlying assumptions. First, viewing African Americans within the *minority* construct fosters a notion of inferiority and powerlessness (Aponte et al., 1995). Second, the idea of being in a racial minority remains closely linked to ideas of being *disadvantaged* and a *victim* (Clark, 1965). As a result, there is a tendency to downplay the idea that African Americans have developed successful coping responses to stress exposure. But many of the issues this chapter presents are fundamentally concerned with the human capital that individuals draw upon to defend against the personally damaging insults of discrimination (Neighbors, Braithwaite, & Thompson, 1995). Thus a better driving question for psychiatric epidemiology is, Given that African Americans are exposed to greater stress than whites, why do they *not* experience higher levels of mental disorder?

The field of African American mental health currently faces an interesting dilemma. We know that among African Americans, symptoms of disorder often go unrecognized, and as a result, disorders like depression and anxiety are undertreated (Sussman, Robins, & Earls, 1987). This underutilization of professional services results in a large amount of unrelieved pain and suffering among African Americans. This raises the important question of how to redirect African American perspectives on mental illness. There is a strong need for mental health education programs targeted specifically toward African Americans. The means of reaching African Americans and the specific content of these messages remain unclear, but certainly the reduction of the stigma attached to mental health should be one of the first issues tackled by mental health educators (DHHS, 1999).

Understanding black-white differences in mental heath is important because analyses that compare race are part of the foundation upon which the existence of racial inequality is made evident. It will be even more useful to address racial differences in mental disorder through more comprehensive studies that incorporate factors that can account for both exposure and response to stress. We must be careful, however, not to focus exclusively on population group comparisons. The variability in rates of disorders that is revealed when such factors as age and sex are inspected within race is impressive and speaks to the limitations inherent in treating blacks and whites as monolithic groups.

Finally, much of the evidence presented here is based on analyses of data from the Epidemiologic Catchment Area program (a study that although still relevant is now more than fifteen years old). The authors of this chapter were surprised to find that no papers focusing explicitly on issues of race and ethnicity and based on data from the more recent National Comorbidity Survey have been published. It seems likely that the underutilization of this epidemiological resource stems from the relatively low numbers of researchers interested in African American issues who are actively engaged in psychiatric epidemiological investigations. We need more investigators to address the research questions raised by this review. Over twenty years ago, Mildred Cannon and Ben Locke called upon the National Institute of Mental Health to increase its efforts toward training investigators of color so that they might address research questions from a different cultural perspective (Cannon & Locke, 1977). Soon after Cannon and Locke's article was published, the NIMH funded the National Survey of Black Americans (Jackson, 1991), a study that has produced numerous books, articles, and research investigators committed to working on issues of black mental health. The next generation of large epidemiological investigations is beginning, and at least one, the National Survey of American Life, will include a nationally representative sample of African Americans (Jackson, 2000). We cannot afford to neglect these new data resources. It is hoped that the questions raised in this review will stimulate a new wave of psychiatric epidemiological research. Only in this way will we generate the volume of quality work necessary to advance our knowledge and understanding of African American mental health.

References

Adebimpe, V. R. (1981). Overview: White norms and psychiatric diagnosis of black patients. *American Journal of Psychiatry, 138,* 279–285.

Adebimpe, V. R., Hedlund, J. L., Cho, D. W., & Wood, J. B. (1982). Symptomatology of depression in black and white patients. *Journal of the National Medical Association, 74,* 185–190.

American Psychiatric Association. (1994). *Diagnostic and statistical manual of mental disorders* (4th ed.). Washington, DC: Author.

Anthony, J. C., Folstein, M., Romanoski, A. J., Von Korff, M. R., Nestadt, G. R., Chahal, R., Merchant, A., Brown, H., Shapiro, S., Kramer, M., & Gruenberg, E. M. (1985). Comparison of the lay Diagnostic Interview Schedule and a standardized psychiatric diagnosis. *Archives of General Psychiatry, 42,* 667–675.

Aponte, J. F., Rivers, R. Y., & Wohl, J. (Eds.). (1995). *Psychological interventions and cultural diversity.* Needham Heights, MA: Allyn & Bacon.

Baker, F. M. (1988). Suicide attempters in New Haven: A ten-year perspective. *Journal of the National Medical Association, 80,* 889–895.

Banks, J. A. (1996). Measures of assimilation, pluralism, and marginality. In R. Jones (Ed.), *Handbook of tests and measurements for black populations.* Hampton, VA: Cobb & Henry.

Bell, C., & Mehta, H. (1980). The misdiagnosis of black patients with manic-depressive illness. *Journal of the National Medical Association, 72,* 141–145.

Bell, C., & Mehta, H. (1981). Misdiagnosis of black patients with manic-depressive illness. *Journal of the National Medical Association, 73,* 101–107.

Berry, J. W., Poortinga, Y. H., Segall, M. H., & Dasen, P. R. (1992). *Cross-cultural psychology: Research and applications.* New York: Cambridge University Press.

Blazer, D. G., Hughes, D., George, L. K., Swartz, M., & Boyer, R. (1991). Generalized anxiety disorder. In L. N. Robins & D. A. Regier (Eds.), *Psychiatric disorders in America: The Epidemiologic Catchment Area study* (pp. 180–203). New York: Free Press.

Bowman, P. J. (1992). Coping with provider strain: Adaptive cultural resources among black husband-fathers. In A.K.H. Burlew, W. C. Banks, H. P. McAdoo, & D. A. Azibo (Eds.), *African American psychology: Theory, research, and practice* (pp. 135–154). Thousand Oaks, CA: Sage.

Brown, C., Schulberg, H. C., & Madonia, M. J. (1996). Clinical presentation of major depression by African Americans and whites in primary medical care practice. *Journal of Affective Disorders, 41,* 181–191.

Brown, D., Ahmed, F., Gary, L., & Milburn, N. (1995). Major depression in a community sample of African Americans. *American Journal of Psychiatry, 152,* 373–378.

Brown, D., Eaton, W. W., & Sussman, L. (1990). Racial differences in prevalence of phobic disorders. *Journal of Nervous and Mental Disease, 178,* 434–441.

Cannetto, S. S., & Lester, D. (1995). Gender and the primary prevention of suicide mortality. *Suicide and Life-Threatening Behavior, 25,* 58–69.

Cannon, M. S., & Locke, B. Z. (1977). Being black is detrimental to one's mental health: Myth or reality? *Phylon, 38,* 408–428.

Centers for Disease Control and Prevention. (1998). Suicide among black youth: United States, 1980–1995. *Morbidity and Mortality Weekly Report, 47,* 193–196.

Clark, K. (1965). *Dark ghetto: Dilemmas of social power.* New York: HarperCollins.

Cose, E. (1995). *A man's world: How real is male privilege and how high is its price?* New York: HarperCollins.

Dana, R. H. (1993). *Multicultural assessment perspectives for professional psychology.* Needham Heights, MA: Allyn & Bacon.

Davis, R. (1979). Black suicide in the seventies: Current trends. *Suicide and Life-Threatening Behavior, 9,* 131–140.

Dohrenwend, B. P., & Dohrenwend, B. S. (1969). *Social status and psychological disorder: A casual inquiry.* New York: Wiley.

Dohrenwend, B. P., Shrout, P. E., Egri, G., & Mendelsohn, F. S. (1980). Nonspecific psychological distress and other dimensions of psychopathology: Measures for use in the general population. *Archives of General Psychiatry, 37,* 1229–1236.

Dressler, W. W. (1988). Social consistency and psychological distress. *Journal of Health and Social Behavior, 29,* 79–91.

Dressler, W. W. (1991). *Stress and adaptation in the context of culture.* Albany: State University of New York Press.

Early, K. E. (1992). *Religion and suicide in the African American community.* Westport, CT: Greenwood Press.

Eaton, W. (2000). A comparison of self-report and clinical diagnostic interviews for depression: Diagnostic Interview Schedule and schedules for clinical assessment in neuropsychiatry in the Baltimore Epidemiologic Catchment Area follow-up. *Archives of General Psychiatry, 57,* 217–222.

Edwards, A., & Polite, C. K. (1992). *Children of the dream: The psychology of black success.* New York: Doubleday.

Fabrega, H., Jr., Mezzich, J. E., & Ulrich, R. F. (1988). Black-white differences in psychopathology in an urban psychiatric population. *Comprehensive Psychiatry, 29,* 285–297.

Fabrega, H., Jr., Mulsant, B. M., Rifai, A. H., & Al, E. (1994). Ethnicity and psychopathology in an aging hospital-based population: A comparison of African American and Anglo-American patients. *Journal of Nervous and Mental Disease, 182,* 136–144.

Farone, S. V., & Tsaung, M. T. (1995). Methods in psychiatric genetics. In M. T. Tsaung, M. Tohen, & G.E.P. Zahner (Eds.), *Textbook in Psychiatric Epidemiology* (pp. 81–131). New York: Wiley-Liss.

Fellin, P. (1996). *Mental health and mental illness: Policies, programs, and services.* Itasca, IL: Peacock.

Fischer, C. S., Hout, M., Jankowski, M. S., Lucas, S. R., Swidler, A., & Voss, K. (1996). *Inequality by design: Cracking the bell curve myth.* Princeton, NJ: Princeton University Press.

Fischer, J. (1969). Negroes and whites and rates of mental illness: Reconsideration of a myth. *Psychiatry, 32,* 428–446.

Forman, T. A., Williams, D. R., & Jackson, J. S. (1997). Race, place, and discrimination. In C. Gardner (Ed.), *Perspectives on social problems* (pp. 231–261). Greenwich, CT: JAI Press.

Frances, A. (1998). Problems in defining clinical significance in epidemiological studies. *Archives of General Psychiatry, 55,* 109–119.

Franklin, A. J., & Jackson, J. S. (1990). Factors contributing to positive mental health among black Americans. In D. S. Ruiz (Ed.), *Handbook of mental health and mental disorder among black Americans.* Westport, CT: Greenwood Press.

Gaw, A. C. (1982). *Cross-cultural psychiatry.* Boston: Wright.

Gibbs, J. T. (1997). African-American suicide: A cultural paradox. *Suicide and Life-Threatening Behavior, 27*(1, Special issue: Suicide: Individual, cultural, international perspectives), 68–79.

Good, B. (1993). Culture, diagnosis, and comorbidity. *Culture, Medicine, and Psychiatry, 16,* 427–446.

Green, V. (1978). The black extended family in the United States: Some research suggestions. In D. B. Shimkin, E. M. Shimkin, & D. A. Frate (Eds.), *The extended family in black societies* (pp. 378–387). The Hague: Mouton DeGruyter.

Grier, W. H., & Cobbs, P. M. (1968). *Black Rage.* New York: Basic Books.

Gurin, P., Gurin, G., Lao, R. C., & Beattie, M. (1969). Internal-external control in the motivational dynamics of Negro youth. *Journal of Social Issues, 25,* 29–53.

Halpern, D. (1993). Minorities and mental health. *Social Science and Medicine, 36,* 597–607.

Helzer, J. E., Robins, L. N., McEvoy, L. T., Spitnagel, E. L., Stoltzman, R. K., Farmer, A., & Brockington, I. F. (1985). A comparison of clinical and Diagnostic Interview Schedule diagnoses. *Archives of General Psychiatry, 42,* 657–666.

Hendricks, L., & Bayton, J. (1983). The NIMH's Diagnostic Interview Schedule: A test of its concurrent validity in a population of black adults. *Journal of the National Medical Association, 75*(7), 667–671.

Hill, R. B. (1983, May). *Comparative socio-economic profiles of Caribbean and non-Caribbean blacks in the United States.* Paper presented at the International Conference on Immigration and the Changing Black Population in the United States, Center for Afro-American and African Studies, Ann Arbor, MI.

Hughes, M., & Demo, D. H. (1989). Self-perceptions of black Americans: Self-esteem and personal efficacy. *American Journal of Sociology, 95,* 132–159.

Hughes, M., & Thomas, M. E. (1998). The continuing significance of race revisited: A study of race, class, and quality of life in America, 1972 to 1996. *American Sociological Review, 63,* 785–795.

Hybels, C., Kaplan, B., Blazer, D., Samsa, G., Schoenbach, V., & Wing, S. (1997, November). *Phobic disorder in a community population: The role of social and personal resources.* Paper presented at the annual meeting of the American Public Health Association, Indianapolis, IN.

Hyman, H. H. (1953). The relation of the reference group to judgments of status. In R. Bendix & S. M. Lipset (Eds.), *Class, status, and power: A reader in social stratification.* New York: Free Press.

Jackson, J. S. (1991). *Life in black America.* Thousand Oaks, CA: Sage.

Jackson, J. S. (2000, June). *The National Survey of American life.* Paper presented at the Summer Training Workshop on African American Aging Research, University of Michigan, Ann Arbor, School of Social Work.

Jackson, J. S., Brown, T. B., Williams, D. R., Torres, M., Sellers, S. L., & Brown, K. B. (1996). Racism and the physical and mental health status of African Americans: A thirteen-year national panel study. *Ethnicity and Disease, 6,* 132–147.

Jackson, P. B., & Lassiter, S. P. (in press). Self-esteem and race. In T. Owens, S. Stryker, & N. Goodman (Eds.), *Extending self-esteem theory and research: Social and psychological currents.* New York: Cambridge University Press.

Jaco, E. G. (1960). *Social epidemiology of mental disorders.* New York: Russell Sage Foundation.

Jahoda, M. (1958). *Current concepts of positive mental health.* New York: Basic Books.

James, S. A. (1994). John Henryism and the health of African Americans. *Culture of Medicine and Psychiatry, 18,* 163–182.

Jones, B. E., & Gray, B. A. (1986). Problems in diagnosing schizophrenia and affective disorders among blacks. *Hospital and Community Psychiatry, 37,* 61–65.

Kachur, S. P., Potter, L. B., James, S. P., & Powell, K. E. (1995). *Suicide in the United States, 1980–1992.* Atlanta, GA: National Center for Injury Prevention and Control.

Kessler, R. C., McGonagle, K., Zhao, S., Nelson, C., Hughes, M., Eshleman, S., Wittchen, H., & Kendler, K. (1994). Lifetime and 12-month prevalence of DSM-III-R psychiatric disorders in the United States: Results from the National Comorbidity Survey. *Archives of General Psychiatry, 51,* 8–19.

Kessler, R. C., Mickelson, K. D., & Williams, D. R. (1999). The prevalence, distribution, and mental health correlates of perceived discrimination in the United States. *Journal of Health and Social Behavior, 40,* 208–230.

Kessler, R. C., & Neighbors, H. W. (1986). A new perspective on the relationships among race, social class, and psychological distress. *Journal of Health and Social Behavior, 27,* 107–115.

Kessler, R. C., & Zhao, S. (1999). The prevalence of mental illness. *A handbook for the study of mental health: Social contexts, theories, and systems* (pp. 58–78). New York: Cambridge University Press.

Kleinman, A. (1996). How is culture important for DSM-IV? In J. E. Mezzich, A. Kleinman, H. Fabrega Jr., & D. L. Parron (Eds.). *Culture and psychiatric diagnosis: A DSM-IV perspective* (pp. 15–25). Washington, DC: American Psychiatric Press.

Kleinman, A., & Good, B. (1985). *Culture and depression: Studies in the anthropology and cross-cultural psychiatry of affect and disorder.* Berkeley: University of California Press.

Kramer, M., Rosen, B., & Willis, E. (1973). *Definitions and distributions of mental disorders in a racist society.* Pittsburgh: University of Pittsburgh Press.

Landrine, H., & Klonoff, E. A. (1996a). *African American acculturation: Deconstructing race and reviving culture.* Thousand Oaks, CA: Sage.

Landrine, H., & Klonoff, E. A. (1996b). The schedule of racist events: A measure of racial discrimination and a study of negative physical and mental health consequences. *Journal of Black Psychology, 22,* 144–168.

Lawson, W. B. (1986). Racial and ethnic factors in psychiatric research. *Hospital and Community Psychiatry, 37,* 50–54.

Lawson, W. B. (1990). Biological markers in neuropsychiatric disorders: Racial and ethnic factors. In E. Sorel (Ed.), *Family culture and psychobiology.* New York: Leyas.

Lawson, W. B. (1996). The art and science of the psychopharmacotherapy of African Americans. *Mount Sinai Journal of Medicine, 63,* 301–305.

Lefley, H. P., & Pedersen, P. B. (1986). *Cross-cultural training for mental health professionals.* Springfield, IL: Thomas.

Leo, R. J., Narayan, D. A., Sherry, C., Micchalek, C., & Pollock, D. (1997). Geropsychiatric consultation for African American and Caucasian patients. *General Hospital Psychiatry, 19,* 216–222.

Lester, D. (1998). *Suicide in African Americans.* Commack, NY: Nova Science.

Lin, K., Poland, R. E., & Silver, B. (1993). *Overview: The interface between psychobiology and ethnicity.* Washington, DC: American Psychiatric Press.

Lin, K. M., Poland, R. E., & Wallaski, G. (1993). *Psychopharmacology and psychobiology of ethnicity.* Washington, DC: American Psychiatric Association.

Link, B. G. (1987). Understanding labeling effects in the area of mental disorders: An assessment of the effects of expectations of rejection. *American Sociological Review, 52,* 96–112.

Link, B. G., Streuning, E., Cullen, F. T., Shrout, P. E., & Dohrenwend, B. P. (1989). A modified labeling theory approach to mental disorders: An empirical assessment. *American Sociological Review, 54,* 400–423.

Magee, W. J. (1993). *Psychological predictors of agoraphobia, simple phobia, and social phobia onset in a U.S. national sample.* Ann Arbor: University of Michigan.

Magee, W. J., Eaton, W. W., Wittchen, H., McGonagle, K. A., & Kessler, R. C. (1996). Agoraphobia, simple phobia, and social phobia in the National Comorbidity Survey. *Archives of General Psychiatry, 53,* 159–168.

Majors, R., & Billson, J. (1993). *Cool pose: The dilemmas of black manhood in America.* New York: Simon & Schuster, Touchstone Books.

Marger, M. N. (1997). *Race and ethnic relations: American and global perspectives* (4th ed.). Belmont, CA: Wadsworth.

Marsella, A. J., & Pedersen, P. B. (1981). *Cross-cultural counseling and psychotherapy*. New York: Pergamon Press.

McCarthy, J., & Yancey, W. (1971). Uncle Tom and Mr. Charlie: Metaphysical pathos in the study of racism and personal disorganization. *American Journal of Sociology, 76*, 648–672.

Mechanic, D. (1999). Mental health and mental illness: Definitions and perspectives. In A. V. Horwitz & T. L. Scheid (Eds.), *A Handbook for the study of mental health: Social contexts, theories, and systems* (pp. 12–28). New York: Cambridge University Press.

Mezzich, J. E., Kleinman, A. E., Fabrega, H., Jr., & Parron, D. L. (1996). *Culture and psychiatric diagnosis: A DSM-IV perspective*. Washington, DC: American Psychiatric Press.

Mirowsky, J., & Ross, C. E. (1980). Minority status, ethnic culture, and distress: A comparison of blacks, whites, Mexicans, and Mexican Americans. *American Journal of Sociology, 86*, 479–495.

Molock, S. D., Kimbrough, R., Lacy, M. B., & McClure, K. P. (1994). Suicidal behavior among African American college students: A preliminary study. *Journal of Black Psychology, 20*, 234–251.

Neeleman, J., Wessely, S., & Lewis, G. (1998). Suicide acceptability in African and white Americans: The role of religion. *Journal of Nervous and Mental Disease, 186*, 12–16.

Neighbors, H. W. (1984). The distribution of psychiatric morbidity in African Americans: A review and suggestions for research. *Community Mental Health Journal, 20*, 5–18.

Neighbors, H. W. (1996, November). *Qualitative methods in examining black male perceptions of mental health and mental illness*. Paper presented at the annual meeting of the National Association of Social Workers, Cleveland, OH.

Neighbors, H. W., Bashshur, R., Price, R., Selig, S., Donabedian, A., & Shannon, G. (1992). Ethnic minority mental health service delivery: A review of the literature. *Research in Community and Mental Health, 7*, 55–71.

Neighbors, H. W., Braithwaite, R. L., & Thompson, E. L. (1995). Health promotion and African Americans: From personal empowerment to community action. *American Journal of Health Promotion, 9*, 281–287.

Neighbors, H. W., Jackson, J. S., Broman, C. L., & Thompson, E. L. (1996). Racism and the mental health of African Americans. *Ethnicity and Disease, 6*, 167–175.

Neighbors, H. W., Jackson, J. S., Campbell, L., & Williams, D. (1989). The influence of racial factors on psychiatric diagnosis: A review and suggestions for research. *Community Mental Health Journal, 25*, 301–311.

Neighbors, H. W., & Lumpkin, S. (1990). The epidemiology of mental disorder in the black population. In D. Ruiz (Ed.), *Handbook of mental health and mental disorder among black Americans*. Westport, CT: Greenwood Press.

Neighbors, H. W., & Sellers, S. (2000). *Effects of goal-striving stress on the mental health of black Americans*. Ann Arbor: University of Michigan, Institute for Social Research.

Neighbors, H. W., Trierweiler, S. J., Munday, C., Thompson, E. L., Jackson, J. S., Binion, V. J., & Gomez, J. (1999). Psychiatric diagnosis of African Americans: Diagnostic divergence in clinician-structured and semistructured interviewing conditions. *Journal of the National Medical Association, 91*, 601–612.

Nisbet, P. A. (1996). Protective factors for suicidal black females. *Suicide and Life-Threatening Behavior, 26*, 325–341.

Parker, M. N., & Jones, R. T. (1999). Minority status stress: Effect on the psychological and academic functioning of African American students. *Journal of Gender, Culture, and Health, 4*, 61–82.

Parker, S., & Kleiner, R. J. (1966). *Mental illness in the urban Negro community*. New York: Free Press.

Pasamanick, B. (1963). Some misconceptions concerning differences in the racial prevalence of mental disease. *American Journal of Orthopsychiatry, 33*, 72–86.

Peterson, C. (1999). Psychological approaches to mental illness. In A. V. Horwitz & T. L. Scheid (Eds.), *A handbook for the study of mental health: Social contexts, theories, and systems* (pp. 104–120). New York: Cambridge University Press.

Pettigrew, T. F. (1964). The Negro American personality: Why isn't more known? *Journal of Social Issues, 20,* 4–23.

Porter, J. R., & Washington, R. E. (1979). Black identity and self-esteem: A review of studies of black self-concept, 1968–1978. *Annual Review of Sociology, 5,* 53–74.

Porter, J. R., & Washington, R. E. (1993). Minority identity and self-esteem. *Annual Review of Sociology, 19,* 139–161.

Ren, X. S., Amick, B., & Williams, D. (1999). Racial/ethnic disparities in health: The interplay between discrimination and socioeconomic status. *Ethnicity and Disease, 9,* 151–165.

Robins, L. N., Helzer, J. E., Croughan, J., & Ratcliff, L. (1981). The NIMH Diagnostic Interview Schedule: Its history, characteristics, and validity. *Archives of General Psychiatry, 38,* 381–389.

Robins, L. N., & Regier, D. A. (Eds.). (1991). *Psychiatric disorders in America: The Epidemiologic Catchment Area study.* New York: Free Press.

Rogler, L. H. (1999). Methodological sources of cultural insensitivity in mental health research. *American Psychologist, 54,* 424–433.

Rogler, L. H., Cortes, D. E., & Malgady, R. G. (1991). Acculturation and mental health status among Hispanics: Convergence and new directions for research. *American Psychologist, 46,* 585–597.

Schermerhorn, R. A. (1956). Psychiatric disorders among Negroes: A sociological note. *American Journal of Psychiatry, 112,* 878–882.

Seiler, L. H. (1973). The 22-item scale used in field studies of mental illness: A question of method, a question of substance, and a question of theory. *Journal of Health and Social Behavior, 14,* 252–264.

Sellers, S. (2000). *Dreams delivered, dreams deferred: Mental and physical health consequences of social mobility.* Unpublished doctoral dissertation, University of Michigan, Ann Arbor.

Singh, G. K., Kochanek, K. D., & MacDorman, M. F. (1996). Advance report of final mortality statistics, 1994. *National Vital Statistics Reports* (Vol. 43, No. 3, Suppl.). Hyattsville, MD: National Center for Health Statistics.

Smith, J. A., & Carter, J. H. (1986). Suicide and black adolescents: A medical model. *Journal of the National Medical Association, 78,* 1061–1064.

Snowden, L. R., & Cheung, F. K. (1990). Use of inpatient mental health services by members of ethnic minority groups. *American Psychologist, 45,* 347–355.

Snowden, L. R., & Hines, A. M. (1999). A scale to assess African American acculturation. *Journal of Black Psychology, 25,* 36–47.

Somervell, P. D., Leaf, P. J., Weissman, M. M., Blazer, D. G., & Bruce, M. L. (1989). The prevalence of major depression in black and white adults in five United States communities. *American Journal of Epidemiology, 130,* 725–735.

Steele, C. M. (1992, April). Race and the schooling of black Americans. *The Atlantic,* pp. 68–78.

Steele, C. M. (1999, August). Thin ice: Stereotype threat and black college students. *The Atlantic,* pp. 44–54.

Strakowski, S. M., McElroy, S. L., Keck, P. E., & West, S. A. (1996). Racial influence on diagnosis in psychotic mania. *Journal of Affective Disorders, 39,* 157–162.

Sue, S., Chun, C., & Gee, K. (1995). Ethnic minority intervention and treatment research. In J. F. Aponte, R. Y. Rivers, & J. Wohl (Eds.), *Psychological interventions and cultural diversity* (pp. 266–282). Needham, MA: Allyn & Bacon.

Summerville, M. B., Kaslow, N. J., & Doepke, K. J. (1996). Psychopathology and cognitive and family functioning in suicidal African-American adolescents. *Current Directions in Psychological Science, 5,* 7–11.

Sussman, L., Robins, L., & Earls, F. (1987). Treatment-seeking for depression by black and white Americans. *Social Science and Medicine, 24,* 187–196.

Taylor, J., Henderson, D., & Jackson, B. B. (1991). A holistic model for understanding and predicting depressive symptoms in African-American women. *Journal of Community Psychology, 19,* 306–320.

Taylor, J., & Jackson, B. B. (1990). Factors affecting alcohol consumption in black women: Pt. 2. *International Journal of Addictions, 25,* 1415–1427.

Taylor, J., & Jackson, B. B. (1991). Evaluation of a holistic model of mental health symptoms in African American women. *Journal of Black Psychology, 18,* 19–45.

Taylor, S. E. (1992). The mental health status of black Americans: An overview. In R. L. Braithwaite & S. E. Taylor (Eds.), *Health Issues in the Black Community.* San Francisco: Jossey-Bass.

Thomas, A., & Sillen, S. (1972). *Racism and psychiatry.* New York: Bruner/Mazel.

Thompson, V. L. (1996). Perceived experiences of racism as stressful life events. *Community Mental Health Journal, 32,* 223–233.

Tomes, E., Brown, A., Semenya, K., & Simpson, J. (1990). Depression in black women of low socioeconomic status: Psychological factors and nursing diagnosis. *Journal of the National Black Nurses Association, 4,* 37–46.

U.S. Department of Health and Human Services. (1999). *Mental health: A report of the surgeon general.* Rockville, MD: Substance Abuse and Mental Health Services Administration.

U.S. Department of Health and Human Services. Task Force on Black and Minority Health. (1985). *Report of the Secretary's Task Force on Black and Minority Health* (Vol. 1, Executive Summary). Washington, DC: U.S. Government Printing Office.

Vega, W. A., & Rumbaut, R. G. (1991). Ethnic minorities and mental health. *Annual Review of Sociology, 17,* 351–383.

Vickerman, M. (1999). *Crosscurrents: West Indian immigrants and race.* New York: Oxford University Press.

Wakefield, J. C. (1999). The measurement of mental disorder. In A. V. Horwitz & T. L. Scheid (Eds.), *A handbook for the study of mental health: Social contexts, theories, and systems* (pp. 29–57). New York: Cambridge University Press.

Warheit, G. J., Bell, R. A., Schwab, J. J., & Buhl, J. M. (1986). An epidemiologic assessment of mental health problems in the Southeastern United States. In M. M. Weissman, J. K. Myers, & C. E. Ross (Eds.), *Community surveys of psychiatric disorders* (pp. 191–208). New Brunswick, NJ: Rutgers University Press.

Warheit, G. J., Holzer, C. E., & Arey, S. A. (1975). Race and mental illness: An epidemiologic update. *Journal of Health and Social Behavior, 16,* 243–256.

Weissman, M. M., Bruce, M. L., Leaf, P. J., Florio, L. P., & Holzer, C. (1991). Affective disorders. In L. N. Robins & D. A. Regier (Eds.), *Psychiatric disorders in America: The Epidemiologic Catchment Area study* (pp. 53–80). New York: Free Press.

Whaley, A. L. (1997). Ethnicity/race, paranoia, and psychiatric diagnoses: Clinician bias versus sociocultural differences. *Journal of Psychopathology and Behavioral Assessment, 19,* 1–20.

Whaley, A. L. (1998). Cross-cultural perspectives on paranoia: A focus on the black American experience. *Psychiatric Quarterly, 69,* 325–343.

Williams, D. R. (2000). Race, stress, and mental health: Findings from the Commonwealth Minority Health Survey. In C. Hogue, M. Hargraves, & K. Scott-Collins (Eds.), *Minority health* (pp. 209–243). Baltimore: Johns Hopkins University.

Williams, D. R., & Chung, A. M. (in press). Racism and health. In R. Gibson & J. S. Jackson (Eds.), *Health in black America.* Thousand Oaks, CA: Sage.

Williams, D. R., & Harris-Reid, M. (1999). Race and mental health: Emerging patterns and promising approaches. In A. V. Horwitz & T. L. Scheid (Eds.), *A handbook for the study of mental health: Social contexts, theories, and systems* (pp. 295–314). New York: Cambridge University Press.

Williams, D. R., Takeuchi, D. T., & Adair, R. K. (1992a). Marital status and psychiatric disorders among blacks and whites. *Journal of Health and Social Behavior, 33,* 140–157.

Williams, D. R., Takeuchi, D. T., & Adair, R. K. (1992b). Socioeconomic status and psychiatric disorders among blacks and whites. *Social Forces, 7,* 179–194.

Williams, D. R., Yu, Y., Jackson, J. S., & Anderson, N. (1997). Racial differences in physical and mental health: Socioeconomic status, stress, and discrimination. *Journal of Health Psychology 2,* 335–351.

Williams-Flournoy, D. F., & Anderson, L. P. (1996). The Acculturative Stress Scale: Preliminary findings. In R. Jones (Ed.), *Handbook of tests and measurements for black populations.* Hampton, VA: Cobb & Henry.

Wilson, W. J. (1999). *The bridge over the racial divide.* Berkeley: University of California Press.

CHAPTER SEVEN

THE ROLE OF BLACK FAITH COMMUNITIES IN FOSTERING HEALTH

Anne E. Streaty Wimberly

The role of black faith communities in promoting the health and well-being of black people is not new. Historically, these communities have been key promoters of black people's health and vitality through the organizational base they have provided for health and educational resources, emotional support, social activities, financial assistance, community services, and political advocacy (Du Bois, 1903; Mays & Nicholson, 1969; Frazier, 1966; Lincoln & Mamiya, 1990; Billingsley, 1992). This multifaceted role of black churches has been essential in light of the hardships and social inequalities that have resulted from racism. However, the magnitude and complexity of current health issues challenge anew the acceptance by black churches of their indispensable role in black people's "struggle for life" (Billingsley, 1992). Black churches have an obligatory role in addressing this struggle. To understand this role we must look backward as well as forward, answering the questions: How have black churches responded in the past, How are churches now responding, and, How must they yet respond?

This chapter summarizes background information on the historical obligatory faith and health movement of black churches. Second, it attends to challenges to black churches in the emerging faith and health movement. Third, it summarizes key practices of black churches and presents exemplary church-based models. The final section proposes steps to develop broad-based church partnerships in the faith and health movement.

Background

Because of historical barriers to health care for black Americans, resulting from discriminatory practices in the larger social arena, organized black religion has consistently carried on a mandatory faith and health movement on behalf of black people. This task of the black church has meant tackling any problem black people face and has invariably required the use of the church's religious beliefs, experiences, and practices and its resources for caring and curative purposes in every aspect of people's lives. This approach has been undergirded by the assumption that black religion, ways of practicing it, and participation in it are significantly linked to spiritual health and to the whole spectrum of the physical health concerns of black people.

Health and the Practices of Faith

The black church worship tradition has been a central means by which black people have come into the presence of God with joys and troubles to praise God; to obtain guidance through sermon, prayer, song, and testimony; and to experience spiritual vitality and healing. Prayer, especially, has continued to be a dominant way of seeking God's healing in the midst of suffering. Prayer has manifested black people's belief in God's intimate presence and healing activity in them, in others, and in the affairs of life (Washington, 1994).

The black cultural reference to the *prayer warrior* epitomizes the importance of ardent prayer in a turbulent existence. Wimberly's (1990, 1996) emphasis on prayer in pastoral counseling stresses its vital relationship with spirituality and health. In fact, prayer is receiving new attention from black clergy, who are emphasizing its role in endeavors focused on holistic health and healing. The valuable contribution of prayer was a topic at the First National African American Health, Healing, and Spirituality Conference in Cleveland, Ohio, November 3 to 5, 1999 (G. Durley, personal communication, November 15, 1999). The conference was sponsored by Olivet Institutional Baptist Church, Olivet Housing and Community Development Corporation, and the Olivet Health and Education Institute. With this emphasis, the black church stands in the center of a growing revolutionary trend toward active inclusion of prayer in the work of the health professions (Epperly, 1995; Elkins, 1987; Dossey, 1993).

Music is a historical aspect of black worship that has continued as "an important means of helping people confront their struggles and to move toward healing" (Wimberly, 1997b). Through song, black people have told and listened to stories of joy and struggle, accounts of God's activity in life, and proposed responses to life situations. The therapeutic impact of music in black churches correlates with similar contemporary findings about uses of music in the practice of medicine, psychotherapy, and alternative medical practices (Scarantino, 1987). Testimonies are also a historical aspect of black worship. Hoyt (1997) describes them as therapeutic and salvific expressions in sermon, song, and storytelling through which affirmation, encouragement, catharsis, and healing occur.

Albert Raboteau's historical study (1986) of black church involvement in matters of health also documents the importance of faith healing that followed the early-twentieth-century Azuza Street Revival in Los Angeles and that became a pivotal part of Holiness-Pentecostal church life. Black Pentecostal churches did not shun the help of scientific medicine, although the latter was not always available to the members. Rather, faith healing (including the use of intercessory prayer and laying on of hands) was and still is central to the religious life of Pentecostal Christians and a growing number of black Christians in mainline churches, and this healing activity reflects their belief in the amazing work of God. However, Pentecostal churches gave equal importance to the role of sanctification, or growing in holiness, which requires members to refrain from the health inhibiting uses of tobacco, alcohol, narcotics, gambling, and other "worldly" amusements. Holy living meant making healthy lifestyle choices based on ethical rules set by the sanctified community. This emphasis continues today.

The religious tenets of the Nation of Islam have similarly informed the Nation's emphasis on healthy diets and a lifestyle of sobriety, cleanliness, honesty, and industry at the same time as the Nation has consistently promoted the use of medical science, even amid its critique of the commercialization of medicine (Raboteau, 1986).

Part of the black faith tradition also includes the presumption of a curative impact of emotional expression on black congregants during church worship. Raboteau suggests that during the nineteenth-century Protestant revival movement, black "shouting" churches served as agents of health for slaves and free black people. This shouting included ecstatic behavior that took the form of weeping, hollering, singing, jerking, dancing, and fainting. This freedom of expression in black worship was understood to be the external evidence of spiritual healing. At the same time, black religious expressionism was considered to be a means of ameliorating stressful life events and countering the destructive effects of racism on physical, social, and psychological health (Raboteau, 1986). Although more sedate forms of worship became the norm in many twentieth-century black urban churches where members had higher educational attainment levels, in many other cases the "old-time" religion endured (Raboteau, 1986). In recent years, there has been a revival of emotional expressiveness in mainline black churches.

By the mid-twentieth century, black churches had gained prominence as community centers and outreach agencies. In this role the churches attempted to address the needs in every facet of black life. Churches provided spiritual uplift through worship; relationship enhancement in the form of boys', girls', and mothers' clubs; psychological support through encouragement; educational assistance through church-sponsored lectures, classes, and schools; economic resources through savings banks and employment bureaus; social services in the form of child care, relief programs for the unemployed, and burial societies to ease the cost of care for the dead; recreational opportunities through church athletic activities and gyms; and political advocacy on behalf of civil rights and just treatment in society (Mays & Nicholson, 1969; Frazier, 1966; Spear, 1969). Through the continuation of these endeavors over the twentieth century, the black church demonstrated a holistic understanding of the connection between faith and health (George, Richardson, Lakes-Matyas, & Blake, 1989; Billingsley & Caldwell, 1991; Lincoln & Mamiya, 1990; Brown, Ndubuisi, & Gary, 1990).

Church Attendance and Health Promotion

A number of studies document findings that connect faith and health with black people's participation in church life. Studies show that the frequency and quality of black people's church involvement is correlated with health promoting informal support, opportunities for self-expression, contacts with revered religious symbols and beliefs, guidance from sermons, and participation in rituals such as prayer (Graham et al., 1978; Sata, Perry, & Cameron, 1979; Griffith, English, & Mayfield, 1980; Taylor, 1989; Chatters & Taylor, 1989b).

Data further point to specific effects that black people's involvement in church and other religious activities has; it correlates with the reduction of depressive symptoms, with older adults' life adjustment and positive evaluation of health, and with access to health promotion information and intervention programs focused on cardiovascular health, cancer diagnosis and treatment, good nutrition, and other healthy behaviors (Brown, Ndubuisi, & Gary, 1990; Levin, 1984; Hatch, 1992; Smith & Merritt, 1997; Paskett, Case, Tatum, Velez, & Wilson, 1999; Williamson, 1999).

Challenges to Black Churches in the Emerging Faith and Health Movement

Black churches constitute a major institutional presence in the United States. There are approximately 190 distinctly black-oriented and black-controlled church bodies and church networks, with more than seventy-five thousand black congregations including parishes in predominantly white denominations (Billingsley, 1992; Dilulio, 1998). It is also estimated that more than 40 percent of the total black population attends church, with seven out of ten in this group attending one or more times per month and two out of three holding church membership (Scandrett, 1996; Staples & Johnson, 1993). Moreover, the majority of black laity "believes that part of the church's mission is to liberate individuals from economic, political, and physical suffering" (Staples & Johnson, 1993, p. 217).

Because of the prevalence of black churches and the active pattern of black people's church attendance, black churches are regarded as indispensable participants in the current burgeoning national and worldwide faith and health movement. The present movement results from increasing broad-based awareness that health and well-being are influenced by more than scientific strategies and treatment. Health professionals and the general public recognize that science and technology are limited in addressing the broad spectrum of health and ethical issues that people currently face. Black churches have a special stake as partners in this movement because of black people's continuing "struggle for life" in a society that has often given less than adequate care to them.

The partnership of black churches in the broader faith and health movement does not come without challenges. Partnership requires them to gain the fullest possible awareness of critical health and well-being issues confronting the black community, awareness of the overall role of black churches in the movement, and awareness of the dimensions of health and well-being. Such awarenesses provide a basis for determining the healing practices that the churches can best implement.

Awareness of Health and Well-Being Issues

Black people of all ages, both male and female, experience critical deficits in health and well-being. Black children are more likely than white children "to be born in poverty, . . . to die in the first year, . . . to live in substandard housing, . . . to be unemployed as teenagers, . . . to be murdered before one year of age or as a teenager, . . . or to be incarcerated between fifteen and nineteen years of age" (Edelman, 1987, pp. 2–3). Both black males and black females are disproportionately represented in the prison population. Many are parents whose children are at risk for substance abuse, delinquency, and cross-generational incarceration. Moreover, many of the imprisoned do not receive visits from family or friends (Staples & Johnson, 1993; Beatty, 1997).

Being at increased risk for problematic health is also indicated by the continuing high concentration of poverty and unemployment rates in central cities where people of color are in the majority. Moreover, health and well-being are jeopardized in one out of three young black women aged sixteen to twenty-three because of their disconnection from support and resources for at least a year as a result of not being in school, in a job, in the military, or married to someone who is connected in any of these ways (Brown & Emig, 1999).

Compared to the rest of the population, black elderly are poorer and experience higher rates of multiple chronic illnesses such as hypertension, obesity, and diabetes. For a disproportionate number in this group, economic insufficiencies and low educational attainment levels result in insufficient awareness of agencies and available services and reduced access to health care resources (Jackson, 1988; Calsyn & Winter, 1999). With both elders and those of younger ages, situations of dying and death raise complex bioethical concerns. Needs arise for careful attention to patients' rights, to informed consent in medical testing and experimental treatment, and to ensured care for terminally ill patients that is unhampered by economic insufficiency (Bullard, 1994; Wimberly, 1992–1993).

Black women are less likely than their white counterparts to show awareness of breast cancer risks and to access breast cancer screening. Likewise, black men do not show adequate degrees of awareness of prostate cancer risks and do not seek regular prostate screening. In another extremely critical and growing area of health concerns, according to 1997–1998 CDC reports, 47 percent of all reported AIDS cases in 1997 were non-Hispanic black Americans. The incidence of substance abuse adds to the devastating impact of the AIDS epidemic and is regarded as a major destructive force in the black community alongside its dramatic impact on crime, violence, mental disorders, and school and job-related problems (Billingsley, 1992). Moreover, community leaders are sounding an alarm about the incidence of death by suicide, which, according to U.S. census data, occurs at the highest rate among black adults between the ages of twenty and thirty-four and in the eighty-five-plus group. The black teen suicide rate has tripled since 1980 (Billingsley, 1992; Hewlett & West, 1998).

Disparities in the distribution of transportation benefits are borne to a greater degree by people of color. Moreover, people of color in low-income communities are more likely than their white counterparts to be exposed to the environmental health risks associated with close proximity to hazardous waste sites, crumbling infrastructure, deteriorating housing, inadequate schools, and chronic unemployment (Bullard, 1993). These people "bear a disproportionate share of the nation's environmental and health problems" (Bullard & Johnson, 1997, p. 10).

These risks to health and well-being are only part of the extensive and complex situation to which faith communities may direct attention and help. They must also be concerned with the impact of gender and age differences in church involvement on the health and well-being of black people. Females tend to have greater access to health benefits that derive from church involvement. Moreover, there is evidence that the health-related functions of the church do not affect females and males in the same way. Data show that black females are more apt than black males to draw directly and regularly on the self-expressive, social support, and friendship mechanisms of church life that buffer the impact of stressful life events on their mental health. Black males are less likely to attend church; and when they do attend, they rely less upon the self-expressive, social support, and friendship mechanisms of church life, except during crises or in times of acute stress in their lives (Brown, Ndubuisi, & Gary, 1990).

The young tend to be less involved than their elders in organized group modes of religious activities, especially in mainline black churches. In fact, "for the first time in black history, a generation of unchurched youths is emerging from northern and western urban areas and, to a lesser extent, southern cities" (Staples & Johnson, 1993, p. 217). This tendency challenges the role of the church as a health resource for them. On the opposite end of the age spectrum, even though churches provide caring networks, spiritually nurturing activities, and coping resources to elderly churchgoers, this help lessens or ceases as the elders' involvement wanes due to debilitating health (Taylor, 1989; Chatters, 1988; Chatters & Taylor, 1989a; Wimberly & Wimberly, 1995; Chadiha et al., 1996).

Awareness of the Role of Black Churches

Of course it is unrealistic to assume that all black churches are able to address competently the myriad health issues faced by their members and community residents. However, each congregation can discover its strengths and resources. Moreover, churches exist in a new climate that promotes interaction between medical treatment and faith and partnerships between health professionals and churches. Such partnerships are guided by a premise that Gunderson (1997) summarizes: "The faith-and-health movement reflects an idea underlying much contemporary health science, which tells us that no magic bullet, no one pill or plan, no one action is capable of bringing health to a community. There is no way to fix all problems, cure all diseases, or patch up all injuries. The movement is instead about prevention and connection. It is not defined by what we can do by ourselves but by what we must do together. This act shapes our strategy and the tools we choose" (p. xiv).

The quest of the movement is for an integrated and holistic approach to health and well-being that emphasizes the interrelationship of spiritual, mental, physical, relationship, economic, recreational, and environmental dimensions. This approach is a familiar and important one for black churches. Because of the historical exclusion of black people from functions of mainstream society, black churches and their constituents tended to embrace a holistic frame of reference that differed from the dominant culture's Cartesian model.

The black holistic philosophical system drew from the African communal, religious worldview that focused on the interpenetration of all of life's dimensions rather than on the compartmentalized, or mind-centered and individualistic, orientation of Western culture that was inherited from Cartesian philosophy. Moreover, black churches have functioned on the theological premise that God desires health and wholeness for all people, that all human life is made in God's image and is a precious and valuable gift, and that all God's people yearn for love, honor, respect, and care, which contribute to health and well-being. These tenets of black religion can be turned into action through the black churches' reaffirmation of, overt claim to, and systematic activity on behalf of the holistic orientation. The holistic orientation is an important theological guidepost for black churches in the faith and health movement.

Awareness of Dimensions of Health and Well-Being

Descriptions of health and well-being emphasize the view that "health is the complete and successful functioning of every part of the human being, in harmonious relationship with every other part and with the relevant environment" (Weatherhead, 1952, p. 315). Moreover, any interruption or impairment in this harmonious relationship results in disease. These descriptions connect health and well-being with unity of body, mind, and spirit and with the communal and natural environment in which people live (Weatherhead, 1952; Benson & Stuart,

1992). Howard Clinebell (1997) presents a comprehensive catalogue of dimensions of well-being that is useful for the intentional formation and evaluation of church goals in a faith and health ministry. The following summarizes the seven dimensions presented by him:

1. *Spiritual well-being* is viewed as the heart of all well-being because it consists of beliefs, values, meanings, and commitments that allow people to go on with their purpose in life in the midst of hardship and loss. Spiritual well-being guides people's choices and the quality of their relationships and actions in every aspect of well-being.

2. *Mental well-being* derives from people's use of intellectual, problem-solving, creative, and productive capacities for the good of oneself and others. Underlying this description of mental well-being is the assumption that the ways in which people seek out and access opportunities to confront life issues and use their minds can contribute to their overall health. Conversely, lack of attention to opportunities to address the heart's hurts can hinder overall health.

3. *Physical well-being* is the experience of the effective functioning, sensual aliveness, and relatively pain-free condition of the human body. This dimension of well-being is informed by every other dimension of well-being and is promoted through the care of self and others.

4. *Relationship well-being* arises from the positive and growth-producing qualities of people's social networks, especially family and friends, who are critical to health and wholeness. Relationship well-being can be nurtured, particularly by religious communities.

5. *Work and economic well-being* comes from people's access to economic resources and support; their ability to sustain themselves and others for whom they are responsible economically; and their sense of achievement, life purpose, and self-worth resulting from what they do. From a religious perspective, this dimension relates to having a sense of vocation that fulfills some purpose in God's intentions.

6. *Recreational (or play) well-being* comes through achieving a balance between productive and economically sustaining work and revitalizing recreation; it is supported by readily available, accessible, and safe recreational facilities and options.

7. *Environmental well-being (well-being of our world)* happens through our proactive care for all God's creations including the natural environment and the health and just functioning of society and its institutions (work settings, churches, health care institutions, labor unions, social and service agencies, and political and economic structures).

Part of the importance of the holistic paradigm of health and well-being lies in the direction it offers black churches in determining and evaluating present and future practices that address the interrelated dimensions.

Faith and Health in Prospect: Key Practices of Black Churches

Black faith communities in the third millennium faith and health movement will need to be intentional catalysts with the capacity for stimulating health promoting expectations, encouraging health promoting actions, building helping systems, and bringing resources to bear on the all too often denied health needs of black people, especially the poor. Black churches must engage intentionally in practices through which this catalytic role may come to life. The remainder of this section presents five interconnected practices that support the interrelated dimensions of health and well-being presented in the foregoing section and that black churches historically have undertaken to various degrees. They are caring practices, educating practices, mediating practices, sustaining practices, and advocating practices (summarized in Table 7.1).

Caring Practices

Caring practices are the primary entry point for black church participation in the third millennium faith and health movement. At the center of caring practices is black churches' vision of the activities to be undertaken on behalf of their members and the wider community. The question then is, What is the connection of caring practices to spiritual, mental, physical, relationship, work and economic, recreational, and environmental health and well-being?

Caring practices are those intentional efforts of black churches to create a space in which faith and healing can connect. Churches help black people make the connection between their identified religiocultural beliefs and values and their priorities and lifestyle commitments that affect health and well-being. Included in this effort is the churches' affirmation of the healing gifts of black church tradition, found in prayer, song, testimony, open emotional expression, and the healing rituals of laying on of hands and anointing with oil. Through caring practices, churches also encourage critical consideration of individuals' assessment of folk medicine and remedies as well as beliefs in God that cause people to refuse or delay medical care (Paskett et al., 1999).

Caring practices reflect the view that all persons are persons of worth. Caring means showing concern for self-esteem, self-worth, and well-being by treating people with honor and respect and by seeking ways within and outside the faith community to reach people in crisis to give hope where there is anger, fear, pain, and depression. Staples and Johnson (1993) call this kind of caring the provision of "a refuge in times of severe trouble . . . [and] reinforcement in resisting personal and social stressors" (pp. 213–214). Caring practices also include instruction and ceremonies that assist youths in the transition into responsible adulthood and that find and respond to cases of illiteracy and the needs of children and adults for educational support. Examples of these caring practices include the lay

TABLE 7.1. FIVE INTERCONNECTED PRACTICES OF BLACK CHURCHES IN THE FAITH AND HEALTH MOVEMENT.

Dimensions of Well-Being	Caring Practices	Educating Practices	Mediating Practices	Sustaining Practices	Advocating Practices
Spiritual well-being	Provide an environment that nurtures development of health enhancing values, priorities, and lifestyle commitments.	Give moral direction and invite examination of beliefs and spiritual values that distort or diminish holistic health and wellness.	Use worship, sermons, prayer, healing services, scripture, music, testimony, and other forms of expressivity to promote people's connection with the source of life, a guiding overarching story, life-giving values; help people grasp their worthiness of love and life and ability to act responsibly in life on their own and other's behalf.	Assure a variety of ongoing celebrative, meditative, and spiritually uplifting activities in and beyond the church, such as prayer and Bible study groups; children's, youth, men's and women's groups; support groups; choirs that contribute to renewal and healing.	Constantly seek new and creative ways to contribute to spiritual renewal, growth, and ethically informed action on behalf of self and others; form church committees on faith and health practices and have them form goals and strategies for making the practices work.
Mental well-being	Regard everyone as a person of worth, treat all with honor and respect, and reach out to people in crisis to give hope where there is anger, fear, pain, and depression.	Help people across the life cycle to tell their stories of pain and struggle and to explore inner strengths and abilities and ways to address health diminishing attitudes and actions; sponsor forums that help people build health promoting and crisis management skills.	Connect or refer people to support groups or competent mental health caregivers when more than informal or self-help measures are needed; identify and announce available community mental health resources.	Encourage all ages and stages to engage as much as possible in activities in and beyond the church that contribute constructively to self-esteem and confidence and that use the mind, talents, emotions, and energies constructively and creatively on behalf of self and others.	Look in the community mental health structures for affordable support forums and esteem-building programs and activities that cannot be provided by the church; push for community mental health supports where few or none are found.

Physical well-being	Promote body care and a lifestyle that helps maintain the best possible physical fitness and health.	Provide spiritual foundations for body care, concrete information on health care management and intervention programs, and forums on life and death issues.	Motivate use of healthy habits, replacement of unhealthy habits, participation in wellness programs, and regular medical assessment and support plans; cosponsor or provide space for health clinics and health fairs.	Constantly encourage people to make body care a high priority, and attend to families in life and death matters; use motivating devices such as flyers and other health awareness announcements to promote healthy lifestyles.	Press for and intercede for adequate access to health care, nutritious food for low-income families, and needed social and economic supports within and beyond the faith community.
Relationship well-being	Create a positive environment for affirming regard for others and accepting responsibility for one another.	Teach meaning and methods of attaining relational health, and train volunteers to reach out to the sick, the hungry, the naked, the lonely, the imprisoned, the hurting, and the needy.	Create bridges from within and beyond the faith community to address difficult relationships and circumstances such as abuse, violence, abandonment, and family crises.	Keep abreast of people and places where relationship breakdowns and crises exist, and maintain a support system in tandem with community agencies; assess the adequacy of the system.	Partner with community agencies for professional expertise in providing communications, tools, conflict management, family counseling, parenting skills, and marital enrichment.
Employment and economic well-being	Identify and ensure responses to needy individuals and families in and beyond the church.	Make people aware of job opportunities, job readiness workshops, government entitlement programs, money management seminars, affordable quality housing, home maintenance projects, and cost-effective and nutritious food purchases.	Help individuals access needed programs that aid economic sufficiency; cosponsor with community agencies or provide space for programs; organize clothes closets, food banks, feed the homeless initiatives, and economic support funds.	Maintain contact with individuals and families in need and with community and self-help programs and strategies that work; develop follow-up plans to determine ongoing needs of individuals and families and levels of need satisfaction.	Mobilize political and community action to ensure governmental, employer, and school responsibility for and investment in programs and strategies resulting in occupational and educational equity that can foster economic viability especially for the poor.

(Continued on page 140)

TABLE 7.1. (*Continued*)

Dimensions of Well-Being	Caring Practices	Educating Practices	Mediating Practices	Sustaining Practices	Advocating Practices
Recreational (leisure) well-being	Emphasize the necessary balance between work and play and the importance of recreation in nurturing spirituality and overall health.	Inform people of health-promoting purposes of play (the renewal of persons spiritually, mentally, physically, and relationally); engage people in exploring forms of play that promote health and the churches' role in recreation provision.	Promote, organize, cosponsor, or refer people to age and stage-appropriate recreation that provides exercise, emotional release, positive participation, cooperation, friendly competition, and uses for creativity, skills, and talents.	Structure time for recreation in the total program of the church; help people of all ages and stages to recognize negative, unsafe, or harmful recreational activities; and sponsor, cosponsor, or refer people to programs that address issues of substance abuse and other forms of addiction resulting from faulty and health negating assumptions about play.	Raise awareness of needs for available, adequate, and safe community-based recreation facilities and programs; and establish strategies for addressing the needs.

Environmental well-being	Affirm environmental justice principles set forth by the multinational People of Color Environmental Leadership Summit, including the sacredness of the earth; the right of all to live, go to school, and work in healthy environments; and the need for policies that ensure the cleaning up and rebuilding of hazardous living environments, adequacy of access for all to the full range of resources, and enforcement of informed consent in medical practice.	Make people aware of social and environmental issues; provide information about informed consent in medical practice and about hazards such as lead paint, pesticides, asbestos, tobacco use, and dumpsites and other health risks in and around home, neighborhood, wider community, and globe; raise people's consciousness about lifestyles that promote present and future human and environmental health and about mechanisms for addressing service inequities.	Propose strategies for individual, family, church, and community support of environmental justice principles; encourage people to assess their lifestyles and make lifestyle changes that support and advance a healthy environment.	Keep before members and community residents the importance of their vigilance and their ability to act to ensure safe and clean environments wherever they live, go to school, work, or play.	Urge people's participation in public hearings on environmental issues; strategize action to deal with dilapidated housing, unsafe playgrounds, unsanitary and illness-producing workplaces, and neighborhood redlining by realty companies; join coalitions and environmental groups to form a unified voice.

care ministry of Ben Hill United Methodist Church in Atlanta, Georgia, which trains the laity to be present with and give guidance to individuals and families in crisis, and the Orita Rites of Passage program of Union Temple Baptist Church in Washington, D.C., which uses instruction and ceremonies to facilitate the transition of black youths to responsible manhood and womanhood (Billingsley, 1992).

Caring practices promote body care, physical fitness, and care of the critically and terminally ill. These practices highlight concerns such as nutrition, medical screening, substance abuse, suicide prevention, safe sex, and response to the AIDS crisis. Examples of some of these emphases are found in the North Carolina Churches United for Better Health project, which began with the express purpose of reducing cancer and other health risks through improved nutrition; the fitness center of Holy Ghost Roman Catholic Church in rural Opelousas, Louisiana, a full-service fitness center intended "to enhance the physical development of children and adults in rural areas" (Billingsley, 1992, p. 370); the Alcohol and Drug Counseling program of Union Temple Baptist Church in Washington, D.C., which provides weekly individual and group counseling and support to help substance abusers overcome their addiction (Billingsley, 1992); and the Black Infant Health Project at Bethel African Methodist Episcopal Church in Fontana, California, which is working to reduce the infant mortality rate (Hill, 1999).

Relationship health and well-being is an aim of caring practices in black churches. These practices emphasize people's positive regard for one another and their acceptance of responsibility for one another. Through these practices the black church functions as the modern-day equivalent of the ancestral African tribe or village and "welds community and unrelated families to each other" (Staples and Johnson, 1993, p. 211). Attention is directed toward black parenting and grandparenting; disconnected teens and young adults; homebound elders and people in long-stay medical or mental health facilities; gangs; violence in homes, schools, and the community; and incarcerated individuals. Examples of relationship caring practices are the Ecumenical Families Alive Project, based at the Interdenominational Theological Center, which offers services to grandparents raising grandchildren and to homeless families; the Teen Parenting Enrichment Place at Bethel African Methodist Episcopal Church in Baltimore, which seeks to prevent adolescent pregnancy and enhance both male and female teen parenting skills (Billingsley, 1992); and the Crisis Counseling Center at Greater Christ Baptist Church in Detroit, which serves as a resource during marriage and family crises and responds to crisis calls of members and the surrounding community (Perkins, 1999).

Caring practices also direct concern to economic circumstances. The practices highlight interconnectedness, communalism, and the building of health and well-being through black financial empowerment (Perkins, 1999). Models of economic-oriented caring practices include the Detroit Eastside Coalition of

Churches (DECC), an ecumenical initiative directed toward "the issues of crime, lack of affordable housing, inadequate public transportation, and a decline in health care services, . . . all rooted in the economic downturn that is keenly felt by the residents of Detroit" (Perkins, 1999, p. 43); the Quitman County Development Organization and Economic Development Project of Valley Queen Baptist Church in rural Marks, Mississippi, which sponsors a credit union and thrift shop, builds community and economic development leadership, and provides technical assistance to enhance the social and economic well-being of black children, youths, adults, families, and the total community (Billingsley, 1992); the Allen Housing Corporation of Allen African Methodist Episcopal Church in Jamaica in the borough of Queens, New York, which "buys dilapidated houses, hires and trains local citizens to repair them, then arranges low-interest loans from local lenders so that low- and moderate-income families can become home owners" (Billingsley, 1992, p. 362); and the Outreach Program of Ben Hill United Methodist Church in Atlanta, which provides food and care packages to low-income individuals and families and also provides volunteers to homeless shelters, feeding centers, and Habitat for Humanity building teams who construct affordable housing for low-income families.

Recreational health and well-being is also a focus of caring practices in black churches. These practices emphasize the necessary balance between work and play and the importance of recreation in nurturing spirituality and overall health. The practices assume that physical activity, play, and social interaction broaden and enrich the lives of children and adults, enhance relationship skills, and foster creativity and a sense of fair play. Church-sponsored Scout troops and after-school recreation programs for children and youths as well as adult social clubs are among the caring practices in numerous black churches. In addition, churches such as the Faith United Church of Christ in Washington, D.C., and church-based groups such as the Concerned Citizens of South Central Los Angeles and the Gary Clean City Coalition of Gary, Indiana, target the availability and safety of parks and recreation (Bullard, 1994).

Black church caring practices affirm the environmental justice principles that have been set forth by the multinational People of Color Environmental Leadership Summit. These principles address, among other issues, the sacredness of the earth; the right of all people to live, go to school, and work in healthy environments; the need for policies that ensure the cleaning up and rebuilding of hazardous living environments; the adequacy of access for all to the full range of resources; and the enforcement of informed consent in medical practice (Bullard, 1994). Church-based groups that carry out these practices include those groups mentioned earlier as promoting caring practices directed at recreational well-being and also Ascension Parish Residents Against Pollution in Geismar, Louisiana, a group that directs its activities toward preventing toxic and waste seepage into well water in order to combat the high incidence of cancer, and the Brooklyn Council to Eradicate Lead Poisoning (Bullard, 1994).

Educating Practices

Educating practices are integrated to varying degrees with caring practices in black faith communities. Church school classes, workshops, public forums, and other meetings attend to the dimensions of health and well-being in the following ways.

They contribute to spiritual well-being by giving moral direction and inviting people to examine their beliefs and spiritual values that support, distort, or diminish holistic health and well-being. This includes attending to one's bases for decisions in life and death issues (Wimberly, 1992–1993; Wimberly, 1997a).

They contribute to mental well-being by helping people across the life cycle tell their stories of pain and struggle and explore the inner strengths and abilities that they can use to address life circumstances.

Educating practices contribute to relationship well-being through teaching meanings and methods, including conflict resolution skills for building or rebuilding and sustaining positive relationships in the family, school, workplace, and community. In addition, churches and church-based groups may train volunteers to reach out to the needy, sick, hungry, naked, lonely, and imprisoned.

These practices contribute to economic well-being by informing people of job opportunities, government entitlement programs, and affordable quality housing options. Churches may sponsor or cosponsor workshops on job readiness, money management, home maintenance, and cost-effective and nutritious food preparation.

Educating practices contribute to recreational well-being through providing individuals with information about the healthful benefits of balancing work and play; healthy forms of recreation; and safe recreational opportunities.

Finally, these practices contribute to environmental well-being by making people aware of social and environmental issues, by providing information about health hazards and the consequences of exposure to them, and by raising people's consciousness about lifestyles that promote present and future human and environmental health.

Mediating Practices

Mediating practices are those activities of black churches intended to enhance people's spirituality or spiritual resources and to connect black people to resources they need in the larger social sphere to address, promote, and sustain mental, physical, relationship, economic, recreational, and environmental health and well-being. Black faith communities engage in mediating practices as they help link their members and community residents who need assistance with community mental health and medical services and economic support services. Moreover, through mediating practices, people are connected to agencies that can assist them in the areas of family crises; family and community violence; crime; and hazardous environment clean-ups, fix-ups, and removals. Mediating practices also entail black church provision of space for or sponsorship or cosponsorship of needed services or forums that assist individuals with addressing issues important to them.

Sustaining Practices

The sustaining practices of black churches are the variety of means these churches use to ensure the ongoing and maximum functioning of the caring, educating, and mediating practices to the end of producing observable change or difference in each of the dimensions of health and well-being. Sustaining practices focus on ongoing encouragement of people's engagement in health promoting activities. These practices continually raise issues of health and consistently publicize the availability of helping places, programs, and forms of assistance with health awareness announcements in church meetings, with bulletins and flyers, and with special promotions or invitations to health fairs and clinics.

Advocating Practices

Black faith communities must necessarily be advocates on behalf of black people to ensure available, affordable, and adequate medical services, nutrition resources, financial supports, living conditions, and recreational facilities; to work for safe and clean environments; and to promote appropriate public policies, especially for the poor. The fact is that "black churches historically have had a liberation theology dictated by the deprived position of the black population. They have traditionally provided programs designed for the social, political, physical, and spiritual needs of black families and their communities" (Staples & Johnson, 1993, p. 220). Black churches will need to continue their advocacy role into the third millennium, and it will be through intentionally planned advocacy practices that this role will be fulfilled.

Advocacy practices of black churches are those initiatives that push for ethically informed action and that help black people recognize their right and ability to use voice, action, and political clout in areas needing redress. Advocating practices are mobilizing actions that engage people in discussing needs and deficits, in identifying areas that call for self-help, and in fulfilling the helping roles that can be undertaken by the churches. One especially important advocating practice for black churches is to partner with community agencies to seek and offer solutions to issues of black people's health and well-being.

Steps to Broad-Based Church Partnership in the Faith and Health Movement

Use of these interrelated practices in the faith and health movement need not be confined to black churches. These practices are usable across the denominational and ethnic cultural spectrum, but they are particularly vital in churches that embrace and serve other minority ethnic cultural groups, because these groups, especially Latinos and Native Americans, suffer disparities in health and well-being along with black people. Through collaborative and creative efforts, faith communities, community agencies, educational institutions, and health structures can construct a vital base for addressing the comprehensive and inter-acting dimensions of the health and well-being of blacks and other minorities.

Churches who are already participating in collaborations provide important insights on the partnership formation process. Moving into partnership happens, preliminarily, through a church's explicit recognition of itself as "the link between personal, private spirituality and the many social factors that affect community life" (Gunderson, 1997, p. 19). The partnering congregation sees itself as "a com-munity within the larger community, forming, nurturing, and challenging indi-viduals to participate with other humans in social networks" (p. 19). An additional preliminary step the church takes when entering into partnerships is to clearly identify what Snyder calls the narrative or story of faith that undergirds its faith community and that guides that community's formation of values shaped by its faith, or "virtue ethics." The content of the narrative is important because it re-veals a moral guide for the church's decision making about what is important to do and how it will act (Snyder, 1988).

Beyond these preliminary steps, three additional steps assist a faith commu-nity to enter into active participation in a collaborative network. The first of these steps is the identification by designated church personnel of individuals and fam-ilies in the church and community who are confronting crucial issues and the tar-geting of their unaddressed needs and problems of access to resources. For some churches, assistance in this process has come from outside agencies. For example, one of the member churches of the Detroit Eastside Coalition of Churches re-ceived assistance from a state university in conducting a community survey on health and health-related issues (Perkins, 1999).

The second step is for the church to become aware of services or resources that are specifically designed to address the targeted issues, with a focus on lo-cating available lists or compiling a public and private resource list, including the names and telephone numbers of contact persons. Congregations like New Mount Calvary Baptist Church in Los Angeles illustrate this step, which Gun-derson (1997) calls "convening," or opening the doors to potential collaborators. As part of the process, the Mount Calvary pastor builds and maintains a phone list on a Rolodex; the list is information intensive, with the details not only of "'contacts' but of relationships formed over decades of meetings, burials, mar-riages, births, and personal passages" (p. 47).

The third step requires church collaboration teams to actually connect the resources and the persons who need them. In one situation, for example, the Health Ministries Program of Provident Missionary Baptist Church in Atlanta has linked with the Morehouse School of Medicine to increase black men's aware-ness of prostate cancer through organized forums and through outreach into bar-ber shops. Senior pastor Gerald A. Durley reports that connections with local hospitals make possible free prostate cancer screening. The church also links with the Georgia Department of Public Health and the local chapter of the American Cancer Society to confront health risks associated with the use of tobacco and cigarette smoking. Also, through the Center for Cancer Survivorship housed at Provident Missionary Baptist Church under the direction of Joyce Guillory, women are connected with resources to increase their breast cancer awareness, to promote regular screening, and to increase cancer survivorship.

Although churches may be the initiators of collaborative efforts to link people with services, these efforts may also originate in the social service, educational, political, or community agency sector. In the latter case, churches become receptive links in the faith and health movement. One example is the North Carolina–based project Black Churches United for Better Health, which was initiated by the National Cancer Institute in 1991. Fifty churches in ten North Carolina counties participated in the project to help black members reduce cancer risks and reduce health disparities through improved nutrition (Williamson, 1999). In another case the Interdenominational Theological Center's AIDS Project has linked with local churches to provide information, support, and guides to services.

Church connections with existing coalitions and national programs also enhance the process of linking people with needed resources and engaging them in health promoting activities and advocacy. For example, the church-based Coalition for Community Action in Baton Rouge is an environmental advocacy group, as is the Brooklyn Council to Eradicate Lead Poisoning (Bullard, 1994). Balm in Gilead is a national organization headquartered in New York City that works through black churches to confront HIV and AIDS crises in the black community through prayer, education, and advocacy.

In short, these steps are helpful ones that can be undertaken by churches who join the faith and health movement in an effort not simply to promote but to ensure the health and well-being especially of those who "struggle for life" in the midst of disparities in services.

Conclusion

This chapter highlights the issues of health and well-being that black communities confront and the ways that black faith communities have responded in the past and must yet respond. Black faith communities have a substantial history of helping black people meet their needs within and beyond the church, and the currently emerging faith and health movement continues that tradition, actively addressing the ongoing health concerns that challenge blacks. Effective responses of black churches in the third millennium will rest on their awareness of the issues, awareness of the role that black churches must assume, and awareness of the multiple and interrelated dimensions of health and well-being. Moreover, the intentional participation of black churches in the widely evolving faith and health movement will require church consideration of key practices through which issues of health and well-being may be addressed: caring practices, educating practices, mediating practices, sustaining practices, and advocating practices.

References

Beatty, C. (1997). *Parents in prison, children in crisis: An issue brief.* Washington, DC: Child Welfare League of America.

Benson, H., & Stuart, E. M. (1992). *The wellness book.* New York: Simon & Schuster.

Billingsley, A. (1992). *Climbing Jacob's ladder: The enduring legacy of African-American families.* New York: Simon & Schuster.

Billingsley, A., & Caldwell, C. H. (1991). The church, the family, and the school in the African American community. *Journal of Negro Education, 60,* 427–440.

Brown, B. V., & Emig, C. (1999). Prevalence, patterns, and outcomes. In D. J. Besharow (Ed.), *America's disconnected youth.* Washington, DC: Child Welfare League of America.

Brown, D. R., Ndubuisi, S. C., & Gary, L. E. (1990). Religiosity and psychological distress among blacks. *Journal of Religion and Health, 29*(1), 55–68.

Bullard, R. D. (Ed.). (1993). *Confronting environmental racism: Voices from the grassroots.* Boston: South End Press.

Bullard, R. D. (1994). *People of color environmental groups: 1994–1995 directory.* Atlanta, GA: Environmental Justice Resource Center.

Bullard, R. D., & Johnson, G. S. (Eds.). (1997). *Just transportation: Dismantling race and class barriers to mobility.* Stony Creek, CT: New Society.

Calsyn, R. J., & Winter, J. P. (1999). Predicting older adults' knowledge of services. *Journal of Social Services Research, 25*(4), 1–14.

Chadiha, L., Proctor, E., Morrow-Howell, N., Darkwa, O. K., & Dore, P. (1996). Religiosity and church-based assistance among chronically ill African American and white elderly. *Journal of Religious Gerontology, 10*(9), 17–36.

Chatters, L. M. (1988). Subjective well-being among older black adults: Past trends and current perspectives. In J. S. Jackson (Ed.), *The black American elderly: Research on physical and psychosocial health.* New York: Springer.

Chatters, L. M., & Taylor, R. J. (1989a). Age differences in religious participation among black adults. *Journal of Gerontology, 44*(5) 183–189.

Chatters, L. M., & Taylor, R. J. (1989b). Life problems and coping strategies of older black adults. *Social Work, 6,* 313–319.

Clinebell, H. (1997). *Anchoring your well-being: A guide for congregational leaders.* Nashville, TN: Upper Room.

Dilulio, J. J., Jr. (1998). Living faith: The black church outreach tradition. In *The Jeremiah Project: An initiative of the Center for Civic Innovation* (Report No. 98-3, pp. 1–10) [On-line]. Available: www.manhattan.institute.org/html/jrp-98-3.htm

Dossey, L. (1993). *Healing words: The power of prayer and the practice of medicine.* San Francisco: Harper San Francisco.

Du Bois, W.E.B. (1903). *The Negro church.* Atlanta, GA: Atlanta University.

Edelman, M. W. (1987). *Families in peril: An agenda for social change.* Cambridge, MA: Harvard University Press.

Elkins, T. E. (1987). The meaning of prayer: A Christian physician's experience. *Journal of Religion and Health, 26*(4), 286–299.

Epperly, B. G. (1995). To pray or not to pray: Reflection on the intersection of prayer and medicine. *Journal of Religion and Health, 34*(2), 141–148.

Frazier, E. F. (1966). *The Negro church in America.* New York: Schocken Books.

George, Y., Richardson, V., Lakes-Matyas, M., & Blake, F. (1989). *Saving black minds: Black churches and education.* Washington, DC: American Association for the Advancement of Science.

Graham, T. W., Kaplan, B. H., Cornoni-Huntley, J. C., James, S. A., Becker, C., Hames, C. G., & Heyden, S. (1978). Frequency of church attendance and blood pressure elevation. *Journal of Behavioral Medicine, 1,* 37–43.

Griffith, E. H., English, T., & Mayfield, V. (1980). Possession, prayer, and testimony: Therapeutic aspects of the Wednesday night meeting in a black church. *Psychiatry, 43,* 120–128.

Gunderson, G. (1997). *Deeply woven roots: Improving the quality of life in your community.* Minneapolis, MN: Fortress.

Hatch, J. (1992). Empowering black churches for health promotion. *Health Values, 16*(5), 3–11.

Hewlett, S. A., & West, C. (1998). *The war against parents: What we can do for America's beleaguered moms and dads.* Boston: Houghton Mifflin.

Hill, K. (1999, Summer). Be sensitive. *Faith and Health,* p. 12.

Hoyt, T., Jr. (1997). Testimony. In D. C. Bass (Ed.), *Practicing our faith.* San Francisco: Jossey-Bass.

Jackson, J. S. (Ed.). (1988). *The black American elderly: Research on physical and psychosocial health.* New York: Springer.

Levin, J. (1984). The role of the black church in community medicine. *Journal of the National Medical Association, 76,* 477–483.

Lincoln, C. E., & Mamiya, L. H. (1990). *The black church in the African American experience.* Durham, NC: Duke University Press.

Mays, B., & Nicholson, J. (1969). *The Negro's church.* New York: Russell and Russell.

Paskett, E. D., Case, L. D., Tatum, C., Velez, R., & Wilson, A. (1999). Religiosity and cancer screening. *Journal of Religion and Health, 38*(1), 39–51.

Perkins, J. C. (1999). *Building up Zion's walls: Ministry for empowering the African American family.* Valley Forge, PA: Judson.

Raboteau, A. J. (1986). The Afro-American traditions. In R. L. Numbers & D. W. Amundsen (Eds.), *Caring and curing: Health and medicine in the Western religious traditions.* Baltimore: John Hopkins University Press.

Sata, L. S., Perry, D. A., & Cameron, C. (1979). Store-front churches in the inner city. *Mental Hygiene, 54*(2), 256–260.

Scandrett, A., Jr. (1996). Health and the black church. *Journal of Religion and Health, 35*(3), 231–244.

Scarantino, B. A. (1987). *Music power: Creative living through the joys of music.* New York: Dodd, Mead.

Smith, E. D., & Merritt, S. L. (1997, August). Church-based education: An outreach program for African Americans with hypertension. *Ethnicity & Health, 2*(3), 243–253.

Snyder, G. F. (1988). *Tough choices: Health care decisions and the faith community.* Elgin, IL: Brethren.

Spear, A. H. (1969). *Black Chicago: The making of a Negro ghetto, 1890–1920.* Chicago: University of Chicago Press.

Staples, R., & Johnson, L. B. (1993). *Black families at the crossroads: Challenges and prospects.* San Francisco: Jossey-Bass, 1993.

Taylor, R. J. (1989). Religious participation among elderly blacks. *The Gerontologist, 26,* 630–636.

Washington, J. M. (1994). *Conversations with God: Two centuries of prayers by African Americans.* New York: HarperCollins.

Weatherhead, L. D. (1952). *Psychology, religion and healing* (2nd ed.). London: Hodder and Stoughton.

Williamson, D. (1999, August 30). *Study shows black churches can help improve healthy behaviors* (University of North Carolina News Service, No. 511) [On-line]. Available: www.unc.edu/news/newsserv

Wimberly, A. S. (1992–1993). Reverence for life in severe and terminal illness: A theological ethical viewpoint. *Journal of the Interdenominational Theological Center, 20*(1–2), 1–21.

Wimberly, A. S. (Ed.). (1997a). *Honoring African American elders: A ministry in the soul community.* San Francisco: Jossey-Bass.

Wimberly, A. S. (1997b). Music and the promotion of healing in religious caregiving. *Journal of the Interdenominational Theological Center, 25*(2), 99–124.

Wimberly, A. S., & Wimberly, E. P. (1995). Pastoral care of African Americans. In M. Kimble, S. H. McFadden, J. W. Ellor, & J. J. Seeber (Eds.), *Spirituality and religion: A handbook.* Minneapolis, MN: Fortress.

Wimberly, E. P. (1990). *Prayer in pastoral counseling: Suffering, healing, and discernment.* Louisville, KY: Westminster/John Knox.

Wimberly, E. P. (1996). Spirituality and health. *The Caregiver Journal, 12*(4), 1–7.

CHAPTER EIGHT

THE EPIDEMIC OF HOMICIDE AND VIOLENCE

W. Rodney Hammond, Deborah Prothrow-Stith

Individuals and organizations working to stem violence and homicide in the United States have reason for optimism. Violence—defined by the Centers for Disease Control and Prevention (CDC) as the use of physical force or power, threatened or actual, against oneself, against another person, or against a group or community, that either results in or has a high likelihood of resulting in injury, death, psychological harm, mal-development, or deprivation—has been on the wane for the past decade (World Health Organization, 1996).

On close examination of the statistics, however, a "good news, bad news" scenario emerges. The overall decline of homicide and violence masks the rising percentage of African Americans, especially the young, who are victims.

First the Good News . . .

Annual nonfatal and fatal firearm-related injury rates in the United States for all groups peaked in the late 1980s and early 1990s and have declined consistently since 1993 (Hoyert, Kochanek, & Murphy, 1999). From 1993 to 1997, the annual nonfatal firearm-related injury rate decreased 40.8 percent, from 40.5 per 100,000 to 24.0 per 100,000. The annual fatal firearm-related injury rate dropped from 15.4 per 100,000 in 1993 to 12.1 per 100,000 in 1997, a decrease of 21.1 percent. Firearm-related suicide rates declined as well, going from 7.5 per 100,000 to 6.6 per 100,000 during this five-year period, a reduction of 10.9 percent (CDC, 1999).

During these years, nonfatal and fatal firearm-related injury rates declined for members of the vulnerable fifteen to twenty-four age group as well. This group, which had a rate of 138.4 nonfatal firearm-related injuries per 100,000 in 1993, had a rate of 82.6 such injuries per 100,000 in 1997. This represents a decrease of 40.3 percent (CDC, 1999).

Homicide rates for the fifteen to twenty-four age group dropped from 31 per 100,000 to 22.3 per 100,000, a 27.8 percent reduction (CDC, 1999). In addition, results from the 1999 Youth Risk Behavior Survey indicate a 25 percent decline in the number of high school students carrying guns on school property and a 9 percent decline in physical fights on school grounds between 1993 and 1997 (Brener, Simon, Krug, & Lowry, 1999).

Numerous factors may have contributed to these declines: improving economic conditions, an aging population, a decline in the crack cocaine market, changes in legislation and sentencing guidelines, changes in law enforcement practices, and improved violence prevention programs. However, the importance and relative contribution of these factors is not known (CDC, 1999; Hoyert et al., 1999).

. . . And Now the Bad News

The declining rates of homicide and violence, although encouraging, must be placed in perspective. Even with significant decreases in nonfatal and fatal firearm-related injury rates, approximately 96,000 persons in the United States sustained gunshot wounds in 1997 (CDC, 1999). Homicide remains the second leading cause of death for all U.S. youths aged fifteen to twenty-four, accounting for 6,146 deaths in 1997 (CDC, 1999; Hoyert et al., 1999).

Homicide remains the leading cause of death among African American youths of both sexes in the fifteen to twenty-four age group, accounting for 3,529 deaths in 1997. This is three times the number of deaths members of this cohort experienced from all other health problems combined. In 1997, African American males fifteen to twenty-four years of age were nine times more likely to die as a result of homicide than were white males in the same age group. In addition, African American males were three times more likely than the comparable white Hispanic cohorts to die as a result of homicide (Hoyert et al., 1999).

Self-directed violence, in the form of suicide and suicide attempts, has increased dramatically among African American youths. In 1997, suicide was the third leading cause of death among all U.S. youths aged fifteen to twenty-four, regardless of race or ethnicity (Hoyert et al., 1999). A look at trends shows that between 1980 and 1995, the suicide rate for black youths aged ten to nineteen escalated from 2.1 to 4.5 per 100,000, an increase of 114 percent. This was most pronounced in African Americans aged ten to fourteen: their suicide rates increased 233 percent during this fifteen-year period. Furthermore, the suicide rate in the fifteen to nineteen age group grew more rapidly among young black males (146 percent) than among white males (22 percent). Firearm-related suicides accounted for 96 percent of the increased rates for African American youths aged ten to nineteen (CDC, 1998). These figures undergird the continuing efforts to stem violence among all youths and among African American youths in particular.

Contributing Risk Factors for Violence

Violence is a complex issue, and there is no consensus on its ultimate causes. Various conceptual approaches used to explain the high incidence of assaultive violence among African Americans posit (1) a subculture of violence, (2) economic deprivation, or (3) a combination of structural and cultural factors (that is, poverty and lack of opportunity combined with attitudes about violence) (Hammond & Yung, 1993).

The culture of violence theory posits the existence of self-perpetuating community or regional norms that support the use of aggression as a legitimate means of resolving relationship problems (Wolfgang & Ferracutti, 1967, 1982).

Economic deprivation formulations attribute violence to frustration resulting from lack of desired material resources and stimulating feelings of resentment and hostility and aggressive impulses (Agnew, 1990; Bell, 1987; Hampton, 1986; Oliver, 1994; Roberts, 1990).

The structural-cultural perspective focuses on dysfunctional cultural adaptations to environmental pressures (Hammond & Yung, 1993). Poussaint (1972) suggested that self-hatred among some young African American men may prompt them to strike out at others who resemble them. Ramey (1980) referred to "free-floating anger" as a result of disenfranchisement and suggested that African American men experiencing this constant tension strike out at those targets that are most convenient.

All these perspectives have their detractors. Critics of the first note its circular reasoning, failure to give weight to external factors such as poverty and racial discrimination, and overprediction of the number of African Americans who are likely to become involved in violent behavior (Bernard, 1990; Hawkins, 1990; Lester, 1986; Oliver, 1994; Sampson, 1987). Critics of the economic deprivation perspective point out that it does not explain why many African Americans who are poor do not engage in violent behavior (Agnew, 1990; Bell, 1987; Hampton, 1986; Oliver, 1994; Roberts, 1990). Others have noted that global lists do little to establish which causal factors are the most important and offer little guidance for shaping policy or designing interventions (Hawkins, 1990).

It is likely that interactions among risk factors and cumulative effects of multiple risks promote the development and maintenance of violent behavior. The magnitude and impact of lethal and nonlethal violence in America and the impact of this violence on individuals, groups, and the health care system make it essential to address violence as a health problem. The complexity of the social, behavioral, and environmental factors that spawn and perpetuate an increased risk of violence argues persuasively that violence be addressed from a public health perspective.

The Public Health Approach to Violence

The public health approach to preventing violence offers several key contributions. First, and most important, it is a proactive approach committed to changing the social, behavioral, and environmental factors that encourage violence and to identifying policies and programs that help prevent violence (Mercy, Rosenberg, Powell, Broome, & Roper, 1993). As such, it substitutes the reactive stance, so typically seen among the media and public, with a structured approach that produces policies and interventions matched to particular kinds of violence.

Second, this approach advocates a multidisciplinary scientific effort that is directed explicitly toward identifying effective methods of prevention. Public health approaches are defined not by the sector or discipline that carries them out but by whether the prevention strategy or policy has the potential to reduce the physical or mental health consequences of violence (Mercy & Hammond, 1998).

Third, public health's tradition of integrative leadership facilitates the organization of a broad array of scientific disciplines, organizations, and communities to work together. This ability to unify the various scientific disciplines pertinent to violence prevention and establish links with entities representing education, labor, public housing, media, business, medicine, and criminal justice, among others, has an important consequence. It enables the forging of responses to violence that are both more efficient and complementary than traditional approaches, which tend to be fragmented or narrowly focused in the criminal justice sector (Mercy & Hammond, 1998).

Fourth, public health has an essential role in building the scientific foundation for developing effective treatments and therapies to mitigate the physical, psychological, sensory, and cognitive consequences of injury. Among the ways it can do this is to help consolidate the literature on the etiology of interpersonal violence risk and on prevention strategies (Mercy & Hammond, 1998). At present, this literature is compartmentalized into separate bodies of work that study child abuse (Finklehor & Dzuiba-Leatherman, 1994), domestic violence, and youth assaultive violence as discrete phenomena (Hampton, 1987; Jenkins, 1995).

Fifth, public health brings a long-standing commitment to supporting and facilitating the central role of communities in solving health problems (Mercy & Hammond, 1998). For example, successful community-based health promotion efforts have improved dietary habits (Johnson et al., 1993), reduced teenage pregnancy rates (Vincent, Clearie, & Schluchter, 1987), and lowered the prevalence of smoking among adolescents (Bruvold, 1993).

Sixth, a public health approach can facilitate the prevention of violence by helping community members see this violence as a problem that can be understood and changed, not as an inevitable consequence of modern life. It can further help by providing the information and skills individuals need to choose alternatives to violence (Mercy & Hammond, 1998).

Finally, the public health approach offers a breadth of potential solutions from different systems of influence to address the problems of violence simultaneously for various populations.

Implementation of the public health approach involves a four-step process (Mercy & Hammond, 1998):

1. Define the problem by obtaining information such as the demographic characteristics of the persons involved, the times and places where the incidents took place, the relationship of the actors, and the severity and costs of the injuries.
2. Identify why the incidents occurred so as to define populations at high risk and suggest specific interventions.
3. Evaluate the efficacy of existing programs, policies, and strategies, and develop and test new interventions based on the information obtained in steps 1 and 2.
4. Implement interventions and measure their prevention effectiveness. This requires developing guidelines and procedures for putting programs in place, and then continuously improving and assessing them as specific challenges are encountered and addressed.

Step 1 has yielded essential information. A key contribution of the public health sector has been to conceptualize and segment violent behavior into meaningful categories that improve our understanding of various risks, contributing factors, and possible interventions. An emerging consensus distinguishes among at least four types of violence: (1) primary, expressive, or relationship violence; (2) secondary, predatory, or instrumental criminal violence; (3) situational or mob violence; and (4) psychopathological violence associated with severe mental illness (Tolan & Guerra, 1994). Moreover, we know that the first type, expressive violence, is especially prevalent in the United States and that some individuals and groups are disproportionately at risk (Yung & Hammond, 1994; Guerra, Tolan, & Hammond, 1995).

Identification of these four categories of violent behavior has allowed the development of interventions that are appropriate to the risk factors in each category. There is a growing consensus, for example, that interventions aimed at anger management and the development of social skills are particularly suited to addressing expressive or relationship-oriented violence (Yung & Hammond, 1994; Guerra, Tolan, & Hammond, 1995). Because African American youths face an increased risk of death or injury from violence, many initial public health violence prevention efforts have focused on this group and have paid particular attention to developing programs that they will respond to and accept.

Although the late 1980s and early 1990s were characterized by comparatively more action around steps 2 and 3 and very little action around step 4, the past five years have seen considerable progress in implementing prevention-focused programs and in performing ongoing monitoring and evaluation of these programs. Much must still be done, however, to ensure that those programs not yet evaluated will be and to increase the sophistication of program assessment techniques where needed (Mercy & Hammond, 1998).

The thoroughness of the public health process means that it is unlikely to provide a quick fix. But the complexity of the interaction among biological, psychological, and social factors that has produced the current epidemic of violence makes it unlikely that less comprehensive approaches will work.

Youth Violence Prevention Programs

Three programs, each of which exemplifies how public health may be applied to youth violence at the community level, illustrate violence prevention programs. The Boston project is a large-scale, citywide initiative that addresses youth violence at multiple levels. Responding in Peaceful and Positive Ways (RIPP), which targets sixth through eighth graders, teaches conflict resolution, communication skills, and values that foster nonviolent behaviors. Positive Adolescent Choices Training (PACT) specifically addresses African American youths aged twelve to fifteen and focuses on cultural competence as the key to violence prevention. These three programs share the common characteristic of being community based, but each one brings unique qualities and perspectives to youth violence prevention. Although the ability to perform outcome evaluations of each program has varied, all three have made a positive difference in reducing violence. (Readers interested in reviewing other promising and effective programs may want to review Samples and Aber's chapter, "Evaluations of School-Based Violence Prevention Programs," in *Violence in American Schools*, 1998.)

The Boston Project: A Large-Scale Community Intervention

An early example of a community-based program, the Boston project was evaluated on a very basic level by assessing the availability of and people's satisfaction with various aspects of the program. Although the program design and evaluation did not include outcome criteria, declines in violence were associated with implementation of the program, which represents an exciting example of how all segments of a community can come together to address a common problem. However, because the program was multifaceted and had many interventions, involved many segments of the community, and used rudimentary evaluation techniques, it is impossible to know which intervention or combination of interventions was responsible for its success.

What is known is that during the 1980s, the city of Boston experienced an epidemic of adolescent violence. At this epidemic's height, between 1989 and

1991, one homicide a month in Boston involved a child sixteen or younger, and most of these homicides were firearm related. The city's response to this epidemic was to mount a comprehensive prevention effort, using a public health perspective that guided a complex, multidecade effort based on several significant premises and involving many programs from many disciplines (the following description is based on Prothrow-Stith & Spivak, 1992).

The key premises were that

- Youth violence is preventable.
- Youth service professionals across disciplines had to change their responses to violence. The police could no longer just arrest youths who engaged in violence or ignore children who had witnessed their mothers being beaten. Hospital emergency room staff could no longer just stitch youths up and send them back into the old environment. Members of all professions and disciplines had to incorporate violence prevention strategies into their work.
- Everyone, including young people, had a contribution to make.

Clearly, Boston police had a continuing role to play. However, their efforts were incorporated into an existing public health perspective. In 1982, Boston City Hospital became the first hospital in the country to initiate a comprehensive violence prevention program based on public health strategies. By labeling violence as a public health problem, the hospital challenged youth-serving professionals to complement the intervention role of police.

Members from all segments of the community were involved. Violence prevention became a movement in Boston. Educators, youth outreach workers, peer educators, police, lawyers, community agency staff, clergy, probation officers, activists, nurses, doctors, and emergency response teams were trained and challenged to begin new programs and to integrate violence prevention strategies into their existing work. The Boston Public Schools developed the country's first violence prevention curriculum to address peer fighting in the high schools. It also provided in-service training in violence prevention for teachers.

In 1990, staff members at the Boston City Hospital began visiting and providing violence prevention counseling to adolescents who were admitted to the hospital with gunshot or stab wounds and to these youths' friends and family. These staff provided a safety plan and follow-up services as well. Later the hospital expanded its efforts by implementing an exemplary program for children who witness violence.

The Harvard Community Health Plan Foundation developed the Think— Violence Is for Those Who Don't campaign and sponsored parent information brochures about television programs and disciplinary techniques. WBZ-TV's six-year-old Stop the Violence campaign was a concerted media blitz that had a measurable impact on public policy and funding for domestic violence initiatives.

Boston's business community also made important contributions. Efforts included a significant increase in mortgages to people in low- and moderate-income brackets, direct partnerships with schools, and community development projects that included locating bank branches, drugstores, and grocery stores in underserved neighborhoods. Individuals made important contributions, as well, as did Boston's youths. Students participating in the Violence Prevention Curriculum for Adolescents (Prothrow-Stith, 1987) were trained to become peer counselors. These same students then participated in violence prevention training sessions, working with other adolescents.

Several national initiatives were incorporated into Boston's efforts to stem the epidemic of adolescent violence. These included the Squash It campaign, which used the media to send the message that it is acceptable to walk away from fights, the Safe Start initiative of Children's Defense Fund, curriculum and policy efforts of the Center to Prevent Handgun Violence, and brochures and special initiatives of the American Medical Association and the American Academy of Pediatrics. Several publicly funded programs from the CDC, the National Institutes of Justice, and the U.S. Department of Education contributed as well.

Seen in its entirety, the Boston project provides an excellent example of a comprehensive, communitywide effort to address violence prevention. It demonstrates what happens when community support is galvanized into a coordinated effort by both public health and law enforcement.

Responding in Peaceful and Positive Ways: Teaching Health Promotion Behaviors in an Urban Setting

The per capita murder rate in Richmond, Virginia, was routinely ranked fourth or fifth among all U.S. cities. Because risk-taking and violence-related behaviors often surface in middle school, the ongoing Richmond Youth Against Violence project mounted a school-based program it called Responding in Peaceful and Positive Ways (RIPP).

RIPP was one of the first youth violence prevention interventions developed with support from the CDC. The program, which was developed by Farrell and Meyer (and is described in Farrell, Meyer, & Dahlberg, 1996), is a twenty-five-session, sixth-grade primary prevention curriculum grounded in social-cognitive learning theory. Students who received the intervention participated in weekly sessions of twenty-five to fifty minutes for seven to eight months. The program, which is based on Perry and Jessor's health promotion model (Perry & Jessor, 1985), introduces participants to adult role models who teach and encourage conflict resolution behaviors and values that promote nonviolence and foster positive communication.

The RIPP program design includes random assignment of children to treatment and no-treatment control groups. Evaluators, who relied on school disciplinary records and student self-reports, found that the prevalence of school discipline code violations, in-house suspensions, and fight-related injuries was similar for the treatment and control groups during the first three-quarters of the school year.

However, this changed during the fourth quarter. At that point, school disciplinary records showed that students in the control group were charged with fighting more than twice as often as their treatment group peers. Control group youths were also nearly four times more likely to be charged with bringing a weapon to school than were their peers in the treatment group. In addition, the rate of in-house suspensions for control group youths was higher than that among students who received the treatment.

Student self-reports were consistent with these data. They revealed significantly lower frequencies of fighting and fewer fight-related injuries among the treatment group. Preliminary findings at six months postintervention found significantly fewer in-house and out-of-school suspensions among the treatment group.

Responding in Peaceful and Positive Ways was not designed specifically for African American youths. However, more than 90 percent of the students in the city's public school system are black, a fact that is reflected in the curriculum structure. For example, the prevention specialists selected were all African American men with good communication skills and a deep commitment to preventing violence in the black community. In addition, RIPP is an excellent example of a *best practices* program in an urban setting. (Best practices are discussed later in the chapter.)

Positive Adolescent Choices Training: Cultural Sensitivity in Violence Prevention

The Positive Adolescent Choices Training program (PACT), developed by the lead author while he was on the faculty at Wright State University in Ohio and supported by a CDC grant, is an intervention that focuses on cultural sensitivity as a key aspect of a successful violence prevention program. Cultural sensitivity (or cultural competence as it is sometimes called) places the intervention in a context that is acceptable, relevant, and accessible to ethnic minority youths (Dumas, Rollock, Prinz, Hops, & Blechman, 1999). It also incorporates the idea that ethnic-specific influences may contribute to problem behavior.

PACT targets African American youths aged twelve to fifteen (this description is derived from Yung & Hammond, 1998). The goal of the program is to help adolescents learn more appropriate and socially effective ways to interact with others—in short, to get what they want in ways that do not infringe on others' rights and that do facilitate cooperation, not aggression. The program uses a cognitive-behavioral group-training method and incorporates concepts and techniques taken from several programs and curricula for social skills development, anger management, aggression replacement, and violence prevention. The PACT approach has these principal components:

- Violence risk education, which aims to replace violence myths with facts and uses Prothrow-Stith's Word Web Chart Exercise (1987) to help participants link violence risk information to their own lives.

- Training in anger management skills to be used in situations of interpersonal conflict.
- Training in techniques for recognizing anger and for expressing or controlling it constructively.
- Training in three social skills: giving negative feedback, receiving negative feedback, and negotiation.

The program achieves cultural appropriateness by making the setting as pleasant and social as possible, providing community figures who are positive African American role models, stressing the use of familiar expressions that young African American adolescents understand, and employing reality-based scenarios for vignettes and class discussions.

Of particular importance are the beliefs and expectations of program facilitators—doctoral students in clinical psychology who are participating in a formal, supervised practicum. These facilitators are encouraged to examine their own beliefs and assumptions and confront any negative stereotypes about program participants. They are also expected to understand participants' common stressors and neighborhood attributes such as gang activity, to know whether interracial conflict is a major problem in the school or community, and to be aware of other facets of the youngsters' immediate environment. They are also expected to be familiar with broader cultural influences such as images of African American youths in music and the popular media.

Evaluation of the PACT program involves pre- and postintervention ratings of participants by teachers, parents, or other significant adults on the three social skills taught and on other more generic prosocial skills. It also involves pre- and postintervention self-ratings by participants to determine if they are more confident in their ability to perform the three target and the general prosocial skills.

School behavior records and juvenile court records provide additional information. Early evaluations indicated that youths who participated in PACT demonstrated a significant reduction in physical aggression at school. Their behavior improved during the course of the training period and was maintained beyond their participation in the program. Nontreatment youths typically showed either no reduction or an increase in incidents during this time. Juvenile court records provided longer-term follow-up. These records indicated that the untrained comparison youths were two and one-half times more likely to be arrested than were the treatment youths. In addition, untrained youths demonstrated a trend of greater involvement in types of criminal activity that carry a high risk of death or injury to themselves or others. These treatment effects were in evidence two years postintervention.

These results underscore the findings in Dumas, Rollock, Prinz, Hops, and Blechman's review (1999), which suggested intervention programs that strive to be culturally sensitive are more efficacious than those that do not.

Community Health Promotion Programs

Successful public health initiatives rely on the interaction of macro- and micro-level interventions. Community-based health promotion programs aimed at modifying the beliefs and behaviors of individuals must be grounded in a larger effort. Conversely, large-scale multifaceted initiatives such as the Boston project must include community-based programs aimed at individuals if they are to reach the constituents they desire to influence. The Boston model, for example, included the public school system's Violence Prevention Curriculum for Adolescents (Prothrow-Stith, 1987).

Many other examples of community-based programs exist. They include efforts to prevent substance abuse and HIV and AIDS infection as well as violence, and they are directed at Native American, Asian American, and Hispanic youths as well as African American youths (Yung & Hammond, 1998). Yet, until recently, empirical evaluation of community-based health promotion programs was extremely limited. Published research on outcomes of violence prevention efforts was no exception. Outcome research on violence prevention efforts directed to specific ethnic minority adolescents was rarer still.

This situation is slowly changing. In the past decade, evaluation of community-based health promotion programs for preventing violence has increased. These outcome evaluations have provided important clues about the core characteristics of successful violence prevention programs in general and on what does and does not work when implementing a community-based program directed at adolescents.

Setting Standards for Violence Prevention Programs

The experience so far with violence prevention programs suggests some evaluation criteria, best practices, and facilitating techniques that can help communities define and plan successful programs.

Blueprint Criteria

Standards for measuring the effectiveness of violence prevention programs include four *blueprint criteria* (University of Colorado, 2000):

1. Program results must have outcomes clearly associated with aggression.
2. The evaluation must include a comparison group.
3. The effects of the intervention must last at least a year.
4. The intervention must show a benefit in more than one setting.

These criteria were developed at the University of Colorado as part of a cataloging of effective violence prevention interventions funded by the U.S. Department of Justice and the CDC. To date, ten programs have achieved status as blueprint programs, based on a review by a committee of experts at the university. Meeting these criteria is considered essential to a community-based program's success.

Four categories of programs appear to show the most promise for meeting these criteria and preventing youth violence (University of Colorado, 2000):

1. Home-visiting programs in which trained nurses frequently visit at-risk families during the child's first two years of life. These programs, which achieved the *gold standard*—that is, met all of the blueprint criteria—have been associated with sharp reductions in violence and unintentional injuries in the life trajectory of children whose parents received the intervention.
2. Parenting programs that focus on instilling effective discipline skills and remedying poor parental monitoring of children as they grow older. Intervention research suggests that the most effective of these programs are those aimed at helping parents of children aged five to twelve.
3. Mentoring programs that serve children who may not have access to a responsible adult in their lives.
4. Programs aimed at directly teaching youths social and cognitive skills that are incompatible with the development of violent behaviors.

Best Practices

Complementing these criteria is the CDC's list of characteristics, or best practices, shared by successful programs. Eighty violence-prevention experts convened at two national meetings were asked to identify those programs they believed to be most successful. Although reference to the blueprint criteria was implicit in their choices, they also considered other factors (Thornton, Craft, Dahlberg, Lynch, & Baer, 2000). Effective programs, according to a number of experts, share these characteristics: (1) they are comprehensive and include family members, peers, community members, and the media; (2) they begin in the early grades and are reinforced across grade levels; (3) they are tailored to the developmental level of the targeted children and youths; (4) they focus on promoting personal and social competencies; (5) they make use of interactive techniques such as role-playing and behavioral rehearsal; (6) they use culturally sensitive materials; (7) they emphasize program staff development and training; and (8) they operate in schools that have a positive climate and adequate discipline (Dusenbury, Falco, Lake, Brannigan, & Bosworth, 1997).

Practices that appear not to work include using scare tactics that picture violent scenes; imposing violence prevention programs on schools that are overwhelmed with administrative burdens, programs, and paperwork; and segregating students who are actively exhibiting antisocial and aggressive behavior from other at-risk students. Programs unlikely to work also include those that are brief and not supported by a positive climate, those that focus exclusively on self-esteem enhancement, and those that only provide information (Dusenbury et al., 1997).

Program Facilitators

Practices and techniques that appear to facilitate successful adolescent-focused programs—those aimed at teaching adolescents social and cognitive skills that are incompatible with the development of violent behaviors—include the following:

- Establish violence prevention programs on site, where adolescents already gather. Doing so allows easy access to a large pool of potential participants, results in higher levels of attendance and retention, and reduces the need for transportation.
- Make participation voluntary, and provide incentives that encourage compliance and participation. Programs that did so reported better attendance, higher levels of youth participation in program activities, and better retention rates than compulsory programs.
- Employ counselors and outreach workers who are ethnically similar to the participants, and consult with neighborhood or tribal advisory panels. Programs that failed to do so reported lower recruitment and retention rates than programs that did.
- Tailor program content to local cultural norms and circumstances. Programs that did so had better outcomes. Such tailoring might, for example, entail adapting teaching methods for ethnic minority African American or Native American youths, who may have a culturally rooted discomfort with self-disclosure.
- Use multimodal and interactive teaching and learning techniques with liberal use of role-playing, group discussion, video, audio, cartoons, television, music, and newspapers. Again, this has led in practice to better participation.

Conclusion

Although the reduction in fatal and nonfatal firearms violence is welcome and the increased implementation and evaluation of violence prevention programs promising, much remains to be done. African American youths, in particular, remain at extraordinarily high risk of mortality due to homicide and more recently to suicide.

The following initiatives must be undertaken (Mercy & Hammond, 1998). There remains a vital need for widespread adoption and implementation of violence prevention interventions that reflect public health standards and are culturally competent. Parallel to these efforts, there is a need for a greater number of functional surveillance mechanisms at the state and local levels and for more effective ways to obtain information beyond what is available from crime reports about the context of violence-related injuries and homicides.

Also needed is the development of a clear and systematic infrastructure to facilitate the transfer of appropriate violence prevention programs, services, and technology into the community. In addition, the potential roles the private sector could take on and the possibility of combined public-private efforts must be more seriously addressed.

More information about the effects of community structural conditions that contribute to violence is essential as well. Such conditions include the effects of poverty, unemployment, neighborhood socioeconomic isolation, drug trafficking, easy availability of guns, and a low level of safety resources. Finally, it is essential to better understand the conditions in communities, homes, schools, and families that reinforce nonviolent patterns of behavior and other forms of healthy development in various at-risk groups.

This combination of initiatives is most likely to provide the knowledge, infrastructure, and community-based programs needed to reduce the unacceptably high rate of firearm-related fatal and nonfatal injuries among America's youths.

References

Agnew, R. (1990). The origins of delinquent events: An examination of offender accounts. *Journal of Research in Crime and Delinquency, 27,* 267–294.

Bell, C. (1987). Preventive strategies for dealing with violence among blacks. *Community Mental Health Journal, 23,* 217–228.

Bernard, D. (1990). Angry aggression among the "truly disadvantaged." *Criminology, 28,* 73–94.

Brener, N. D., Simon, T. R., Krug, E. G., & Lowry, R. (1999). Recent trends in violence-related behaviors among high school students in the United States. *Journal of the American Medical Association, 282,* 440–446.

Bruvold, W. H. (1993). A meta-analysis of adolescent smoking prevention programs. *American Journal of Public Health, 83,* 872–880.

Centers for Disease Control and Prevention. (1998). Suicide among black youths: United States, 1980–1995. *Morbidity and Mortality Weekly Report, 47,* 193–196.

Centers for Disease Control and Prevention. (1999). Nonfatal and fatal firearm-related injuries: United States, 1993–1997. *Morbidity and Mortality Weekly Report, 48,* 1029–1034.

Dumas, J. E., Rollock, D., Prinz, R. J., Hops, H., & Blechman, E. A. (1999). Cultural sensitivity: Problems and solutions in applied and preventive intervention. *Applied and Preventive Psychology, 8,* 175–196.

Dusenbury, L., Falco, M., Lake, A., Brannigan, R., & Bosworth, K. (1997). Nine critical elements of promising violence prevention programs. *Journal of School Health, 67,* 409–414.

Farrell, A. D., Meyer, A. L., & Dahlberg, L. L. (1996). Richmond youth against violence: A school-based program for urban adolescents. *American Journal of Preventive Medicine, 12,* 13–21.

Finklehor, D., & Dzuiba-Leatherman, J. (1994). Children as victims of violence: A national survey. *Pediatrics, 94,* 413–420.

Guerra, N., Tolan, P. H., & Hammond, W. R. (1995). Prevention and treatment of adolescent violence. In L. D. Eron, J. Gentry, & P. Schlegel (Eds.), *Reason to hope: A psychosocial perspective on violence and youth* (pp. 383–403). Washington, DC: American Psychological Association.

Hammond, W. R., & Yung, B. (1993). Psychology's role in the public health response to assaultive violence among young African American men. *American Psychologist, 48*(2), 142–154.

Hampton, R. (1986). Family violence and homicide in the black community: Are they linked? In U.S. Department of Health and Human Services, Task Force on Black and Minority Health, *Report of the Secretary's Task Force on Black and Minority Health*, Vol. 5, (pp. 69–96). Washington, DC: U.S. Government Printing Office.

Hampton, R. (1987). Family violence and homicide in the black community: Are they linked? In R. Hampton (Ed.), *Violence in the black family* (pp. 135–156). Lexington, MA: Heath.

Hawkins, D. (1990). Explaining the black homicide rate. *Journal of Interpersonal Violence, 5,* 151–163.

Hoyert, D. L., Kochanek, K. D., & Murphy, S. L. (1999). Deaths: Final data for 1997. *National Vital Statistics Reports* (Vol. 47, No. 19). Hyattsville, MD: National Center for Health Statistics.

Jenkins, P. (1995). Threads that link community and family violence: Issues for prevention. In T. Gullotta, R. Hampton, & P. Jenkins (Eds.), *When anger governs: Preventing violence in America* (pp. 33–45). Thousand Oaks, CA: Sage.

Johnson, C. L., Rifkind, B. M., Sempos, C. T., Carroll, M. D., Bachorik, P. S., Briefel, R. R., Gorden, D. L., Burt, V. L., Brown, C. D., Lippel, K., & Cleeman, J. I. (1993). Declining serum total cholesterol levels among U.S. adults: The National Health and Nutritional Examination Survey. *Journal of the American Medical Association, 269,* 3002–3008.

Lester, D. (1986). *The murderer and his murder: A review of the research.* New York: AMS Press.

Mercy, J. A., & Hammond, W. R. (1998). Preventing homicide: A public health perspective. In M. D. Smith & M. A. Zahn (Eds.), *Studying and preventing homicide* (pp. 274–294). Thousand Oaks, CA: Sage.

Mercy, J. A., Rosenberg, M. L., Powell, K. E., Broome, C. V., & Roper, W. L. (1993). Public health policy for preventing violence. *Health Affairs, 12,* 7–29.

Oliver, W. (1994). *The violent social world of black men.* San Francisco: Jossey-Bass.

Perry, C., & Jessor, R. (1985). The concept of health promotion and the prevention of adolescent drug abuse. *Health Education Quarterly, 12*(2), 169–184.

Poussaint, A. (1972). *Why blacks kill blacks.* New York: Emerson Hall.

Prothrow-Stith, D. (1987). *Violence prevention curriculum for adolescents* (Teenage health teaching modules). Newton, MA: Education Development Center.

Prothrow-Stith, D., & Spivak, H. (1992). Homicide and violence: Contemporary health problems for America's black community. In R. L. Braithwaite & S. E. Taylor (Eds.), *Health issues in the black community.* San Francisco: Jossey-Bass.

Ramey, L. (1980). Homicide among black males. *Public Health Reports, 95,* 549–561.

Roberts, S. (1990). Murder, mayhem, and other joys of youth. *Journal of NIH Research, 2,* 67–72.

Samples, F., & Aber, L. (1998). Evaluations of school-based violence prevention programs. In D. S. Elliott, B. A. Hamburg, & K. R. Williams (Eds.), *Violence in American schools* (pp. 217–252). New York: Cambridge University Press.

Sampson, R. (1987). Urban black violence: The effect of male joblessness and family disruption. *American Journal of Sociology, 93,* 348–405.

Thornton, T. N., Craft, C. A., Dahlberg, L. L., Lynch, B. S., & Baer, K. (2000). *Best practices of youth violence prevention: A sourcebook for community action.* Atlanta: Centers for Disease Control and Prevention, National Center for Injury Prevention and Control.

Tolan, P. H., & Guerra, N. (1994). Prevention of delinquency: Current status and issues. *Journal of Applied and Preventive Psychology, 3,* 251–273.

University of Colorado. (2000, August 21). *Blueprints for violence prevention.* [On-line]. Available: www.colorado.edu/cspv/blueprints/about/criteria.htm

Vincent, M. L., Clearie, A. R., & Schluchter, M. D. (1987). Reducing adolescent pregnancy through school and community-based education. *Journal of the American Medical Association, 257,* 3382–3386.

Wolfgang, M., & Ferracutti, F. (1967). *The subculture of violence.* London: Tavistock.

Wolfgang, M., & Ferracutti, F. (1982). *The subculture of violence: Towards an integrated theory in criminology.* Thousand Oaks, CA: Sage.

World Health Organization. (1996). *Violence: A public health priority.* Working document EHA/SPI/POA.2.

Yung, B., & Hammond, W. R. (1994). The positive case for school-based violence prevention programs. *Health Affairs, 13,* 170–173.

Yung, B., & Hammond, W. R. (1998). Breaking the cycle: A culturally sensitive violence prevention program for African American children and adolescents. In J. Lutzker (Ed.), *Handbook of child abuse research and treatment* (pp. 319–340). New York: Plenum.

CHAPTER NINE

THE DILEMMA OF ORGAN
AND TISSUE TRANSPLANTATION

Clive O. Callender, Margruetta B. Hall

Increasing organ and tissue transplant awareness among minorities, increasing the potential donor pool, and promoting disease prevention to reduce the need for transplantation are health care priorities for minority population groups just as they are for the general population in the United States. The donor-recipient disparity has been identified as the number one problem in transplantation today (Callender & Washington, 1997). Initiatives over the past fifteen years have not reached the goal of significantly increasing the supply of available organs to address this health problem. The need for donation continues to increase, with significant gaps between the number of those needing transplants and the number of organs and tissues available for donation. This is an ironic tragedy because advances in immunosuppression, organ preservation, and surgical techniques have made organ and tissue transplantation a viable medical option for those who need transplants to survive and to enhance their quality of life (Oberley, Sacksteder, Curtin, Calder, & Binder, 1991).

Many strategies have been proposed to address the problem of organ recovery. They include professional education, community education, required re-

This chapter describes the work of the Minority Organ/Tissue Transplant Education Program (MOTTEP), based at Howard University Hospital in Washington, D.C. MOTTEP is funded by the National Institutes of Health, Diabetes, and Digestive and Kidney Diseases (Grant number 5R25DK50474-04).

quests (requiring hospitals to report deaths to organ procurement organizations), legislation for presumed consent (allowing removal of organs from cadaveric donors without family consent), and others. Initiatives to address this health problem received support at the state and federal level beginning in 1968 with the Uniform Anatomical Gift Act, which validated the distribution of donor cards throughout the United States. Health education continues to be a significant approach, because this strategy presents the greatest opportunity to establish public awareness and increase knowledge about donation and transplantation and to initiate behavioral change among the public so that people incorporate donation as a cultural value and norm. Several studies have shown that there is a high level of awareness of organ transplantation, yet a significant gap exists between the number of people who are aware of organ donation and the number of people who actually donate (Oberley et al., 1991).

In 1980, a report from the Southeastern Organ Procurement Foundation (SEOPF) indicated that at least 50 percent of all dialysis patients listed were black, yet less than 10 percent of the organ donors were black. At the present time, nearly half of the patients on transplant waiting lists are ethnic minorities, and average time on the waiting list is longer for minorities than for whites. This is a significant problem because African Americans and Hispanics are disproportionately affected by diabetes and hypertension and are more vulnerable than whites to end-stage renal disease (ESRD), a health condition leading to the need for transplantation (Kasiske et al., 1991; United Network for Organ Sharing [UNOS], 1999). Because donation rates among whites are significantly higher than they are among minorities, the process of matching donor and recipient blood groups and the histocompatibility-complex results in most of the available kidneys being allocated to whites rather than to poorly matched minority patients (Partnership for Organ Donation, 1998).

Some studies addressing minorities and organ donation report that willingness to donate is associated with perceived need for transplants among other African Americans. The willingness to accept a transplant among African Americans is associated with the sources of information about donation (Callender, Hall, et al., 1991; Callender, Miles, & Yeager, 1998). Callender, Hall, et al. (1991), Townsend, Rovelli, & Schweizer (1990), Kappel, Whitlock, & Schutte (1993), and Gentry, Brown-Holbert, and Andrews (1997) conducted studies to identify barriers to donation and to identify strategies to increase donation rates among African Americans. Common findings from their studies include the importance of (1) community education, (2) the use of culturally appropriate messengers, (3) having family discussions, and (4) the use of African American coordinators. Across the study groups, two factors were predictive of willingness to donate: (1) having a family discussion about organ donation and (2) understanding that the medical teams that save lives are separate from the transplant medical teams. Among the critical problems identified was that insufficient programs are targeted toward minorities.

The Literature and Study Findings

There were 21,990 transplants performed in 1999, 774 more than in 1998; however, 64,373 patients were on the waiting list at the end of 1998 (see Table 9.1). As of October 28, 2000, the waiting list had increased to 72,585 patients; it was more than 11 percent greater than it had been at the end of 1998 (UNOS, 2000). UNOS policies allow patients to be listed at more than one transplant center; therefore the number of registrants is greater than the actual number of patients. The number of patients who died awaiting an organ transplant in 1999 was slightly more than 6,000, compared to slightly more than 5,000 in 1998.

Nationally, data from the *1999 Annual Report of the U.S. Scientific Registry of Transplant Recipients and the Organ Procurement and Transplantation Network* (UNOS, 1999) show that black cadaveric donors increased from 8.6 percent in 1989 to 11.3 percent in 1998 (see Table 9.1). By the last day in 1998, Hispanics represented

TABLE 9.1. PERCENTAGES OF CADAVERIC AND LIVING DONORS, RECIPIENTS, AND PEOPLE ON THE WAITING LIST BY RACE AND ETHNICITY, 1989 AND 1998.

	1989 (%)	1998 (%)
Donors, cadaveric	($N = 4,011$)	($N = 5,798$)
Asians	1.3	1.7
Blacks	8.6	11.3
Hispanics	7.5	10.3
Other	0.6	0.4
Whites	81.9	76.2
Donors, living	($N = 1,918$)	($N = 4,273$)
Asians	1.8	2.4
Blacks	11.3	12.5
Hispanics	8.8	10.6
Other	2.3	1.6
Whites	75.9	73.0
Recipients	($N = 13,178$)	($N = 21,363$)
Asians	2.2	3.1
Blacks	16.2	16.8
Hispanics	7.7	9.7
Other	2.3	1.6
Whites	71.6	68.8
Waiting list	($N = 19,093$)	($N = 64,373$)
Asians	3.9	4.1
Blacks	27.7	26.5
Hispanics	7.9	8.2
Other	1.0	1.0
Whites	59.5	60.3

Note: Based on data extracted from UNOS, 1998a, 1998b, 1999.

10.3 percent of the cadaveric donors, Asian Americans 1.7 percent, and whites 76.2 percent. Although there was an increase in the percentages of donors and recipients among the minorities from 1989 to 1998, there was also an increase in the number of patients on the transplant waiting list. Thus the gap between those needing transplants and the number of organs available for transplantation widened. This gap is disproportionately more evident for minority groups—especially among blacks. The *1999 Annual Report* data show that between 1989 and 1998, the total number of U.S. organ transplants increased 60 percent—from 13,082 to 20,989. Cadaveric donors increased 45 percent, from 4,011 in 1989 to 5,798 in 1998 (see Figure 9.1).

At the end of 1998, about 39 percent of those waiting for organ transplants were minority (African American, Hispanic, Asians, and others). Of those 25,282 patients, 66.7 percent were African American, 21 percent were Hispanic, and 10.2 percent were Asian. There were 10,071 cadaveric and living donors registered with the United Network for Organ Sharing (UNOS) in 1998 compared to 5,929 donors registered in 1989, a 70 percent increase in donors (according to data from the *1999 Annual Report,* UNOS, 1999). In 1998, 20,989 organs were transplanted, compared to 13,082 in 1989. The 1998 transplant recipient charac-

FIGURE 9.1. NUMBERS OF CADAVERIC DONORS, TRANSPLANTS, AND PEOPLE ON TRANSPLANT WAITING LIST.

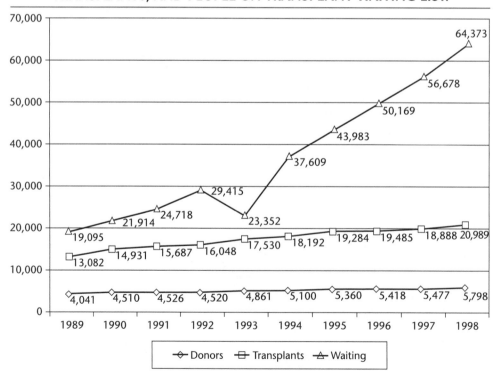

Note: Based on data extracted from UNOS, 1998a, 1998b, 1999.

teristics show that 16.8 percent of recipients were black, 9.7 percent Hispanic, and 3.1 percent Asian. In 1989, 16.2 percent of the transplant recipients were black, 7.7 percent Hispanic, and 2.2 percent Asian. In 1999, UNOS (2000) noted only ten more cadaveric donors than there had been in 1998. The number of transplants increased by 3 percent between 1998 and 1999 primarily because of the increase in the number of living donors and better use of the limited supply of available organs.

The organ in greatest demand for transplant is the kidney. According to U.S. Scientific Registry data (UNOS, 1999), as of September 30, 1999, there were 45,243 patients on the kidney waiting list (35 percent black, 48 percent white, 9 percent Hispanic, and 6 percent Asian). In 1998, there were 8,013 cadaveric kidney recipients (27 percent black, 56 percent white, 11 percent Hispanic, and 4 percent Asian).

These statistics provide compelling evidence of the status of the organ donation and transplantation health problem in our country, especially among black and other minority population groups. Educating the public about the importance of becoming an organ donor and having family discussions on the issue is a continuous need that must be addressed.

The Need for Donation

Current strategies for addressing the problem of insufficient donations in black and other minority communities include donor legislation, education campaigns, driver's license identification of organ donors, distribution of literature and organ donor cards, and community-based health education programs. In 1980, Clive Callender, the lead author of this chapter, implemented a grassroots pilot study at Howard University to identify the primary factors that influenced low donorship in the black community. This study found that after participating in structured interviews, 90 percent of the participants who had been initially unwilling to consent to donation signed organ donor cards. Their initial reluctance was based on several key factors: (1) lack of awareness of the need for organs among blacks, (2) religious beliefs and misperceptions, (3) distrust of the medical establishment, (4) fear of premature death (if they signed a donor card), and (5) a personal belief that blacks would not be the recipients of donated organs. After the interviews, 100 percent of those interviewed signed donor cards. Based on these findings, Callender and his associates (with representatives from local medical, political, educational, business, and religious communities) developed strategies from 1982 to 1988 to change the attitudes and behavior of black communities regarding organ and tissue donation.

Information was presented to African Americans by ethnically or racially appropriately spokespersons (organ donors, recipients, candidates for transplantation, families of cadaveric donors, and professionals). These messengers emphasized the need to increase the rate of organ and tissue donation and the importance of getting blood pressure measurements after the age of twelve. As a result, the number of donor cards signed by African Americans between 1982 and 1989 increased from 25 cards per month to 750 cards per month (Callender, Hall, et al., 1991). Black families were encouraged to hold family discussions about organ donation and transplantation and to include children in these discussions (Callender, Hall, Yeager, Washington, & Smith, 1994).

Results from other studies addressing the health needs of different minority population groups provide additional evidence that supports the need for continuing research to develop effective strategies to gain support for organ and tissue transplantation. Molina and Aguirre-Molina (1994) reported data from the Texas Kidney Health Program for the period 1978 to 1984 showing that Mexican Americans and African Americans were more likely to be treated for end-stage renal disease (ESRD) than whites. They further reported that Haffner et al. found in a 1992 study that Mexican Americans have a greater prevalence of proteinuria with diabetes than whites, an early indicator of renal disease in diabetics progressing to ESRD.

Callender and Washington (1997) reported that the blacks and Hispanics together exceed 40 percent of many dialysis and transplantation waiting lists and totaled more than 60 percent of some urban waiting lists. Kasiske et al. (1991) reported that for adult Native Americans living in the United States, the overall risk of ESRD is approximately threefold higher than it is for whites. Cruz and Hosten (1989) investigated the ESRD program at Howard University Hospital and concluded that black dialysis patients were younger than the average dialysis patient and therefore required more aggressive and less expensive therapies to prevent the premature onset of ESRD. This study suggested that prevention strategies combining educational, social, and economic programs are less costly than treatment and are viable approaches for addressing this kidney disease problem among African Americans.

Models, Approaches, and Interventions to Address Organ and Tissue Donation and Transplantation

As reported by the Lewin Group (1997), Kappel and associates in St. Louis, Missouri, examined efforts to increase organ donation among African Americans in a project with a public education–only component and a component that featured both public education and donation requestors who were also black. Their findings showed an increase in the number of African Americans referred for transplants in a twelve-month period (1988 to 1989) but a decrease in the number of African American donors in the public education-only component. The number of African American donors and the donation consent rates rose between 1989 and 1992 in the public education and minority requestor component of the study, suggesting the complementary nature of these components.

Dow Chemical Company and the National Association for the Advancement of Colored People (NAACP), under the auspices of Dow Chemical's Take Initiative Program (DOW-TIP), sponsored a donor education program in twenty-two cities with significant black populations. Donations increased among African Americans in cities where this program was presented. Levels of awareness and the number of blacks signing organ donor cards increased significantly between 1985 and 1990 (Callender, Hall, et al., 1994). Callender and colleagues further reported that this progress was associated with the development of messages specifically tailored to communities and with using ethnically similar volunteers, collaborative local efforts, and health education activities integrated with other neighborhood and community activities.

Callender, Burston, Burton, and Miles (1994) conducted a preliminary study in 1995 to assess the effectiveness of the Howard University Minority Organ/ Tissue Transplant Education Program (MOTTEP) seminars in changing the levels of knowledge, attitudes, and willingness to donate among audiences exposed to the MOTTEP presentations. Results indicated that statistically significant changes occurred in people's knowledge and attitudes toward organ transplantation after attending program seminars. Willingness to sign donor cards did not change significantly. Callender and Washington suggested community-based education programs as a powerful strategy for educating communities in order to bring about behavioral change that would increase the pool of organ and tissue donors and to promote health-related behaviors that would reduce the need for organ and tissue donations (Callender & Washington 1997). Molina and Aguirre-Molina (1994) also called for community-based health education strategies and considered community involvement critical for increasing awareness of health problems in Latino communities. Health education programs that include the community in program design and implementation, use community volunteers, and apply culturally appropriate strategies have been shown to be effective methods for the delivery of health education programs.

MOTTEP: An Exemplary Community-Based Model for Addressing Organ and Tissue Donation and Transplant Education

The national Minority Organ/Tissue Transplant Education Program, initially targeted to African Americans only, expanded its focus in 1995 to include Latinos (Hispanic), Asian Americans and Pacific Islanders, Alaskan Natives, and Native Americans. This multiyear demonstration research project has a national program and research office at Howard University Hospital in Washington, D.C., and fifteen local sites (Anchorage; Birmingham, Alabama; Los Angeles; Washington, D.C.; Miami, Florida; Atlanta; Honolulu; Chicago; Detroit; Albuquerque; Brooklyn; Cleveland; Nashville; Houston; and Richmond, Virginia). It has been largely funded by the National Institutes of Health (NIH). This program, the first of its kind in the country, was designed to (1) educate minority communities on facts about organ and tissue transplantation, (2) empower minority communities to develop transplant education programs that involve community members in addressing the shortage of donors, (3) increase minority participation in organ and tissue transplant endeavors, including signing organ donor cards, (4) encourage and increase family discussions about organ and tissue donations, (5) increase the number of minority individuals who donate organs and tissues, and (6) promote healthy lifestyle choices to prevent the need for transplantation.

The results of an outcome study on the effectiveness of the MOTTEP provided evidence of the program's ability to increase awareness and knowledge about organ and tissue donation in minority communities. The MOTTEP also contributed to changing the behavioral intentions of program participants, as confirmed by study results. Callender, Jones, Hall, Taylor, & Johnson (1998) conducted a pre- and postintervention study using data collected from a sample of 820 adults and youth who attended MOTTEP presentations on organ and tissue donation and disease prevention at churches, schools, hospitals, and other community settings in twelve cities during 1996 and 1997. These participants completed both a preintervention and a postintervention questionnaire. The preintervention questionnaire addressed six content areas: (1) thoughts on organ and tissue donation, (2) need for organ and tissue donation, (3) beliefs about organ and tissue donation, (4) future plans for organ and tissue donation, (5) disease prevention, and (6) background. The postintervention questionnaire addressed (1) the need for organ and tissue donation, (2) beliefs about organ and tissue donation, and (3) future plans. The objective of the study was to determine whether a culturally specific, community-implemented health education program could affect attitudes, knowledge, and behavior of different ethnic groups. The primary outcome measures were participant perceptions of the need for organ and tissue donation, beliefs about organ and tissue donation, and future plans concerning organ and tissue donation. There were significant increases ($p < .05$) in awareness of the need for organ and tissue donation and in knowledge about the facts concerning organ and tissue donation. The presentations appeared to change participants' beliefs, and participants were significantly more likely to say that they intended to become organ and tissue donors (Callender, Jones, et al., 1998). Additional outcomes based on 1997 to 1998 program data collected from more than 1,500 participants showed findings consistent with those from the previous year's results. Preliminary findings from the first wave of a telephone follow-up study of 258 people who attended MOTTEP presentations at least three months prior to the follow-up interview showed a significant ($p < .5$) difference in those holding family discussions after attending the MOTTEP presentations and those willing to donate their organs and the organs of their loved ones. The MOTTEP model is the first program of its kind to address the specific needs of the minority transplant community.

The MOTTEP successes also included reaching more than four million persons between 1995 and 1999 and inauguration of National Minority Donor Awareness Day in 1996. Held each August 1, this is a day for special efforts in educating minority communities. By 1999, the MOTTEP had generated over three billion impressions in the print, radio, and television media. The number of local volunteers who participate in MOTTEP initiatives has increased from sixty people in 1995 to five hundred people in 1999 (Callender, Miles, and Yeager, 1998; Callender, Hall, & Miles, 2000). The total number of youths reached by MOTTEP in 1999 was 80,245, compared to 19,504 in 1996. This represents an increase of over 300 percent. The MOTTEP model incorporates the delivery of health messages that are culturally appropriate and delivered by ethnically similar messengers recognized by the community. These strategies are consistent with earlier strategies identified by researchers that called for tailoring health messages to target communities and for the use of ethnically similar volunteers, transplant recipients, donors, donor families, and patients awaiting transplantation as the appropriate spokespersons (Callender, Burston, et al., 1994).

This national program includes elements of grassroots community mobilization, health promotion, and social marketing. The grassroots approach was used because of its past effectiveness in organizing, empowering, and mobilizing black communities to address pressing social, political, and civil problems, as in the 1960s civil rights movement and throughout black history (Callender, Hall, et al., 1994). The guiding principles of grassroots strategy include (1) centrally involving key local stakeholders, (2) organizing to discuss issues needing community solutions and strategies, (3) understanding personal and environmental issues (context) initiatives, and (4) using personal and community skills and strengths to effect change. Another characteristic of grassroots strategy is the commonality of language among those involved. Henry (1990) addresses the use of "public language," which means language that reflects shared norms and implicit understanding (a central norm in African American culture), in his discussion of African American culture and politics. The involvement of ethnically similar messengers meets this need for commonality of language and ensures that there is little dissonance between the value of the message and the authenticity of the messenger. More recently, Berger and Neuhaus (1996) have discussed the value, place, and empowerment of neighborhood, family, church, and volunteer associations (that is, mediating structures), in support of the idea that persons in communities are best situated to answer local problems and to order their own lives together. In this model, health care professionals serve in auxiliary and support roles to provide resources and technical assistance as appropriate to local programs. This is especially valuable because minority communities have limited numbers of health care professionals and professionals in related fields. This model supports and uses methods that create an atmosphere that encourages open communication between local organizations and the medical community and creates linkages to other members of the lay community. This strategy encourages the formation of coalitions, ethnically sensitive role models, and localized health messages in ethnically oriented media.

Other theories and studies that focused on addressing community empowerment, capacity building for local action, coalition building, and sustaining organizations and that also influenced the MOTTEP model are Wandersman (1985); Smith and Macaulay (1980); Rothman (1970); Wright, Naylor, Werter, Bauer, and Sutcliffe (1997); and Flora, Schoolar, and Pierson, (1997). Common to all these studies is a focus on community social forces that can influence behavior.

The MOTTEP's grassroots foundation also incorporates social marketing principles as exemplified by the DOW-TIP effort between 1986 and 1992. These were important in designing health promotion activities that emphasize lifestyle changes based on the needs, norms, and values of the target population. The social marketing approach that MOTTEP uses for its activities is similar to the approach addressed in the work of Flora, Schoolar, and Pierson (1997), who examined the role of culture in developing effective health promotion in communities of color using principles of social marketing. The disproportionate morbidity and mortality experienced by underrepresented racial and ethnic groups in the United States highlights the need for more effective health promotion. Flora and associates discuss designing and delivering health messages in light of a racial or ethnic group's history with the health care system, culturally specific views about health issues, and cultural barriers to change. They further state that health messages should be delivered through appropriate channels (community leaders, electronic and print media, and organizations and institutions such as schools, churches and work sites). Social marketing concepts offer a useful framework for the development, implementation, and evaluation of health promotion programs targeted for people of color.

The Structure of the MOTTEP

The national MOTTEP office engages in program marketing and public relations, conducts research studies, designs health messages and disease prevention materials, develops linkages, and collaborates with related organizations addressing organ and tissue donation and transplantation problems. Local MOTTEP sites develop strategic plans to (1) implement locally developed MOTTEP initiatives, (2) establish local advisory boards to guide program development and implementation, (3) collect program evaluation data, and (4) seek additional funding to sustain their programs beyond the program grant period. All local MOTTEP sites adopt the national MOTTEP mission but develop goals and objectives, strategies, and program activities based on local culture and community values.

Community members (volunteers, donor families, transplant recipients, patients on transplant lists, program coordinators, and others) deliver health education messages that are culturally sensitive and targeted to ethnic groups. The community members are ethnically similar to the groups they address. Intervention strategies are designed by the local MOTTEP staff and their advisory boards. Local MOTTEP sites also participate in the MOTTEP cross-site evaluation study designed by the national office in collaboration with an external evaluation team and the local MOTTEP coordinators.

The MOTTEP model integrates the same elements as those considered critical by Bracht and Kingsbury (1990) in their five-stage health promotion model for community-based health education. This health promotion model is based on stimulating conditions for changing and mobilizing citizens and communities for health action. This community organizing process will maintain citizen interest, nurture program participation, and encourage support for sustaining and institutionalizing successful interventions. A fundamental principle of this model is community ownership, allowing community members to shape the direction of the program. Table 9.2 presents some key elements of MOTTEP that fit the stages of the Bracht and Kingsbury model.

TABLE 9.2. MOTTEP COMMUNITY-BASED HEALTH PROMOTION MODEL.

Stages	Some Key Elements
1. Community analysis	Defining the community Assessing community capacities and barriers Assessing community readiness for change
2. Design and initiation	Establishing a core planning group of community members, organizations, and agencies Establishing the local MOTTEP organizational structure Defining the mission and goals of the local MOTTEP Clarifying the roles and responsibilities of the local MOTTEP advisory board members, staff, and volunteers Acquiring appropriate training to enhance local MOTTEP capacity
3. Implementation	Generating community participation Developing a strategic plan for intervention activities Using multiple strategies with the potential to influence community norms Integrating community values into program materials and health messages Evaluating the program (data collection for national MOTTEP evaluation research studies) Conducting twice yearly three-day workshops for local program coordinators Carrying out annual site visits to provide ongoing assessment and program improvement
4. Program maintenance and consolidation	Integrating intervention activities into community networks Establishing regular communication links with other local MOTTEP programs Developing strategies for ongoing recruitment of staff and volunteers in long-term projects Disseminating information to the advisory board and community on project activities and evaluation results Functioning as a national minority transplant resource center
5. Dissemination and reassessment	Proposal development for future program funding Reviewing outcomes from program effectiveness studies Updating the community analysis Revising the strategic plan to include new program directions and modifications

Note: Based on the Bracht and Kingsbury (1990) five-stage community health promotion model.

In stages 1 and 2, local MOTTEP sites provide the national MOTTEP office with a comprehensive overview of the local community (values, beliefs, knowledge levels, and norms) to better inform the national staff and to guide the development of the best strategies to promote changes in attitudes and behavior (these are stages of change and motivational influences on behavior). In stage 3, local MOTTEP coordinators work with their advisory boards to ensure that local stakeholders are used as community educators. These and other ethnically similar health messengers generate the interest and involvement of the community in planning programs reflecting community norms and values. The strategies include presenting personal testimonies; participating in health fairs; conducting media campaigns; distributing literature; making presentations to organizations, churches, schools, and businesses; and participating in meetings and conferences. Program maintenance and consolidation initiatives (stage 4) solidify MOTTEP in the community. The primary activities of local MOTTEP sites in stage 5 are planning for the future by identifying funding sources and preparing proposals to sustain their programs beyond the NIH demonstration research period.

The National MOTTEP Office and Its Mandate

The national MOTTEP office serves as a catalytic agent that stimulates and also collaborates with local MOTTEP sites. This office provides technical assistance and national data, it assists local sites in developing their programs, and it supports them in fundraising initiatives. The national office hosts training workshops for all local site coordinators, maintains regular contact with the local national program coordinators, and visits local sites during the program year. The intent is to support capacity building at the local level.

The national office also collaborates with related health organizations to gain MOTTEP recognition in the larger organ and tissue donation community. Other efforts include establishing national minority organ and tissue donation awareness days; providing achievement awards for local MOTTEP programs; honoring organizations and individuals that have contributed significantly to addressing this health issue; and participating in local, national, and international conferences, symposia, and meetings addressing organ and tissue donation and disease prevention.

Rigorous program evaluation, a core value of the national MOTTEP office and integrated throughout the program design, demands that the MOTTEP be systematically planned, bounded, organized, and implemented using theory and best practices to assure the evaluability of the program. The MOTTEP evaluators conduct both process and outcome studies. The process evaluation studies are used for program monitoring, feedback, and planning and for program implementation that details and documents what the program is actually delivering to the communities. The outcome evaluation studies assess whether MOTTEP is making a difference in the local communities. Evaluation studies to date include (1) a preliminary outcome study to determine how audiences responded to MOTTEP seminars and educational materials (Callender, Burston, et al., 1994); (2) a pre-post cross-sectional outcome study to assess changes in attitudes, beliefs, thoughts, behavioral intentions (future plans), and disease prevention activities of participants at selected MOTTEP presentations (Callender, Burston, et al., 1994; Callender, Jones, et al., 1998); and (3) a preliminary follow-up study to examine short-term gains in behavioral change (Callender & Hall, 2000). Figure 9.2 presents the MOTTEP model and highlights the key components in the model.

Local MOTTEP interventions and strategies are designed to contribute to accomplishing expected program outcomes—to significantly increase organ donation, reduce the need for transplantation, and promote good health behaviors in local communities. The program works to achieve the short-term (immediate) and intermediate outcomes that communities must accomplish to achieve desired long-term program outcomes.

FIGURE 9.2. MOTTEP MODEL.

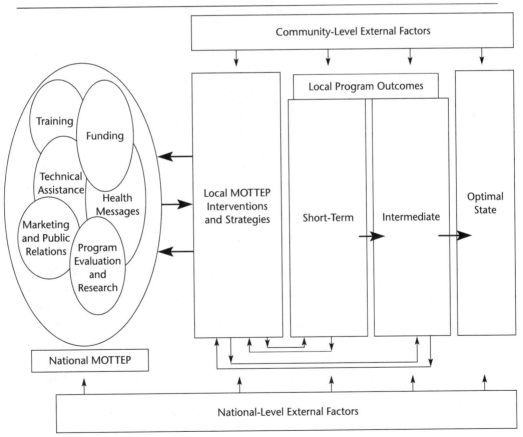

Program Implications for Minority Communities

The MOTTEP model is fundamentally a successful grassroots health promotion model, with theoretical underpinnings found in several behavioral theories and health promotion models. Many of the barriers and challenges that have faced blacks concerning organ donation and transplantation are quite similar to those facing other ethnic minority communities—lack of awareness of the problem, a disproportionately high rate of diabetes and hypertension, religious fears, lack of trust of the medical system, and fear of mutilation. Like blacks, other minorities exhibit significant gaps between the size of the donor pool and the number of minority patients on the waiting lists. Strategies that were being used in MOTTEP prior to 1995 are strategies that have been found effective in other minority communities. Collaboration with members of the Asian American and Pacific Islander, Native American, Alaskan Native, and Latino communities has now resulted in the expansion of the MOTTEP to include a focus on multiple ethnic population groups. Using behavioral objectives has ensured that the enhanced MOTTEP focuses on unique community action to bring about desired health behavior change or the intention to change behavior. At the same time, all MOTTEP sites are connected by adoption of the national MOTTEP mission and supported by all the communities involved.

As a result of this health education, health promotion, and disease prevention program and NIH funding, the national MOTTEP office has successfully initiated and supported fifteen local MOTTEP sites for five years. The evaluation results provide evidence that MOTTEP presentations significantly (1) increased community awareness about the need for organ and donation, (2) increased the knowledge level of program participants on facts about organ and tissue donation, and (3) increased the number of participants who expressed their intentions to become organ and tissue donors in black, Latino, and Asian American and Pacific Islander communities.

MOTTEP is philosophically committed to inclusion—paying close attention to the culture, norms, and values of different ethnic communities—as the basic premise for building successful local programs. The MOTTEP is locally owned yet linked with all other local MOTTEP programs and the national MOTTEP office in a learning community. Community organizations and stakeholders are responsible for planning and implementing local MOTTEP programs (ensuring community buy-in and ownership) with support from the national MOTTEP office. The application of culturally appropriate social marketing principles for community mobilization programs ensures that interventions are appropriately targeted and delivered by messengers who are ethnically similar to and acceptable to the targeted community.

The MOTTEP provides a community-based model for a national program that fits comfortably in local communities through the inclusion of those communities and their stakeholders in the program design, implementation, and assessment process. This program begins to suggest some ways to contribute to closing the gap between the numbers of those needing transplants and the potential donor pool and to promote disease prevention to reduce the need for organ and tissue transplantation among minority population groups.

MOTTEP Summary

This successful grassroots health education model uses community values, assets, and norms for achieving success. Solutions are generated by community members who are most affected by problems—those with no special knowledge or training concerning the problems being addressed (Callender, Hall, et al., 1994). Communities engage in discussions with problem area experts to gain more knowledge to solve community problems using the *community family*, grassroots empowerment, and community organizing. Sabl (1999), in his discussion on community organizing and Tocquevillean politics, describes similar fundamentals for organizing minority communities during the civil rights movement of the 1950s and 1960s. Not unlike those communities and organizations that supported civil rights activities, MOTTEP communities "take in" national MOTTEP staff and program consultants, accepting them as honorary community members. This process legitimizes the outside experts, making them partners with each community in its local effort to develop appropriate strategies and methods for implementing health education and health promotion initiatives.

The MOTTEP also integrates elements from several theories of behavioral change and from social marketing approaches. These include (1) the social marketing and community mobilization model (Middlestadt, Schechter, Peyton, & Tjugum, 1997), (2) the theory of reasoned action and planned behavior (Ajzen & Fishbein, 1980), (3) the transtheoretical model of behavior change (Prochaska, DiClemente, & Norcross, 1992), and (4) the principles of social marketing and the role of culture in effective health promotion (Flora et al., 1997).

Implications of the MOTTEP model are that ultimately, if enough community members practice improved behaviors over time, health indicators will provide evidence of significant increases in the donation rates among minority groups (which is currently the case). Further, health indicators will provide evidence that the need for transplantation has decreased because of improved health (this is not yet the case). However, this model also understands that external factors at both the local and national levels influence community behavior and norms and must therefore be accounted for (or acknowledged) when attempting to determine the influence of MOTTEP on contributing to positive changes in organ and tissue donation and transplantation.

Conclusion: Future Directions for Research and Practice

Insufficient organ and tissue donation is the major barrier to transplantation. Increasing the number of donors in all population groups and emphasizing healthy lifestyles must become a value and priority among all ethnic groups. Much more must be done to educate communities and change their values and behaviors regarding organ and tissue donation and transplantation. Developing effective health education programs at the community level needs to be supported in significant ways in minority communities to increase organ and tissue donation and prevent the need for transplantation. More science-based studies are needed to test the effectiveness of these types of health education, disease prevention, and health promotion models. Demonstration research programs need to be funded at significant levels to provide opportunities for more science-based research studies in minority communities. Current evidence suggests that community-based programs with national support can work to support behavioral change and can change individuals' health and wellness norms and values. Opportunities to discuss the findings in the field and exchange information need to be provided through conferences and media formats. As long as the disparities between donors and recipients remain and as long as the transplant waiting lists continue to grow, the problem remains—for blacks, other minorities, and the population at large.

To date the MOTTEP health education program is the only comprehensive demonstration research study that has examined organ and tissue donation and transplantation across multiple ethnic minority groups. Earlier exploratory studies funded by the Health Resources and Services Administration (Hall, 1991; Harris & Hall, 1990) that focused on the race of the donation requestor and the role of the church in the black community did not produce significant findings. Sustained behavioral changes among participants need to be assessed to determine the model's ability to contribute to achieving long-term outcomes. Longitudinal studies should be conducted to determine whether MOTTEP participants maintained their changed attitudes and behavioral intentions and behaviors over time. Another prevention-oriented strategy that we continue to suggest is checking for hypertension. This is a critical first step toward prevention of kidney failure, heart attacks, and stroke.

A more thorough examination should be undertaken of the MOTTEP model and of other social marketing, health education, and health promotion models that have been applied to implementing community health programs. There is also a need to identify among multi-ethnic people shared or similar values, principles, and beliefs that contribute to improved health and health behavior. Enhanced knowledge of these domains will contribute to developing ethnically appropriate interventions for replication and adaptation in local minority communities. More prevention initiatives, designed to enhance health and prevent the need for donation and transplantation, could be developed. As has been often stated by the authors and their colleagues, this is still the tip of the iceberg; the work to close the gap continues. The appendix to this chapter lists a number of organizations that can be contacted to learn more about organ and tissue donation.

Appendix: Resources

National Minority Organ Tissue Transplant Education Program (MOTTEP)
Howard University Hospital, Ambulatory Care Center
2041 Georgia Avenue, Suite 3100
Washington, DC 20060
Ms. Patrice Miles, Executive Director
(800) 393-2839; (202) 865-4888

Coalition on Donation
1110 Boulders Parkway, Suite 500
Richmond, VA 23225-8770
(804) 330-8620

United Network for Organ Sharing
1100 Boulders Parkway, Suite 500
P.O. Box 13770
Richmond, VA 23225-8770
(888) TXINFO1; (804) 330-8576

Health Resources and Services Administration (HRSA)
Office of Special Programs
Division of Transplantation
5600 Fishers Lane
Rockville, MD 20857

National Kidney Foundation
30 East 33rd Street, Suite 1100
New York, NY 10016
(800) 622-9010; (212) 889-2210

American Kidney Fund
6110 Executive Boulevard, Suite 1010
Rockville, MD 20852
(800) 638-8299

Transplant Recipients International Organization
1000 16th Street NW, Suite 602
Washington, DC 20036-5705
(800) TRIO-386; (202) 293-0980

References

Ajzen, I., & Fishbein, M. (1980). *Understanding attitudes and predicting social behavior*. Upper Saddle River, NJ: Prentice Hall.

Berger, P. L., & Neuhaus, R. J. (1996). *To empower people* (2nd ed.). Washington, DC: American Enterprise Institute.

Bracht, N., & Kingsbury, L. (1990). Community organization principles in health promotion: A five-stage model. In N. Bracht (Ed.), *Health promotion at the community level* (pp. 66–83). Thousand Oaks, CA: Sage.

Callender, C. O., Burston, B. W., Burton, L. W., & Miles, P. (1994). *An assessment of the impact of the national Minority Organ Tissue Transplant Education Program* (Annual report for HIDDK, NIH). Washington, DC: Howard University Hospital, Ambulatory Care Center.

Callender, C. O., & Hall, M. B. (2000). *Sustained change among youth and adults participating in MOTTEP presentations: A follow-up study*. Unpublished MOTTEP research report, Howard University, Washington, DC.

Callender, C. O., Hall, M. B., & Miles, P. V. (2000). *A national public education campaign to promote disease prevention and minority donor awareness*. Unpublished MOTTEP slide presentation, Howard University, Washington, DC.

Callender, C. O., Hall, L. E., Yeager, C. L., Barber, J. B., Dunston, G. A., & Pinn-Wiggins, V. S. (1991). Special report, organ donation and blacks: A critical frontier. *New England Journal of Medicine, 324*, 442–444.

Callender, C. O., Hall, L. E., Yeager, C. L., Washington, A. W., & Smith, P. G. (1994). The anatomy of a black community-based transplant education program: A model for community empowerment. In A. Dula & S. Goerin (Eds.), *It just ain't fair: The ethics of health care for African Americans* (pp. 234–243). Westport, CT: Praeger.

Callender, C. O., Jones, D. J., Hall, M. B., Taylor, R., & Johnson, R. (1998). *Assessing the effectiveness of the MOTTEP program, 1996–1997 data* (Unpublished research report by MBH Limited under contract to the MOTTEP project). Washington, DC: Howard University.

Callender, C. O., Miles, P., & Yeager, C. L. (1998, January–February). Organ transplantation in cardiovascular and related disease. *ABC Digest of Urban Cardiology*, pp. 8–15.

Callender, C. O., & Washington, A. W. (1997). Organ/tissue donation the problem! Education the solution: A review. *Journal of the National Medical Association, 89*, 878–893.

Cruz, I. A., & Hosten, A. O. (1989). An update of the end-stage renal disease program at Howard University. *Transplant Procedures, 21*, 3892–3894.

Flora, J. A., Schoolar, C., & Pierson, R. M. (1997). Effective health promotion among communities of color: The potential of social marketing. In M. E. Goldberg, M. Fishbein, & S. E. Middlestadt (Eds.), *Social marketing: Theoretical and practical perspectives* (pp. 353–368). Mahwah, NJ: Erlbaum.

Gentry, D., Brown-Holbert, J., & Andrews, C. (1997). Racial impact: Increasing minority consent rate by altering the racial mix of an organ procurement organization. *Transplant Procedures, 29*(8), 3758–3759.

Hall, M. B. (1991). Organ/tissue donation: Does the race of the requestor make a difference? Final report to the Department of Transportation, Health Resources, and Services Administration. Contract to HMR, Inc., Landover, MD.

Harris, J., & Hall, M. B. (1990). The role of the church and clergy in organ/tissue donation in African American communities. Final report to the Department of Transportation,

Health Resources, and Services Administration. Contract to ROW Sciences, Inc., Rockville, MD.

Henry, C. P. (1990). *Culture and African American politics.* Bloomington: Indiana University Press.

Kappel, D. F., Whitlock, M. E., & Schutte, L. (1993). Increasing African American organ donation: The St. Louis experience. *Transplant Procedures, 25*(4), 2489–2490.

Kasiske, B. L., Neylan, J. F., III, Riggio, R. R., Danovitch, G. M., Kahana, L., Alexander, S. R., & White, M. G. (1991). The effect of race on access and outcome in transplantation. *New England Journal of Medicine, 324,* 302–307.

The Lewin Group. (1997). *Evaluability of organ donation strategies: Literature review.* Unpublished technical report prepared under contract HHE-1097-100-10097-0012 for the U.S. Department of Health and Human Services, Office of the Assistant Secretary for Planning and Evaluation.

Middlestadt, S. E., Schechter, C., Peyton, J., & Tjugum, B. (1997). Community involvement in health planning: Lessons learned from practicing social marketing in a context of community control, participating and ownership. In M. E. Goldberg, M. Fishbein, & S. E. Middlestadt (Eds.), *Social marketing: Theoretical and practical perspectives* (pp. 45–76). Mahwah, NJ: Erlbaum.

Molina, C. W., & Aguirre-Molina, M. (Eds.). (1994). *Latino health in the U.S.: A growing challenge.* Washington, DC: American Public Health Association.

Oberley, E. T., Sacksteder, P. A., Curtin, R. B., Calder, A. E., & Binder, D. J. (1991). *Public education in organ and tissue donation: Review and recommendations.* Washington, DC: Medical Media Publishing.

Partnership for Organ Donation. (1998). *Organ donation and ethnicity: Predictors of support for organ donation among ethnic groups.* Boston: Author.

Prochaska, J. O., DiClemente, C.F.C., & Norcross, J. C. (1992). In search of how people change: Applications to addictive behavior. *American Psychologist, 47,* 1102–1114.

Rothman, J. (1970). Three models of community organization practice. In F. M. Cos, J. L. Erlich, J. Rothman, & J. E. Trotman (Eds.), *Strategies of community organization* (pp. 20–36). Itasca, IL: Peacock,

Sabl, A. (1999). *Community organizing as Tocquevillean politics: The art of association and the overcoming of democratic servility.* Unpublished paper, Vanderbilt University, Nashville, TN.

Smith, D. H., & Macaulay, J. (1980). *Participation in social and political activities: A comprehensive analysis of political involvement, expressive leisure time and helping behavior.* San Francisco: Jossey-Bass.

Townsend, M. E., Rovelli, M. A., Schweizer, R. T. (1990). Value of discussion groups in educating blacks about organ donation and transplantation. *Transplant Procedures, 22* (2), 324–325.

United Network for Organ Sharing. (1998a). *Snapshot of patient registrations on the National Transplant Waiting List* [On-line]. Available: www.unos.org/newsroom/critdata-htm

United Network for Organ Sharing. (1998b). *UNOS Update: Data Highlights.* [On-line]. Available: www.unos.org

United Network for Organ Sharing. (1999, April 27). *Annual Report of the U.S. Scientific Registry of Transplant Recipients and the Organ Procurement and Transplantation Network: Transplant Data 1989–1998* [On-line]. Available: www.unos.org.Data/anrpt_main.htm

United Network for Organ Sharing. (2000, April 18). *News Release.* [On-line]. Available: www.unos.org/Newsroom/archive_newsrelease_20000418_donornumbers.htm

Wandersman, A. (1985). Psychology and community. In K. Heller (Ed.), *Psychology and community change: Challenges of the future* (pp. 337–339). Homewood, IL: Governance.

Wright, A. L., Naylor, A., Werter, R., Bauer, M., & Sutcliffe, E. (1997). Using cultural knowledge in health promotion: Breastfeeding among the Navajo. *Health Education and Behavior, 24,* 626–639.

PART THREE

CHRONIC DISEASES

CHAPTER TEN

HYPERTENSION AND OTHER RISK FACTORS FOR STROKE

John M. Flack, Navdeep K. Mann,
Preeti Ramappa, Jaiwant K. Rangi

Stroke is the third leading cause of death in the United States, after coronary heart disease and cancer. Among African Americans, stroke is the third and sixth leading cause of death in men and women, respectively (Gillum, 1999). Overall risk of stroke is higher among African Americans than among whites (Figure 10.1) (Gillum, 1999). The excess relative risk for African Americans, relative to whites, is greatest at the younger to middle ages and declines progressively until the stroke mortality rates for the two groups cross over in the ninth decade of life (Howard, Anderson, et al, 1994; National Center for Health Statistics, 1998). The Atherosclerosis Risk in Communities (ARIC) Study (Rosamond et al., 1999) found, among 15,792 men and women aged forty-five to sixty-four, that ischemic stroke incidence rank-ordered as African American men > African American women > white men > white women. However, the overall 141 percent excess in African Americans relative to whites attenuated to a 38 percent excess after adjustment for baseline hypertension, diabetes, educational level, smoking status, and prevalent coronary heart disease. These data highlight the importance of potentially modifiable risk factors as contributors to the excess stroke among African Americans. For unclear reasons, African Americans appear to suffer relatively fewer strokes attributable to extracranial carotid atherosclerosis than whites (Wityk et al., 1996). Also, Gillum and coworkers have reported that stroke case-fatality rates are higher among African Americans than whites (Gillum, 1999; Qureshi et al., 1997). African Americans also have higher rates of intracranial and subarachnoid hemorrhage than non-Hispanic whites (Rosamond et al., 1999; Broderick, Brott, Tomsick, Miller, & Huster, 1993; Sacco, Boden-Albala, et al., 1998; Broderick et al., 1998; Qureshi et al., 1997).

FIGURE 10.1. STROKE DEATH RATES BY RACE AND SEX, 1996.

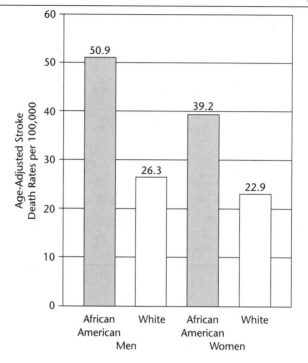

Source: Adapted from Gillum, 1999, pp. 1711–1712.

The long-term secular decline in stroke risk in the African American and white populations has slowed considerably since the mid-1980s (Cooper, McGee, Liao, & Durazo-Arvizu, 1996). Moreover, the absolute number of stroke deaths in African Americans increased by more than 8 percent between 1992 and 1996 (Gillum, 1999). Furthermore, the risk of stroke recurrence in first-time stroke survivors is 140 percent greater in African Americans and 190 percent greater in Hispanics compared to whites (Sheinart et al., 1998). Hispanics also have higher stroke rates than whites (Sacco, Boden-Albala, et al., 1998). Other populations manifesting high stroke rates are those in China, Japan, and Eastern European countries such as Hungary and Czechoslovakia (He, Klag, Wu, & Whelton, 1995; Gillum, 1996). Interestingly, stroke mortality is much higher among Czechoslovakian men and women than among same-sex African Americans (Gillum, 1999).

Modifiable or Potentially Modifiable Risk Factors

This section examines the relationship of high blood pressure to stroke, especially ischemic stroke, and discusses what is known about modifying this risk. It also looks at a number of other risk factors including lifestyle factors.

Blood Pressure

In numerous epidemiological studies hypertension has been shown to be the most important modifiable risk factor linked to increased risk of stroke (Kannel et al., 1981; Cutler, 1996; MacMahon et al., 1990; Strandgaard, 1996; American Heart Association, 1995). Table 10.1 displays the major stroke subtypes and their relative frequency of occurrence, and Table 10.2 lists the risk factors for the most common subtype, ischemic strokes.

Hypertension is a major risk factor for ischemic stroke, subarachnoid hemorrhage, and intracranial hemorrhage. Hypertension is more prevalent, manifests an earlier onset, and is associated with more cardiovascular-renal target-organ injury and mortality in African Americans than in whites in the U.S. adult population—even at similar levels of blood pressure (Burt et al., 1995; Flack, Gardin, Yunis, & Liu, 1999; Flack, Neaton, Daniels, & Esunge, 1993). The age-adjusted prevalence of hypertension among adult African Americans is 32.4 percent compared with 23.3 percent for non-Hispanic whites and 22.6 percent for Mexican Americans (Burt et al., 1995). The stroke risk gradient is incrementally greater at higher levels of both systolic and diastolic blood pressure, though the gradient is steeper for systolic blood pressure. Nevertheless, stroke mortality risk is ten- to twelvefold higher in the highest levels of diastolic blood pressure compared to the lowest (MacMahon & Rodgers, 1994). Systolic blood pressure rises with advancing age whereas diastolic blood pressure falls progressively after the mid-sixth decade of life. Thus, not surprisingly, isolated systolic hypertension (systolic blood pressure ≥ 160 and diastolic blood pressure < 90 mmHg) is the most common hypertension phenotype after seventy years of age. Isolated systolic hypertension shows a predilection for older females, particularly African American women (Cornoni-Huntley, LaCroix, & Havlik, 1989). Though stroke risk rises

TABLE 10.1. CLASSIFICATION OF STROKE.

Ischemic (85% of Cases)

• Thrombotic
   Large-artery
   Small-artery (lacunar type)
• Embolic
   Cardiogenic
   Artery-to-artery
   Aortic arch atheroma

Hemorrhagic (15% of Cases)

• Intracranial
• Subarachnoid
   Aneurysmal rupture
   Arteriovenous malformation

Source: Adapted from Adams, R. D., Victor, M., & Ropper, H. (Eds.) (1997). *Principles of Neurology,* (p.807). NY: McGraw-Hill.

TABLE 10.2. RISK FACTORS FOR ISCHEMIC STROKE.

Nonmodifiable	Modifiable and Well Documented
• Age	• Hypertension
• Male sex	• Atrial fibrillation
• Race/ethnicity	• Mitral stenosis
African American	• Recent myocardial infarction
Hispanic	• Infective endocarditis
Japanese	• Left ventricular hypertrophy
Chinese	• Cigarette smoking
• Heredity	• Diabetes mellitus
• Previous atherothrombotic	• TIA/history of stroke
brain infarction	• Asymptomatic carotid stenosis

Not as Well Documented

• Cardiac diseases	• Physical inactivity
Cardiomyopathies	• Hypercoagulability
Mitral annular calcification	• Hyperinsulinemia
Mitral valve prolapse	• Elevated hematocrit
Valvular strands	• Dietary salt
Aortic stenosis	• Obesity
Patent foramen ovale	• Low HDL cholesterol
Atrial septal aneurysm	• Raised triglycerides
Nonbacterial endocarditis	• Low dietary magnesium
• Elevated cholesterol	• Low dietary calcium
• Oral contraceptives	• Low dietary potassium
• Heavy alcohol consumption	

Source: Adapted from Sacco, Benjamin, et al., 1997.

exponentially with age, the relative risk associated with hypertension declines progressively from an odds ratio of 4 at age fifty to an odds ratio of 1 by age ninety.

The identification of blood pressure as a risk factor for stroke would be less meaningful if hypertension treatment had not been shown to reduce stroke risk (Joint National Committee . . ., 1997). Pharmacological treatment of hypertension in African Americans has been shown to reduce stroke risk (Hypertension Detection and Follow-up Program Cooperative Group, 1979), an observation that is consonant with the results of numerous other placebo-controlled hypertension treatment trials (Collins et al., 1990; Gueyffier, Bulpitt, et al., 1999; Fagard & Staessen, 1999; Systolic Hypertension in the Elderly Program [SHEP] Cooperative Research Group, 1991; Lisheng, 1996; Staessen et al., 1997). The majority of individuals in these trials had either combined systolic and diastolic hypertension or isolated systolic hypertension. The reduction of stroke risk with hypertension treatment has not only been proven for the primary prevention of stroke but has also been demonstrated to reduce the risk of stroke in persons surviving their initial stroke (secondary prevention) (Gueyffier, Boissel, et al., 1997).

There are no data, however, available regarding the solitary influence of dietary and lifestyle modifications (that is, sodium restriction, dietary potassium augmentation, reduced saturated fat intake, weight loss, or increased physical activity), alone or in combination with one another, on stroke risk. However, there are experimental data that are consonant with epidemiological data in suggesting a plausible role for high levels of dietary sodium and low intake of potassium, calcium, and magnesium in the pathogenesis of blood pressure elevation or vascular injury potentially leading to stroke (Iso, Stampfer, et al., 1999; Xie, Sasaki, Joossens, & Kesteloot, 1992; Fang, Madhavan, & Alderman, 2000). Therefore it seems prudent to encourage the aforementioned, multifaceted lifestyle interventions to lower both blood pressure and cholesterol levels, given the ability of both of these interventions to lower stroke risk.

Though the majority of the aforementioned epidemiological and clinical trial data were not derived specifically from African Americans, there seems to be no convincing reason not to extrapolate the benefits of treatment of either hypertension or hypercholesterolemia to the high-risk African American population. Thus, successful hypertension treatment represents perhaps the major pharmacological intervention strategy for stroke risk reduction. Only 25 percent of the almost six million African American hypertensives have achieved blood pressure levels < 140/90 mmHg (Burt et al., 1995). Moreover, fewer than 50 percent of drug-treated hypertensive African Americans have attained blood pressure levels < 140/90 mmHg (Burt et al., 1995). Lack of systolic blood pressure control has been the predominant reason that adults have not reduced blood pressure levels to < 140/90 mmHg. We recently reported from the National Health and Nutrition Examination Survey (NHANES) III data set that 63 percent of hypertensive adults with blood pressure levels ≥ 140/90 mmHg have elevated systolic blood pressure; 49.7 percent of these individuals had only systolic blood pressure elevations (Flack et al., 2000).

Blood Pressure and Geography

The influence of hypertension on stroke risk in African Americans may, to a degree, be confounded by geography (Obisesan, Vargas, & Gillum, 2000; Cushman et al., 2000; Perry & Roccella, 1998). The African American population lives preferentially in the Southeastern United States. Approximately one-half of the thirty million African American U.S. residents live in thirty Southeastern states. Stroke mortality rates are higher for African American as well as for white men and women residing in the Southeast compared to rates for race and sex matched individuals living outside this geographic region (Pickle, Mungiole, & Gillum, 1997). Nevertheless, stroke mortality risk is not uniform among Southeastern U.S. African Americans; both men and women, residing in nonmetropolitan areas (both within and outside of the Southeastern United States) have higher stroke mortality rates than their metropolitan counterparts do (Gillum & Ingram, 1996).

Does hypertension have a role in this geographic disparity? Hypertension prevalence is greater among African American women and men who reside in the Southeastern United States than it is among race and sex matched individuals residing elsewhere (Obisesan et al., 2000) (Figure 10.2); a similar observation has been made for middle-aged non-Hispanic white men and older non-Hispanic white men. Both within and outside the Southeastern United States, African American men, but not women, residing in nonmetropolitan areas manifest borderline higher odds of hypertension (odds ratio = 1.38; 95 percent confidence internal, 0.97 to 1.68) relative to same-sex metropolitan residents (Gillum & Ingram, 1996). Nevertheless, hypertension awareness and treatment rates for African American men and women living in the Southeast are either similar to awareness and rates outside that region or favor the nonmetropolitan regions in regard to predicting a lower stroke risk (Obisesan et al., 2000). Paradoxically, blood pressure control rates were actually higher for Southeastern African American nonmetropolitan residents aged sixty to seventy-nine than for outside residents of that age, being ~ 2-fold higher in men and ~ 1.5-fold higher among women.

How are these data to be interpreted, given that the highest risk group of African Americans (nonmetropolitan residents) has significantly higher blood pressure control rates? These data suggest a greater burden of severe hypertension in the Southeastern United States, with the prevalence of these extreme

FIGURE 10.2. RISK OF HYPERTENSION ASSOCIATED WITH SOUTHERN RESIDENCE, NHANES III, 1988–1994.

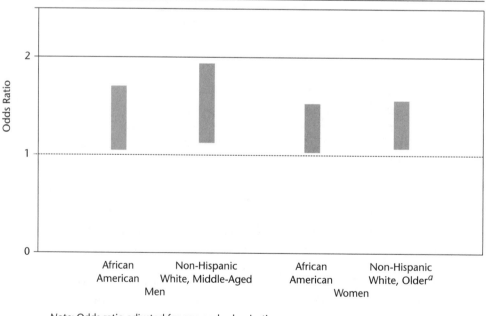

Note: Odds ratio adjusted for age and urbanization.

[a]Nonmetropolitan residents only.

Source: Adapted from Obisesan, Vargas, & Gillum, 2000.

blood pressure readings being greater in nonmetropolitan than in metropolitan areas. Indeed, Roccella and Lenfant (1989) previously reported a higher prevalence of severe hypertension among Southern residents. Nevertheless, data are lacking to document higher blood pressure levels in Southeastern African Americans residing in nonmetropolitan compared to metropolitan areas. Contemporary data do, however, suggest that Southeastern African Americans have higher blood pressures than their same region white counterparts as well as higher systolic blood pressure levels than African Americans residing elsewhere (Gillum & Ingram, 1996). In fact, Southeastern African American women had much higher average blood pressures in comparison to Southeastern white women (159.7 versus 142.2 mmHg) as well as to African American women residing outside this geographic region.

Risk Factors Other Than Blood Pressure

As Table 10.2 illustrates, there are a number of risk factors for stroke in addition to hypertension.

Prior Stroke or Transient Ischemic Attack. A prior history of clinically detectable ischemic cerebrovascular disease—stroke or transient ischemic attack (TIA)—predicts a heightened future risk for stroke. The average annual stroke risk among individuals with a history of TIA is ~ 4 percent (Howard, Evans, et al., 1994). A prior history of stroke, however, portends even greater risk of stroke. Among persons with prior stroke, long-term recurrence rates vary from 4 percent to 14 percent. The recurrence rate approximates 6.1 percent and 9 percent, respectively, for those with a history of major and minor stroke.

Asymptomatic Carotid Stenosis Extracranial carotid stenosis should be suspected when cervical bruits are auscultated on physical exam, when there are carotid pulse deficits, and in persons with evidence of coronary or peripheral vascular disease. Cervical bruits are present in 4 percent to 5 percent of persons older than forty-five and prevalence increases with advancing age. Annual stroke risk is 1.3 percent in those with < 70 percent stenosis and 3.3 percent in those with ≥ 70 percent stenosis (Chambers & Norris, 1986; Wolf, Kannel, Sorlie, & McNamara, 1981). Extracranial carotid artery stenosis as determined by B-mode ultrasonography has been linked to high levels of systolic blood pressure and low diastolic blood pressure (<75 mmHg) in older adults with isolated systolic hypertension (Sutton-Tyrrell, Alcron, Wolfson, Kelsey, & Kuller, 1993). In fact, in Sutton-Tyrrell et al.'s study, an association of low diastolic blood pressure with carotid artery stenosis was present despite a somewhat weaker, though positive, association of carotid artery stenosis with systolic blood pressure. Moreover diuretic-based antihypertensive therapy in older persons with isolated systolic hypertension slows the rate of progression and more often regresses extracranial carotid artery atherosclerosis than does placebo therapy (Sutton-Tyrrell,

Wolfson, & Kuller, 1994). These observations have potentially important diagnostic and therapeutic implications for physicians and other health care practitioners caring for African American patients. Though African Americans have less often been found to have extracranial carotid atherosclerosis than whites, such disparities do not validate an automatic assumption that extracranial carotid atherosclerosis is absent among this high-risk population.

Cigarette Smoking. Cigarette smoking nearly doubles the risk of ischemic stroke, with a clear dose-response relationship. Moreover, cigarette smoking is perhaps the most important risk factor for subarachnoid hemorrhage. Cessation of smoking leads to reduction of stroke risk; the majority of this reduction is seen in two to five years (Shinton & Beevers, 1989; Wolf, D'Agostino, Kannel, Bonita, & Belanger, 1988; Wannamethee, Shaper, Whincup, & Walker, 1995). The linkage of cigarette smoking to stroke risk has important implications for African Americans given that African Americans are more likely than whites to smoke, though they tend to smoke fewer cigarettes per day (Wagenknecht et al., 1990; Gillum, 1999), and given the typically early age of initiation of the smoking habit and the tremendous difficulty in cessation of the habit.

Diabetes Mellitus. The relative risk of ischemic stroke for persons with diabetes mellitus is from 1.8 to 3.0. In addition, persons with diabetes mellitus also experience greater morbidity and mortality than others as the result of stroke (Burchfiel et al., 1994; Abbott, Donahue, MacMahon, Reed, & Yano, 1987). Though some of the stroke risk in persons with diabetes mellitus can be attributed to the association of glucose intolerance with other risk factors such as dyslipidemia and hypertension, epidemiological studies have confirmed that diabetes mellitus is indeed an independent stroke risk factor. In addition, both hyperinsulinemia and insulin resistance have been linked to increased stroke risk in persons with normal glucose levels (Shinozaki et al., 1996; Howard, O'Leary, et al., 1996). These data too potentially have profound implications for African Americans given the excessive prevalence of diabetes mellitus, especially type 2, and the high burden of diabetes mellitus type 2 antecedents such as obesity and physical inactivity.

Atrial Fibrillation. Atrial fibrillation is a powerful risk factor for stroke (Wolf, Abbott, & Kannel, 1991). Approximately one-half of all cardioembolic strokes occur as a consequence of atrial fibrillation. The incidence and prevalence of stroke increase with advancing age (Wolf, Benjamin, et al., 1996). Accordingly, the risk of stroke doubles with each successive decade of life above age fifty-five. In the Framingham Study (Wolf, Abbott, et al., 1991), nonvalvular atrial fibrillation was independently associated with a threefold to fivefold risk of stroke. Annual stroke risk averages ~ 5 percent among persons with atrial fibrillation. However, for patients younger than sixty-five who have no other stroke risk factors, annual stroke risk ranges between 0.5 and 1 percent. However, when three other proven stroke risk factors are present, annual stroke risk approximates 15 percent. Chemical or electrical cardioversion to normal sinus rhythm after an appropriate period of anticoagulation is the optimal treatment for atrial fibrillation—assuming no easily reversible cause such as hyperthyroidism can be identified and corrected. When normal sinus rhythm cannot be attained, stroke risk can be reduced up to 70 percent using oral anticoagulation with warfarin when the international normalized ratio is maintained between 2.0 and 3.0 (Hart & Halperin, 1999; Atrial Fibrillation Investigators, 1994).

Myocardial Infarction. Transmural myocardial infarction, particularly of the anterior wall, is an important stroke risk factor. The pathophysiology involves a large area of ventricular injury leading to stasis of blood within the ventricle, subsequent coagulation, and finally, cerebral embolization. The risk of stroke is greatest in the first few weeks after transmural infarction. In the Framingham Study, risk of stroke was increased twofold by coronary heart disease, more than threefold by hypertension, and more than fourfold by heart failure (Wolf, Abbott, et al., 1991).

Hyperlipidemia. Though hypercholesterolemia has been identified as an important risk factor for coronary heart disease, the link to ischemic stroke has been controversial. At a minimum the relationship is complex. A positive relationship between serum cholesterol and death from nonhemorrhagic stroke has been observed. However, among these same Multiple Risk Factor Intervention Trial male screenees followed for six years, an inverse relationship was observed between serum cholesterol levels and hemorrhagic stroke, though only among men with diastolic blood pressure > 90 mmHg (Iso, Jacobs, Wentworth, Neaton, & Cohen, 1989). Other epidemiological studies in diverse populations have confirmed the link of hypercholesterolemia to stroke incidence and mortality (Haheim, Holme, Hjermann, & Leren, 1993; Yamori, Nara, Mizushima, Sawamura, & Horie, 1994). Accordingly, there also has been a positive correlation of total and LDL cholesterol and an inverse relationship of HDL cholesterol with extracranial carotid atherosclerosis (Furberg et al., 1994). In the Scandinavian simvastatin study, strokes and transient ischemic attacks were reduced by 30 percent among persons with hypercholesterolemia and coronary artery disease treated with simvastatin, an HMG-CoA reductase inhibitor (Scandinavian Simvastatin Survival Study, 1994). Moreover, post-myocardial infarction patients, both men and women with average cholesterol levels, treated with pravastatin also had significant reductions in stroke risk (Plehn et al., 1999). These data are consistent with the findings of a recent overview of all statin trials where an overall 29 percent reduction of risk in stroke was documented, with the greatest reductions occurring in secondary prevention studies; results from primary and mixed primary and secondary prevention studies were more variable (Hebert, Gaziano, Chan, & Hennekens, 1997; Weinberger & Terashita, 1999).

Alcohol. There is a dose-dependent, though J-shaped, relationship between alcohol consumption and ischemic stroke. Moderate to heavy alcohol consumption has been linked to a higher risk of stroke whereas light drinkers have a lower stroke risk compared to nondrinkers (Camargo, 1989; Sacco, Lin, et al., 1997). Heavy alcohol consumption also increases risk of intracranial hemorrhage.

Lifestyle Factors. Obesity, particularly central obesity, is an independent risk factor for stroke. Epidemiological evidence also suggests that moderate physical activity has a protective effect against stroke (Kiely, Wolf, Cupples, Beiser, & Kannel, 1994; Gillum, Mussolino, & Ingram, 1996). Dietary sodium intake has been positively linked with stroke risk (Perry & Beevers, 1992; Xie et al., 1992), whereas low dietary potassium intake has been linked to ischemic stroke risk (Xie et al., 1992; Iso, Stampfer, et al., 1999; Fang et al., 2000) as has low intake of dietary calcium and of magnesium (Iso, Stampfer, et al., 1999). These lifestyle observations, in aggregate, have potentially profound implications for African Americans given the high rates of obesity (particularly among women) and the relatively high dietary sodium and low dietary potassium intakes in African Americans, especially among those residing in the Southeastern United States. In addition, the Treatment of Mild Hypertension Study has documented higher urinary sodium/potassium ratios among lower-socioeconomic status hypertensive African Americans (Ganguli et al., 1997).

Oral Contraceptives. Earlier oral contraceptive preparations containing more than 50 micrograms (< 50 μg) of estrogen were strongly associated with risk for stroke. However, recently, studies of low-dose oral contraceptives (< 50 μg estrogen) document no increase in stroke risk (Petitti et al., 1996).

Homocysteine. Serum homocysteine was related in NHANES III to physician-diagnosed ischemic stroke risk among African American and white adults, even after adjustment for traditional stroke risk factors (Giles, Croft, Greenlund, Ford, & Kittner, 1998). Moreover, the adjusted odds ratio (highest versus lowest quartile) did not differ by race, being 2.5 in whites and 1.4 in African Americans. A smaller epidemiological study linked plasma homocysteine levels to risk of ischemic stroke as well (Eikelboom et al., 2000; Perry et al., 1995). Oral supplementation with folate or pyridoxine (or both), both B vitamins, can lower circulating homocysteine levels (Boushey, Beresford, Omenn, & Motulsky, 1995).

Fibrinogen. Fibrinogen and tissue plasminogen activator has been linked to increased stroke risk (Wilhelmsen et al., 1984). This observation has been confirmed for the relation of fibrinogen and risk of stroke mortality in hospitalized consecutive cohorts of African stroke survivors (Longo-Mbenza et al., 2000).

Illicit Drug Use. Cocaine is the illicit drug most commonly associated with stroke. Other illicit drugs associated with an increased stroke risk include amphetamines, heroin, LSD, and marijuana (Kelly, Gorelick, & Mirza, 1992).

Intracranial Hemorrhage Risk Factors

Intracranial hemorrhage (ICH) is more than twice as common as subarachnoid hemorrhage and is much more likely to result in death or disability than subarachnoid hemorrhage (Broderick, Brott, Tomsick, Miller, & Huster, 1993). Table 10.3 displays the risk factors for subarachnoid and intracranial hemorrhage.

The risk for intracranial hemorrhage increases exponentially with advancing age. Intracranial hemorrhage is more common in men than women and occurs more commonly in African Americans than whites (Rosamond et al., 1999; Broderick, Brott, Tomsick, Miller, & Huster, 1993; Systolic Hypertension in the Elderly Program [SHEP] Cooperative Research Group, 1991; Broderick, Brott, Tomsick, Huster, & Miller, 1992; Klatsky, Armstrong, & Friedman, 1991). In a series of 403 African American ICH patients, men were younger at diagnosis than women (fifty-four versus sixty years old). Qureshi et al. (1997) also reported that women and older ICH survivors were more likely to be "dependent" at the time of discharge. Amyloid angiopathy in the elderly is an important risk factor for spontaneous lobar hemorrhage.

Hypertension is the most powerful modifiable risk factor for ICH (Qureshi et al., 1997). Indeed, pharmacological treatment trials in hypertensive persons

TABLE 10.3. RISK FACTORS FOR SUBARACHNOID AND INTRACRANIAL HEMORRHAGE.

Factor	Subarachnoid Hemorrhage	Intracranial Hemorrhage
Age	+	+ +
Female sex	+	−
Ethnicity	+	+
Heredity	+	0
Hypertension	+	+
Cigarette smoking	+ +	?
Heavy alcohol use	+ +	+
Oral contraceptives	0	?
Anticoagulation	?	+ +
Diabetes	0	0
Hypercholesterolemia	0	0
Amyloid angiopathy	0	+ +
Cocaine use	+	+
Glucocorticoid remedial aldosteronism	−	+

+ + Strong evidence

+ Moderate evidence

− Moderate inverse evidence

0 No relation

? Equivocal

Source: Adapted from Sacco, Benjamin, et al., 1997.

have shown a decreased incidence of ICH after pharmacological blood pressure lowering. In the Systolic Hypertension in the Elderly Program (SHEP) study, the treatment of isolated systolic hypertension in persons aged sixty and older (the average age was seventy-two) lowered the combined risk of ICH and subarachnoid hemorrhage by 54 percent (Perry et al., 2000).

Anticoagulation and antithrombotic therapies are also associated with increased risk of ICH (Hylek & Singer, 1994; Johnston, Selvin, & Gress, 1998). Among individuals receiving anticoagulation therapy, the risk for ICH is increased when the INR exceeds 3. Therefore, careful monitoring and control of the intensity of anticoagulation during warfarin therapy should decrease the risk of subsequent ICH. Heavy alcohol consumption and use of cocaine and sympathomimetic amines also increase the risk of ICH. Cigarette smoking and elevated cholesterol are not definitively proven ICH risk factors.

Subarachnoid Hemorrhage Risk Factors

Subarachnoid hemorrhage (SAH) less commonly causes stroke than cerebral infarction or intracranial hemorrhage. Aneurysms and arteriovenous malformations are the most commonly identified causes of SAH. The incidence of SAH increases with age and is 57 percent higher in women than in men (Ingall, Whisnant, Wiebers, & O'Fallon, 1989). African Americans have approximately 1.6 to 2 times the age-adjusted risk for SAH that whites do (Johnston et al., 1998). According to data from the National Center for Health Statistics spanning the years 1979 to 1994, SAH mortality rates have declined 1 percent annually, and there has been a slight rise in the median age of death from fifty-seven to sixty years of age (Johnston et al., 1998). In this same data set the median age for death from SAH was fifty-nine years—fourteen years younger than the median age for death from ICH and twenty-two years younger than the median age of death from ischemic stroke. Therefore, despite the much lower incidence of subarachnoid hemorrhage (4.4 percent) compared to ischemic stroke, the former causes only slightly less premature mortality than the latter. In fact, 27.3 percent of the stroke-related years of potential life lost prior to sixty-five years of age is attributable to SAH compared to 38.5 percent attributable to ischemic stroke and 34.2 percent to intracranial hemorrhage (Johnston et al., 1998).

Cigarette smoking is perhaps the most important modifiable risk factor for SAH (Bromberg et al., 1995; Juvela, Hillbom, Numminen, & Koskinen, 1993; Canhao, Pinto, Ferro, & Ferro, 1994; Knekt et al., 1991; Teunissen, Rinkel, Algra, & Van Gijn, 1996), manifesting a dose-dependent risk that appears to be maximal within three hours of smoking a cigarette. Cessation of smoking decreases the risk; however, it may not completely eliminate it (Kawachi et al., 1993). Hypertension is another important modifiable risk factor for SAH (Knekt et al., 1991; Teunissen et al., 1996). Excess alcohol intake (>150 g/week) is a significant although less constant risk factor (Donahue, Abbott, Reed, & Yano,

1986; Gill et al., 1991). The linkage of oral contraceptives with SAH has been controversial. Older studies on oral contraceptives with higher estrogen composition than current ones had shown increased risk; however, recent studies do not support this finding (Hannaford, Croft, & Kay, 1994; Inman, 1979). On the contrary, hormone replacement therapy appears protective against SAH (Longstreth, Nelson, Keopsell, & Van Belle, 1994). Diabetes and cholesterol do not appear to be risk factors for SAH (Iso, Jacobs, et al., 1989; Yano, Reed, & MacLean, 1989). A positive family history for cerebral aneurysm further augments the risk of cerebral aneurysm between two- and sevenfold (Ronkainen et al., 1997; Bromberg et al., 1995). Several genetic syndromes that have been associated with increased risk of SAH are (1) Ehlers-Danlos syndrome type IV, (2) autosomal dominant polycystic disease (ADPKD), (3) Marfan's syndrome, (4) coarctation of the aorta, and (5) other vascular collagen disorders.

Screening, Diagnosis, and Treatment

Data from the National Hospital Discharge Survey (1980 to 1993) showed that African American stroke patients were less likely than whites to undergo both cerebral angiography and carotid endarterectomy, a disparity that was greater for cerebral angiography than for carotid endarterectomy (Gillum, 1995). Nevertheless, before 1988 carotid endarterectomy rates were 50 percent higher in African Americans than in whites but only 20 percent higher from 1988 to 1992 (Gillum, 1995). These data have been somewhat replicated in the Veterans Administration system, where low-income African American veterans with stroke, TIA, or other conditions that made them likely candidates for carotid angiography underwent fewer carotid angiograms and carotid endarterectomies than similar white veterans (Oddone, Horner, & Lipscomb, 1998). However, African Americans also more often expressed a willingness to avoid surgical revascularization than whites at the expense of accepting a greater hypothetical risk of death.

The treatment of acute cerebral ischemic syndromes is beyond the scope of this chapter. Aspirin has proven useful in reducing stroke risk among persons presenting with transient ischemic attacks who are at high risk for subsequent ischemic stroke. The optimal dose of aspirin for stroke prevention has been the focus of contentious debate. However, current recommendations for secondary prevention are for aspirin doses ranging from 50 to 325 mg per day (Albers, Easton, Sacco, & Teal, 1998; "Internal Analgesic, Antipyretic, and Antirheumatic Drug Products . . . ," 1998), although benefit, albeit at higher risk for gastrointestinal upset and bleeding, has been documented at doses of up to 1,200 mg per day (Algra & van Gijn, 1996). Dipyridamole, another antiplatelet agent, is similar to low-dose aspirin monotherapy in lowering risk of stroke and death. The combination of aspirin with dipyridamole in patients with symptomatic atherosclerosis reduces the composite of stroke, myocardial infarction, and vascular death by 28 percent and reduces stroke and TIA risk by 37 percent relative to placebo therapy (Diener et al., 1996; Hankey, 1998); moreover, this combination reduces stroke risk 23 percent more than aspirin alone. Clopidogrel, more than aspirin alone, lowers the risk of vascular death, stroke, myocardial infarction, re-hospitalization for ischemic events, or bleeding among individuals with recent ischemic stroke, myocardial infarction, or symptomatic peripheral vascular disease (Bhatt et al., 2000). Clopidogrel and ticlopidine have similar efficacy, although the former has a better safety profile and can be dosed once daily (Weinberger & Terashita, 1999).

Summary

Stroke is a cardiovascular disease condition of significant clinical and public health importance with several proven and reversible risk factors, and perhaps even more suspected. Comprehensive CVD risk factor management of blood pressure (especially systolic blood pressure), hypercholesterolemia, hyperglycemia, and smoking cessation are therapeutic maneuvers proven to lower stroke risk. Moreover, the prevalence of these potentially modifiable risk factors is at least equally if not more prevalent in African American than white populations. Fruitful areas of future research will relate to nutritional and genetic influences on stroke risk. Nevertheless, there is much that can be accomplished today if strategies already proven to lower stroke risk are more effectively implemented in the population at large.

References

Abbott, R. D., Donahue, R. P., MacMahon, S. W., Reed, D. M., & Yano, K. (1987). Diabetes and the risk of stroke. *Journal of the American Medical Association, 257,* 949–952.

Adams, R. D., Victor, M., & Ropper, H. (Eds.). (1997). *Principles of Neurology.* NY: McGraw-Hill, p. 807.

Albers, G. W., Easton, J. D., Sacco, R. L., & Teal, P. (1998). Antithrombotic and thrombolytic therapy for ischemic stroke. *Chest, 114,* 683S–698S.

Algra, A., & van Gijn, J. (1996). Aspirin at any dose above 30 mg offers only modest protection after cerebral ischemia. *Journal of Neurology, Neurosurgery and Psychiatry, 60,* 197–199.

American Heart Association. (1995). *Heart and stroke facts, 1996 statistical supplement.* Dallas, TX: Author.

Atrial Fibrillation Investigators. (1994). Risk factors for stroke and efficacy of antithrombotic therapy in atrial fibrillation: Analysis of pooled data from five randomized controlled trials. *Archives of Internal Medicine, 154,* 1449–1457.

Bhatt, D. L., Hirsch, A. T., Ringleb, P. A., Hacke, W., & Topol, E. J. (2000). Reduction in the need for hospitalization for recurrent ischemic events and bleeding with clopidogrel instead of aspirin. *American Heart Journal, 140*(1), 67–73.

Boushey, C. J., Beresford, S. A., Omenn, G. S., & Motulsky, A. G. (1995). A quantitative assessment of plasma homocysteine as a risk factor for vascular disease: Probable benefits of increasing folic acid intakes. *Journal of the American Medical Association, 274,* 1049–1057.

Broderick, J. P., Brott, T., Kothari, R., Miller, R., Khoury, J., Pancioli, A., Gebel, J., Mills, D., Minneci, L., & Shukla, R. (1998). The Greater Cincinnati/Northern Kentucky Stroke Study: Preliminary first-ever and total incidence rates of stroke among blacks. *Stroke, 29,* 415–421.

Broderick, J. P., Brott, T., Tomsick, T., Huster, G., & Miller, R. (1992). The risk of subarachnoid and intracerebral hemorrhage in blacks as compared with whites. *New England Journal of Medicine, 326,* 733–736.

Broderick, J. P., Brott, T., Tomsick, T., Miller, R., & Huster, G. (1993). Intracerebral hemorrhage more than twice as common as subarachnoid hemorrhage. *Journal of Neurosurgery, 78,* 188–191.

Bromberg, J. E., Rinkel, G. J., Algra, A., Greebe, P., Van Duyn, C. M., Hasan, D., Limburg, M., Ter Berg, H. W., Wijdicks, E. F., & Van Gijn, J. (1995). Subarachnoid hemorrhage in first- and second-degree relatives of patients with subarachnoid hemorrhage. *British Medical Journal, 311,* 288–289.

Burchfiel, C. M., Curb, J. D., Rodriguez, B. L., Abbott, R. D., Chiu, D., & Yano, K. (1994). Glucose intolerance and 22-year stroke incidence: The Honolulu Heart Program. *Stroke, 25,* 951–957.

Burt, V. L., Whelton, P., Roccella, E. J., Brown, C., Cutler, J. A., Higgins, M., Horan, M. J., & Labarthe, D. (1995). Prevalence of hypertension in the U.S. adult population: Results from the Third National Health and Nutrition Examination Survey, 1988–1991. *Hypertension, 25,* 305–313.

Camargo, C. A., Jr. (1989). Moderate alcohol consumption and stroke: The epidemiologic evidence. *Stroke, 20,* 1611–1626.

Canhao, P., Pinto, A. N., Ferro, H., & Ferro, J. M. (1994). Smoking and aneurysmal subarachnoid hemorrhage: A case-control study. *Journal of Cardiovascular Risk, 1,* 155–158.

Chambers, B. R., & Norris, J. W. (1986). Outcome in patients with asymptomatic neck bruits. *New England Journal of Medicine, 315,* 860–865.

Collins, R., Peto, R., MacMahon, S., Hebert, P., Fiebach, N. H., Eberlein, K. A., Godwin, J., Qizilbash, N., Taylor, J. O., & Hennekens, C. H. (1990). Blood pressure, stroke, and coronary heart disease: Pt. 2. Short-term reductions in blood pressure: Overview of randomized drug trials in their epidemiological context. *Lancet, 335,* 827–838.

Cornoni-Huntley, J., LaCroix, A. Z., Havlik, R. J. (1989). Race and sex differentials in the impact of hypertension in the United States. The National Health and Nutrition Examination Survey I Epidemiologic Follow-Up Study. *Archives of Internal Medicine, 149,* 780–788.

Cooper, R., McGee, D., Liao, Y., & Durazo-Arvizu, R. (1996). Patterns of comorbidity and mortality risk in blacks and whites. *Annals of Epidemiology, 6,* 381–385.

Cushman, W. C., Reda, D. J., Perry, H. M., Williams, D., Abdellatif, M., & Materson, B. J. (2000). Regional and racial differences in response to antihypertensive medication use in a randomized controlled trial of men with hypertension in the United States: Department of Veterans Affairs Cooperative Study Group on Antihypertensive Agents. *Archives of Internal Medicine, 160,* 825–831.

Cutler, J. A. (1996). High blood pressure and end organ damage. *Journal of Hypertension, 14*(6, Suppl.), S3–S6.

Diener, H. C., Cunha, L., Forbes, C., Sivenius, J., Smets, P., & Lowenthal, A. (1996). European Stroke Prevention Study 2: Dipyridamole and acetylsalicylic acid in secondary prevention of stroke. *Journal of Neurological Science, 143,* 1–13.

Donahue, R. P., Abbott, R. D., Reed, D. M., & Yano, K. (1986). Alcohol and hemorrhagic stroke: The Honolulu Heart Program. *Journal of the American Medical Association, 225,* 2311–2314.

Eikelboom, J. W., Hankey, G. J., Anand, S. S., Lofthouse, E., Staples, N., & Baker, R. I. (2000). Association between high homocysteine and ischemic stroke, large- and small-artery disease but not other etiologic subtype ischemic stroke. *Stroke, 31,* 1069–1075.

Fagard, R. H., & Staessen, J. A. (1999). Treatment of isolated systolic hypertension in the elderly: The Syst-Eur Trial (Systolic Hypertension in Europe [Syst-Eur] Trial Investigation). *Clinical and Experimental Hypertension, 21,* 491–497.

Fang, J., Madhavan, S., & Alderman, M. H. (2000). Dietary potassium intake and stroke mortality. *Stroke, 31,* 1532–1537.

Flack, J. M., Doyle, J., Casciano, R., Arocho, R., Casciano, J., & Gonzalez, M. A. (2000). The health economic impact of failure to reach blood pressure goals. *American Journal of Hypertension, 13,* 17A–19A.

Flack, J. M., Gardin, J. M., Yunis, C., & Liu, K. (1999). Static and pulsatile blood pressure correlates of left ventricle structure and function in black and white young adults: The CARDIA Study. *American Heart Journal, 138,* 856–864.

Flack, J. M., Neaton, J. D., Daniels, B., & Esunge, P. (1993). Ethnicity and renal disease: Lessons from the Multiple Risk Factor Intervention Trial and the Treatment of Mild Hypertension Study. *American Journal of Kidney Diseases, 21*(4, Suppl. 1), 31–40.

Furberg, C. D., Adams, H. P., Jr., Applegate, W. B., Byington, R. P., Espeland, M. A., Hartwell, T., Hunninghake, D. B., Leftkowitz, D. S., Probstfield, J., & Riley, W. A. (1994). Effect of lovastatin on early carotid atherosclerosis and cardiovascular events. *Circulation, 90,* 1679–1687.

Ganguli, M. C., Grimm, R. H., Jr., Svendsen, K. H., Flack, J. M., Grandits, G. A., & Elmer, P. J. (1997). Higher education and income are related to a better Na:K ratio in blacks: Baseline results of the Treatment of Mild Hypertension Study (TOMHS) data. *American Journal of Hypertension, 10,* 979–84.

Giles, W. H., Croft, J. B., Greenlund, K. J., Ford, E. S., & Kittner, S. J. (1998). Total homocysteine concentration and the likelihood of nonfatal stroke: Results from the Third National Health and Nutrition Examination Survey, 1988–1994. *Stroke, 29,* 2473–2477.

Gill, J. S., Shipley, M. J., Tsementzis, S. A., Hornby, R. S., Gill, S. K., Hitchcock, E. R., & Beevers, D. G. (1991). Alcohol consumption: A risk factor for hemorrhagic and non-hemorrhagic stroke. *American Journal of Medicine, 90,* 489–497.

Gillum, R. F. (1986). Cerebrovascular disease morbidity in the United States, 1970–1983: Age, sex, region, and vascular surgery. *Stroke, 17,* 656–661.

Gillum, R. F. (1995). Epidemiology of carotid endarterectomy and cerebral arteriography in the United States. *Stroke, 26,* 1724–1728.

Gillum, R. F. (1996). Epidemiology of hypertension in African American women. *American Heart Journal, 131,* 385–395.

Gillum, R. F. (1999). Stroke mortality in blacks: Disturbing trends. *Stroke, 30,* 1711–1715.

Gillum, R. F., & Ingram, D. D. (1996). Relation between residence in the Southeast region of the United States and stroke incidence. The NHANES 1 Epidemiologic Follow-Up Study. *American Journal of Epidemiology, 144,* 665–673.

Gillum, R. F., Mussolino, M. E., & Ingram, D. D. (1996). Physical activity and stroke risk in men and women: The NHANES I Epidemiologic Follow-Up Study. *American Journal of Epidemiology, 143,* 860–869.

Gueyffier, F., Boissel, J. P., Boutitie, F., Pocock, S., Coope, J., Cutter, J., Ekbom, T., Fagard, R., Friedman, L., Kerlikowske, K., Perry, M., Prineas, R., & Schron, E. (1997). Effect of antihypertensive treatment in patients having already suffered from stroke: Gathering the evidence (INDANA [Individual Data Analysis of Antihypertensive Intervention Trials] project collaborators). *Stroke, 28,* 2557–2562.

Gueyffier, F., Bulpitt, C., Boissel, J. P., Schron, E., Ekbom, T., Fagard, R., Casig, K., & Coope, J. (1999). Antihypertensive drugs in very old people: A subgroup meta-analysis of randomised controlled trials (INDANA group). *Lancet, 353,* 793–796.

Haheim, L. L., Holme, I., Hjermann, I., & Leren, P. (1993). Risk factors of stroke incidence and mortality: A 12-year follow up of the Oslo Study. *Stroke, 24,* 1484–1489.

Hankey, G. J. (1998). One year after CAPRIE, IST and ESPS2: Any change in concept? *Cerebrovascular Disease, 8*(Suppl. 5), 1–7.

Hannaford, P. C., Croft, P. R., & Kay, C. R. (1994). Oral contraception and stroke: Evidence from the Royal College of General Practitioners' Oral Contraception Study. *Stroke, 25,* 935–942.

Hart, R. G., & Halperin, J. L. (1999). Antithrombotic therapy to prevent stroke in patients with atrial fibrillation: A meta-analysis. *Annals of Internal Medicine, 131,* 492–501.

He, J., Klag, M. J., Wu, Z., & Whelton, P. K. (1995). Stroke in the People's Republic of China: Geographic variations in incidence and risk factors. *Stroke, 26,* 2222–2227.

Hebert, P. R., Gaziano, J. M., Chan, K. S., & Hennekens, C. H. (1997). Cholesterol lowering with statin drugs, risk of stroke and total mortality: An overview of the randomised trials. *Journal of the American Medical Association, 278,* 313–321.

Howard, G., Anderson, R., Sorlie, P., Andrews, V., Backlund, E., & Burke, G. L. (1994). Ethnic differences in stroke mortality between non-Hispanic whites, Hispanic whites, and blacks: The National Longitudinal Mortality Study. *Stroke, 25,* 2120–2125.

Howard, G., Evans, G. W., Crouse, J. R., 3rd, Toole, J. F., Ryu, J. E., Tegeler, C., Frye-Pierson, J., Mitchell, E., & Sanders, L. (1994). A prospective reevaluation of TIAs as a risk factor for death and fatal and nonfatal cardiovascular events. *Stroke, 25,* 342–345.

Howard, G., O'Leary, D. H., Zaccaro, D., Haffner, S., Rewers, M., Hamman, R., Selby, J. V., Saad, M. F., Savage, P., & Bergman, R. (1996). Insulin sensitivity and atherosclerosis (The Insulin Resistance Atherosclerotic Study Investigators [IRAS]). *Circulation, 93,* 1809–1817.

Hylek, E. M., & Singer, D. E. (1994). Risk factors for intracranial hemorrhage in outpatients taking warfarin. *Annuals of Internal Medicine, 120,* 897–902.

Hypertension Detection and Follow-up Program Cooperative Group. (1979). Five-year findings of the Hypertension Detection and Follow-Up Program. II. Mortality by race-sex and age. *Journal of the American Medical Association, 242,* 2572–2577.

Ingall, T. J., Whisnant, J. P., Wiebers, D. O., & O'Fallon, W. M. (1989). Has there been a decline in subarachnoid hemorrhage mortality? *Stroke, 20,* 718–724.

Inman, W. H. (1979). Oral contraceptives and fatal subarachnoid hemorrhage. *British Medical Journal, 2,* 1468–1470.

Internal analgesic, antipyetic, and antirheumatic drug products for over-the-counter human use: Final rule for professional labeling aspirin, buffered aspirin, and aspirin in combination with antacid drug products, 63 Fed. Reg. 56802–56819 (1998).

Iso, H., Jacobs, D. R., Jr., Wentworth, D., Neaton, J. D., & Cohen, J. D. (1989). Serum cholesterol levels and six-year mortality from stroke in 350,977 men screened for multiple risk factor intervention trial. *New England Journal of Medicine, 320,* 904–910.

Iso, H., Stampfer, M. J., Manson, J. E., Rexrode, K., Hennekens, C. H., Colditz, G. A., Speizer, F. E., & Willett, W. C. (1999). Prospective study of calcium, potassium, and magnesium intake and risk of stroke in women. *Stroke, 30,* 1772–1779.

Johnston, S. C., Selvin, S., & Gress, D. R. (1998). The burden, trends, and demographics of mortality from subarachnoid hemorrhage. *Neurology, 50,* 1413–1418.

Joint National Committee on Prevention, Evaluation, and Treatment of High Blood Pressure. (1997). Sixth report of the Joint National Committee on Prevention, Evaluation, and Treatment of High Blood Pressure (JNC VI). *Archives of Internal Medicine, 157,* 2413–2446.

Juvela, S., Hillbom, M., Numminen, H., & Koskinen, P. (1993). Cigarette smoking and alcohol consumption as risk factors for aneurysmal subarachnoid hemorrhage. *Stroke, 24,* 639–646.

Kannel, W. B., Wolf, P. A., McGee, D. L., Dawber, McNamara, P., & Castelli, W. P. (1981). Systolic blood pressure, arterial rigidity, and risk of stroke: The Framingham Study. *Journal of the American Medical Association, 245,* 1225–1229.

Kawachi, I., Colditz, G. A., Stampfer, M. J., Willett, W. C., Manson, J. E., Rosner, B., Speizer, F. E., & Hennekens, C. H. (1993). Smoking cessation and decreased risk of stroke in women. *Journal of the American Medical Association, 269,* 232–236.

Kelly, M. A., Gorelick, P. B., & Mirza, D. (1992). The role of drugs in etiology of stroke. *Clinical Neuropharmacology, 15,* 249–275.

Kiely, D. K., Wolf, P. A., Cupples, L. A., Beiser, A. S., & Kannel, W. B. (1994). Physical activity and stroke risk: The Framingham Study. *American Journal of Epidemiology, 140,* 608–620.

Klatsky, A. L., Armstrong, M. A., & Friedman, G. D. (1991). Racial differences in cerebrovascular disease hospitalizations. *Stroke, 22,* 299–304.

Knekt, P., Reunanen, A., Aho, K., Heliovaara, M., Rissanen, A., Aromaa, A., & Impivaara, O. (1991). Risk factors for subarachnoid hemorrhage in a longitudinal population study. *Journal of Clinical Epidemiology, 44,* 933–939.

Lisheng, L. (1996). Effects of hypertension control on stroke incidence and fatality: Report from Syst-China and post-stroke antihypertensive treatment. *Journal of Human Hypertension, 10*(Suppl. 1), S9–S11.

Longo-Mbenza, B., Tonduangu, K., Muyeno, K., Phanzu, M., Kebolo Baku Muvova, D., Lelo, T., Odio, W., Lukoki, L., Bikangi Nkiabungu, F., Kilembe Tshiamala, P., Katalay, L., Mwema, M., & Muyembe, T. (2000). Predictors of stroke-associated mortality in Africans. *Revue D Epidemiologie et de Sante Publique, 48*(1), 31–39.

Longstreth, W. T., Nelson, L. M., Keopsell, T. D., & Van Belle, G. (1994). Subarachnoid haemorrhage and hormonal factors in women: A population-based case-control study. *Annuals of Internal Medicine, 121,* 168–173.

MacMahon, S. (1994). The epidemiological association between blood pressure and stroke: Implications for primary and secondary prevention. *Hypertension Research, 17*(Suppl. 1), S23–S32.

MacMahon, S., Peto, R., Cutler, J., Collins, R., Sorlie, P., Neaton, J., Abbott, R., & Stamler, J. (1990). Blood pressure, stroke, and coronary heart disease: Pt. 1. Prolonged differences in blood pressure: Prospective observational studies corrected for the regression dilution bias. *Lancet, 335,* 765–774.

MacMahon, S., & Rodgers, A. (1994). Blood pressure, antihypertensive treatment and stroke risk. *Journal of Hypertension, 12*(Suppl.), S5–S14.

National Center for Health Statistics. (1998). *Health, United States, 1998, with Socioeconomic Status and Health Chartbook.* Hyattsville, MD: Public Health Service.

Obisesan, T. O., Vargas, C. M., & Gillum, R. F. (2000). Geographic variation in stroke risk in the United States: Region, urbanization, and hypertension in the Third National Health and Nutrition Examination Survey. *Stroke, 31,* 19–25.

Oddone, E. Z., Horner, R. D., & Lipscomb, J. (1998). Understanding racial variation in the use of carotid endarterectomy: The role of aversion to surgery. *Journal of the National Medical Association, 90,* 25–33.

Perry, H. M., Jr., Davis, B. R., Price, T. R., Applegate, W. B., Fields, W. S., Guralnik, J. M., Kuller, L., Pressel, S., Stamler, J., & Probstfield, J. L. (2000). Effect of treating isolated systolic hypertension on the risk of developing various types and subtypes of stroke. *Journal of the American Medical Association, 284,* 465–471.

Perry, H. M., & Roccella, E. J. (1998). Conference report on stroke mortality in the Southeastern United States. *Hypertension, 31,* 1206–1215.

Perry, I. J., & Beevers, D. G. (1992). Salt intake and stroke: A possible direct effect. *Journal of Human Hypertension, 6,* 23–25.

Perry, I. J., Refsum, H., Morris, R. W., Ebrahim, S. B., Ueland, P. M., & Shaper, A. G. (1995). Prospective study of total serum homocysteine concentrations and risk of stroke in middle-aged British men. *Lancet, 346,* 1395–1398.

Petitti, D. B., Sidney, S., Bernstein, A., Wolf, S., Quesenberry, C., & Ziel, H. K. (1996). Stroke in users of low dose oral contraceptives. *New England Journal of Medicine, 335,* 8–15.

Pickle, L. W., Mungiole, M., & Gillum, R. F. (1997). Geographic variation in stroke mortality in blacks and whites in the United States. *Stroke, 28,* 1639–1647.

Plehn, J. F., Davis, B. R., Sacks, F. M., Rouleau, J. L., Pfeffer, M. A., Bernstein, V., Cuddy, T. E., Moye, L., Rutherford, J., Simpson, L. M., & Braunwald, E. (1999). Reduction of stroke incidence after myocardial infarction with pravastatin: The Cholesterol and Recurrent Events (CARE) Study (The CARE investigators). *Circulation, 99,* 216–223.

Qureshi, A. I., Suri, M. A., Safdar, K., Ottenlips, J. R., Janssen, R. S., & Frankel, M. R. (1997). Intracerebral hemorrhage in blacks: Risk factors, subtypes, and outcome. *Stroke, 28,* 961–964.

Roccella, E. J., & Lenfant, C. (1989). Regional and racial differences among stroke victims in the United States. *Clinical Cardiology, 12*(12, Suppl. 4), 18–22.

Ronkainen, A., Hernesniemi, J., Puranen, M., Niemitukia, L., Vanninen, R., Ryynanen, M., & Kuivaniemi, H. (1997). Familial intracranial aneurysms. *Lancet, 349,* 380–384.

Rosamond, W. D., Folsom, A. R., Chambless, L. E., Wang, C. H., McGovern, P. G., Copper, L. S., & Shahar, E. (1999). Stroke incidence and survival among middle-aged adults: 9-year follow-up of the Atherosclerosis Risk in Communities (ARIC) cohort. *Stroke, 30,* 736–743.

Sacco, R. L., Benjamin, E. J., Broderick, J. P., Dyken, M., Baston, J. D., Feinberg, W. M., Goldstein, L. B., Gorelick, P. B., Howard, G., Kittner, S. J., Mardio, T. A., Whisnant, J. P., Wolf, P. A. (1997). American Heart Association prevention conference. IV. Prevention and rehabilitation of stroke. Risk factors. *Stroke, 28,* 1507–1517.

Sacco, R. L., Boden-Albala, B., Gan, R., Chen, X., Kargman, D. E., Shea, S., Paik, M. C., Hauser, W. A., & Gertrude, H. (1998). Stroke incidence among white, black, and Hispanic residents of an urban community: The Northern Manhattan Stroke Study. *American Journal of Epidemiology, 147,* 259–268.

Sacco, R. L., Lin, I. F., Boden-Albala, B., Kargman, D. E., Gan, R., Roberts, J. K., Elkind, M. S., Shea, S., Hauser, W. A., & Paik, M. (1997). Alcohol and the risk of ischemic stroke: Verification of a J-shaped relationship from the Northern Manhattan Stroke Study. *Stroke, 28,* 250.

Scandinavian Simvastatin Survival Study. (1994). Randomized trial of cholesterol lowering in 4,444 patients with coronary heart disease. *Lancet, 344*(8934), 1383–1389.

Sheinart, K. F., Tuhrim, S., Horowitz, D. R., Weinberger, J., Goldman, M., & Godbold, J. H. (1998). Stroke recurrence is more frequent in blacks and Hispanics. *Neuroepidemiology, 17*(4), 188–198.

Shinozaki, K., Naritomi, H., Shimizu, T., Suzuki, M., Ikebuchi, M., Sawada, T., & Harano, Y. (1996). Role of insulin resistance associated with hyperinsulinemia in ischemic stroke. *Stroke, 27,* 37–43.

Shinton, R., & Beevers, G. (1989). Meta-analysis of relationship between cigarette smoking and stroke. *British Medical Journal, 298,* 789–794.

Staessen, J. A., Fagard, R., Thijs, L., Celis, H., Arabidze, G. G., Birkenhager, W. H., Bulpitt, C. J., De Leeuw, P. W., Dollery, C. T., Fletcher, A. E., Forette, F., Leonetti, G., Nachev, C., O'Brien, E. T., Rosenfeld, J., Rodicio, J. L., Tuomilehto, J., & Zanchetti, A. (1997). Randomised double blind comparison of placebo and active treatment for older patients with isolated systolic hypertension in Europe (Syst-Eur) Trial Investigation. *Lancet, 350,* 757–764.

Strandgaard, S. (1996). Hypertension and stroke. *Journal of Hypertension, 14*(Suppl. 3), S23–S27.

Sutton-Tyrrell, K., Alcron, H. G., Wolfson, S. K., Jr., Kelsey, S. F., & Kuller, L. H. (1993). Predictors of carotid stenosis in older adults with and without isolated systolic hypertension. *Stroke, 24,* 355–361.

Sutton-Tyrrell, K., Wolfson, S. K., Jr., & Kuller, L. H. (1994). Blood pressure treatment slows the progression of carotid stenosis in patients with isolated systolic hypertension. *Stroke, 25,* 44–50.

Systolic Hypertension in the Elderly Program Cooperative Research Group. (1991). Prevention of stroke by antihypertensive drug treatment in older persons with isolated systolic hypertension: Final results of the Systolic Hypertension in the Elderly Program (SHEP). *Journal of the American Medical Association, 265,* 3255–3264.

Teunissen, L. L., Rinkel, G. J., Algra, A., & Van Gijn, J. (1996). Risk factors for subarachnoid hemorrhage: A systematic review. *Stroke, 27,* 544–549.

Wagenknecht, L. E., Perkins, L. L., Cutter, G. R., Sidney, S., Burke, G. L., Manolio, T. A., Jacobs, D. R., Jr., Liu, K. A., Friedman, G. D., & Hughes, G. H. (1990). Cigarette smoking behaviour is strongly related to educational status: The CARDIA Study. *Preventive Medicine, 19,* 158–169.

Wannamethee, S. G., Shaper, A. G., Whincup, P. H., & Walker, M. (1995). Smoking cessation and the risk of stroke in middle-aged men. *Journal of the American Medical Association, 274,* 155–160.

Weinberger, J., & Terashita, D. (1999). Drug therapy of neurovascular disease. *Heart Disease, 1,* 163–178.

Wilhelmsen, L., Svardsudd, K., Korsan-Bengtsen, K., Larsson, B., Welin, L., & Tibblin, G. (1984). Fibrinogen as a risk factor for stroke and myocardial infarction. *New England Journal of Medicine, 311,* 501–505.

Wityk, R. J., Lehman, D., Klag, M., Coresh, J., Ahn, H., & Litt, B. (1996). Race and sex differences in the distribution of cerebral atherosclerosis. *Stroke, 27,* 1974–1980.

Wolf, P. A., Abbott, R. D., & Kannel, W. B. (1991). Atrial fibrillation as an independent risk factor for stroke: The Framingham Study. *Stroke, 22,* 983–988.

Wolf, P. A., Benjamin, E. J., Belanger, A. J., Kannel, W. B., Levy, D., & D'Agostino, R. B. (1996). Secular trends in the prevalence of atrial fibrillation: The Framingham Study. *American Heart Journal, 131,* 790–795.

Wolf, P. A., D'Agostino, R. B., Kannel, W. B., Bonita, R., & Belanger, A. J. (1988). Cigarette smoking as a risk factor for stroke: The Framingham Study. *Journal of the American Medical Association, 258,* 1025–1029.

Wolf, P. A., Kannel, W. B., Sorlie, P., & McNamara, P. (1981). Asymptomatic carotid bruit and risk of stroke: The Framingham Study. *Journal of the American Medical Association, 245,* 1442–1445.

Xie, J. X., Sasaki, S., Joossens, J. V., & Kesteloot, H. (1992). The relationship between urinary cations obtained from the INTERSALT study and cerebrovascular mortality. *Journal of Human Hypertension, 6,* 17–21.

Yamori, Y., Nara, Y., Mizushima, S., Sawamura, M., & Horie, R. (1994). Nutritional factors for stroke and major cardiovascular diseases: International epidemiological comparison of dietary prevention. *Health Reports, 6*(1), 22–27.

Yano, K., Reed, D. M., & MacLean, C. J. (1989). Serum cholesterol and hemorrhagic stroke in the Honolulu Heart Program. *Stroke, 20,* 1460–1465.

CHAPTER ELEVEN

CANCER

Lovell A. Jones, María A. Hernández-Valero,
Angelina Esparza, Donella J. Wilson

This chapter reviews and provides information on the current cancer data collection system as that information relates to African Americans, racial and ethnic differences, the epidemiology of the five leading cancers (bronchus, breast, prostate, colon, and rectum) with emphasis on the status of African Americans, and prevention and early detection. We also recommend future actions and present a list of cancer resources.

The data in this chapter were acquired from the most current cancer information sources. Incidence, survival, and some mortality data were obtained from the Surveillance, Epidemiology, and End Results (SEER) Program of the National Cancer Institute (NCI), and the majority of the mortality data from the National Center for Health Statistics (NCHS). Information from the American Cancer Society (ACS) Surveillance Program was also used, including the web site of the ACS Cancer Resource Center (CRC) (www3.cancer.org.cancerinfo) and the ACS's *Cancer Facts and Figures* (ACS, 2000a).

Cancer Data Collection System: Limitations of Data

The NCHS is the primary source for U.S. mortality data, and cancer incidence data are collected primarily by SEER registries via surveys, personal interviews, additional record abstraction, and the collection of biological materials.

There have been attempts to coordinate efforts in cancer data collection to develop a more precise measure of rates and trends. Yet many problems still exist in data collection methods as they pertain to minority groups such as African Americans. In 1998, through the combined efforts of the ACS, SEER, NCHS, and Centers for Disease Control (CDC), a report entitled *Cancer Incidence and Mortality, 1973–1995: A Report Card for the United States* (Wingo, Ries, Rosenberg, Milles, & Edwards, 1998) was issued. This report reiterated what much of the data had previously shown, that minority populations suffered disproportionately from cancer incidence (for some sites) and mortality. The data, however, over-looked Native Americans and the rural poor (for example, in Appalachia and the rural South) and overgeneralized data for Asian American populations, high-lighting the limitations of current data collection methods. Because many of the data seen in this chapter are taken from the SEER Program, these limitations should be discussed. The SEER Program provides an oversampling of minority populations to ensure adequate statistical numbers for evaluation based on num-bers from the Census. Even with this oversampling, data from smaller popula-tions are less precise and must be viewed with caution (Haynes & Smedley, 1999). It is also worth noting that although ethnic and racial determination on the cen-sus is by self-report, such identification for the purposes of the SEER Program in extracting data from medical records and death certificates is made by clinicians or intake workers. The use of surnames as identifiers may also skew results. Even with these limitations, significant trends and patterns can be identified.

In terms of the African American population, too much emphasis is often placed on the racial classification with little regard to the ethnic or geographic differences within the population that might affect health. Jones and Laufman (1999) offer an evaluative perspective of the deficiencies in the current system for collecting cancer data on the African American population. Historically, the system has excluded the geographic areas with the highest concentration of African Americans (for example, Alabama, Arkansas, east Texas, Louisiana, and Mississippi). The SEER Program's African American population is more evenly distributed across the country (28 percent in Los Angeles, 25 percent in Detroit, 19 percent in Atlanta, and 12 percent in San Francisco). Unfortunately, data collection for rural communities is limited to ten counties in the state of Georgia. Numbering approximately 50,000 individuals, these black communities are poorer and less educated than the white communities in the same counties (Haynes & Smedley, 1999).

The diversity of the African American community also must be recognized. Liberal classifications are used in order to facilitate the creation of minority group-ings. However, intra-ethnic differences may be more significant than interethnic differences. African Americans are as diverse as Hispanics and other ethnic and racial populations, as reflected by Americans of African heritage from Nigeria, Ethiopia, South Africa, or the West Indies. Levels of socioeconomic status, edu-cation, and access to quality health care vary in the African American commu-nity as they do for all people in this country. It can also be argued that differences among U.S. communities in different geographic areas can have significant im-pact on outcomes, resources available, and standard of care. An African Ameri-can in rural west Alabama experiences a different variety of circumstances than does an African American in the urban San Francisco area or in Atlanta. The current data collection system does not satisfactorily elucidate these racial, ethnic, and geographic differences observed in variant African American populations. In addition, the states with the greatest number of African Americans (states in the Southeast) are omitted by most collection services and therefore not considered in overall evaluation of the problem of cancer (Jones & Laufman, 1999).

Just recently, the NCI proposed the creation of a national cancer surveillance plan that would extend the area of coverage and form partnerships among organizations such as the ACS, the American College of Surgeons, the North American Association of Central Cancer Registries, and the National Cancer Registrar's Association to further their cancer surveillance and control efforts (NCI, 2000). It is hoped that this expansion will ameliorate the present data exclusion problem.

Racial and Ethnic Differences

Racial and ethnic minority groups in the United States are at a disadvantage relative to whites in access to and availability of health care and preventive services (NCHS, 1994). In addition to limited access to appropriate care, other reasons may contribute to poorer outcomes, such as dietary practices, environmental exposure, language differences, and socioeconomic and educational status (Schottenfeld & Fraumeni, 1996). These factors, along with an excess of employment in high-risk occupations, prejudice, and discrimination, may contribute to the increased cancer incidence and mortality and to the survival disparities experienced among all minority and disadvantaged populations (Baquet & Ringen, 1986; Jones & Newell, 1989).

However, due to the limitations of data collection mentioned earlier and the limited cancer research targeted to minority populations, the existing cancer disparities are not yet fully understood. For instance, many barriers still prevent African Americans and other minority populations from participating in cancer research (CDC, 1998; Mouton, Harris, Rovi, Solorzano, & Johnson, 1997; Paskett, DeGraffinreid, Tatum, & Margitic, 1996). Overall, African Americans have more negative attitudes than whites do toward participating in cancer studies due to the mistrust they may have of the scientific community. Many African Americans and other minority groups believe that scientists who conduct health research should not be trusted because their main interest lies in conducting research and not in helping those they are studying (Mouton et al., 1997). These negative beliefs and attitudes held by many African Americans and members of other minority groups may stem from their own negative experiences or from the mistrust that the scientific community has instilled in these populations through the years. For example, the African American community still mistrusts the scientific community due to the way black men were abused by the unethical Tuskegee syphilis study. These negative perceptions held by minority populations need to be changed; otherwise they will continue to limit the recruitment, participation, and retention of African Americans and other minorities in cancer research.

As illustrated in Tables 11.1 and 11.2, cancer incidence and mortality statistics differ notably among racial and ethnic groups in the United States, with

African Americans experiencing the highest rates of incidence per 100,000 (men, 598.0; women, 335.6) and mortality (men, 308.8; women, 168.1), whereas Native Americans experience the lowest incidence (men, 177.8; women, 136.8) and mortality rates (men, 123.3; women, 90.2) among all racial and ethnic groups. The cancer incidence rates for Hispanics (men, 326.6; women, 243.2) and Asians and Pacific Islanders (men, 325.5; women, 244.9) are similar to each other, and the same similarity is observed when comparing mortality rates (Hispanic men, 131.8, women, 83.3; Asian and Pacific Islander men, 129.2, women, 83.5). The only exception in this picture is for breast cancer—white women obtained a higher incidence rate (113.2) than African American women (99.3).

Table 11.3 illustrates that overall, African Americans have the poorest five-year survival rate for all cancer sites (48 percent) when compared to whites (61 percent) or to all groups combined (59 percent).

Figure 11.1 shows the ratios by which the death rates for African American men and women exceed the death rates for the white population for many

TABLE 11.1. CANCER INCIDENCE RATES PER 100,000 BY SITE, GENDER, RACE, AND ETHNICITY, 1990–1996.

Incidence	White	African American	Asian and Pacific Islander	American Indian	Hispanic*
All sites					
Males	480.2	598.0	325.5	177.8	326.9
Females	351.6	335.6	244.9	136.8	243.2
Total*	402.9	442.9	279.1	153.4	275.4
Prostate	147.3	222.9	81.5	46.5	102.8
Breast (female)	113.2	99.3	72.6	33.9	69.4
Lung and bronchus					
Males	73.1	112.3	52.4	25.3	38.8
Females	43.3	46.2	22.5	13.5	19.6
Total*	55.9	73.9	35.8	18.6	27.6
Colon and rectum					
Males	53.2	58.1	47.5	21.5	35.7
Females	36.8	44.9	31.4	12.4	24.0
Total*	43.9	50.4	38.6	16.4	29.0

Note: Age-adjusted to the 1970 U.S. standard population. It should be noted that the denominator can include multiple primary cancers occurring in one individual. This rate can be computed for each type of cancer as well as for all cancers combined. Rates are for invasive cancers only, unless otherwise specified. Data are from ten SEER areas (San Francisco, Connecticut, Detroit, Iowa, New Mexico, Seattle, Utah, Atlanta, San Jose-Monterey, and Los Angeles).

*Hispanic does not exclude membership in an additional racial or ethnic group.

Source: Ries, Kosary, Hankey, Miller, Clegg, & Edwards (1999). Reprinted by the permission of the American Cancer Society, Inc.

TABLE 11.2. CANCER MORTALITY RATES PER 100,000 BY SITE, GENDER, RACE, AND ETHNICITY, 1990–1996.

Mortality	White	African American	Asian and Pacific Islander	American Indian	Hispanic*
All sites					
Males	208.8	308.0	129.2	123.3	131.8
Females	139.8	168.1	83.5	90.2	83.3
Total*	167.5	223.3	103.4	104.0	104.9
Lung and bronchus					
Males	70.1	100.8	34.9	40.5	32.0
Females	33.8	32.8	14.9	19.8	11.0
Total*	49.3	60.5	23.7	28.8	19.9
Prostate	23.7	54.8	10.7	14.3	16.7
Breast (female)	25.7	31.4	11.4	12.3	15.3
Colon and rectum					
Males	21.5	27.8	13.4	11.0	13.2
Females	14.5	20.0	9.0	8.9	8.4
Total*	17.4	23.1	10.9	9.9	10.4

Note: Age-adjusted to the 1970 U.S. standard population. It should be noted that mortality rates can be computed for each type of cancer as well as for all cancers combined. Data for Hispanics do not include deaths that occurred in Connecticut, Louisiana, New Hampshire, and Oklahoma.

*Hispanic does not exclude membership in an additional racial or ethnic group.

Source: Ries, Kosary, Hankey, Miller, Clegg, & Edwards, 1999. Reprinted by the permission of the American Cancer Society, Inc.

TABLE 11.3. TRENDS IN FIVE-YEAR RELATIVE SURVIVAL RATES BY SELECTED SITES AND RACE, 1989–1995.

Survival	White (%)	African American (%)	All Races* (%)
All sites	61	48	59
Prostate	93	84	92
Breast (female)	86	71	85
Uterine corpus	86	56	84
Uterine cervix	71	59	70
Colon	62	52	62
Rectum	60	51	60
Esophagus	13	9	12
Liver	6	3	5
Pancreas	4	4	4

Note: Percentage rates are adjusted for normal expectancy and are based on cases diagnosed from 1989 and followed through 1996.

*Includes Hispanics, Asians and Pacific Islanders, and Native Americans as well as African Americans and whites.

Source: Data adapted from ACS, 2000. Reprinted by the permission of the American Cancer Society, Inc.

FIGURE 11.1. CANCER SITE RATIOS WHERE AFRICAN AMERICAN MORTALITY EXCEEDS WHITE MORTALITY, 1992–1996.

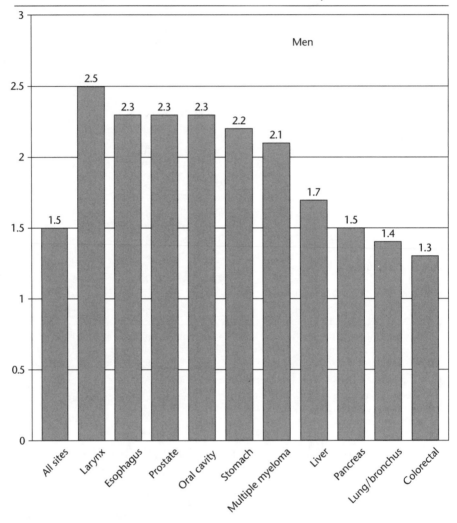

Note: Rates are age adjusted to the 1970 U.S. standard population.

Source: Ries et al., 1999. Reprinted by the permission of the American Cancer Society, Inc.

FIGURE 11.1. CANCER SITE RATIOS WHERE AFRICAN AMERICAN MORTALITY EXCEEDS WHITE MORTALITY, 1992–1996.

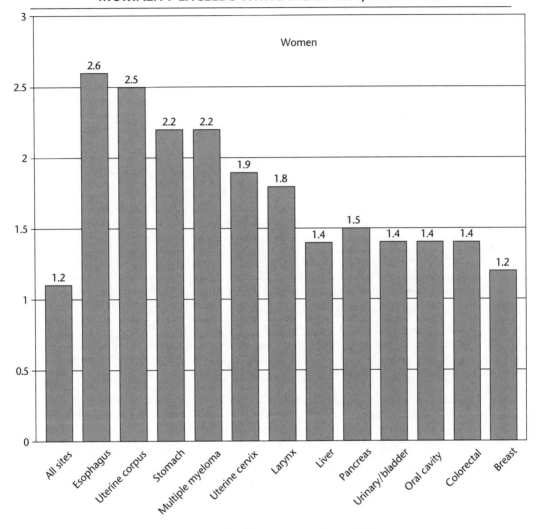

Note: Rates are age adjusted to the 1970 U.S. standard population.

Source: Ries et al., 1999. Reprinted by the permission of the American Cancer Society, Inc.

cancer sites. These cancers are not only the cancers with poor survival rates overall, where the mortality rates are close to the incidence rates (esophagus, liver, pancreas), but also the cancers with better survival rates overall (uterine corpus and cervix, prostate, and breast [female]) (Schottenfeld & Fraumeni, 1996; Ries, Kosary, et al., 1998, 1999). There are a few cancers for which African Americans have a better survival rate compared to white Americans, including cancer of the nervous system and the brain, myelocytic leukemia, and non-Hodgkin's lymphoma (females) (Schottenfeld & Fraumeni, 1996; Ries, Miller, et al., 1994).

The following sections look more closely at racial and ethnic differences for specific cancers.

Lung Cancer

Both incidence and mortality rates for lung cancer in African American men are higher than the rates among their white and Hispanic counterparts. Researchers have tried to discover reasons for the high incidence of lung and bronchus cancers in African Americans by hypothesizing different causation. For example, Perez-Stable, Herrera, Jacob, and Benowitz (1998) concluded that African Americans could be at a higher risk of developing lung and bronchus cancer because they tend to metabolize serum cotinine (a major metabolite of nicotine) at a lower rate than other racial or ethnic groups, thus suggesting it is more difficult for this population to quit smoking. Other studies that have examined the role of genetics as a predisposing factor for lung and bronchial cancer have found that smoking patterns and not polymorphic gene variance were a greater determining factor for the increased risk among the African American population (Haynes & Smedley, 1999). These biological and inherited differences warrant further investigation before definite conclusions are made. Smoking rates among African American youngsters have been on the increase since the mid-1990s, and at the same time, approximately 45,000 African Americans die each year from smoking-related diseases. If these patterns continue, an estimated 1.6 million African American teenagers will become regular smokers, and about 500,000 will die from smoking-related diseases (CDC, 1998).

Prostate Cancer

More African American men develop and die of prostate cancer than do men in any other racial or ethnic group. African American men with advanced prostate cancer are less likely than white men to receive surgical treatment, and this lack of treatment options plus the inability to obtain the best treatments may result in the higher mortality rate observed in African American men with advanced disease (Ries, Kosary, et al., 1999). This indicates that the health care industry may also contribute to the poor outcomes observed in the racial and ethnic minority populations in regard to cancer survival. It has also been postulated that one of the reasons prostate cancer is more prevalent in African American men than in white men may be hormonal differences, even in utero. Henderson, Bernstein, Ross, Depue, and Judd (1988) have reported that pregnant African American women have significantly higher serum testosterone levels than pregnant white women. In addition, this group has also reported a significant difference between the non-protein bound testosterone serum fraction in young African American men and that in their white male counterparts (Ross, Bernstein, Judd, Hanisch, Pike, & Henderson, 1986).

Breast Cancer

African American women suffer from the highest mortality rate for breast cancer and are less likely than white women to survive five years postdiagnosis (see Table 11.3). Seventy-five percent of the survival differences observed among these two racial groups might be attributed to stage at diagnosis, tumor characteristics, comorbidity, and socioeconomic factors. Thus increased screening and the availability of a continuum of care among African American women may help improve their survival rates (Schottenfeld & Fraumeni, 1996).

Compared with white women in the United States, African American women have similar incidence rates for some cancers; nevertheless, their mortality rates are much higher. Another unexplainable difference between African American women and white women is that even when breast cancer is diagnosed at the same stage, African American women have larger tumors and lymph nodes are usually affected (Seidman, Silverberg, & Holleb, 1976; Walker, Figgs, & Zahm, 1995).

Assumptions have been made that the reasons for the excessive cancer incidence and mortality experienced by African American women include lack of access to medical care, comparatively lower socioeconomic status, improvements in case finding, census underenumeration of African Americans in general (which would inflate incidence rates), smoking, alcohol consumption, diet, negative social behavior, and urban living (President's Cancer Panel, 1999). However, the majority of the studies are descriptive and not analytic to explain the findings (Jones & Laufman, 1999).

It is often stated that both white and African American women (and other women) share many of the same cancer risk factors, but this does not explain the differences in cancer morbidity and mortality rates. Although the previously mentioned factors may be related to cancer etiology, precise associations with increased risk have not been examined (Jones & Laufman, 1999).

The factors affecting African American men (for example, lack of treatment options and the inability to obtain the best treatments) may also result in the higher mortality rate observed in African American women with advanced breast cancer.

A national breast cancer survey study conducted by the American College of Surgeons that compared data from 2,400 African American women and 24,000 white women with breast cancer (Natarjan, Nemoto, Mettlin, & Murphy, 1985) indicated that African American women were less likely to have positive estrogen receptors in their primary tumors. In addition, it also concluded that African American women have poorer survival rates when matched with white women with the same tumor stage and estrogen receptor status. Significant differences were also observed between African American and white female patients for family history of breast cancer, age at first pregnancy, number of pregnancies, and age at menopause. This has led to the question of whether there is a difference between these groups on other variables, such as oncogene patterns. Unpublished data from a study conducted by Jones et al. (1995) indicates that non-protein bound and albumin bound estradiol serum fractions may be higher in young African American women compared to white women. It is possible that all of these hormonal differences may be related to cultural variables such as diet (Jones & Newell, 1989). Therefore, it is evident that a study of African American–white cancer rate differences that incorporates nutritional factors has the potential to provide new insight into the etiology of cancer for the entire population (Jones & Newell, 1989).

Colorectal Cancer

African Americans have a higher risk of colorectal cancer than any other racial group, 30 percent higher than the risk among whites and about twice as much as the risk among Native Americans or among Asians and Pacific Islanders. Comparison of incidence rates among racial and ethnic populations in the United States reveals the influence of cultural and socioeconomic differences (for example, lifestyle practices, dietary habits, use of tobacco and alcohol consumption, physical activity, and high-risk occupations) (Schottenfeld & Fraumeni, 1996). There is evidence of possible genetic and environmental interactions, as there is for most cancers.

Cancer Prevention and Early Detection

Early in the twentieth century, cancer was the leading cause of death in the United States, but presently it is the second leading cause of death, killing 23.3 percent of the population and surpassed only by cardiovascular diseases (which account for 31.4 percent of deaths) (Weinberg, 1996). That is, one of every four deaths in the United States is attributable to cancer. If this trend continues, cancer will be the leading cause of death in this country in the twenty-first century (Weinberg, 1996). The ACS Cancer Resource Center (1999) reports that approximately 50 percent of men and 30 percent of women in the United States will develop cancer during their lifetime. Since 1990, approximately 5 million Americans have died from cancer, and almost 13 million were diagnosed with the disease. The ACS (1999, 2000a, 2000b) predicts that by the year 2000, around 1,220,100 new cancer cases will occur in the United States (619,700 in men and 600,400 in women); during the same year, 552,000 Americans will die from the disease (284,100 men and 268,100 women), and approximately 124,400 of these cancer deaths will occur among African Americans. The five cancers with the highest five-year survival rates by stage and diagnosis are cancers of the testes and thyroid (95 percent), prostate (92 percent), melanoma (88 percent), and breast (85 percent); whereas those with the poorest five-year survival rates are cancers of the pancreas (4 percent), liver (5 percent), esophagus (12 percent), lung and bronchus (14 percent), and stomach (21 percent) (ACS, 2000).

A risk factor is "anything that increases a person's chance of developing a disease, including cancer" (ACS, 2000b). Different cancers have different risk factors. For example, smoking is a risk factor for cancers of the lungs, mouth, throat, larynx, bladder, and several other organs. Although risk factors increase a person's chance of developing a disease, they do not always cause the disease. Many people with one or more risk factors never develop cancer, whereas others with this disease have no known risk factors. It is important, however, to know about risk factors so that appropriate vigilant action can be taken, such as changing one's health behavior or receiving close monitoring for a potential cancer (ACS Prostate Cancer Resource Center, 2000).

Cancer sometimes does not cause overt symptoms until it has spread so far that it is impossible for the patient to be cured. However, when prompt attention is given to the signs and symptoms that do appear, this may lead to an early diagnosis and treatment that can result in a cure for patients (ACS Lung Cancer Resource Center, 2000).

The only cancers that currently have recommended guidelines for screening and early detection for asymptomatic individuals are cancers of the breast, prostate, colon and rectum, and uterine cervix. Table 11.4 summarizes the ACS recommendations for the screening and early detection of these cancers in asymptomatic individuals, including a general cancer-related checkup.

Because there are no screening tests for lung and bronchus cancer available for the general population, it is logical to assume that periodic surveillance of high-risk groups, including sputum cytology, may be the only mode available to detect early-stage cancers (Schottenfeld & Fraumeni, 1994). Nevertheless, studies conducted among asymptomatic individuals have not shown a reduction in lung cancer mortality (Fontana, 1986). Primary prevention is the only major preventive measure—for example, the avoidance of cigarette smoking could be the most important available preventive measure for lung and bronchus cancer (Wynder, 1989), followed by antismoking laws governing the workplace and public places (Environmental Protection Agency, 1992).

TABLE 11.4. DETECTION OF CANCER IN ASYMPTOMATIC PEOPLE.

Site	Recommendation
General	A cancer-related checkup is recommended every 3 years for people aged 20 to 40 and every year for people aged 40 and older. This exam should include health counseling and, depending on a person's age, might include examinations for cancers of the thyroid, oral cavity, skin, lymph nodes, testes, and ovaries, as well as for some nonmalignant diseases.
Breast	Women 40 and older should have an annual mammogram and an annual clinical breast examination (CBE) by a health care professional. They should also perform a monthly breast self-examination. The CBE should be conducted close to the scheduled mammogram. Women aged 20 to 39 should have a CBE by a health care professional every 3 years and should perform a monthly breast self-examination.
Colon and rectum	Beginning at age 50, men and women should follow one of these examination schedules: a fecal occult blood test every year and a flexible sigmoidoscopy every 5 years, a colonoscopy every 10 years, or a double-contrast barium enema every 5 to 10 years. A digital rectal exam should be done at the same time as the sigmoidoscopy, colonoscopy, or double-contrast barium enema. People who are at moderate or high risk for colorectal cancer should talk with a doctor about a different testing schedule.
Prostate	The ACS recommends that both the prostate-specific antigen (PSA) blood test and the digital rectal examination be offered annually, beginning at age 50, to men who have a life expectancy of at least 10 years and to younger men who are at high risk. Men in high-risk groups, such as those with a strong familial predisposition to this cancer (that is, two or more affected first-degree relatives) or blacks, may begin at a younger age (45).
Cervix-uterus	All women who are or have been sexually active or who are 18 years old and older should have an annual Pap test and pelvic examination. After 3 or more consecutive satisfactory examinations with normal findings, the Pap test may be performed less frequently. Discuss the matter with your physician. Women at high risk for cancer of the uterus should have a sample of endometrial tissue examined when menopause begins.

Source: American Cancer Society Cancer Resource Center, 2000. Reprinted by permission of the American Cancer Society, Inc.

Recommendations and Needed Action

Many issues need to be addressed in order to better understand the causes of cancer, to reduce its incidence and mortality rates, and to improve the survival rates among the African American population. One of the important issues that needs to be addressed in research is using special strategies that speak to the unique barriers, beliefs, and concerns of the African American population. These strategies need to be culturally sensitive in order to attract African American participants into clinical and epidemiological cancer studies (Paskett et al., 1996). Many barriers still prevail that prevent African Americans and other minority populations from participating in cancer research (CDC, 1998; Mouton et al., 1997; Paskett et al., 1996). Overall, African Americans have more negative attitudes toward participating in cancer studies than whites. They are more likely to mistrust scientists' motives, and they are aware of such harsh events in the past as the unethical Tuskegee study. These beliefs need to be changed to open the way for the recruitment and participation of African Americans in cancer studies and ultimately in cancer control. Optimally, the cancer institutions conducting research need to employ investigators who reflect the racial or ethnic composition of their study participants in order to improve trust between researcher and patient and to create a perception of a caring attitude toward minority populations (Mouton et al., 1997).

In addition, they must

- Restructure the current cancer data collection system by expanding its sampling base to include the regions with high concentrations of African Americans.
- Increase the types and number of variables in the current surveillance system.
- Conduct better descriptive and analytic cancer studies, recognizing that African Americans are not all alike, either genetically or culturally, and collecting data from a number of different groups.
- Develop culturally sensitive methodologies to provide accurate cancer information about the African American population.
- Examine the relationship between cancer and the cancer risks associated with the African American population by conducting quality behavioral and epidemiological research.
- Disseminate research findings in a manner that makes them available to the African American community at large.

If the design of cancer research among African Americans takes into consideration all of these points, accurate cancer information may be obtained that ultimately will decrease the high incidence and mortality and increase the survival rates of the African American population. Once the newly proposed national cancer surveillance program directed by the NCI in collaboration with other agencies and institutions begins, more cancer registries will be available in regions with a high concentration of African Americans and more accurate data from this minority population will be collected.

Appendix: Resources

The following are a few of the agencies and organizations dealing with cancer. They may also provide information about available services in specific communities.

African-American Breast-Cancer Alliance
P.O. Box 8981
Minneapolis, MN 55408
(612) 825-3675

American Cancer Society National Headquarters
599 Clifton Road NE
Atlanta, GA 30329
(404) 320-3333
Fax: (404) 636-2317
Cancer Information Center: (800) ACS-2345
Web site: www.cancer.org

American Lung Association
1840 York Road, Suite M
Timonium, MD 21093
(800) LUNG-USA
Fax: (202) 682-5874

Cancer Care
1180 Avenue of the Americas
New York, NY 10036
(212) 302-2400; (800) 813-HOPE
Fax: (212) 719-0263

Colon Cancer Alliance
175 Ninth Avenue
New York, NY 10011
(212) 627-7451; (877) 422-2030
Fax: (425) 940-6147

Intercultural Cancer Council
PMB-C

1720 Dryden Street
Houston, TX 77030
(713) 798-4617
Fax: (713) 798-3990
E-mail: icc@bcm.tmc.edu
Web site: http://icc.bcm.tmc.edu

National Cancer Institute
International Cancer Information Center
9030 Old Georgetown Road
Bethesda, MD 20814-1519
(800) 624-7890
Fax: (301) 402-5874

National Coalition for Cancer Survivorship
1010 Wayne Avenue, Suite 770
Silver Spring, MD 20910-5600
(877) 633-7937
Fax: (301) 565-9670
E-mail: info@cansearch.org
Web site: www.cansearch.org

References

American Cancer Society (1999). *Cancer facts and figures, 1999* [On-line]. Available: www.cancer.org/statistics

American Cancer Society. (2000a). *Cancer facts & figures: 2000* [On-line]. Available: www.cancer.org/statistics

American Cancer Society. (2000b). *Cancer facts & figures for African Americans: 2000–2001* [On-line]. Available: www.cancer.org/statistics

American Cancer Society Cancer Resource Center. (1999). *Cancer Resource Center* [On-line]. Available: www3.cancer.org.cancerinfo

American Cancer Society Cancer Resource Center. (2000). *Cancer Resource Center* [On-line]. Available: www3.cancer.org.cancerinfo

American Cancer Society Lung Cancer Resource Center. (2000). *Lung cancer* [On-line]. Available: www3.cancer.org.cancerinfo

American Cancer Society Prostate Cancer Resource Center. (2000). *Prostate cancer* [On-line]. Available: www3.cancer.org.cancerinfo.

Baquet, C., & Ringen, K. (1986). *Cancer among blacks and other minorities.* Washington, DC: National Institutes of Health.

Centers for Disease Control and Prevention. (1998). Provisional estimates from the National Health Interview Survey Supplement on cancer control. *Morbidity and Mortality Weekly Report, 37,* 417–420.

Environmental Protection Agency. (1992). *Respiratory health effects of passive smoking: Lung cancer and other disorders.* Washington, DC: Author.

Fontana, R. S. (1986). Screening for lung cancer: Recent experience in the United States. In H. Hansen (Ed.), *Lung cancer: Basic and clinical aspects.* Boston: Nijhoff.

Haynes, M. A., & Smedley, B. D. (Eds.). (1999). *The unequal burden of cancer: An assessment of NIH research and programs for ethnic minorities and the medically underserved.* Washington, DC: National Academy Press.

Henderson, B. E., Bernstein, L., Ross, R. K., Depue, R. H., & Judd, K. L. (1988). The early in utero estrogen and testosterone environment of blacks and whites: Potential effects on male offspring. *British Journal of Cancer, 57*(2), 216–218.

Jones, L. A. (Ed.). (1989). Minorities and cancer. New York: Springer-Verlag.

Jones, L. A., Dipaolo, D., Insull, W., Johnston, D. C., Mitchell, M. F., Vogel, V., Berkowitz, A., Shallelberger, R., Klish, W., Yick, J., & Johnston, D. (1995). The effects of a low-fat diet on bioavailable estrogen levels in an ethnically diverse population [Extended abstract]. In Proceedings: American Association for Cancer Research (Vol. 36, p. 686).

Jones, L. A., & Laufman, L. (1999). Data collection in African American communities: Discussion and recommendations. *Journal of Registry Management, 26*(4), 149–152.

Jones, L. A., & Newell, G. R. (1989). Introduction to section 1. (pp. 03–04). In L. A. Jones (Ed.), *Minorities and cancer.* New York: Springer-Verlag.

Mouton, C. P., Harris, S., Rovi, S., Solorzano, P., & Johnson, M. S. (1997). Barriers to black women's participation in cancer clinical trials. *Journal of the National Medical Association, 89,* 721–727.

Natarjan, N., Nemoto, T., Mettlin, C., & Murphy, G. P. (1985). Race-related differences in breast cancer patients. *Cancer, 56*(7) 1704–1709.

National Cancer Institute. (1998, April 6). Breast cancer prevention trial shows major benefit, some risks [Press release]. Bethesda, MD: National Institutes of Health.

National Cancer Institute. (2000, March 17). President's Cancer Panel, January 1, 1997–December 31, 1999. Cancer care issues in the United States: Quality of care, quality of life. (Report of the chairman, President's Cancer Panel, 1999.) Bethesda, MD: National Institutes of Health, Office of Cancer Communications.

National Center for Health Statistics. (1994). *Health, United States, 1993* (DHHS Publication No. PHS 94-1232). Hyattsville, MD: Author.

Paskett, E. D., DeGraffinreid, C., Tatum, C. M., & Margitic, S. E. (1996). The recruitment of African Americans to cancer prevention and control studies. *Preventive Medicine, 25,* 547–553.

Perez-Stable, E. J., Herrera, B., Jacob, P., & Benowitz, N. L. (1998). Nicotine metabolism and intake in black and white smokers. *Journal of the American Medical Association, 280,* 152–156.

President's Cancer Panel, January 1, 1997–December 31, 1998. (1999). *Cancer care issues in the United States: Quality of care, quality of life. Report of the chairman, president's cancer panel 1999.* Bethesda, MD: National Cancer Institute, National Cancer Program. Available: http://deainfo.nci.nih.gov/advisory/pcp/pcp97-98rpt/pcp97-98rpt.htm

Ries, L.A.G., Kosary, C. L., Hankey, B. F., Miller, B. A., & Edwards, B. K. (Eds.). (1998). *SEER cancer statistics review, 1973–1995* (NIH Publication No. 98-2789). Bethesda, MD: National Cancer Institute.

Ries, L.A.G., Kosary, C. L., Hankey, B. F., Miller, B. A., Clegg, L. X., & Edwards, B. K. (Eds.). (1999). *SEER cancer statistics review, 1973–1996* (NIH Publication No. 99-2789). Bethesda, MD: National Cancer Institute.

Ries, L.A.G., Miller, B. A., Hankey, B. F., Kosary, C. L., Harras, A., & Edwards, B. K. (Eds.). (1994). *SEER cancer statistics review, 1973–1991: Tables and graphs* (NIH Publication No. 94-2789). Bethesda, MD: National Cancer Institute.

Ross, R., Bernstein, L., Judd, H., Hanisch, R., Pike, M., & Henderson, B. (1986). Serum testosterone levels in healthy young black and white men. *Journal of the National Cancer Institute, 76,* 45–48.

Schottenfeld, D., & Fraumeni, J. F. (Eds.). (1994). *Cancer epidemiology and prevention.* New York: Oxford University Press.

Schottenfeld, D., & Fraumeni, J. F. (Eds.). (1996). *Cancer epidemiology and prevention* (2nd ed.). New York: Oxford University Press.

Seidman, H., Silverberg, E., & Holleb, A. I. (1976). Cancer statistics: A comparison of white and black populations. *Cancer, 26,* 2–29.

Walker, B., Figgs, L., & Zahm, S. H. (1995). Differences in cancer incidence, mortality, and survival between African Americans and whites. *Environmental Health Perspectives, 8,* 275–281.

Weinberg, R. A. (1996). *Racing to the beginning of the road.* New York: Harmony Books.

Wingo, P. A., Ries, L.A.G., Rosenberg, H. M., Milles, D. S., & Edwards, B. K. (Eds.). (1998). *Cancer incidence and mortality, 1973–1995: A report card for the United States.* Atlanta, GA: American Cancer Society, National Cancer Institute, and Centers for Disease Control and Prevention.

Wynder, E. L. (1989). Lung cancer and smoking: The science of applying intervention strategies. *Journal of the National Cancer Institute, 81,* 388–389.

CHAPTER TWELVE

DIABETES

M. Joycelyn Elders, Frederick G. Murphy

Diabetes mellitus is a major clinical and public health problem in the African American community. The impact of the problem in terms of prevalence, quality of life, death, and disability is greatly magnified in African American communities. Diabetes mellitus was relatively uncommon among African Americans at the beginning of this century. It is now the third leading cause of death from disease in African Americans. According to the U.S. Bureau of the Census, African Americans constituted 12.2 percent of the U.S. population in 1988, a 14 percent increase since 1980. By 2005, almost 50 percent of the population will be other than white—51 percent white; 26 percent Hispanic; 14 percent African American (more than thirty-four million people); and 8 percent Asian (U.S. Department of Health and Human Services [DHHS], 1998).

Surveillance data from the Centers for Disease Control and Prevention (CDC) have shown that the prevalence of diabetes is substantially higher among blacks than whites. Black men have a prevalence of diabetes that is 80 percent higher than that for white men, and black women have a prevalence 90 percent higher than that for white women. During the 1980s, age-adjusted diabetes mortality among black men and women increased 36 percent and 16 percent, respectively. In 1990, the age-adjusted rate of hospitalizations related to diabetes for black women (183 per 10,000) was 22 percent higher than for black men (150 per 10,000), 213 percent higher than for white women (85 per 10,000), and 213 percent higher than for white men (86 per 10,000). In 1990, the age-adjusted rate for hospital discharges for diabetic ketoacidosis among black men with diabetes was 34 per 1,000. This was more than three times higher than the corresponding rate of 10 per 1,000 for white men with diabetic ketoacidosis. Similar disparities exist between black and white women with diabetes mellitus.

The United States has made positive gains toward improving the health status of its citizens over the past generation. However, not all segments of the population have fully benefited from these improvements. The country's poor and ethnic minority populations continue to be plagued by disproportionately high rates of death and disability. In 1984, the secretary of the Department of Health and Human Services formed the Task Force on Black and Minority Health to analyze the disparities in health status. The task force identified six health areas that account for more than 90 percent of excess deaths among U.S. minorities; diabetes mellitus was cited as one of the six and continues to be on the list, along with HIV.

Defining Diabetes

For the purposes of this chapter, it is important to first define diabetes in the most practical terms possible. Diabetes mellitus comprises a group of metabolic diseases characterized by hyperglycemia resulting from defects in insulin secretion, insulin action, or both (De Courten, Hodge, & Zimmet, 1998). It is a common, chronic, systemic disease characterized by glucose intolerance or the inability of the body to properly use glucose, and it has no cure. A person develops diabetes because his or her pancreas does not make enough insulin or stops making insulin entirely or because the cells in his or her body are resistant to insulin action. As a result, too much sugar begins to build up in the blood and another source of energy has to be sought. Any of these conditions leads to problems that seriously threaten the body's health. Some of the frequent clinical manifestations of diabetes are unusual thirst, frequent urination, excessive eating, weight loss, fatigue, and a constant feeling of being ill. The chronic hyperglycemia of diabetes is associated with long-term damage. Organ and other complications related to diabetes are found in the blood vessels, heart, nerves, feet, eyes, and kidneys; it also causes problems with pregnancy.

In 1997, the Expert Committee on the Diagnosis and Classification of Diabetes Mellitus issued its latest classifications for diabetes mellitus and other categories of glucose regulation. Diabetes was classified into four major categories based on etiology:

1. *Type 1 diabetes.* Beta cell destruction is present, usually leading to absolute insulin deficiency. Type 1 diabetes may be immune mediated or idiopathic.
2. *Type 2 diabetes.* This disease may range from predominantly insulin resistant with relative insulin deficiency to a predominantly secretory defect with insulin resistance.
3. *Other specific types* (De Courten et al., 1998). These include (a) genetic defects of the beta cell, (b) genetic defects in insulin action, (c) diseases of the exocrine pancreas, (d) endocrinopathies, (e) drug- or chemical-induced diabetes,

(f) viral infections, (g) uncommon forms of immune-mediated diabetes, and (h) other genetic syndromes sometimes associated with diabetes.

4. *Gestational diabetes mellitus.*

Type 1 diabetes is an autoimmune disease that results in damage or destruction of the beta cells of the pancreas in which insulin is produced, leading to partial or complete insulin deficiency. Type 2 diabetes is a metabolic disorder that has the consequence of insulin resistance occurring at the tissue level, with little or no impairment of insulin synthesis or release. These forms of diabetes differ in their age of onset, occurrence in the population, clinical manifestations, degree of inheritability, and treatment.

Type 1 diabetes (previously known as insulin-dependent diabetes mellitus [IDDM] or juvenile-onset diabetes [JODM]) may occur at any age but typically develops in children or young adults under thirty years of age. Type 1 diabetes accounts for approximately 5 percent of the diabetic population in the United States (DHHS, 1998). In this country, it is less common in blacks than in whites. Some clinical manifestations of type 1 diabetes involve modest hyperglycemia for several days, weeks, or even months before hyperglycemia becomes severe. Patients usually develop diabetic ketoacidosis and coma, and die if not treated with insulin (Plotnick, 1994). Type 1 diabetes is characterized by low levels or a total absence of insulin; individuals with this kind of diabetes must inject insulin for diabetes control and in order to live.

Other complications may manifest gradually during the course of the disease and are often associated with control of the disease. Examples are limited joint mobility, growth failure, delayed puberty, and cataracts. Chronic complications include retinopathy, nephropathy, neuropathy, and coronary disease. The risk of developing type 1 diabetes is higher than the risk for virtually all other severe chronic diseases of childhood, with peak incidence occurring during puberty (American Diabetes Association [ADA], 2000).

Type 2 diabetes (previously known as non-insulin dependent diabetes mellitus [NIDDM] or maturity-onset diabetes [MOD]) is the most common type of diabetes, accounting for 90 to 95 percent of all cases. It most often affects adults, usually over age forty, seems to run in families, and is more common in women than in men. Type 2 is more common among blacks than whites, with many studies suggesting a ratio of 2 to 1 or less. The black to white ratio is higher for women than for men. The prevalence of diabetes among black men and women increases with age, as it does among whites, but the age of peak onset among blacks appears to be lower. People with the disease are often obese. They may have high, normal, or low levels of insulin, but their ability to use it effectively is impaired. Individuals with type 2 diabetes often can manage the disease through diet, weight control, and exercise, although some may require treatment with oral hypoglycemic agents or insulin. The most distressing difficulties with type 2 diabetes are related to the chronic complications of cardiovascular disease, retinopathy, neuropathy, and nephropathy.

The incidence of type 2 diabetes in childhood and adolescence is increasing, especially in minority populations (from 4 percent in 1982 to 16 percent in 1994), and may be as high as 33 percent of newly diagnosed diabetes in minorities. The increase in the prevalence of this disorder at younger ages is thought to be related to a more sedentary lifestyle than children had in the past and an increased prevalence of obesity. In addition to the hyperglycemia, these children usually manifest obesity as opposed to weight loss, mild hypertension, acanthosis nigricans, and a family history of type 2 diabetes mellitus. Their diabetes is usually controlled with diet, exercise, and oral hypoglycemic agents. They do not require insulin for control as most are hyperinsulinemic and they are not ketosis prone under basal conditions (Pihoker, Scott, Lensing, Craddock, & Smith, 1998; Stuart, Gilkison, Smith, Keenan, & Nagamani, 1998).

Impaired glucose tolerance constitutes a heterogeneous grouping of patients who fit neither into the type 1 nor the type 2 category. These patients have abnormal glucose metabolism, which may be demonstrated by their impaired ability to dispose of a glucose load, or fasting hyperglycemia. However, inadequate insulin secretion or action is not the primary pathogenic abnormality.

Maturity-onset diabetes mellitus of youth (MODY), a very specific genetic form of carbohydrate intolerance, has an autosomal dominant mode of inheritance and has been shown to be due to an abnormality of the insulin molecule.

Gestational diabetes (GDM) is a mild form of diabetes that affects women only during pregnancy. The prevalence of GDM has been stated to range from 2 percent to 5 percent of all nondiabetic pregnant women. In select patient populations, the incidence rate is 2 to 7 percent of pregnant women, with no significant differences among black, white, and Hispanic populations. Approximately 40 percent of women with GDM who have been obese before pregnancy develop type 2 diabetes within four years. GDM identifies health risks to the fetus and the newborn (ADA, 2000; DHHS, 1998).

Pregnant women with diabetes are usually seen by a physician or nurse more often during their pregnancy than other women who are pregnant. The National Diabetes Advisory Board and the CDC recommend that pregnant women with diabetes be cared for jointly by an obstetrician, pediatrician, health educator, and primary care practitioner or internist familiar with diabetes. With the new knowledge, skills, and equipment available today, the probability of delivering a healthy baby, even when the mother or baby has developed a medical problem, is much greater than in previous years (CDC, 1991).

Overview of the Problem

Diabetes mellitus remains the seventh leading cause of death in the United States, primarily from the cardiovascular disease it causes. According to death certificate data, diabetes contributed to 198,140 deaths in 1996 (ADA, 2000). Type 2 diabetes and the complications associated with it are increasing substantially in the

United States and throughout the world. The number of individuals with diabetes is steadily increasing, especially in minority communities (Flegal et al., 1991), to the point that it is now considered a common disease, with approximately 800,000 new cases diagnosed per year in the general population (DHHS, 1998; Clark, 1998; Vinicor, 1994).

There are 15.7 million people, or 5.9 percent of the population, in the United States who have type 2 diabetes. Approximately half of the estimated 10.3 million individuals who have diabetes mellitus are not aware they have the disease. African Americans are 1.7 times as likely to have type 2 diabetes as the general population. An estimated 2.3 million African Americans, or 10.8 percent, have diabetes. Twenty-five percent of African Americans between the ages of sixty-five and seventy-four have diabetes. One in four African American women over fifty-five years of age has diabetes (ADA, 2000).

In 1997, the per capita cost of health care for all persons without diabetes was $2,699 compared to $10,071 for those with diabetes. The total economic cost of diabetes in 1997 was estimated to be $98 billion (ADA, 2000). Many persons learn they have diabetes, dubbed the *silent killer* and the *hidden disease,* only when a life-threatening complication occurs (Expert Committee, 1997; Eastman & Vinicor, 1997). Here is a closer look at these complications.

Cardiovascular disease. Heart disease is present in 75 percent of diabetes-related deaths, more than 77,000 deaths per year. People with diabetes are two to four times more likely to have heart disease, and two to four times more likely to suffer a stroke (ADA, 2000). Not all the connections are clear, but it is apparent that the higher incidence among persons with diabetes (PWDs) of coronary risk factors such as hypertension, cigarette smoking, increased body fat, and elevated blood cholesterol contributes to their chances of developing heart disease. Coronary artery disease alone claims 38,000 diabetics annually, and it is estimated that preventive (risk reduction) measures could reduce this mortality rate by 45 percent (DHHS, 1998). Because high blood pressure is a major risk factor for stroke, the correlation between stroke and diabetes may be largely due to the increased prevalence of hypertension, especially in African American PWDs. Controlling high blood pressure might prevent a vast majority of strokes from occurring among this population.

Blindness. Diabetes is the leading cause of new cases of blindness in individuals aged twenty to seventy-four. Approximately 20,000 persons lose their sight each year due to diabetes (CDC, 1997b; DHHS, 1998). The primary vision disorder affecting diabetics is retinopathy, a condition in which enlarged and damaged capillaries lead to swelling and hemorrhaging in the retina, often impairing the portion of the eye specializing in detail vision. As capillaries become closed off, new blood vessels form, breaking through and leaking into the inner surface of the retina and seriously interfering with vision. Retinopathy can be detected before damage is evident, and a variety of treatments, including laser therapy and surgery, can improve vision and slow retinal damage. However, many African

Americans cannot obtain or afford such care. Consequently, a disproportionate number may lose their vision because of this barrier to eye care. African Americans are twice as likely to suffer from blindness due to diabetic retinopathy (ADA, 2000). These numbers could be substantially reduced by an increase in access to care for PWDs.

Kidney disease. Kidney diseases occur among PWDs when high blood sugar forces the kidney to filter more blood than is actually needed in an effort to keep wastes in the blood low. This overwork initially leads to hypercellularity of the glomeruli followed by a gradual degeneration of the kidneys' vital cleaning system. Known as diabetic nephropathy, this condition develops with diabetes. End-stage renal disease (ESRD), the most severe form of kidney disease, requires dialysis or transplantation for survival. Diabetes is the leading cause of end-stage renal disease, resulting in approximately 40 percent of new cases each year. In 1995, this translated into approximately 27,900 people (DHHS, 1998; ADA, 2000). African Americans with diabetes are 2.6 to 5.6 times more likely than whites to experience end-stage renal disease; this means more than 4,000 new cases of end-stage renal disease each year (ADA, 2000).

Nerve disease and amputations. According to the Public Health Service, diabetes is the leading cause of nontraumatic amputations in the United States (approximately 57,000 per year). Most individuals (60 to 70 percent) with diabetes have mild to severe forms of diabetic nerve damage, which when severe can lead to amputations. African Americans are 1.5 to 2.5 times more likely than whites to have lower limb amputations (ADA, 2000). Forty-five percent of amputations not caused by injury occur as complications of diabetes. Most often, these amputations—usually of the foot or lower leg—are necessitated by gangrene and ulceration or by peripheral arterial disease. This condition, which is four times more common in PWDs than in those without the disease, involves both hardening of the normally elastic arterial walls and deposits of plaque in the artery. Among diabetics, 60 percent of the new cases of peripheral arterial disease are estimated to be preventable.

The minority communities of African Americans, Hispanics, American Indians and Alaskan Natives, and Asians and Pacific Islanders are vulnerable, high-risk populations constituting a worsening major diabetic disease challenge for the United States (DHHS, 1998; Clark, 1998; CDC, 1997a, 1997c). Two factors contribute substantially to this chronic disease epidemic.

Improper nutrition. Increasing numbers of persons are overweight in the United States, especially in minority communities and in association with a diet high in high-fat and processed foods (CDC, 1997a; Kuczmarski, Flegal, Campbell, & Johnson, 1994). Obesity, improper nutrition, and lack of physical activity now occur in persons younger than fifteen years of age, perhaps explaining the reporting of type 2 diabetes in young teenagers (Christoffel & Ariza, 1998; DHHS, 1998).

Decreased physical activity. Physical activity in the United States is decreasing steadily for all segments of the population (DHHS, 1996, 1998).

African Americans have a higher prevalence of obesity than other population groups than whites do, a strong risk factor for type 2 diabetes. Among people with diagnosed diabetes, 82 percent of adult African American women are obese compared with 62 percent of white women; among men, 45 percent of African Americans are obese compared with 39 percent of whites. African Americans are also known to have a higher prevalence of hypertension, which is associated with retinopathy and renal and cardiovascular complications—major complications in African American diabetic patients. Studies are needed to elucidate the disease processes involved in these conditions and to develop better methods of prevention and treatment.

Studies of dietary habits of African Americans indicate that they consume less fiber and more cholesterol-rich foods than whites, although their total caloric consumption and fat intake are lower. African Americans tend to have less access to financial, social, health, and educational resources that would help improve their health status and health awareness. Educational resources—including materials and programs—are needed that take the lifestyles, interests, and cultural and economic considerations of the African American population into account (Murray & Lopez, 1997; DHHS, 1998).

Building a Research Agenda and Taking Current Action

Working with data from the Human Genome Project, researchers have already identified single genes associated with a number of diseases. As research progresses, investigators will also uncover the mechanisms for diseases caused by several genes or by a gene interacting with environmental factors. Genetic components have been implicated in both type 1 and type 2 diabetes (Pozilli, 1996; O'Rahilly, 1997). For type 1 diabetes, genetic markers that indicate a greater risk for this condition have been identified that are sensitive but not specific. Type 2 diabetes, especially in vulnerable minority populations, may be associated with a *thrifty gene* that promotes fat deposition and confers a survival advantage when the food supply is irregular (Neel, 1996). The possible identification of these genes and their proteins may pave the way to more effective therapies and preventive measures (Diabetes Control and Complications Trial [DCCT] Study Group, 1995; National Institutes of Health [NIH], 1993; DHHS, 1998).

In basic, clinical, applied, epidemiological, psychological, economic, and genetic engineering investigations, important observations have been made and will continue to occur concerning diabetes. It is clear that future scientific results will greatly influence the prevention and management of diabetes (Weatherall, 1995; DHHS, 1998).

Future research developments from the laboratory cannot be the sole hope for PWDs, however. There are many other avenues of prevention, diagnosis, and treatment that can be addressed immediately. Patient education and close monitoring by knowledgeable medical personnel are key to maintaining control of this multisystem chronic disease right now. Employment, security, education, and availability of health care are social issues that must be addressed and improved to reduce individuals' likelihood of developing type 2 diabetes and to promote the effective control of both types of diabetes (McDonald, 1997; Smith, 1997; DHHS, 1998).

Quality of life and degree of disability are important indicators for chronic diseases such as diabetes. Both medical professionals and nonmedical professionals such as clergy, government officials, and employers are all involved in critical decisions affecting chronic diseases. The degree to which we are able to incorporate nonmedical professionals into the lives of PWDs and accurately measure their quality of life will dictate our ability to both recognize and deal with a disease such as diabetes (Erickson, Wilson, & Shannon, 1997; Murray & Lopez, 1997; DHHS, 1998).

The availability of a responsive and effective health care system will determine our capability to ensure access to quality care, especially for secondary and tertiary prevention. At the present, about 90 percent of all PWDs receive their continuous care from their primary care community rather than from diabetic specialists. The relationship between primary care providers and specialists needs to improve to provide greater quality of care (Smith, 1997; DHHS, 1998).

Concrete recommendations must be brought to the forefront through the use of innovative yet appropriate strategies and methodologies. The importance of cultural and linguistic variables cannot be overemphasized when health interventions and medical research initiatives are being planned for minority communities. Special considerations must be taken into account, particularly in the African American community, when attempting to introduce concepts or programs that deal with primary and secondary prevention, risk reduction, community empowerment, community ownership, and infrastructure building. Without such cultural attention, research efforts will prove irrelevant, and preventive interventions will be short lived with little or no substantive impact or outcome. Prevention and primary care strategies and methodologies for the African American community must, above all, be designed with effectiveness and longevity in mind. This is not an easy task, especially considering the socioeconomic, psychosocial, ecological, environmental, political, and religious determinants that dynamically coexist in the African American community today. This constellation of critical determinants could make the development and implementation of appropriate methodologies a lifelong task for the dedicated health professional.

Chronic diseases such as diabetes mellitus must be battled forthrightly in African American communities. Health professionals must begin to spend more time on the identification and development of appropriate health intervention strategies to reduce the risk factors, morbidity, and mortality associated with diabetes. These interventions must prove effective, translatable, and replicable. Reputable institutions, both private and public, must continually develop and publish research findings and develop policies focusing on diabetes and other chronic diseases. However, this must be done with the assurance that these policies have been formulated on sound research principles and designed with cultural sensitivity. Only then will they be feasible, acceptable, and usable by professionals and agencies involved in the delivery of community-level primary, secondary, and tertiary health care. Any attempt to do otherwise will prove futile, wasting dollars.

Here are a number of specific recommendations for current practice and for research.

Personnel

- Establish the number and types of health professionals, including those in allied and associated public health fields, needed to accomplish the practice, education, and research that will manage diabetes more successfully and reduce its incidence.
- Provide an appropriate curriculum on diabetes and chronic disabling conditions in all schools and programs that prepare students for careers in the health professions, including allied and associated public health fields, and ensure that all graduates of such schools and programs demonstrate knowledge of these subjects.
- Increase the number of continuing education programs on chronic and disabling conditions that are offered by national professional associations whose members have roles in this area.
- Promote the training of more minority health professionals.

Data Collection

- Establish national and state surveillance systems that can monitor the prevalence, complications, mortality, and major risk factors associated with diabetes.
- Establish racial and ethnic identifiers in national databases, and statistically reliable samples of high-risk minority populations in national surveys.
- Collect more detailed information on the race and ethnicity recorded on hospital discharge abstracts and ESRD treatment forms.
- Improve diabetes reporting on birth certificates to monitor reproductive and birth outcomes among women with diabetes.
- Establish mechanisms for tracking blindness in general and due to diabetes specifically.

Research

- Conduct basic and clinical research to better understand the etiology and pathogenesis of diabetes and its complications.
- Conduct research to develop optimal capabilities for the diagnosis, treatment, cure, and prevention of diabetes and its complications.

Intervention Programs: Identifying Persons for Diabetes Care and Management

The 1997 Expert Committee on the Diagnosis and Classification of Diabetes Mellitus suggested these criteria for diabetes testing:

- Testing for all individuals aged ≥ 45 years
- Testing more frequently for individuals who (1) are obese, (2) have relatives with diabetes, (3) are members of high-risk ethnic groups, (4) have delivered a baby weighing ≥ 9 lb. or have been diagnosed with GDM, (5) are hypertensive, (6) have HDL cholesterol ≤ 35 and (7) had impaired glucose tolerance or impaired fasting glucose at previous testing

The factors leading to these recommendations include (1) the steep rise in the incidence of the disease after age forty-five, (2) the finding that blood glucose control is more effective in preventing the initial development of microvascular complications than in preventing the progression of complications once they have become established, (3) the negligible likelihood of developing any of the complications of diabetes in the three-year interval following a negative screening test, and (4) knowledge of the well-documented risk factors for the disease.

Although the evidence for early detection of and intervention in diabetes mellitus does not indicate that such detection is overwhelmingly successful, it does suggest some benefits from community-based screening (Bennett & Knowler, 1984; Hawthorne & Crowe, 1984). Another study, the Diabetes Control and Complications Trial (DCCT), provides some definitive data about the importance of screening for the effects of blood glucose control on the complications of diabetic retinopathy and for early detection of nephropathy (DCCT Research Group, 1990).

In recent years, several community-based diabetes intervention and study programs were designed and implemented that focused upon such specific areas as (1) decreasing the prevalence of untreated diabetic risk factors and complications in the intervention population, (2) increasing knowledge and changing attitudes and high-risk behaviors among the intervention population, and (3) improving diabetes care including patient adherence and compliance. For example, the DCCT looked at diabetes nutrition education, glucose monitoring, and insulin administration. Results of this intervention indicated the need for early detection through testing and screening of blood glucose, insulin adjustment, maintenance of normal glucose without hypoglycemia, and glycosylated hemoglobin (HgbA).

Guidelines reported in *The Prevention and Treatment of Complications of Diabetes Mellitus: A Guide for Primary Care Practitioners* recommend annual dilated eye exams for all persons with diabetes except those with insulin-dependent diabetes mellitus of less than five years duration (CDC, 1991). This practitioner's guide also recommends screening for early detection and control of hemoglobin A1c, foot problems, retinopathy, cardiovascular disease, adverse outcomes of pregnancy, periodontal disease, kidney disease, neuropathy, and acute glycemic complications.

Intervention programs focusing upon nutrition and exercise for persons with and at risk for diabetes have resulted in positive protective effects. Health intervention programs that address prevention and control of diabetes among other health issues have been more effective when based on social learning and self-directed changes than when based on the more traditional method of imparting knowledge alone (Bandura, 1986; Meyer & Henderson, 1974). Programs that provide not only the information needed to change knowledge and attitudes but also instruction on how to monitor change and achieve gradual incremental changes in dietary habits have been successful, for example, in lowering blood cholesterol level. An increasing number of small-group studies with high-risk adults have been conducted among different cultural groups in various countries and have reported effecting lasting changes in dietary habits (Institute of Medicine, 1991). An important consideration is that individuals were motivated to participate in these programs through screening tests that identified risk factors for cardiovascular disease.

Diabetes Education and Evaluation Programs

According to Hiss, Frey, and Davis (1986), persons with diabetes see their physician about three times per year and each visit lasts approximately twelve minutes. Therefore, on the average, a person with diabetes has thirty-six minutes of physician contact each year. The nonreimbursable nature of a lot of diabetes care (such as education), the lack of primary care physician time to deal with the complex aspects of diabetes education and counseling, and the poor fit of diabetes in an acute care health system collectively create a situation in which most persons with diabetes are significantly undertreated (Greene & Kreuter, 1992).

Several programs have documented the feasibility of conducting community-based evaluation centers or programs for persons with diabetes (Baker, Vallbona, Pavlik, Armbruster, & Higgins, 1991; McGill, Yue, Plehwe, Wiley, & Turtle, 1991). This is a model of how hospitals and primary care physicians can share in diabetes management based on resource availability.

Fink and Ross (1991) have also shown the effectiveness of diabetes education centers in Canada where the staff includes ophthalmologists in order to screen for and control the risk factors for vision associated with the diabetic complications.

Fink and Ross (1991) and Deeb, Wolfe, Freeman, and Wise (1991) used a standardized medical record as an evaluation-of-care instrument, entering data from a systematic random sample of diabetics each quarter. This form of surveillance program can serve as a template for collecting data and conducting an ongoing evaluation on a comprehensive system of care.

Strategies to Increase Adherence and Compliance to Treatment

Numerous intervention programs have been applied to improve patient management and treatment outcomes in diabetes mellitus. Attempts to provide information about diabetes generally have had little effect on adherence-related behaviors. Enhanced educational programs intended to inform people about their treatment, either alone or in combination with teaching behavioral strategies, have met with moderate success. A number of strategies to enhance patients' involvement in their care have been introduced.

There is substantial evidence that patients have specific desires for information and for involvement in clinical interaction (Anderson, DeVellis, Boyles, & Feussner, 1989). Moreover, patients report more dissatisfaction with information given to them by physicians in the course of the medical visit than with any other aspect of their medical care (Pendleton, 1983). Mason (1985) found that when patients' perceptions of their diabetes were in conflict with what they were told by the physician, patients expressed considerable uncertainty and anxiety about the illness and its management.

D'Eramo-Mekus and Demas (1989) surveyed twenty-five patient-physician pairs to assess the congruence of the participants' perceptions of treatment goals. Patient participants were adults being treated in private practice for non-insulin dependent diabetes mellitus. More than one-half of the patient-physician pairs did not agree on a single treatment goal. The largest discrepancy was found in perceptions of a defined weight loss goal; patients were far less likely than physicians to believe that a specific goal had been set.

Advocates of patient consumerism encourage patient involvement in medical interactions and more active participation in medical care in general. Although there is no clear consensus on the effect of this involvement, when patients are more active in their medical interactions they generally tend to be more satisfied with their care. As a result a number of interventions have focused upon coaching patients to be more assertive through asking more questions of their provider or disclosing more information about their own needs (Anderson & Sharpe, 1991; Greenfield, Kaplan, Ware, Yano, & Frank, 1988).

Some studies suggest that physicians who are "warm and friendly" are preferred by patients, although other studies indicate that physicians who are "serious and intense" have more satisfied patients (Anderson & Sharpe, 1991). In general, patients appear to be more consistently satisfied when interacting with physicians who are perceived as being involved in the interaction and who appear to be concerned about them (Pendleton, 1983). Another approach to improving diabetes care is to provide patients with good problem-solving skills so they can cope better with ongoing barriers to adherence.

In the context of diabetes education and compliance, empowerment has been defined as "an interactive process that enables persons with diabetes to acquire and enhance social, problem-solving techniques and communication skills necessary to manage their own diabetes care in a variety of life situations" (Funnel et al., 1991). This approach to diabetes care is a more appropriate model for certain racial and ethnic populations than is the more conventional compliance approach. In the traditional adherence and compliance approach to diabetes control, clients are directed by health care providers to perform specific diabetes self-care. Beliefs, expectations, and capability to perform these treatment behaviors are often not given adequate consideration (Murphy, Satterfield, Anderson, & Lyons, 1993). This approach to diabetes care and education may be especially problematic for persons from a background that differs in cultural values from the background of the provider. Because health care providers often are unaware of the cultural values meaning of prescribed diabetes care regimens, the likelihood of noncompliance is significantly increased.

The health care delivery system may require alterations in order to improve diabetes care and compliance. Major recommended interventions in the health care delivery system include changing the office-based system and reorganizing existing health care services and professionals into consultative programs, and introducing new policies such as managed care initiatives.

Despite the belief of many primary care physicians that preventive measures should be performed on a regular basis, in many settings they are not performed as recommended (Romm, Fletcher, & Hulka, 1981). Several studies have shown that computer-generated reminders (Ornstein, Garr, Jenkins, Rust, & Arnon, 1991; Harris, O'Malley, Fletcher, & Knight, 1990; McDonald et al., 1984; Tierney, Hui, & McDonald, 1986), nurse-initiated reminders (Davidson, Fletcher, Retchin, & Duh, 1984; Mandel, Franks, & Dickerson, 1985), health promotion checklists (Cohen, Littenberg, Wetzel, & Neuhauser, 1982), flow sheets (Madlon-Kay, 1987), mailed reminders (Thompson, Michnich, Gray, Friedlander, & Gilson, 1986), and administrative changes (Frame, Kowlich, & Liewellyn, 1984) can result in improved adherence and compliance to preventive services recommended by physicians. In addition, reminders to patients (Brimberry, 1988) improved adherence and compliance to preventive service recommendations in primary care settings. However, as indicated by Belcher (1990), campaigns directed at patients encouraging them to ask for services are not likely to be effective unless reinforced and encouraged in practice settings.

Conclusion

Diabetes mellitus is a major clinical and public health problem in the African American community that appears to be increasing. The fight against diabetes in African Americans must incorporate cultural sensitivity, community organization and development, infrastructure building, and community empowerment. Such structuring will enable linkages to be formed between providers and recipients and will create an atmosphere conducive to reciprocity. Without the creation of appropriate forums in which translation activities between institutions and communities, communities and individuals, and the different individuals within a community can take place, interventions will have only a minimal chance of success, and risk factors, morbidity rates, and mortality rates will continue to rise throughout the twenty-first century.

References

American Diabetes Association. (2000). *Diabetes facts and figures* [On-line]. Available: www.diabetes.org/ada/facts.asp

Anderson, L., DeVellis, R., Boyles, B., & Feussner, J. R. (1989). Patients' perceptions of their clinical interactions: Development of multidimensional desire for control scales. *Health Education Research, 4,* 383–397.

Anderson, L., & Sharpe, P. (1991). Improving patient and provider communication: A synthesis and review of communication interventions. *Patient Education and Counseling, 17,* 99–134.

Baker, S., Vallbona, C., Pavlik, B., Armbruster, M., & Higgins, C. (1991). Adult-onset diabetes control programs in a public healthcare setting. *Diabetes, 40*(Suppl. 1), 358A.

Bandura, A. (1986). *Social learning theory.* Upper Saddle River, NJ: Prentice Hall.

Belcher, D. (1990). Implementing preventive services. *Archives of Internal Medicine, 150,* 2533–2541.

Bennett, P., & Knowler, W. (1984). Early detection and intervention in diabetes mellitus: Is it effective? *Journal of Chronic Diseases, 37,* 653–666.

Brimberry, R. (1988). Vaccination of high-risk patients for influenza: A comparison of telephone and mail reminder methods. *Journal of Family Practice, 26,* 397–400.

Centers for Disease Control and Prevention. Division of Diabetes Translation. (1991). *The prevention and treatment of complications of diabetes mellitus: A guide for primary care practitioners.* Atlanta, GA: Author.

Centers for Disease Control and Prevention. (1997a). *Diabetes Surveillance, 1997.* Atlanta, GA: Author.

Centers for Disease Control and Prevention. (1997b). *National diabetes fact sheet: National estimates and general information on diabetes in the United States.* Atlanta, GA: Author.

Centers for Disease Control and Prevention. (1997c). Trends in the prevalence and incidence of self-reported diabetes mellitus: United States, 1980–1994. *Morbidity and Mortality Weekly Report, 46,* 1014–1018.

Christoffel, K., & Ariza, A. (1998). The epidemiology of overweight in children: Relevance for clinical care. *Pediatrics, 101,* 103–105.

Clark, C. (1998). How should we respond to the worldwide diabetes epidemic? *Diabetes Care, 21,* 475–476.

Cohen, D., Littenberg, B., Wetzel, C., & Neuhauser, D. (1982). Improving physician compliance with preventive medicine. *Medical Care, 20,* 1040–1045.

Davidson, R., Fletcher, S., Retchin, S., & Duh, S. (1984). A nurse-initiated reminder system for the periodic health examination. *Archives of Internal Medicine, 144,* 2167–2170.

De Courten, M., Hodge, A., & Zimmet, P. (1998). Epidemiology of diabetes: Lessons for the endocrinologist. *The Endocrinologist, 8,* 62–70.

Deeb, L., Wolfe, L., Freeman, G., & Wise, J. (1991). Development of an evaluation strategy for primary care. *Diabetes, 40* (Suppl. 1), 311A.

D'Eramo-Mekus, G., & Demas, P. (1989). Patient perceptions of diabetes treatment goals. *Diabetes Educator, 15*(5), 440–443.

Diabetes Control and Complications Trial Research Group. (1990). Diabetes control and complication trial (DCCT). *Diabetes Care, 13,* 427–433.

Diabetes Control and Complications Trial Study Group. (1995). The diabetes prevention trial: Type 1 diabetes (DCCT-1): Implementation of screening and staging of relative intervention. *Transplant Process, 27,* 3377.

Eastman, R., & Vinicor, F. (1997). Science: Moving us in the right direction. *Diabetes Care, 20,* 1057–1058.

Erickson, P., Wilson, R., & Shannon, I. (1997). *Years of Healthy Life* (Statistical Notes No. 7). Hyattsville, MD: National Center for Health Statistics.

Expert Committee on the Diagnosis and Classification of Diabetes Mellitus. (1997). Report of the Expert Committee on the Diagnosis and Classification of Diabetes Mellitus. *Diabetes Care, 20,* 1183–1197.

Fink, G., & Ross, S. (1991). Failure to treat high-risk foot ulceration: Causing diabetes complication. *Diabetes, 40*(Suppl. 1), 470A.

Flegal, K., Ezzati, T., Haynes, S., Juarez, R., Knowler, W., Perez-Stable, E., & Stern, M. (1991). Prevalence of diabetes in Mexican Americans, Cubans and Puerto Ricans from the Hispanic Health and Nutritional Examination Survey, 1982–1984. *Diabetes Care, 14,* 628–638.

Frame, P., Kowlich, P., & Liewellyn, A. (1984). Improving physician compliance with a health maintenance protocol. *Journal of Family Practice, 19,* 341–344.

Funnel, M., Anderson, R., Arnold, M., Bart, P., Donnelly, M., Johnson, P., Taylor-Moon, D., & White, N. (1991). Empowerment: An idea whose time has come in diabetes education. *The Diabetes Educator, 17*(1), 37–41.

Greene, L., & Kreuter, N. (1992). *Health promotion planning: An educational and environmental approach.* Mountain View, CA: Mayfield.

Greenfield, S., Kaplan, S. H., Ware, J. E., Yano, E. M., & Frank, N.I.L. (1988). Patients' participation in medical care: Effects on blood sugar control and quality of life in diabetes. *Diabetes Spectrum, 3*(4), 220–229.

Harris, R., O'Malley, M., Fletcher, S., & Knight, B. (1990). Prompting physicians for preventive procedures: A five-year study of manual and computer reminders. *American Journal of Preventive Medicine, 6,* 145–152.

Hawthorne, V., & Crowe, C. (1984). Some thoughts on early detection and intervention in diabetes mellitus. *Journal of Chronic Diseases, 37,* 667–669.

Hiss, R., Frey, M., & Davis, W. (1986). Diabetes patient educating in the office setting. *Diabetes Education, 12,* 281–285.

Institute of Medicine. (1991). *Improving America's diet and health: From recommendations to action: A report of the Committee on Dietary Guidelines Implementation, Food and Nutrition Board, Institute of Medicine.* Washington, DC: National Academy Press.

Kuczmarski, R. J., Flegal, K. M., Campbell, S. M., & Johnson, C. L. (1994). Increasing prevalence of overweight among U.S. adults: National Health and Nutrition Examination Survey, 1960–1991. *Journal of the American Medical Association, 272,* 206–211.

Madlon-Kay, D. (1987). Improving the periodic health examination: Use of a screening flow chart for patients and physicians. *Journal of Family Practice, 25,* 470–473.

Mandel, I., Franks, P., & Dickerson, J. (1985). Improving physician compliance with preventive medicine guidelines. *Journal of Family Practice, 21,* 223–224.

Mason, C. (1985). The production and effects of uncertainty with special reference to diabetes mellitus. *Social Science and Medicine, 21,* 1329–1334.

McDonald, C., Hui, S., Smith, D., Tierney, W. M., Cohen, S. J., Weinberger, M., & McCabe, G. P. (1984). Reminders to physicians from an introspective computer medical record: A two-year randomized trial. *Annals of Internal Medicine, 100,* 130–138.

McDonald, R. (1997). The evolving care of diabetes: Models, managed care and public health. *Annals of Internal Medicine, 20,* 685–686.

McGill, M., Yue, D., Plehwe, W., Wiley, K., & Turtle, J. (1991). Single-visit screening of diabetic complications: A new concept. *Diabetes Care, 12,* 599–600.

Meyer, A., & Henderson, J. (1974). Multiple risk factor reduction in the prevention of cardio-vascular disease. *Preventive Medicine, 3*, 225–236.

Murphy, F., Satterfield, D., Anderson, R., & Lyons, A. (1993). Diabetes education as cultural translation. *The Diabetes Educator, 19*(2), 113–115.

Murray, C., & Lopez, A. (1997). Alternative projections of mortality and disability by cause, 1990–2020: Global burden of disease study. *Lancet, 349*, 1498–1504.

National Institutes of Health. (1993). Non-insulin dependent diabetes primary prevention trial. *NIH Guide to Grants and Contracts, 22*, 1–20.

Neel, J. (1996). At mid-point in the molecular revolution. *Bioessays, 18*, 943–944.

O'Rahilly, S. (1997). Diabetes in midlife: Planting genetic time bombs. *Nature Medicine, 3*, 1080–1081.

Ornstein, S., Garr, D., Jenkins, R., Rust, P., & Arnon, A. (1991). Computer-generated physician and patient reminders. *Journal of Family Practice, 32*, 82–90.

Pendleton, D. (1983). Doctor-patient communication: A review. In D. Pendleton & J. Hasler (Eds.), *Doctor-patient communication* (pp. 5–53). Orlando, FL: Academic Press.

Pihoker, C., Scott, C., Lensing, S., Craddock, M., & Smith, J. (1998). Non-insulin dependent diabetes mellitus in African American youths of Arkansas. *Clinical Pediatrics, 37*, 97–102.

Plotnick, L. (1994). Insulin dependent diabetes mellitus. In F. Oski (Ed.), *Principles and practices of pediatrics*, pp. 1991–1992. Philadelphia: Lippincott.

Pozilli, P. (1996). Prevention of insulin-dependent diabetes. *Diabetes Metabolism Review, 12*, 27–136.

Romm, F., Fletcher, S., & Hulka, B. (1981). The periodic health examination: Comparison of recommendations and internists' performance. *Southern Medical Journal, 74*, 265–271.

Smith, D. (1997). Toward common ground. *Diabetes Care, 20*, 467–468.

Stuart, C., Gilkison, C., Smith, M., Keenan, B., & Nagamani, M. (1998). Acanthosis nigricans as a risk factor for non-insulin dependent diabetes mellitus. *Clinical Pediatrics, 37*, 73–80.

Thompson, R., Michnich, M., Gray, J., Friedlander, L., & Gilson, B. (1986). Maximizing compliance with hemocult screening for colon cancer in clinical practice. *Medical Care, 24*, 904–914.

Tierney, W. M., Hui, S. I., & McDonald, C. (1986). Delayed feedback of physician performance versus immediate reminders to performance. *Medical Care, 24*, 659–660.

U.S. Department of Health and Human Services. Centers for Disease Control and Prevention. National Center for Chronic Disease Prevention and Health Promotion. (1996). *Physical activity and health: A report of the surgeon general.* Atlanta, GA: Author.

U.S. Department of Health and Human Services. Public Health Service. (1998). *Healthy people 2010* (IV—016-0497-221). Washington, DC: Author.

Vinicor, F. (1994). Is diabetes a public health disorder? *Diabetes Care, 17*(Suppl. 1), 22–27.

Weatherall, D. (1995). *Science and the quiet art: The role of medical research in health care.* New York: Norton.

CHAPTER THIRTEEN

SICKLE CELL ANEMIA

Charles F. Whitten

The purpose of this chapter is to provide sufficient details about sickle cell conditions to enable an understanding of the challenges these conditions engender and the progress that has been made in addressing them. It covers the origin and basis for the conditions, how they are acquired, and the manifestations and management of the disease as well as the service needs of the carriers. This chapter also discusses the status of research to prevent or cure the disease and to prevent or ameliorate its effects, and the role governmental entities and the black community have played in addressing the challenges. An appendix lists some organizations that are information resources.

Discovery of Sickle Cell Anemia

In 1904, a black student from Grenada who was attending the Chicago College of Dental Surgery became ill. On examining his blood under a microscope, his physician discovered that some of his red blood cells were sickle shaped rather than round as is normal (Herrick, 1910). This was the beginning of the medical profession's recognition of sickle cell anemia (SCA), but there is evidence that the disease has been present for centuries. In several West African ethnic groups, there are indigenous names for the disease that reflect some of its characteristics. For example, for the Ga of Ghana, the name Chwechweechwe reflects the relentless, repetitious, and gnawing nature of the pain that individuals with SCA experience (Konotey-Ahulu, 1968). A Ghanaian sickle cell specialist has established through oral history that SCA has probably been present in nine generations of his family dating back to 1670 (Konotey-Ahulu, 1974).

The Sickle Cell Condition

The basis for the occurrence of sickle-shaped red blood cells is the presence of a special type of hemoglobin called sickle hemoglobin. Red blood cells contain hemoglobin, a substance that carries oxygen from the lungs to the various organs and tissues that require oxygen to live and carry out their functions. Red blood cells that contain normal hemoglobin remain round when they release oxygen, whereas cells that contain sickle hemoglobin can assume a sickle shape. On the release of oxygen, the millions of minute hemoglobin particles (molecules) in these cells tend to join together, forming *rods* that can distort each cell into the shape of a sickle.

Sickle cells have two undesirable characteristics—they are rigid and fragile. Normal red blood cells are soft and pliable and are easily deformable enough to be propelled through small blood vessels, whereas sickle cells, because of their rigidity, tend to plug blood vessels, thereby obstructing the flow of blood from time to time. This can result in tissue and organ damage. Normal red blood cells have a life span of about 120 days. Because they are fragile, sickle cells survive only six to thirty days, and the bone marrow cannot make cells fast enough to completely replace those that are destroyed. The result is a constant anemia, that is, a smaller than normal quantity of red blood cells and hemoglobin.

Sickle cell anemia is a genetic disease that is determined by genes that govern the type of hemoglobin that will be produced. For the purpose of understanding sickle cell conditions, what one needs to know about these genes is that the type of hemoglobin one has is determined by two hemoglobin genes, one from each parent. Those who have inherited a gene for sickle hemoglobin from both parents have SCA. Virtually all of their hemoglobin is sickle hemoglobin, and rod formation and sickling readily occurs in many cells when oxygen is released to the organs and tissues.

There are three other major types of sickle cell disease: sickle cell-hemoglobin C disease, a condition in which the individual has inherited the gene for sickle hemoglobin from one parent and for hemoglobin C (another abnormal hemoglobin) from the other; and sickle cell-Beta$^+$ and Beta$^\circ$ thalassemia disease, conditions in which the individual has inherited the gene for sickle hemoglobin from one parent and the gene for thalassemia from the other. The thalassemia gene decreases or prevents the production of normal hemoglobin. These three diseases tend to be milder in severity than SCA. For simplicity's sake, this chapter uses the term *sickle cell anemia* to mean all four diseases.

Inheritance of the gene from only one parent results in sickle cell trait (SCT), in which only about one-half of the hemoglobin is sickle hemoglobin. This amount is too small for rod formation and sickling to occur when oxygen is released to organs and tissues. Thus SCT is a carrier state and not a disease.

In the United States, sickle cell conditions occur primarily in blacks. Approximately one of every twelve black Americans is born with SCT and about one of every six hundred with SCA. Far less frequently, sickle cell conditions occur in other U.S. populations, primarily those who have black African ancestry: for example, Puerto Ricans and Cubans.

The Effects of Sickle Cell Anemia

There are significant health problems that occur primarily from the two factors just described (the obstruction of blood flow and anemia). These problems include recurrent, unpredictable pain attacks that may be severe enough to require narcotics and hospitalization. (This is the only disease with a lifetime propensity for pain attacks.) The pain most frequently involves the extremities, the abdomen, and the chest but may be generalized. Additional problems are anemia; a lowered tolerance for exercise; the plugging of blood vessels and acute infection in the lungs (acute chest syndrome); painful swelling of hands and feet in infancy; sudden pooling of blood in the spleen in infancy (which can be a cause of sudden death); a susceptibility to overwhelming pneumococcal infections; leg ulcers; the breakdown of the head of the femur (the major bone in the hip joint); the tendency to tire easily; growth retardation; delayed onset of puberty; prolonged, painful erection of the penis; gallstones; and strokes.

Individuals with SCA also may have to cope with a number of psychosocial stresses that include a lifetime of unpredictable occurrences of pain, growth retardation, delayed onset of puberty, repeated hospitalizations (most frequently for pain management), unpredictable interruption of important activities, unavailability of a cure, decreased life expectancy, limited job opportunities, and uncertainties about the desirability of marriage and having children. The psychosocial effects were first reported by Whitten and Fischhoff (1973).

It needs to be emphasized that no one experiences all of these physical and psychosocial problems. There is a wide and varied spectrum in the clinical expression of SCA with respect to the frequency, duration, and severity of pain attacks; the incidence of complications; the impact on psychosocial and functional status; and the effect on the life span. Furthermore, there is no basis for predicting the severity of the disease. Even the past history of an individual with SCA is unreliable for predicting his or her future course (see also National Institutes of Health, 1995; Whitten & Bertles, 1989).

Basic Elements in Managing the Physical Health Problems

The management of sickle cell disease has two components: managing the physical health problems and managing the psychosocial effects. The goal of each component is to enable individuals with SCA to live lives that to the extent possible, are not compromised by alterable aspects and effects of the disease.

Physicians have not had the ability to accomplish any of the following rational and potentially effective objectives: (1) preventing cells from sickling, (2) converting sickle cells to normal blood cell shape, (3) giving sickle cells a normal life span, (4) preventing sickle cells from plugging blood vessels, and (5) unplugging blood vessels blocked with sickle cells. The thrust of medical care with respect to the physical manifestations of the disease has been basically limited to treating health problems when they occur and making efforts to minimize physical disability. These limited goals have been accomplished by prompt treatment of pain with whatever pain killer is necessary up to and including morphine, by giving blood transfusions when anemia is severe or there is sudden pooling of blood in the spleen, by treating infections with antibiotics, by removing gallstones, by replacing destroyed hip joints, by preventing recurrent strokes with regularly administered transfusions, and by preventing infections with vaccines and antibiotics. One recent finding that goes beyond the aims of this limited management armamentarium is the evidence that administration of hydroxyurea (to be discussed later) has the ability to decrease the frequency of some health problems in some individuals.

Medical care can be satisfactorily provided by interested primary care physicians (family medicine specialists, pediatricians, and internists) who, when the health problems warrant it, consult with or refer patients to specialists in specific fields such as diseases of the blood (hematologists), lung (pulmonologists), and central nervous system (neurologists).

Basic Elements in Managing the Psychosocial Effects

The health care field recognizes that the lives of individuals with chronic illnesses are frequently more negatively affected by psychosocial factors than by the physical manifestations. That is true of SCA. Thus management has included efforts to prevent or ameliorate the debilitating psychosocial effects of the disease. The services have included patient and parent sickle cell education, genetic counseling, adjustment counseling, anticipatory guidance (informing them of what might occur and how they should respond), tutoring, career development assistance, job retention counseling, assistance in obtaining scholarships for education and vocational training, and social work services.

As these tasks suggest, there are a number of specifically trained individuals whose services are needed and of value in the prevention and management of the adverse psychosocial effects of SCA: individuals such as educators, vocational and rehabilitation counselors, social workers, and mental health professionals.

Sickle Cell Trait Service Needs

Sickle cell trait is not a disease, and the knowledge that one has it is of no value to one's own health status or care, but couples who both have SCT have a 25 percent chance in *each* pregnancy of having a child with SCA. In the absence of any intervention that gives individuals an opportunity to exercise options with respect to mate selection or to taking the risk, the first child of one out of approximately every six hundred black couples with sickle cell trait will have SCA. These parents will be faced with the psychological, emotional, social, and economic burden of caring for a child with an illness that is currently incurable and that reduces life expectancy.

The technology is available to diagnosis SCT, and individuals with this trait deserve to have the option of being made aware that they have SCT and to have the ability to make informed decisions that they believe are in their best interest about the possibility of having children with this disease. To state that they deserve to be tested and counseled is perhaps an understatement. For the failure to provide adequate services can be viewed as an abridgment of two fundamental rights: the right to know and the right to decide—in this case the right to know about the potential health care status of their children if that is knowable and the right to decide (to make personal choices about the health care status of their children) if options are available.

The service need relative to sickle cell trait is to identify individuals with the condition and then to counsel them. The counseling, which is better called education because advice should never be given, consists of providing the following information:

- The health status of individuals with SCT.
- The possible outcomes of sickle cell conditions in each pregnancy for trait $\times$ trait and trait $\times$ nontrait.
- The health problems, psychosocial problems, and basic management of SCA.
- The variability and unpredictability of health problems in SCA.
- The family planning options for SCT couples.
- The racial groups that have sickle cell conditions.
- The prevalence of SCT and SCA in the United States in the counselee's racial group.

Satisfactory education or counseling requires that sessions be conducted by trained individuals who use a format or protocol and who are periodically monitored to assure adherence to the protocol (see, for example, Whitten, Thomas, & Nishiura, 1981).

Status of Research and Research Implementation

Although important basic discoveries about sickle cell disease were made early in the first two-thirds of the twentieth century, it is only recently that we have begun to see the real possibility of not only controlling the disease but also curing and preventing it.

Early Research Findings

From 1910, when the disease was first reported in the medical literature, to 1940, sickle cell research was largely characterized by efforts of patient care specialists to gain a better understanding of what constituted SCA and how to differentiate it from other diseases.

From 1941 to 1970, biochemists and geneticists became involved, and three major discoveries were made. First was the recognition of the genetic difference between SCT and SCA; that is, one sickle hemoglobin gene is inherited in SCT and two in SCA (Beet, 1949; Neel, 1949). Second was the discovery by Nobel Laureate Linus Pauling that there is a chemical difference in the hemoglobin molecule of those who have a sickle cell condition (Pauling, Itano, Singer, & Wells, 1949). Indeed, SCA has a prominent place in medical history as the first identified molecular disease in that the hemoglobin molecule is the causative agent.

Third was the recognition that there has been an advantage to having sickle cell trait in West African countries (Allison, 1954). We can assume that at some point in history everyone made normal hemoglobin, then a change in the hemoglobin genes occurred in some, and some individuals began making sickle hemoglobin instead of normal hemoglobin. This is called gene mutation. When it occurred in individuals in West African countries where a form of malaria had been responsible for thousands and thousands of deaths, it was beneficial. Young children who have SCT are less likely to contract and die from malaria and hence are more likely to live and ultimately pass the gene on to their children. This survival of the fittest has been the major factor in the development of a high frequency of SCT among black West Africans who lived in countries where malaria was prevalent and among their descendants wherever they live. The sickle cell gene is present also in the populations of other countries with malaria zones (Sicily, Italy, and Greece, for example). Obviously, however, although having one sickle cell gene and SCT has been advantageous, having two genes and SCA has not been advantageous.

Despite those three landmark advances, the period from 1941 to 1970 has been characterized as one of benign neglect—few dollars were available for research, and little effort was made to inform the black population of what was known about the inheritance of the disease so that individuals could benefit from this knowledge. For example, during those thirty years no effort was made to detect and educate trait carriers so that they could decide whether they wished to take the chance of having a child with SCA. As late as the early 1970s, virtually every parent who had a child with SCA became aware of his or her potential for having an affected child only after the birth of his or her first child with the disease.

Subsequent Research Findings

Since 1970 there has been significant support for and progress in sickle cell research. These research endeavors can be classified into three groups.

Group 1. The projects in this group have been designed to identify the chemical and physical factors that promote the formation of sickle cells and the obstruction of blood flow. These investigations are absolutely essential to provide the basis for the development of drugs and chemicals that can accomplish the goals of preventing or treating SCA health problems. Description or discussion of these highly technical studies is beyond the scope of this chapter, but the progress in this research has been outstanding.

Group 2. This group involves data from one large project, the Comprehensive Study of Sickle Cell Disease (CSSCD), which was established by the National Institutes of Health (NIH) to gain an understanding of the natural history of the disease. Designed and supported by the NIH, the study collected data on over four thousand patients over a period of twenty years. The study was conducted in twenty-two sickle cell centers. Through over forty publications, it has provided physicians with useful documented information about a number of disease aspects, such as the age-related incidence, frequency, and progress of the various health problems.

Group 3. This group comprises projects designed to be of immediate benefit to patients. They include research to prevent the disease; to achieve a cure; to prevent or decrease the incidence of complications; to improve the management of the health problem; and to prevent, ameliorate, or resolve the adverse psychosocial effects. Following is a brief description of each study with comments on the accessibility and availability of the treatment involved. It needs to be recognized that in some instances the studies are so new that the research deals only with one individual and in other instances further perfection is necessary and expensive funding has to be provided before universal application of the work is possible.

Prevention of SCA Through the Diagnosis of Sickle Cell Anemia in the First Four Months of Pregnancy.

Since 1983, we have had the ability to diagnose SCA within four months after the onset of pregnancy. This is accomplished by DNA analysis of cells obtained from the placenta at nine weeks or from the amniotic fluid (bag of waters) at fifteen weeks. For this testing to be implemented, pregnant women have to be tested first to ascertain whether they have SCT and, if they do, whether the father of the unborn child also has SCT. If both parents have SCT, then of course there is a 25 percent chance that the developing unborn child has SCA. A DNA analysis under these circumstances enables the parents to find out whether the unborn has SCA and, if so, to decide whether they wish to continue or terminate the pregnancy.

This is an extremely valuable advance because prior to its development, SCT couples that wished to be absolutely certain that they would not have a child with SCA had to forego having their own biological children. As will be discussed under the challenges, the implementation of this process should but has not become a standard of care for pregnant women who are at risk for having a child with SCA.

Prevention of SCA Through Preimplantation Genetic Diagnosis.

In 1999, a second approach to prevention was reported (Kangpu, Zhong, Veeck, Hughes, & Rosenwaks, 1999). Eggs from a mother who had SCT were removed from one of her ovaries and tested for the sickle cell gene. Seven eggs that did not have the gene for SCT were then fertilized in a test tube with sperm from the father who had sickle trait. Three fertilized eggs that did not have the SCT gene and one that did were implanted in the mother's womb. The mother later gave birth to fraternal twins neither of whom have SCT or SCA. This couple had previously elected to terminate two pregnancies when prenatal testing indicated that the fetus had sickle cell anemia. The procedure, called preimplantation genetic diagnosis, has been used in cases involving several other genetic diseases in the past. This was the first effort to implement it for sickle cell anemia.

Cure of SCA Through Bone Marrow Transplantation. Red blood cells are manufactured in the bone marrow. So one approach to a cure is to destroy all of the patient's bone marrow and replace it with bone marrow from a donor who does not have SCA. The procedure is called bone marrow transplantation. There are problems associated with this procedure. First, the donor must have cells that match the recipient's cells in many respects; otherwise the donor bone marrow will be destroyed after transplantation. Bone marrow transplants usually require a suitable sibling, who frequently does not exist. Second, the donor cells, even though compatible, might not grow in the recipient. As in the first case this leaves the recipient with the potential for an inability to make red blood cells to carry oxygen, white blood cells to fight infections, and platelets that are necessary for blood to clot. Third, the donor cells might attack the recipient's body cells. This is called graft versus host disease, which is serious and potentially lethal. Because the procedure can result in unpredictable graft rejection and graft versus host disease, decisions have to be made about the advisability of undergoing this procedure. The basic question is whether the risks in allowing the disease to continue its unpredictable course are greater than the risks of graft rejection or graft versus host disease. Currently, the best resolution for this dilemma is to recommend for bone marrow transplantation those children who have already had severe SCA complications, such as a stroke or acute chest syndrome.

Until further progress is made in preventing or substantially reducing the risk of graft rejection and graft versus host disease, bone marrow transplantation will continue to be offered primarily to children who have had severe complications. To date, only about 120 bone marrow transplantations for SCA have been done worldwide (Walters, 1999).

Cure of SCA Through Cord Blood Transplantation. Red blood cells start out as stem cells. Stem cells can also develop into platelets or white blood cells. Bone marrow from donors contains these multipotential cells. Stem cells are also present in umbilical cord blood. In addition to altering the manufacture of red blood cells in the bone marrow through bone marrow transplantation, this alteration can be accomplished by transplanting cord blood stem cells.

In 1998, Yeager et al. used umbilical cord blood to transplant stem cells to a twelve-year-old boy. He had suffered a stroke with residual partial paralysis and was on a chronic transfusion program. At the time of the report, some eighteen months after the transplant, his bone marrow was producing red blood cells without sickle hemoglobin. Umbilical cord blood was used because a suitable bone marrow donor was not available.

The use of umbilical cord blood rather than bone marrow for the transplant has several advantages. First, the compatibility match does not have to be as complete, and second, umbilical cord blood is more readily available than bone marrow as it is being collected and stored by several institutions. Third, the incidence of graft versus host disease is lower. This was the first report of an umbilical cord stem cell transplantation.

Prevention of Recurrence of Stroke Through Chronic Blood Transfusions.

Strokes in people with SCA result primarily from the plugging of blood vessels in the brain that have been narrowed by the effects of sickle cells on the walls of these vessels. Children who have had one stroke are then highly likely to have repeated strokes. They may completely recover from the first incident but may then be permanently paralyzed and have mental retardation or may die from subsequent occurrences.

Since 1972, children who have had a stroke have been placed on a transfusion program to prevent recurrences. They are given transfusions every three to four weeks. This procedure prevents stroke recurrence because it gives them a high percentage of normal red blood cells that cannot sickle. But transfusion therapy is not free of disadvantages. Hemoglobin contains iron and, when the transfused red blood cells break down, iron is released. Unfortunately, the human body does not have an effective mechanism for eliminating iron and eventually the retained iron damages the heart, liver, and pancreas. There are drugs called chelators that when combined with iron, form a complex readily excreted by the kidneys. The chelators are administered through a needle inserted in the thigh and are pumped in while the child sleeps. Both the transfusions and chelation therapy are difficult to maintain and impair the quality of life. But they are now the standard of care and thus are universally used in the management of children with SCA who have had a stroke.

Prevention of a Lethal Complication in Infants Through Penicillin Prophylaxis.

At as early as three months of age, infants with SCA are prone to the development of pneumococcal (bacterial) infections that proceed rapidly and can result in death in as few as two hours after the onset of fever. When the infants have not had health problems associated with the disease, the infections and outcome can occur before a diagnosis of SCA is made. The vulnerability to pneumococcal infections occurs because a normal mechanism for the destruction and prevention of the spread of bacteria is deficient in infants with SCA. The responsible organ, the spleen, does not effectively filter out and destroy the bacteria as it does in infants who do not have the disease because the flow of blood in the spleen is compromised by sickle cell plugging.

In a 1983 study of children with SCA designed and supported by the National Institutes of Health (Gaston et al., 1986), 105 children (three to thirty-six months old) were given penicillin twice daily, and 110 children received a noneffective substance. Two of the 105 children who received penicillin developed pneumococcal infections, whereas 13 out of the 110 children did, and there were three deaths in the group that did not receive penicillin, yet no deaths in the penicillin group. This conclusively established the value of giving penicillin to prevent pneumococcal infections. Because the diagnosis of SCA needs to be made before the third month of life for this treatment to be most effective, a consensus conference in 1986 adopted the position that all newborns should be screened for sickle cell disease (American Medical Association, 1987).

The results of the penicillin study and the consensus conference recommendations were so definitive that thirty-four states currently require all or selective (those susceptible to SCA) newborns to be tested for SCA and have provided procedures and funds for the necessary follow-up. Minimally, the follow-up consists of obtaining a confirmatory test, starting infants on daily penicillin, monitoring penicillin compliance, and resolving problems that are barriers to complete compliance. Currently, penicillin is administered daily through at least the first five years of life.

Although the conference participants recognized the value of community sickle cell organizations, few states are using this resource for follow-up programs. When one considers that for some families, aggressive but sensitive and skillful efforts are required to maintain the penicillin compliance necessary to gain the desired benefits, it is apparent that the experience, credibility, and acceptability of the staffs of community organizations could enhance the probability of achieving that high level of compliance.

The identification of SCA in newborns provides a golden opportunity to save their lives. In addition, it provides an opportunity to influence their development and adjustment early enough and over a long enough period that the individuals with SCA in this generation have the potential to become adults who are economically self-sufficient and who have lifestyles and a quality of life that are not unduly compromised by having SCA.

Reduction of Complication Frequency Through the Administration of Hydroxyurea. In a study by Charache, Moore, and Terrin (1995), 152 adults with SCA were treated with hydroxyurea, and 147 received a placebo (a noneffective substance). The treatment group experienced a significant reduction in the frequency of painful episodes, acute chest syndrome, and the need for transfusions. The results were so definitive that the study was discontinued after a follow-up of only eight months. Although not effective in all individuals, hydroxyurea is now being widely used for adults, and studies are in progress to determine if it is effective and safe for children.

Prevention of Stroke Through the Identification of Children Who Are Vulnerable. In 1996, a study was conducted by Adams et al. (1998) in which the rate of flow of blood in the large vessels that supply blood to the brain was measured in a group of 2,000 children by transcranial doppler (TCD) ultrasonography.

When blood vessels are narrowed, the blood flows through them at a faster rate than it does when the vessels are of normal size.

The study was further designed to determine whether the children who had narrowed vessels and were also placed on a transfusion program had fewer strokes than those with narrowed vessels who were not treated. The results were positive. One of every sixty-five children who had narrowed vessels and received transfusions had a stroke, compared to ten of out of every seventy who did not receive transfusions. As previously stated, children who are receiving transfusions on a long-term basis must also be treated with a chelator to prevent iron damage. Although the results of the study were positive, various aspects of the procedure require additional investigation before it can become a standard practice.

Augmentation of Our Knowledge About the Psychosocial Effects. There is now a substantial body of literature that deals with four dimensions of the psychosocial effects of SCA. Over one hundred articles have been published in this area since the first by Whitten, Thomas, and Nishiura (1974). The foci of the studies are further delineation of the psychosocial effects; identification of factors that contribute to the effects; identification of factors that contribute to the achievement of satisfactory psychosocial adjustment; and identification of methodologies that can be of value in the prevention, amelioration, or resolution of the effects (see, for example, Barbarin, 1994; Baskin et al., 1998; Chavis & Norman, 1993; Hurtig, Koepler, & Park, 1989; Midence, Fuggle, & Davies, 1993; Nash, 1994; Telfair, 1994; Thompson, Gil, Abrams, & Phillips, 1996).

Challenges

The ultimate challenge, of course, is to discover and implement methods to prevent and cure sickle cell anemia. Until that final goal is achieved, we also face a challenge to develop and implement methodologies to minimize the effects of the disease. A brief overview of the current status of these first two challenges was provided in the previous section on research. A third level of challenge is to remedy service deficits that are correctable now. A brief discussion of six of these service challenges follows (see also Whitten & Nishiura, 1985).

Challenge 1: Implement Satisfactory Emergency Room Protocol. Some patients have pain attacks that occur very frequently over a period of time and require narcotics for relief. When they seek care at emergency rooms, all too often they are suspected or accused of being drug abusers, and this suspicion affects attitudes toward them and how they are managed. This is a universally voiced complaint. The problem is compounded by the fact that we have no objective way to determine whether the pain the person is complaining of exists and, if it does, whether it is sickle cell related, for unquestionably there are a few substance abusers in the adult sickle cell population. There is a need to develop a universally practiced sensitive approach to patients who seek relief of pain in hospital emergency rooms (see also American Pain Society, 1999).

Challenge 2: Resolve Barriers to Employment. Optimally, individuals with SCA would be gainfully employed and thereby economically independent. However, the socioeconomic status of adults with SCA is deplorable. A 1985 study by Farber, Kosby, and Kinney found that 45 percent of adults with SCA were unemployed. A 1998 to 1999 study in Detroit revealed that for 127 of 250 adults (51 percent), the sole source of income was Supplemental Security Income (SSI). Some adults with SCA have unpredictable, disabling pain episodes frequently enough to prohibit gainful employment because their absenteeism during these episodes exceeds employers' ability to accommodate them. These individuals then apply for SSI, and for some that becomes their major or only source of income. However, the maximum that anyone receives on SSI is below the poverty level.

Others have somewhat less frequent disabling pain episodes; they could work, and the frequency of the resulting absenteeism would be acceptable. However, they opt to obtain SSI benefits because the entry-level jobs that many in this group are qualified for usually do not provide essential health benefits; their SSI support includes Medicaid. Thus these individuals who also are living on income lower than the poverty level are not motivated to seek full-time employment. It obviously would be helpful if individuals in the latter group could become full-time employees and retain Medicaid coverage. The Social Service Administration has designed work incentive programs to achieve this (see also Davis, 1995).

Challenge 3: Expand Individuals' Ability to Make Informed Decisions About Mate Selection and Family Planning. As previously stated, individuals with SCT and of childbearing age should be aware they have this trait so they can make informed decisions that are in their best interest about their possibility of having children with sickle cell anemia.

With the advent of mandatory newborn screening, we can anticipate that at some point the sickle cell status of the vast majority of U.S.-born blacks of childbearing age will have been identified. The exceptions will be among the few who were born in states that are sparsely populated by blacks and that do not provide mandatory screening. If we use 1991 as a baseline for the time when the vast majority of states had implemented mandatory sickle cell testing for newborns and sixteen years as the age at which young men and women may begin planned parenthood, then by 2007 and thereafter the overwhelming majority of individuals when they reach the childbearing age will be aware of their sickle cell status. Perhaps it would be more realistic to state that their parents will have been notified; whether and the extent to which the children are eventually informed is, of course, problematic.

In the interim, there is a major opportunity for some who are already of childbearing age to become aware of their status and to be educated and counseled.

A by-product of newborn screening for SCA is the identification of newborns that have SCT. This of course means that at least one parent also has SCT. Follow-up testing of those parents will identify couples who both have SCT and who could benefit from educational counseling if they intend to have more children. Unfortunately, only a few states fund efforts to contact and provide testing and counseling for these parents (see also U.S. Department of Health and Human Services, 1993).

Challenge 4: Expand the Ability of Pregnant Women with SCT to Decide Whether to Continue or Terminate the Pregnancy. As previously stated, we have had the ability since 1983 to diagnose SCA within four months after the onset of pregnancy. The Scientific Advisory Committee of the Sickle Cell Disease Association of America (1988) has developed a position paper on prenatal diagnosis that includes goals, guidelines, and implementation steps and procedures. The recommendations have been endorsed by three national black professional organizations: the Obstetrics and Gynecology Section of the National Medical Association, the Association of Black Psychologists, and the National Association of Black Social Workers. It was not accepted for inclusion in a technical bulletin published by the American College of Obstetrics and Gynecology.

The committee proposes that the goal of sickle cell prenatal diagnosis should be to enable all women who are pregnant with a child with SCA to make informed decisions that they believe are in their best interest with respect to continuing or terminating the pregnancy. Although there is an inherent preventive by-product in prenatal testing in that it can prevent the birth of children with SCA to parents who elect to avoid that outcome, the goal of such testing is entirely based upon the principle of self-determination. The goal is not intended to be articulated or perceived as preventive. It follows from this goal that successful prenatal diagnosis and counseling should not be determined by the number of pregnancies that are terminated, that is, the decline in the birth of children with SCA, but rather by the extent to which informed self-interest decisions are made.

It is apparent that belief in the right to life versus belief in the pro-choice view has played a role in the failure of some physicians to offer this service. Physicians are entitled to their personal views on the abortion issue, but it is not acceptable for physicians who believe in the right to life to fail to enable women to exercise self-determination by following the recommended procedures or by referring women to a physician who will.

Concerns may also be expressed about the extent to which physicians who do offer testing are conducting the decision-making counseling sessions necessary to help parents arrive at a decision that they believe is in their best interest. This requires parents to examine such factors as their coping abilities, feelings, personal cultural values, and religious beliefs and their need and desire to have children. Of course the counseling session must be nondirective, for the counselor's role is not to give advice but to impart knowledge and to facilitate examination and clarification of feelings, beliefs, and values.

It should be accepted that some women will elect to terminate and others to continue the pregnancy. A number of noncognitive or affective factors are likely to influence or determine the decision. On the one hand some women will elect to continue the pregnancy for one or more of the following reasons: they find abortion to be unacceptable; they have a fatalistic approach to life (what will be will be); they have a great desire and need to have their own children; they are optimists and believe a cure will be discovered soon; they are risk takers, which leads them to feel they will be lucky enough to have a child who will have a mild course; they have confidence and pride in their ability to cope with adversity; the father of the child or significant others in their lives advises, advocates, or demands continuation of the pregnancy; and finally, their religion requires them to adjust to their lot (God's will) or it promotes a positive value in suffering or it is opposed to abortion. On the other hand the converse of these positions will be among the factors that will be responsible for some women electing to terminate their pregnancies.

Decision-making counseling requires individuals who have been specifically trained for this function. Currently medical geneticists, genetic counselors, and some obstetricians and family practitioners are qualified. Training programs are needed to enable primary care physicians, social workers, public health nurses, and others with appropriate backgrounds to become qualified. The individual who conducts the decision-making counseling should also be available to conduct postabortion counseling.

The primary care physician has the obligation to provide recommended services to pregnant women who are at risk for having a child with sickle cell anemia, or to refer them to another provider who can provide these services. The services include sickle cell testing for these women, the provision of basic information about the disease, sickle cell testing for the father, and decision-making counseling.

Challenge 5: Identify the Quality of Life of Individuals with SCA. In the vast body of literature that deals with the psychosocial effects of SCA and methods to prevent, alleviate, or resolve these effects, substantial attention is paid to what constitutes adequate or optimal psychosocial adjustment. However, there is an aspect of the psychosocial effects of SCA that has not been addressed—the quality of the lives of individuals with SCA. Quality of life refers to the individual's own assessment of his or her life satisfaction, sense of well-being, and happiness, and this is distinctly different from psychosocial adjustment. In the assessment of psychosocial adjustment, the evaluator determines the status of the individual's mental health, coping skills and strategies, family relationships, social functioning, treatment compliance, and self-esteem. In the assessment of quality of life, the evaluator reports on the individual's sense of well-being, happiness, and life satisfaction. It is clear that individuals who have achieved objectively determined excellent psychosocial adjustment could simultaneously believe or perceive that they have a poor quality of life, and vice versa.

Although quality of life assessments have been published for a large number of diseases and a journal (*Quality of Life Research*) is solely devoted to the topic, there has been no study of the quality of life of individuals with SCA. This should be done, for the findings could have implications for the services that we currently provide that are designed to achieve a different goal, that is, optimal psychosocial adjustment.

Challenge 6: Provide Sickle Cell Services in Small Communities. As previously described, we now have a clear picture of the medical and psychosocial services that individuals with SCA and their families need and deserve and an understanding of how these services can be provided. However, these services are not universally available. Comprehensive service programs are provided in the ten NIH-supported comprehensive sickle cell centers and in some hospitals in cities with black populations of over fifty thousand. But in the thousands of cities with small black populations, comprehensive sickle cell services are not available. The number of individuals with SCA in those communities is too small to warrant the development of comprehensive centers, leaving individuals with SCA in those communities largely dependent on their physicians to provide care that usually does not include the psychosocial components of optimal comprehensive care. At times an interested social worker in hospitals where these individuals receive inpatient care provides some services. Also, in a few of these communities, sickle cell organizations provide some educational and counseling services. We can and should develop a battery of minimal services and the mechanisms for their delivery for individuals in these small-sized communities.

Contributions of Governmental Entities

Substantive federal interest in and funding for sickle cell conditions was a by-product of the civil rights movement. That thrust led President Nixon in 1972 to propose and Congress to pass the National Sickle Cell Anemia Control Act. The act authorized expenditure of $10 million for sickle cell conditions. Congress, however, never appropriated specific dollars under that authorization. Instead, the National Institutes of Health funded fifteen comprehensive sickle cell centers and twenty-six screening and educational projects.

Through the years, NIH has, through its various divisions such as the Sickle Cell Branch, been the primary source of funding for research. The support has included funding the current ten comprehensive sickle cell centers, whose programs consist of basic and patient-oriented research and related patient care, investigator-initiated research projects, and grants for research projects conceptualized by the Sickle Cell Branch and then awarded to investigators who compete for them.

Congress, through the Orphan Drug Act passed in 1982, mandates the ten sickle cell comprehensive centers. However the funding is flexible, and although the level of NIH funding has been substantial, it has not kept pace with the increase in monies available to the key division. For fiscal year 1998–99, total NIH support for research was approximately $50 million.

State governments have provided the basic support for newborn screening programs, support supplemented in some cases by grants from the Genetic Disease Division of the U.S. Health and Human Services Department.

Contributions of the Black Community

A successful and effective approach to the resolution of a multifaceted health problem such as sickle cell conditions present requires more than research initiatives and the direct provision of services. Some entity has to be responsible for direction, coordination, policy setting, presentation of credible and respected positions on controversial issues, continual assessment and refinement of needs, and overall advocacy.

The need for such an entity is particularly strong in the case of sickle cell anemia because this is the first disease for which there has been a national effort to identify genetic carriers of the disease prior to the birth of an affected child and to provide counseling thereafter. As is to be expected, making this program acceptable and effective has required the resolution of a number of sensitive social and ethical issues.

The development of programs to serve the needs of the sickle cell population was one strong focus of the 1960s civil rights movement. A number of black voluntary groups began to provide public education and testing. Their interest and commitment were laudable, but some of their efforts were misguided. Owing to a lack of adequate information, there was, for example, some use of inaccurate and misleading literature, misinterpretation of test results, and use of an inadequate sickle cell test. However, even though these community group efforts were frequently flawed, it needed to be recognized that their interest and desire to be helpful was laudable and that rather than rejecting them we in the sickle cell disease movement needed to ensure that they were properly informed and trained to make appropriate contributions to the movement. We needed to harness, coordinate, and direct those efforts into an appropriate unified program so that they would be maximally beneficial and effective.

This need surfaced the issue of leadership. We in the sickle cell disease movement learned that the March of Dimes had plans under way to establish a sickle cell component in its branches throughout the country and that its plan had been endorsed by the National Medical Association, an organization of black physicians. Three of us met with the March of Dimes's leadership and argued that because the first national screening for a genetic disease was occurring in the black population, there would be racially sensitive issues to be addressed. Any program was more likely to be acceptable and effective if black leaders decided how that program should be conceptualized, designed, and presented to the black community. The March of Dimes accepted our arguments, dropped its plans, and provided some funding to assist us in establishing a national office.

In 1991, the author of this chapter and Dorothye H. Boswell cofounded the National Association for Sickle Cell Disease (NASCD) to assume the necessary leadership role. Beginning with thirteen community organizations, the organization, known today as the Sickle Cell Disease Association of America (SCDAA), now has over sixty full member organizations and twenty honorary member organizations.

The contributions of the SCDAA to serving the needs of those with SCA and SCT can be classified under eight headings: resolution of untoward thrusts, development of educational materials, achievement of visibility, establishment of standards and guidelines, provision of training programs and conferences, provision of technical assistance, development of a program to encourage scientific careers among youths, and provision of postdoctoral fellowships.

Resolution of untoward thrusts. SCDAA played a major role in achieving the following changes. If the actions and attitudes in question had been allowed to continue, they could have prevented achievement of some major program goals.

- The Department of Defense no longer restricts the military assignments of individuals with SCT.
- The identification and counseling of individuals with SCT is no longer viewed as being genocidal by elements of the black community.
- State laws that required black couples to have a sickle cell test before issuance of a marriage license have been repealed.
- Community organizations no longer use inadequate sickle cell screening tests or inappropriate literature.

Development of educational materials. SCDAA has developed and made available for free distribution and purchase an extensive library of educational materials (written and audiovisual) for the public at large, patients and their families, and health professionals. One of these publications, *Viewpoints,* is unique and free. Whenever the media announce a breakthrough that has treatment implications, patients and their families immediately want to know about its availability and whether they may be denied the potential benefit because of their location or socioeconomic status. As soon as possible after such announcements, an issue of *Viewpoints* is developed that interprets the status of the research. It is written in lay language, and mailed to over twenty thousand recipients. No other national health organization provides this service. There have been fourteen issues of the newsletter to date.

Achievement of visibility. The SCDAA has presented its annual National Poster Child to five U.S. presidents (Carter, Reagan, Ford, Bush, and Clinton). It has developed public service announcements featuring such black celebrities as Bill Cosby, Magic Johnson, Jayne Kennedy, and T. Boz. And it has had as its honorary chairman and spokesperson such black celebrities as Danny Glover, Robert Guillaume, and T. Boz.

Establishment of standards and guidelines. The SCDAA has developed standards for educational, testing, and counseling programs for its member organizations.

Provision of training programs and conferences. SCDAA has conducted ten three-day regional training sessions for sickle cell program staff, underwritten by the NIH and with a total attendance of over five hundred people. It has also conducted three-day SCT counselor training sessions for personnel of Veterans' Administration hospitals and of organizations throughout the United States and in the Bahamas and the Virgin Islands. In conjunction with the NIH Sickle Cell Branch and the New York Academy of Sciences, it has conducted a three-day sickle cell conference and published the proceedings (Scientific Advisory Committee of the SCDAA, 1988). The over three hundred attendees included researchers, patient care specialists, educators, counselors, and program directors. In addition, the SCDAA has conducted a three-day national conference on employment issues for individuals with sickle cell disease.

Provision of technical assistance. SCDAA has prepared a number of program development manuals for community sickle cell organizations.

Development of a program to encourage scientific careers among youths. The SCDAA has sponsored a program that allows promising black high school graduates to spend a summer in the laboratory of a sickle cell investigator to expose them to research methodology and potential role models.

Provision of postdoctoral fellowships. Finally, SCDAA sponsors a postdoctoral fellowship program to support young investigators in sickle cell disease research.

Moreover, the SCDAA's value to the black community extends beyond its contributions to the resolution of sickle cell problems experienced by individuals. The health, social, and economic problems confronting the black community are so extensive and interrelated that program efforts must extend beyond resolution of individual problems. One mission of those who undertake program development must be to deal with problems in a manner that in every way possible also enhances the overall development and well-being of the black community. The SCDAA has a proud record of accomplishment in that regard. There is an ongoing need to demonstrate the capabilities of black leadership, and SCDAA has done so. There is an ongoing need for blacks to establish effective models for dealing with problems that primarily or disproportionately affect the black community, and SCDAA has done so. It is the only national black health organization. There is an ongoing need to expand job opportunities for blacks, and SCDAA has done so through promoting the employment of black individuals by its member organizations to serve as program directors, social workers, career development and tutorial coordinators, trait counselors, secretaries, and data entry clerks.

The SCDAA has also made a contribution to society at large. Increasingly, we will have the ability to identify carriers of genetic diseases that occur predominantly in other racial groups. The SCDAA has shown how to resolve some of the issues that can threaten the acceptability and vitality of screening and counseling programs.

Conclusion

Unquestionably, tremendous progress has been made in addressing the challenges of the sickle cell conditions. As a result of research, ways to prevent and cure the disease have been pilot-tested, and our knowledge of the sickling process and factors related to its adverse effects has been significantly improved. Medical management has improved, and we have a better understanding of how to help individuals and their families make the best possible adjustment to the disease.

There has not been notable progress in genetic engineering (the replacement of disease-producing genes with normal genes) for SCA, which is the best ultimate technique for a cure. But we are fortunate in that we are not dependent solely on sickle cell genetic engineering research expenditures. Genetic engineering is a goal for all genetic diseases, and millions are invested in this endeavor. When techniques for genetic engineering are perfected, they will be applicable to sickle cell anemia.

Given the high cost of the currently piloted techniques for prevention and cure, it is clear that we are going to be faced with a monumental financial challenge if these techniques are to become universally available. We must also have the financial resources to keep up with the doable opportunities to improve services for the sickle cell population.

Appendix: Resources

Sickle Cell Disease Association of America
200 Corporate Pointe, Suite 495
Culver City, CA 90230-7633

Sickle Cell Disease Scientific Research Group
National Heart, Lung, and Blood Institute
6701 Rockledge Drive, MSC 750
Bethesda, MD 20892-7950

Sickle Cell Disease Association of America
Michigan Chapter
18516 James Couzens Highway
Detroit, MI 48235

Georgia Comprehensive Sickle Cell Center
Grady Health System
Emory University School of Medicine
Department of Pediatrics
Atlanta, GA 30322

Psychosocial Research Division of Duke University and the University of North Carolina
309 Battle Hall
Chapel Hill, NC 27599

References

Adams, R., McKie, V., Hsu, L. Files, B., Vichinsky, E., Pegelow, C., Abboud, M., Gallagher, D., Kutlar, A., Nichols, F., Bonds, D. R., & Brambilla, D. (1998). Prevention of a first stroke by transfusion in children with sickle cell anemia and abnormal results on transcranial doppler ultrasonography. *New England Journal of Medicine, 339,* 5–11.

Allison, A. (1954). Protection afforded by sickle cell trait against subtertian malarial infection. *British Medical Journal, 1,* 290–294.

American Medical Association. (1987). Consensus conference: Newborn screening for sickle cell disease and other hemoglobinopathies. *Journal of the American Medical Association, 254,* 1205–1209.

American Pain Society. (1999). *Guidelines for the management of acute and chronic pain in sickle cell disease.* Glenview, IL: Author.

Barbarin, O. (1994). Risk and resilience in adjustment to sickle cell disease: Integrating focus groups, case reviews and quantitative methods. *Journal of Health and Social Policy, 5,* 97–121.

Baskin, M., Collins, M., Brown, F., Griffith, R., Samuels, D., Moody, A., Thompson, M., Echman, J., & Kaslow, N. (1998). Psychosocial considerations in sickle cell disease (SCD): The transition from adolescence to young adulthood. *Journal of Clinical Psychology in Medical Settings, 5,* 315–341.

Beet, E. (1949). The genetics of the sickle cell trait in a Bantu tribe. *Annals of Eugenics, 14,* 279–284.

Charache, S., Moore, R., & Terrin, M. (1995). Effect of hydroxyurea on the frequency of painful crises in sickle cell anemia. *New England Journal of Medicine, 332,* 1317–1327.

Chavis, W., & Norman, G. (1993). Sexuality and sickle cell disease. *Journal of the National Medical Association, 85,* 113–116.

Davis, C. (1995). Sickle cell anemia: An overview posing an employment quandary. *Vocational Evaluation and Work Adjustment Bulletin, 28*(1), 20–23.

Farber, M., Kosby, M., & Kinney, T. (1985). Cooperative study of sickle cell disease: Demographic and socioeconomic characteristics of patients and families with sickle cell disease. *Journal of Chronic Diseases, 38,* 495–505.

Gaston, M., Verter, J., Woods, G., Woods, G., Pegelow, C., Kelleher, J., Presbury, G., Zarkowsky, H., Vichinsky, E., Iyer, R., & Lobel, J. (1986). Prophylaxis with oral penicillin in children with sickle cell anemia. *New England Journal of Medicine, 314,* 1593–1599.

Herrick, J. (1910). Peculiar elongated and sickle shaped red blood corpuscles in a case of severe anemia. *Archives of Internal Medicine, 6,* 517–521.

Hurtig, A., Koepler, D., & Park, K. (1989). Relation between severity of chronic illness and adjustment in children and adolescents with sickle cell disease. *Journal of Pediatric Psychology, 14,* 117–132.

Kangpu, X., Zhong, M., Veeck, L., Hughes, M., & Rosenwaks, Z. (1999). First unaffected pregnancy using preimplantation genetic diagnosis for sickle cell anemia. *Journal of the American Medical Association, 281,* 1701–1706.

Konotey-Ahulu, F. (1968). Hereditary qualitative and quantitative erythrocyte defects in Ghana: A historical and geographical survey. *Ghana Medical Journal, 7,* 118–119.

Konotey-Ahulu, F. (1974). The sickle cell diseases: Clinical manifestations including the "sickle cell crisis." *Archives of Internal Medicine, 133,* 611–619.

Midence, K., Fuggle, P., & Davies, S. (1993). Psychosocial aspects of sickle cell disease (SCD) in childhood and adolescence: A review. *British Journal of Clinical Psychology, 32,* 271–280.

Nash, K. (Ed.). (1994). *Psychological aspects of sickle cell disease: Past, present and future directions of research.* Binghamton, NY: Haworth.

National Institutes of Health. National Heart, Lung, and Blood Institute. Division of Blood Diseases and Resources. (1995). *Management and Therapy of Sickle Cell Disease* (NIH Publication No. 95-2117). Bethesda, MD: National Institutes of Health.

Neel, J. (1949). The inheritance of sickle cell anemia. *Science, 110,* 64–66.

Pauling, L., Itano, H., Singer, S., & Wells, I. (1949). Sickle cell anemia: A molecular disease. *Science, 110,* 543–548.

Scientific Advisory Committee of the Sickle Cell Disease Association of America. (1988). *Prenatal diagnosis* [Position paper].: Author.

Telfair, J. (1994). Factors in the long term adjustment of children and adolescents with sickle cell disease: Conceptualizations and review of the literature. *Journal of Health and Social Policy, 5,* 69–96.

Thompson, R., Jr., Gil, K., Abrams, M., & Phillips, G. (1996). Psychological adjustment of adults with sickle cell anemia: Stability over 20 months, correlates, and predictors. *Journal of Clinical Psychology, 52,* 253–261.

U.S. Department of Health and Human Services. Public Health Service. (1993). *Sickle cell disease: Screening, diagnosis, management and counseling in newborns and infants: Clinical practice guidelines* (DHHS Publication No. DHHS 93-0563). Rockville, MD: Public Health Service.

Walters, M. (1999). Bone marrow transplantation for sickle cell disease: Where do we go from here? *Journal of Pediatric Hematology/Oncology, 21,* 467–474.

Whitten, C., & Bertles, J. (Eds.). (1989). Sickle cell disease. *Annals of the New York Academy of Sciences, 565.*

Whitten, C., & Fischhoff, J. (1973). Psychosocial effects of sickle cell disease. *Archives of Internal Medicine, 133,* 681–689.

Whitten, C., & Nishiura, E. (1985). Sickle cell anemia: Public policy issues. In N. Hobbs & J. Perrin (Eds.), *Issues in the care of children with chronic illness.* San Francisco: Jossey-Bass.

Whitten, C., Thomas, J., & Nishiura, E. (1981). Sickle cell trait counseling: Evaluation of counselors and counselees. *American Journal of Human Genetics, 33,* 802–816.

Yeager, A., et al. (1998, December 9). *Emory physicians perform the first, unrelated umbilical cord blood transplant for high-risk sickle cell anemia* [Press release]. Atlanta, GA: Emory University School of Medicine.

CHAPTER FOURTEEN

TUBERCULOSIS

Herman M. Ellis, Robert S. Levine

At the turn of the nineteenth century, one in five people developed tuberculosis (TB), making TB the number one killer in the world (McCray, Weinbaum, Braden, & Onorato, 1997). African Americans were not immune. As early as 1831, researchers were reporting on particularly striking instances of what was termed *Negro poison* or *Negro consumption* (Yandell, 1831; Torchia, 1977). But progress was slow. It was not until the end of the nineteenth century that clinicians in the United States agreed that tuberculosis in African Americans appeared to be more severe than it was among whites (Torchia, 1977). Nearly one hundred years after this consensus had been reached, a working group of the U.S. National Heart, Lung, and Blood Institute (NHLBI Working Group, 1995) continued to remark about the "unfavorable incidence, prevalence, and mortality data on TB in minorities," with particular reference to blacks and Hispanics (pp. 1380–1392).

Moreover, the Secretary's Task Force on Black and Minority Health found that TB mortality was nearly nine times higher among persons forty-five years of age and dying of an infectious disease, thereby leading a list of forty key causes of death (U.S. Department of Health and Human Services [DHHS], 1985, 1998). Finally, U.S. public health planning documentation for the twenty-first century predicts that TB will continue to be one of the conditions for which racial and ethnic disparities exist and exceed 25 percent (DHHS, 1998).

The languid pace of nearly two centuries of inquiry was, as noted by Polednak (1997) and Freiden (1994), compounded by public health stewardship of a double standard for community diagnosis. For example, in 1980, when it was widely assumed that TB had been controlled in the United States, there were rates of 50 per 100,000 in Central Harlem, New York City; by 1991, when widespread concern about TB emerged upon documentation of a citywide rate of 50 per 100,000, the rate in Central Harlem had increased to 221 per 100,000. "If public health officials had been as alarmed about Central Harlem in 1980 as they were about all of New York in 1991, 'much of the city's epidemic might have been avoided'" (Freiden, 1994, p. 1721; Sibley, 1930/1969). In sum, even though it is a preventable and curable disease, TB persists as an important public health problem that disproportionately affects African Americans. The study of TB may therefore provide both important historical information and lessons for the future.

Epidemiology

National morbidity surveillance for tuberculosis did not begin in the United States until 1953. At that time it was mandated under the Public Health Act, to be managed by what are now the U.S. Centers for Disease Control and Prevention (CDC) (McCray et al., 1997). Before 1953, public health officials and population researchers had to rely on variably standardized mortality data (Yandell, 1831). As Eldbridge Sibley (1930/1969) said many years ago in his book on differential mortality in Tennessee: "The source of most of our data is the private physician. In view of the often very limited facilities at his disposal, especially in country districts, it is far from being a reflection upon his skill to assert that in many cases his diagnosis of disease is not exact. Moreover, he does not witness every fatal case of illness, and he does not always report every death" (p. 5).

Thus efforts to estimate the true magnitude of tuberculosis were impaired. A key element of the national surveillance system was its implementation of a standard case definition. As currently modified, that definition states that a case of TB may be confirmed by demonstrating that a clinical specimen contains either *Mycobacterium tuberculosis* or acid-fast bacilli; alternatively, all of the following criteria must be met: (1) positive reaction to a tuberculin skin test, (2) signs and symptoms compatible with TB, (3) treatment with two or more drugs that act against TB, and (4) a completed diagnostic evaluation (McCray et al., 1997; CDC, 1990). Patients who fail to meet these criteria but who are treated with two or more anti-TB drugs for a complete course of therapy are also traditionally included in the CDC surveillance database and in its national reports (McCray et al., 1997). In 1995, only 2 percent of reported cases did not meet the case definition, although the corresponding figure for children under fifteen years of age was 29 percent (McCray et al., 1997; CDC, 1996).

Even with the availability of national surveillance, questions remain about the completeness of the reporting. In Washington, D.C., heavily populated by African Americans, a 1977 review of discharge records from eleven hospitals found that 37 percent of persons with discharge diagnosis codes of tuberculosis had not been reported (McCray et al., 1997; Marier, 1977). However, the medical records themselves had not been checked for confirmation (McCray et al.,

1997). A systematic study of reporting completeness for the national surveillance system as a whole has not been done.

The following sections examine specific factors of importance in understanding current conditions: time (the long-term trends in TB cases); the places where TB is prevalent; some issues of culture, socioeconomic status, and genetics; the rates of TB at specific ages; the increasing numbers of individuals with both tuberculosis and HIV/AIDS; and the spread of drug-resistant tuberculosis.

Time: Long-Term Trends

Figure 14.1 shows the long-term pattern of TB cases and deaths in the United States from the beginning of national surveillance in 1953 to 1997. From 1953 through 1984, reported TB cases decreased 73.6 percent, from 84,304 to 22,255, and the annual incidence decreased from 53.0 to 9.4 per 100,000 population (CDC, 1996). The decline was more pronounced among whites than nonwhites, however; the annual risk for TB among nonwhites increased from 2.9 to 5.3 during this period (Rieder, Cauthen, Kelly, Bloch, & Snider, 1989). Trend analyses by age, race, and gender suggested little difference by either race or gender for children under five years of age or for those five to fourteen years of age, so most

FIGURE 14.1. TUBERCULOSIS CASES AND DEATHS, 1953–1997.

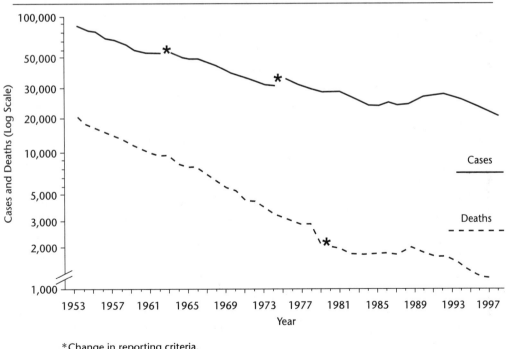

*Change in reporting criteria.

Source: CDC, 1999a, Figure 2.

of the recorded white-nonwhite disparity occurred among adults. By 1985, however, the decline had nearly halted, with a decrease of only fifty-four cases from the previous year (Rieder et al., 1989).

Beginning in 1986, there was a period of slow but steady resurgence, such that in 1992 the yearly number of cases reported was up 20 percent, to 26,673 (Rieder et al., 1989). Possible reasons for the increase included the human immunodeficiency virus (HIV) epidemic (Jereb, Kelly, & Dooley, 1991; CDC, 1992b), which increased the risk for active tuberculosis among persons with latent TB infection (CDC, 1999b), deteriorating socioeconomic conditions and tuberculosis control programs (Brundney & Dobkin, 1991; Friedman et al., 1995), poor understanding of tuberculosis among high-risk groups (Wolfe et al., 1995), increased immigration from countries with a high prevalence of TB (CDC, 1997), transmission of TB in congregate settings such as hospitals and prisons (Cantwell, Snider, Cauthen, & Onorato, 1994), and the development of multidrug-resistant disease (Pablos-Mendez, Raviglione, Battan, & Ramos-Zuniga, 1990).

Then, in 1993, the pattern of decline reappeared. Reductions of 5 percent, 4 percent, and 6 percent, respectively, were noted relative to each preceding year in 1993, 1994, and 1995 (McCray et al., 1997). In 1998, 18,361 cases were reported for a case rate of 6.8 per 100,000. In part, the renewed declines may have reflected stabilization in the impact of HIV, because from 1992 to 1996 it was observed that the incidence of HIV-associated TB remained at 18 percent (Leff & Leff, 1997). Additionally, tuberculosis control programs were becoming more effective in terms of prompt identification of TB-infected individuals, institution of appropriate treatment, and attention to treatment programs such as directly observed therapy that ensured completion of therapy (CDC, 1999b; Weis, 1997).

Place: States and Cities

As illustrated by Figure 14.2, tuberculosis was not uniformly distributed by place in the United States in 1998, and this has been generally true. Similarly, neither the increases nor the decreases in tuberculosis that occurred between 1986 and the present followed a uniform geographic pattern. From 1985 to 1992, for example, five states (New York, New Jersey, California, Florida, and Texas) witnessed 92 percent of the national increase; after 1992, these same states accounted for more than half of the decrease (McCray et al., 1997).

In these states and across the rest of the country, urban areas were the focus of TB's resurgence (CDC, 1996). New York City, Jersey City, Newark, Miami, Tampa, and San Francisco were particularly hard hit (CDC, 1992b, 1996). Even within the urban areas, however, there was diversity of distribution. In New York City, for example, case rates approaching or exceeding 300 per 100,000 were noted in Central Harlem (CDC, 1992b). Similarly, when TB rates began to decline, three health districts (Central Harlem, the Lower East Side, and the Lower West Side), all located in Manhattan (one of New York City's five boroughs) and

FIGURE 14.2. TUBERCULOSIS CASES REPORTED BY U.S. COUNTY, 1998.

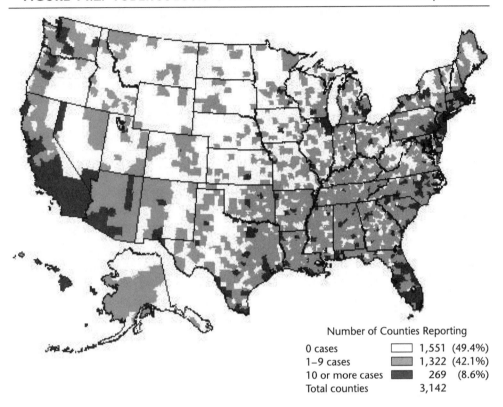

Number of Counties Reporting

0 cases	☐	1,551 (49.4%)
1–9 cases	▨	1,322 (42.1%)
10 or more cases	■	269 (8.6%)
Total counties		3,142

Source: CDC, 1999a, Figure 3.

accounting for only 8.9 percent of the city's population, yielded 52.1 percent of the early reduction (Davidow, Marmor, & Acabes, 1997).

Culture, Socioeconomic Status, and Genetic Factors

Both mortality and morbidity surveillance in the United States have consistently documented higher proportions of TB among members of racial and ethnic minority groups (McCray et al., 1997; Polednak, 1997; Freiden, 1994; Sibley, 1930/ 1969; Rieder et al., 1989; Cantwell, Snider, et al., 1994; Haas & Des Prez, 1989). So, when TB became resurgent between 1986 and 1992, it was not surprising that racial and ethnic minorities bore the brunt of the increase. In 1995, for example, the aforementioned NHLBI Working Group (1995) noted that 70 percent of all cases of TB occurred among members of minority groups. Reported TB cases by race and ethnicity in the United States for 1998 are shown in Figure 14.3. African Americans make up 31.8 percent of the patients (5,831 people), the largest percentage for any racial or ethnic group represented. This figure also

FIGURE 14.3. REPORTED TUBERCULOSIS
CASES BY RACE AND ETHNICITY, 1998.

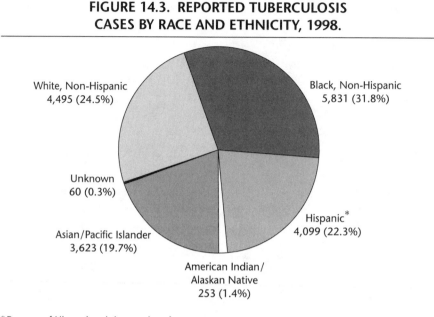

White, Non-Hispanic
4,495 (24.5%)

Black, Non-Hispanic
5,831 (31.8%)

Unknown
60 (0.3%)

Hispanic*
4,099 (22.3%)

Asian/Pacific Islander
3,623 (19.7%)

American Indian/
Alaskan Native
253 (1.4%)

*Persons of Hispanic origin may be of any race.
Source: CDC, 1999a, Figure 4.

illustrates that *minority group* is not a homogeneous term. Still, the epidemiology of TB among minorities consistently evokes two prominent themes. One pertains to immigrants from countries with a high prevalence of TB, and the other relates to African Americans.

As previously noted, one of the reasons for the resurgence of TB in the United States was increased immigration from high-risk countries. As shown in Figure 14.4, the percentage of cases among persons born outside the United States increased steadily from 1986 until it reached a plateau in 1995. During the same period, the number of cases classified as foreign-born nearly doubled. Throughout this period, rates of occurrence among persons born overseas were dramatically higher than those for persons born in the United States (Figure 14.5).

The increasing contribution of foreign-born patients has tempered the recent success in TB control (CDC, 1999b). The countries from which the high-risk arrivals come (Asia, Africa, and Latin America) have tuberculosis rates that are five to thirty times higher than U.S. rates (CDC, 1999b; Zuber, McKenna, Binkin, Onorato, & Castro, 1998). An interesting observation by McKenna, McCray, and Onorato (1995) has been that TB among immigrants generally occurs within five years of arrival. Consistent with this, Davidow et al. (1997) failed to detect an association between TB trends among the foreign-born and the relative number of foreign-born cases treated with directly observed therapy (DOT). They concluded that although DOT appeared to reduce the incidence of secondary cases

FIGURE 14.4. TRENDS IN TB CASES
IN FOREIGN-BORN PERSONS, 1986–1998.

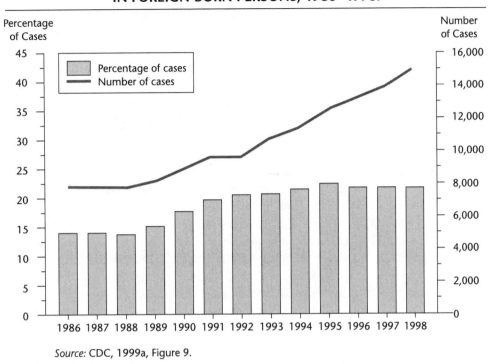

Source: CDC, 1999a, Figure 9.

FIGURE 14.5. TUBERCULOSIS CASE RATES BY ORIGIN, 1986–1998.

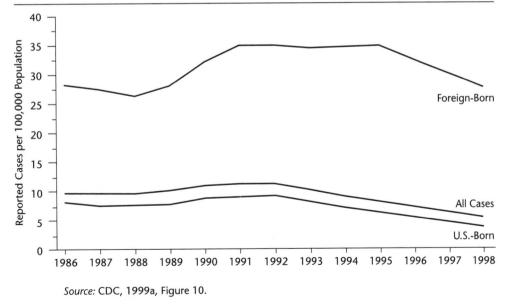

Source: CDC, 1999a, Figure 10.

(Davidow et al., 1997; Reichman, date n/a), it did not halt the portion of the TB epidemic originating in persons from other countries (Haas & Des Prez, 1989).

Chin et al. (1998) were able to use molecular epidemiologic approaches to explore differences between U.S.-born and foreign-born persons with TB in San Francisco. They identified 367 patients with a genetically typed strain of *M. tuberculosis* that was new to the population in 1993. They then traced the transmission of TB from these cases forward for two years. In all, 252 of the 367 cases occurred among the foreign-born, and 115 cases among the U.S.-born. Although patterns in each group were parallel in terms of time, the groups showed different mechanisms of development. Specifically, most if not all foreign-born persons appeared to have been infected prior to their arrival in the United States. Thus their illnesses represented reactivation of the disease. In contrast, U.S.-born patients were more likely to have developed the disease after contact with another infected individual in the United States. Thus, although none of the 252 foreign-born cases appeared to have acquired their disease from a known U.S. source, 19 of the 115 U.S.-born cases were so classified, with 17 of the 19 having been acquired from contact with U.S.-born patients and two from foreign-born persons. Also, in these data only U.S.-born patients showed clustering due to high-risk factors such as HIV/AIDS, illicit drug use, or homelessness.

Mechanisms of development have also been the object of inquiry about TB among African Americans. Two theories predominate. One is that blacks are especially sensitive to TB infection for genetic reasons (for example, increased susceptibility due to poor absorption of vitamin D because of skin color (Long, 1941) or due to as yet undefined inherited factors also related to immunity (Stead, Senner, Reddick, & Lofgran, 1990; Stead, 1997; Crowle & Elkins, 1990; McPeek, Salkowitz, Laufman, Pearl, & Zwilling, 1992; Trump & DiStasio, 1990; "Genetics—NRAMP1 Gene," 1998). The other primary hypothesis is that race is mainly a surrogate for cultural and environmental factors, with low socioeconomic status playing a prominent role in the environmental considerations (Freiden, 1994; Sibley, 1930/1969; Rosenman, 1990; Aoki, 1990; Felton, Smith, & Ehrlich, 1990; Morse & DiFernando, 1990; Bates; 1982; Cantwell, McKenna, McCray, & Onorato, 1998).

Stead et al. (1990) analyzed data from 25,398 residents of Arkansas nursing homes and from three tuberculosis outbreaks among prison inmates in Arkansas and Minnesota. Nursing home residents over the age of fifty who were tuberculin skin test negative on entry into the nursing home, lived in one of 165 homes that were racially mixed, and underwent retesting at least sixty days after their initial two-step skin test, were included. Conversion at the time of the retest was taken as evidence of new infection. It was observed that blacks were 1.9 times more likely than whites to become infected with a new case of TB (95 percent confidence interval 1.7 to 2.1). The difference was found whether the source case was white or black, but there was no corresponding difference in the percentage of blacks or whites who were later found to have clinical TB in the absence of preventive therapy. Data from the prison outbreaks also suggested that blacks were about twice as likely to become infected as whites. A response to Stead et al.'s findings presented a similar observation based on data from an outbreak of tuberculosis on a large U.S. Navy vessel (Trump & DiStasio, 1990).

Stead et al. (1990) felt that their observations were consistent with genetically determined differences in susceptibility between blacks and whites. Stead (1997) argued for the biologic plausibility of this explanation by citing evidence from Crowle and Elkins (1990) to the effect that macrophages from black donors permit significantly more bacillary replication than do those from white donors, and from McPeek et al. (1992) that monocytes have a pattern of HLA-DR expression consistent with innate resistance to *M. tuberculosis* in 70 percent of whites but only 30 percent of blacks. Stead (1997) also pointed out the well-known genetic advantage against malaria possessed by some African Americans due to the formation of sickle cells, and suggested that linkage between the gene encoding for Tay-Sachs disease and the gene that encodes for TB resistance may be an analogous example, one that is consistent with observations of a low incidence of TB among Ashkenazi Jews, who have high rates of Tay-Sachs disease. Additionally, Stead (1997) suggested that differential resistance between races might reflect differences in the duration of experience with TB. White Europeans, with hundreds of years of exposure (promoted by sharing their homes with cattle), had the advantage of many generations of natural selection that African Americans lacked. Finally, Stead et al. (1990) offered the hope, consistent with elimination of racial disparity, that further research might result in the ability to enhance preinfection defenses, thereby preventing tuberculosis infection at its root.

In addition to this work of Stead and his colleague, recent West African research has also supported the genetic hypothesis, suggesting that variation in the NRAMP1 gene may affect susceptibility to TB and help explain why African Americans are at increased risk ("Genetics—NRAMP1 Gene," 1998).

Contrary to these arguments, most workers in the field have suggested that race is a surrogate for environmental factors, particularly those related to culture (Freiden, 1994; Sibley, 1930/1969) and socioeconomic status (Aoki, 1990; Bates, 1982; Cantwell, McKenna, et al., 1998). Medical comorbidity (Rosenman, 1990), external environmental influences in nursing homes and prisons (Rosenman, 1990; Aoki, 1990), and delayed boosting of tuberculin skin tests (Morse & DiFernando, 1990) have also been proposed as alternative explanations for Stead and his colleagues' observations. Doubt has arisen, in part because of the disparity between Stead et al.'s (1990) detection of increased racial susceptibility to TB infection without racial differences in the occurrence of clinical TB once infection has been established (Felton et al., 1990). The HLA phenotype data has been questioned because of the nonspecificity of these halotypes within and across ethnic groups (NHLBI Working Group, 1995). Finally, a study of tuberculosis in children has failed to confirm differences in racial susceptibility (Ussery et al., 1996).

Regarding cultural factors, many researchers have tended to equate *culture* with *minority culture,* thereby putting the cart before the horse. In contrast, Polednak (1997) has emphasized the primary role of majority culture in producing racial disparity. He observes that even after accounting for economic differences, majority discrimination, manifested by segregation in employment and housing, appears to have adversely affected African American health. He notes that segregation may contribute to both the lack of proper medical follow-up for patients with tuberculosis and the crowded conditions that aid the spread of tuberculosis. He also suggests that public health officials may have had a double standard when it came to interpreting tuberculosis surveillance data. Though admitting the difficulty of measuring such issues, Polednek notes that high rates in an "incorrigible," segregated, minority area such as Central Harlem were ignored, whereas the same rates occurring in segregated majority areas were identified as an "epidemic" needing immediate attention (see also Freiden, 1994).

Cantwell, McKenna, et al. (1998), pursued the question of environmental determinants in terms of six indicators of socioeconomic status as tabulated in the 1990 census: crowding (median number of persons per room per household), income (median household income), poverty (percentage of persons living below the poverty level), public assistance (percentage of persons receiving public assistance), unemployment (percentage of persons aged sixteen to sixty-five who were unemployed), and education (percentage of persons twenty-five years old or older who had completed high school). The researchers matched 159,070 cases of TB reported to the CDC from 1987 to 1993 (92.8 percent of all cases reported) with the census database by zip code and four demographic variables (age, gender, race and ethnicity, and place of birth). They then assigned proxy values for the six socioeconomic indicators corresponding to the calculated value for each demographic and zip code–specific group. Using their model to adjust race and ethnic associations for socioeconomic status, they found that race and ethnicity accounted for about half of the increased risk for TB among African Americans, Hispanics, and Native Americans. Further adjustment for interaction between crowding and race and ethnicity accounted for some additional risk but not all.

To date, neither those who favor an interpretation based on cultural factors nor those who favor a genetic interpretation have settled these issues. In part this may explain why neither direct confrontation with cultural factors such as white racism nor interventions based on differential genetic susceptibility are generally included in national public health recommendations for TB control.

Age

During the resurgence of tuberculosis, the overall incidence of TB in the United States increased by about 13 percent, but the rate among children younger than fifteen years of age increased by 35 percent (CDC, 1989; Ussery et al., 1996). Increases in pediatric TB are the hallmark of recent infection because most pediatric cases occur as a result of rapid progression and a short incubation period (Correa, 1997). In untreated children under four years of age, TB develops within the first year of infection in 60 percent (McCray et al., 1997).

The disproportionate burden of TB among young people during the recent resurgence is reflected in part by the decline of the median age for TB cases from forty-nine years of age in 1985 to forty-three in 1992 (McCray et al., 1997). Children, however, were not the largest source of the increase. That unfortunate statistic went to twenty-five- to forty-four-year-olds. They experienced a 54.5 percent increase, due primarily to the higher rates of HIV/AIDS and recent immigration in this group (CDC, 1989). When TB began to decline, the largest drop was seen among twenty-five- to forty-four-year-olds (21.1 percent), primarily because of success in controlling transmission in communities at high risk for HIV/AIDS (McKenna et al., 1995). In contrast, TB rates among the age group comprising persons sixty-five and older, in which TB is most often due to reactivation, were generally stable (CDC, 1989).

Tuberculosis and HIV/AIDS

Before 1993, information linking tuberculosis and HIV/AIDS was available only from cross-matching AIDS and TB case registries. In one study the percentage of TB cases that matched with AIDS cases was shown to have increased steadily from 1981 (9.1 percent) to 1990 (9.5 percent) [McCray et al., 1997; CDC, 1992a). Based on mathematical modeling, an estimated 28,040 excess cases of TB were attributed to HIV between 1985 and 1990 alone (McCray et al., 1997; Burwen et al., 1995; CDC, 1994). In 1993, the case definition of HIV/AIDS for adolescents and adults was expanded to include pulmonary TB (McCray et al., 1997; Burwen et al., 1995), and the national TB surveillance form was modified to include information on the HIV status of each case. During that year, there were 54,432 new cases of AIDS reported based on the expanded definition, among which 3,988 (7 percent) were added solely because of TB diagnosed since 1978 (McCray et al., 1997; Bloom & Murray, 1992).

Additional evidence linking tuberculosis and HIV relates to overlapping epidemiological characteristics: (1) the timing of the increase in TB paralleled the onset of the AIDS epidemic; (2) the age group most affected by AIDS (twenty-five- to forty-four-year-olds) was the same group experiencing the greatest increase in TB from 1986 to 1992; (3) geographically, the large urban areas of California, Florida, New York, and Texas were hardest hit by both diseases (McCray et al., 1997); and (4) both diseases are characterized by racial and ethnic disparities, with African Americans faring worse than other groups.

Drug-Resistant Tuberculosis

The resurgence of TB in the United States was accompanied by increasing numbers of patients whose disease was resistant to the antibiotics used for treatment (McCray et al., 1997). These patients are important not only because they are so vulnerable themselves but also because they tend to remain infectious for longer periods of time than do patients whose disease responds to treatment. For this reason, they have the potential to expand both the number of people infected in a community and the number of people infected with resistant organisms (Gobles, Iseman, & Madsen, 1993).

Two types of drug resistance have been defined—primary and secondary. The former refers to persons whose initial infection is resistant, and the latter indicates the development of resistance from either inadequate treatment or nonadherence to treatment recommendations (McCray et al., 1997). Drug-resistant cases are more common in urban, indigent, and minority populations (McCray et al., 1997). Among the foreign-born, several studies have documented increased frequencies of drug resistance associated with immigration from Haiti, Latin America, and Southeast Asia (McCray et al., 1997; CDC, 1991; Kleeburg & Olivier, 1984; Nolan & Elarth, 1988; Pitchenik et al., 1982; Riley, Arathoon, & Loverde, 1989; Scalcini, Carre, & Jean-Baptiste, 1990; Sandman, Schluger, Davidow, & Bonk, 1999; Pablos-Mendez et al., 1990). Factors other than immigration that have been observed more frequently among persons with drug-resistant disease include the presence of cavitary TB, an age of less than forty-four years, residence in New York City (McCray et al., 1997), and HIV (Sandman et al., 1999).

The question of how race and ethnicity relate to drug resistance may need further investigation. The NHLBI Working Group (1995) commented that there was no race-based difference in the effectiveness of anti-TB medications. However at least one group of researchers, who studied 132 patients admitted to a single hospital in New York City, observed that "resistance was exceedingly rare in white patients (2.2 percent) [McCray et al., 1997; Ussery et al., 1996] and remarkably common in black patients (26.2 percent) [CDC, 1996; Ussery et al., 1996]" (Pablos-Mendez et al., 1990). In addition, Friedman et al. (1995) observed that persons with recent (that is, exogenous) infection were more likely to be seropositive for the HIV virus, U.S.-born, non-Hispanic blacks with multidrug-resistant tuberculosis. The question of whether there are racial and ethnic differences in drug resistance has important implications for the debate over genetic versus environmental explanations for differences in the vulnerability of African Americans to tuberculosis and ultimately for public health policy.

Exemplary Programs, Failures, and Future Directions

The resurgence of tuberculosis and the emergence of multidrug-resistant TB elicited a national response designed to strengthen TB surveillance, improve laboratory capacity for identifying mycobacteria and conducting reliable drug sensitivity testing, expand directly observed therapy, and expedite investigation of individuals who are close contacts of TB patients (CDC, 1999b). All these factors played an important role in the reductions that occurred after 1992. Increases in the capacity for training health care providers in the new advances in diagnosis and treatment also contributed. This training has gone on, for example, at three model TB centers (the Frances J. Curry National Tuberculosis Center, the Charles P. Fenton National Tuberculosis Center at Harlem Hospital, and the New Jersey Medical School National Tuberculosis Center, CDC, 1999b) and through a burgeoning list of sites on the Internet. The CDC, for example, provides major recommendations at www.cdc.gov/nchstp/tb/pubs/mmwrhtml/maj_guide.htm, and from "a small room in suburban Kathmandu, Nepal," via tb.med (www.south-asia.com/ngo-tb), there are links with the Stanford Center for Tuberculosis Research, Princeton Project 55, the New Jersey Medical School model center for tuberculosis, the Centers for Disease Control and Prevention, the World Health Organization, the Case Western Reserve University Tuberculosis Research Unit, the New York City Department of Health, the National Jewish Center of Immunology and Respiratory Medicine, the Center for Pulmonary Infectious Disease Control at the University of Texas Health Center, and others.

Examples of successes that have occurred since the resurgence of TB was recognized include the development of methods that reduce the time needed to detect the growth of *M. tuberculosis* in diagnostic specimens (CDC, 1999b; Crawford, 1994), rapid methods for identifying drug-resistant TB (CDC, 1999b; Drobniewski & Wilson, 1998), a new test for latent TB infection (CDC, 1999b; Streeton, Desem, & Jones, 1998), serodiagnosis (CDC, 1999b; Lyashchenko et al., 1998; Samanich et al., 1998), and DNA fingerprinting (CDC, 1999b; Behr & Small, 1997). In 1997, the CDC established a TB clinical trials consortium to enhance the development of new classes of therapeutic agents (CDC, 1999b). The consortium provided some of the data used in obtaining approval from the U.S. Food and Drug Administration for rifapentine, the first new TB drug approved in more than twenty-five years (CDC, 1999b). There is also a major research effort underway aimed at developing new TB vaccines (CDC, 1998).

In the area of disease control, directly observed therapy (DOT) has become the benchmark. Successful programs have been characterized by strong leadership and extensive coalition building, and the development of intense personal bonds between patients and members of the health care team (Freiden, 1994; Sbarbaro, 1997). In New York City's DOT program (Fujiwara, Larkin, & Freiden, 1997), for example, two key operational strategies have been the setting of specific, measurable goals for treatment and the establishment of DOT as the standard of care for all patients rather than a procedure of last resort. Also, DOT is to be administered with respect for all concerned: the physician, primary DOT provider, and patient all sign a DOT contract outlining goals, expectations, and rights of all involved.

There are two main components of this program: field based and clinic based. In the field, each DOT worker is responsible for up to twelve households and covers the patient's home, street corners, parks, train or ferry stations, crack dens, or any other possible venue for delivering DOT. As with other successful programs, patient incentives are used. In the field these include one can of food supplement drink daily, a $5 food coupon weekly if the patient is adherent with 80 percent or more of the doses, and an extra food coupon if adherent for the month. Once a patient is less than 80 percent adherent, a senior outreach worker or nurse visits the patient to identify barriers. Infected household contacts are offered directly observed preventive therapy.

In the clinic-based program, there is an enriched package of incentives, based in part on recognition of the effort needed to come daily or twice weekly to the clinic. These patients receive transportation tokens, a can of food supplement drink, and breakfast or lunch daily; food coupons are given as they are in the field package. In addition, clinic-based DOT patients who are 100 percent adherent receive a graduated package of additional monetary incentives: $30 worth of public transportation support the first month, $30 the second month, and $60 at the end of the third month. Then the three-month cycle is repeated. DOT programs are also offered in a TB shelter for men, for patients with dual TB/HIV infection, and in the prison system. After release, former prisoners are provided a $25 *show-up voucher* to encourage completion of treatment. Further, this program, like other successful programs (Schecter, 1997; Chaulk & Pope, 1997), has included the capacity for forced detention and treatment of infectious patients. The availability of a locked hospital detention ward gives credence to this component (Fujiwara et al., 1997), even though detention is usually not needed (Gasner, Maw, Feldman, Fujiwara, & Freiden, 1999).

Finally, in addition to the material rewards and the threat of detention, there is the specific quality possessed by the successful DOT worker: the ability to build a trusting, reliable relationship. Patients are often observed to depend upon DOT workers as "friendly visitors who are available for support in times of need as well as for observing medication ingestion" (Fujiwara et al., 1997).

In sum, although the program is complex, it has been relatively inexpensive (about $2,200 per patient cured) and has had a positive public health impact. New cases of TB decreased by 55 percent and cases of multidrug-resistant TB by 87 percent between 1992 and 1997 after institution of the program and its attendant controls on treatment adherence (Gasner et al., 1999). A savings of $6,000 per patient cured could be credited to the program based solely on rehospitalizations avoided (Fujiwara et al., 1997).

Despite successes such as these, the TB experience has also provided evidence that leadership, coalition building, and teamwork do not always add up to success. In Atlanta, for example, a tuberculin screening and isoniazid preventive therapy program, developed in consultation with the Atlanta TB Prevention Coalition, was able to establish tuberculin screening centers in a large public hospital serving inner-city residents, at the city jail, in clinics and mobile vans run by a community-based organization serving homeless populations, at shelters and soup kitchens, and in collaboration with AIDS education workers, on the street (Bock, Metzger, Tapia, & Blumberg, 1999). Coalition members included representatives from two county health department tuberculosis programs, administrators of the local public hospital, the American Lung Association of Georgia, an independent health care program for the homeless, two schools of medicine, and the state health department.

This broad base of participation by key organizations paved the way for access to high-risk populations, and attention to the engagement and orientation of staff from the participating organizations enabled delivery of screening services (a tuberculin skin test) to 7,246 persons between 1994 and 1996, including 6,321 who were members of racial and ethnic minorities. But follow-through was meager. Thirty-five percent of those receiving a skin test did not return to have the test read. In all, 809 (17 percent) had a positive skin test, but 24 percent of those referred for a chest radiograph were lost to follow-up at that point. Of the 409 patients identified as needing isoniazid preventive therapy, only 84 actually completed this treatment. Thus the Atlanta group mirrored the experience of a similar program attempted in Washington, D.C., about thirty years before (Khoury, Theodore, & Platte, 1969).

Conclusion

In truth, for all the successes in tuberculosis control in the United States during the past few years, it could be argued that TB still remains one of the most significant failures of modern medicine. It is preventable, curable, and relatively inexpensive to treat (about $2,000 per case, if not multidrug resistant) (Fujiwara et al., 1997); yet it remains the leading infectious cause of death throughout the world—killing more than 3 million people per year.

Thirty-three percent of the world's population is already infected, and someone new is infected every second of every day; it is estimated that between the end of this century and the start of the third decade of the next, 1 billion more people will be newly infected, 200 million will get sick, and 70 million will die if conditions remain as they are (Adab, Fielding, & Castan, 1999). In 1997, for example, only 32 percent of the world's population resided in an area where effective TB control programs were fully implemented and operational (CDC, 1999b; Netto, Dye, & Raviglione, 1999). Because cases of TB among foreign-born persons residing in the United States will soon outnumber cases of TB among U.S.-born persons, it is unlikely that TB in the United States will be eliminated without substantial worldwide progress (CDC, 1999b).

With respect to African American health, the issue is not that the foreign-born pose a particular hazard. As suggested by Chin et al. (1998), TB cases among the U.S.-born rarely appear to be attributable to a foreign-born individual. Instead, the issue is whether cultural factors related to *both* majority and minority populations can be addressed as part of the solution. Will residential segregation and labor discrimination continue to force people of color into crowded, unsanitary housing? Will marginal health insurance and the placement of poor people into managed care plans whose capacity for providing optimal TB surveillance, reporting, treatment, and prevention is yet untested serve to perpetuate disparities in access to care (CDC, 1999b)? If the numbers of TB cases continue to decrease, will "isolated" epidemics affecting people of color be ignored and tantalizing fields of research lie fallow? Will U.S. programs dwindle as cases decrease, even though global TB remains severe?

If so, it will probably mean that public health programs will continue to exempt remediation of harmful aspects of majority culture from the national treatment plan. Unless other programs can compensate, this in turn may mean that TB will persist as a disproportionate killer of members of low-income populations, including many African Americans. Perhaps, however, the future will not repeat the past. Perhaps instead the majority will recognize that by directly, promptly, and comprehensively addressing all factors that may adversely affect the poor, everyone will benefit.

References

Adab, P., Fielding, R., & Castan, S. (1999). *Epidemiology of tuberculosis* [On-line]. Available: http://supercourse.tmc.edu.tw

Aoki, S. K. (1990). [Letter to the Editor]. *New England Journal of Medicine, 322,* 1670.

Bates, J. H. (1982). Tuberculosis: Susceptibility and resistance. *American Review of Respiratory Diseases, 125,* 20–24.

Behr, M. A., & Small, P. M. (1997). Molecular fingerprinting of *Mycobacterium tuberculosis:* How can it help the clinician? *Clinical Infectious Diseases, 56,* 607–616.

Bloom, B. R., & Murray, C.J.L. (1992). Tuberculosis: Commentary on a re-emergent killer. *Science, 257,* 1055–1064.

Bock, N. N., Metzger, B. S., Tapia, J. R., & Blumberg, H. M. (1999). A tuberculin screening and isoniazid preventive therapy program in an inner-city population. *American Journal of Respiratory and Critical Care Medicine, 159,* 295–300.

Brundney, K., & Dobkin, J. (1991). Resurgent tuberculosis in New York City: Human immunodeficiency virus, homelessness, and the decline of tuberculosis control programs. *American Review of Respiratory Diseases, 144,* 745–749.

Burwen, D. R., Bloch, A. B., Griffen, L. D., Ciesielski, C. A., Stern, H. A., & Onorato, I. M. (1995). National trends in the concurrence of tuberculosis and acquired immunodeficiency syndrome. *Archives of Internal Medicine, 155,* 1281–1286.

Cantwell, M. F., McKenna, M. T., McCray, E., & Onorato, I. M. (1998). Tuberculosis and race/ethnicity in the U.S. *American Journal of Respiratory and Critical Care Medicine, 157,* 1016–1020.

Cantwell, M. F., Snider, D. E., Cauthen, G. M., & Onorato, I. M. (1994). Epidemiology of tuberculosis in the U.S., 1985 through 1992. *Journal of the American Medical Association, 272,* 535–539.

Centers for Disease Control and Prevention. (1989). A strategic plan for the elimination of tuberculosis in the United States. *Morbidity and Mortality Weekly Report, 38*(SS-3), 1–25.

Centers for Disease Control and Prevention. (1990). Case definitions for public health surveillance. *Morbidity and Mortality Weekly Report, 39*(RR-13), 39–40.

Centers for Disease Control and Prevention. (1991). Drug resistance among Indochinese refugees with tuberculosis. *Morbidity and Mortality Weekly Report, 30,* 272–275.

Centers for Disease Control and Prevention. (1992a). 1993 revised classification system for HIV infection and expanded surveillance case definition for AIDS among adolescents and adults. *Morbidity and Mortality Weekly Report, 41*(RR-17), pamphlet inclusive.

Centers for Disease Control and Prevention. (1992b). Prevention and control of tuberculosis in U.S. communities with at-risk minority populations and control of tuberculosis among homeless persons. *Morbidity and Mortality Weekly Report, 41*(RR-5), 1–23.

Centers for Disease Control and Prevention. (1994). Update: Impact of the expanded AIDS surveillance case definition for adolescents and adults on case reporting: United States, 1993. *Morbidity and Mortality Weekly Report, 43,* 160–161, 167–170.

Centers for Disease Control and Prevention. (1996). *Reported tuberculosis in the U.S., 1995.* Washington, DC: U.S. Public Health Service.

Centers for Disease Control and Prevention. (1997). Tuberculosis morbidity: United States, 1996. *Morbidity and Mortality Weekly Report, 46,* 695–700.

Centers for Disease Control and Prevention. (1998). Development of new vaccines for tuberculosis: Recommendations of the Advisory Council for the Elimination of Tuberculosis. *Morbidity and Mortality Weekly Report, 47*(RR-13), pamphlet inclusive.

Centers for Disease Control and Prevention. (1999a). *Reported tuberculosis in the United States, 1998.* Atlanta, GA: Author.

Centers for Disease Control and Prevention. (1999b). Tuberculosis elimination revisited: Obstacles, opportunities, and a renewed commitment (Advisory Committee for the Elimination of Tuberculosis, ACET). *Morbidity and Mortality Weekly Report, 48*(RR-9), pamphlet inclusive.

Chaulk, C. P., & Pope, D. S. (1997). The Baltimore City Health Department program of directly observed therapy for tuberculosis. *Clinical Chest Medicine, 18,* 149–154.

Chin, D. P., Derimer, K., Moss, A. R., Paz, A., Jasmer, R. M., Agasino, C. B., & Hopewell, P. C. (1998). Differences in contributing factors to tuberculosis incidence in U.S.-born and foreign-born persons. *American Journal of Respiratory and Critical Care Medicine, 158,* 1797–1803.

Correa, A. G. (1997). Unique aspects of tuberculosis in the pediatric population. *Clinical Chest Medicine, 18,* 89–98.

Crawford, J. T. (1994). New technologies in the diagnosis of tuberculosis. *Seminars in Respiratory Infections, 9,* 62–70.

Crowle, A. J., & Elkins, N. (1990). Relative permissiveness of macrophages from black and white people for virulent tubercle bacilli. *Infectious Immunology, 58,* 632.

Davidow, A., Marmor, M., & Acabes, P. (1997). Geographic diversity in 1996: Tuberculosis trends and directly observed therapy: New York City, 1991 to 1994. *American Journal of Respiratory and Critical Care Medicine, 156,* 1495–1500.

Drobniewski, F. A., & Wilson, S. M. (1998). The rapid diagnosis of isoniazid and rifampicin resistance of *Mycobacterium tuberculosis:* A molecular story. *Principles and Practices of Infectious Disease, 47,* 189–196.

Felton, C. P., Smith, J. A., & Ehrlich, M. H. (1990). [Letter to the editor]. *New England Journal of Medicine, 322,* 1671.

Freiden, T. R. (1994). Tuberculosis control and social change. *American Journal of Public Health, 84,* 1721–1723.

Friedman, D. R., Stoeckle, M. Y., Kresswith, B. N., Johnson, W. D., Jr., Manoach, S. M., Berger, J., Sathinathan, K., Hafner, A., & Riley, L. W. (1995). Transmission of multi-drug resistant tuberculosis in a large urban setting. *American Journal of Respiratory and Critical Care Medicine, 152,* 355–359.

Fujiwara, P. I., Larkin, C., & Freiden, T. R. (1997). Directly observed therapy in New York City: History, implementation, results, and challenges. *Clinical Chest Medicine, 18,* 135–148.

Gasner, M. R., Maw, K. L., Feldman, L. E., Fujiwara, P. I., & Freiden, T. R. (1999). The use of legal action in New York City to ensure treatment of tuberculosis. *New England Journal of Medicine, 340,* 359–373.

"Genetics—NRAMP1 gene associated with TB susceptibility." (1998, March 30). *Gene Therapy Weekly, 5,* 1–6.

Gobles, M., Iseman, M. D., & Madsen, L. A. (1993). Treatment of 171 persons with pulmonary tuberculosis resistant to isoniazid and rifampin. *New England Journal of Medicine, 328,* 527–532.

Haas, D. W., & Des Prez. (1989). Mycobacterium tuberculosis. In G. L. Mandell, J. E. Bennett, & R. Dolin (Eds.), *Principles and practice of infectious diseases* (4th ed., pp. 2213–2243). New York: Churchill Livingstone.

Jereb, J. A., Kelly, G. D., & Dooley, D. W. (1991). Tuberculosis morbidity in the U.S.: Final data, 1990 (CDC Surveillance Summaries). *Morbidity and Mortality Weekly Report, 40* (SS-3), 23–27.

Khoury, S. A., Theodore, A., & Platte, V. J. (1969). Isoniazid prophylaxis in a slum area. *American Review of Respiratory Diseases, 99,* 345–353.

Kleeburg, H. H., & Olivier, M. S. (1984). *A world atlas of initial drug resistance* (2nd ed.). Pretoria, South Africa: Tuberculosis Research Council.

Leff, D. R., & Leff, A. R. (1997). Tuberculosis control policies in major metropolitan health departments in the U.S. *American Journal of Respiratory and Critical Care Medicine, 156,* 1487–1494.

Long, E. R. (1941). Constitution and related factors in resistance to tuberculosis. *Archives of Pathology, 32,* 122–162.

Lyashchenko, K., Colangeli, R., Houde, M., Al Jahdali, H., Menzies, D., & Gennaro, M. L. (1998). Heterogeneous antibody responses in tuberculosis. *Infectious Immunology, 66,* 3936–3940.

Marier, R. (1977). The reporting of communicable diseases. *American Journal of Epidemiology, 105,* 587–590.

McCray, E., Weinbaum, C. M., Braden, C. R., & Onorato, I. M. (1997). The epidemiology of tuberculosis in the U.S. *Clinical Chest Medicine, 18,* 99–113.

McKenna, M.T.E., McCray, T. E., & Onorato, I. M. (1995). The epidemiology of tuberculosis among foreign-born persons in the U.S., 1986 to 1993. *New England Journal of Medicine, 332,* 1071–1076.

McPeek, M., Salkowitz, J., Laufman, H., Pearl, D., & Zwilling, B. S. (1992). The expression of HLA-DR by monocytes from black and from white donors: Different requirements for protein synthesis. *Clinical and Experimental Immunology, 87,* 163–168.

Morse, D. L., & DiFernando, G. T., Jr. (1990). [Letter to the editor]. *New England Journal of Medicine, 322,* 1671.

National Heart, Lung, and Blood Institute Working Group. (1995). Respiratory diseases disproportionately affecting minorities. *Chest, 108,* 1380–1392.

Netto, E. M., Dye, C., & Raviglione, M. C. (1999). Progress in global tuberculosis control 1995–1996, with emphasis on 22 high-incidence countries (Report for the Global Monitoring and Surveillance Project). *International Journal of Tuberculosis and Lung Disease, 2,* 310–320.

Nolan, C. M., & Elarth, A. M. (1988). Tuberculosis in a cohort of Southeast Asian refugees. *American Review of Respiratory Diseases, 137,* 805–809.

Pablos-Mendez, A., Raviglione, M. C., Battan, R., & Ramos-Zuniga, R. (1990). Drug resistant tuberculosis among the homeless in New York City. *New York State Journal of Medicine, 90,* 351–355.

Pitchenik, A. E., Russell, B. W., Cleary, T., Pejovic, T., Cole, C., & Snider, D. E., Jr. (1982). The prevalence of tuberculosis and drug resistance among Haitians. *New England Journal of Medicine, 307,* 162–165.

Polednak, A. P. (1997). *Segregation, poverty, and mortality in urban African Americans.* New York: Oxford University Press.

Reichman, L. B. (1996). How to ensure the continued resurgence of tuberculosis. *Lancet, 347,* 175–177.

Rieder, H. L., Cauthen, G. M., Kelly, G. D., Bloch, A. B., & Snider, D. E. (1989). Tuberculosis in the U.S. *Journal of the American Medical Association, 262,* 385–389.

Riley, L. W., Arathoon, E., & Loverde, V. D. (1989). The epidemiologic picture of drug-resistant *Mycobacterium tuberculosis* infections. *American Review of Respiratory Diseases, 132,* 1282–1285.

Rosenman, K. D. (1990). [Letter to the editor]. *New England Journal of Medicine, 322*, 1670.

Samanich, K. M., Gelisle, J. T., Sonnenberg, M. G., Keen, M. A., Zolla-Pazner, S., & Laal, S. (1998). Delineating human antibody responses to culture filtrate antigens of *Mycobacterium tuberculosis. Journal of Infectious Diseases, 178*, 1534–1538.

Sandman, L., Schluger, N. W., Davidow, A. L., & Bonk, S. (1999). Risk factors for rifampin-monoresistant tuberculosis. *American Journal of Respiratory and Critical Care Medicine, 159*, 468–472.

Sbarbaro, J. A. (1997). Directly observed therapy: Who is responsible? *Clinical Chest Medicine, 18*, 131–133.

Scalcini, M., Carre, G., & Jean-Baptiste, M. (1990). Anti-tuberculosis drug resistance in central Haiti. *American Review of Respiratory Diseases, 142*, 508–511.

Schecter, G. F. (1997). Supervised therapy in San Francisco. *Clinical Chest Medicine, 18*, 165–168.

Sibley, E. (1969). *Differential mortality in Tennessee, 1917–1928*. New York: Negro Universities Press. (Originally published in 1930)

Stead, W. W. (1997). The origin and erratic global spread of tuberculosis. *Clinical Chest Medicine, 18*, 65–77.

Stead, W. W., Senner, J. W., Reddick, W. T., & Lofgran, J. P. (1990). Racial differences in susceptibility to infection by *Mycobacterium tuberculosis. New England Journal of Medicine, 322*, 422–427.

Streeton, J. A., Desem, N., & Jones, S. L. (1998). Sensitivity and specificity of a gamma interferon test for tuberculosis infection. *International Journal of Tuberculosis and Lung Disease, 2*, 443–450.

Torchia, M. M. (1977). Tuberculosis among American Negroes: Medical research on a racial disease, 1830–1950. *Journal of the History of Medicine, 51*, 252–279.

Trump, D. H., & DiStasio, A. J. (1990). [Letter to the editor]. *New England Journal of Medicine, 322*, 1671–1672.

U.S. Department of Health and Human Services. Task Force on Black and Minority Health. (1985). *Report of the Secretary's Task Force on Black and Minority Health* (Vol. 1, Executive Summary, pp. 63–86). Washington, DC: U.S. Government Printing Office.

U.S. Department of Health and Human Services. Office of Public Health and Science. (1998). *Healthy people 2010 objectives: Draft for public comment*. Washington, DC: U.S. Government Printing Office.

Ussery, X. T., Valway, S. E., McKenna, M., Cauthen, G. M., McCray, E., & Onorato, I. M. (1996). Epidemiology of tuberculosis among children in the U.S., 1985–1994. *Pediatric Infectious Disease Journal, 15*, 697–704.

Weis, S. E. (1997). Universal directly observed therapy: A treatment strategy for tuberculosis. *Clinical Chest Medicine, 18*, 155–163.

Wolfe, H., Marmor, M., Maslansky, R., Nichols, S., Simberhoff, M., Des Jarlais, D., & Moss, A. (1995). Tuberculosis knowledge among New York City injection drug users. *American Journal of Public Health, 85*, 985–988.

Yandell, L. P. (1831). Remarks on Struma Africana, or the disease usually called Negro poison or Negro consumption. *Transylvania Journal of Medicine, 4*, 83–103.

Zuber, P.L.F., McKenna, M. T., Binkin, N. J., Onorato, I. M., & Castro, K. G. (1998). Long-term risk of tuberculosis among foreign-born persons in the U.S. *Journal of the American Medical Association, 278*, 304–307.

CHAPTER FIFTEEN

PEDIATRIC ASTHMA IN AFRICAN AMERICAN CHILDREN

Joyce Essien, Chanda Nicole Mobley, Marcia Griffith, Thomas L. Creer, Robert L. Geller

In providing a framework and rationale for the nation's health objectives, Healthy People 2010 describes the goal of eliminating racial and ethnic and socioeconomic disparities in health status. More specifically, the disease prevention objectives for asthma establish targeted objectives for (1) reductions in deaths, hospitalizations, school days lost, and work days lost and (2) an increase in the number of persons with asthma who receive appropriate care and education including information about community resources and self-help management and maintenance strategies. The recommendations state that as a priority, the nation needs to (1) intensify efforts to reach primary care providers and school personnel and (2) mobilize community resources for a comprehensive, culturally and linguistically competent approach to controlling asthma among high-risk populations.

Healthy People 2010 (U.S. Department of Health and Human Services, 2000) reports that the number of individuals with asthma has increased by 102 percent between 1979 to 1980 and 1993 to 1994. It further describes that death from asthma is two to six times more likely to occur among African Americans and Hispanics than among whites; that rates of hospitalization for African Americans are almost triple those for whites; and that in 1993 and 1994, African Americans were four times more likely than whites to visit the hospital emergency room for treatment of asthma.

The Faces and the Stories

Lara (1999) describes the impact of pediatric asthma in stories of children who are diagnosed too late; of medications that aren't used appropriately because of confusion about the instructions for administration and use; of families who can't afford to purchase preventive medications and medical equipment; of physical activities restricted due to lack of appropriate medications; and of the difficulty of getting medication at school. Williams et al. (2000) report on a telephone survey of the caregivers of African American children with asthma who had been seen in the emergency room of an inner-city public hospital. Ninety-five percent considered their children's asthma to be among the top third of their daily problems. Many of the stories of these families have been heard and observed by community health workers (CHWs) employed by Zap Asthma Consortium who work with asthmatic children and their families that live in Atlanta's Empowerment Zone. These CHWs describe the complex barriers to health faced by the families with whom they work:

- A single parent is confronted by the siblings of her asthmatic child who complain that their needs and interests are being ignored.
- A caregiver of an asthmatic child, employed in a welfare-to-work program, is warned that if there are any more absences from work, she will be fired.
- A parent whose son dies in status asthmaticus is haunted by guilt and self-incrimination—"Why didn't I act sooner?"
- A family with no health insurance relies on episodic care through the emergency room for an asthmatic child and cannot afford to purchase drugs as prescribed.
- A caregiver and asthmatic child living in housing conditions that are unhealthy and with increased exposure to environmental triggers are unable to locate affordable and safe housing after the demolition of a public housing facility.

The data rarely capture and depict the full consequence and impact of this disease on the family and the community or fully describe the factors and forces that influence the complex strategies and interventions required to ensure conditions in which African American children with asthma can achieve their health potential. The picture of the disease in African American children often includes fragmented health care, the inability to adhere to treatment plans, poor housing conditions and exposure to known triggers of the disease, family dysfunction, disruption of social networks, loss of employment, and other stressors.

Although there are many barriers to effective prevention and treatment, there are also promising approaches to eradicating a number of these barriers. This chapter addresses both the barriers and potential solutions. An appendix offers a list of resources for further information.

A Description of the Disease and Its Pathogenesis

The word *asthma* is derived from a Greek word meaning *panting* (Keeney, 1964). The disease has proven elusive to define, although detailed descriptions of the symptoms associated with the disorder can be traced back to Hippocrates (McFadden & Stevens, 1983; Pearce, Beasley, Burgess, & Crane, 1998). One reason for the confusion is that as Busse and Reed (1988) noted, the disorder is often defined based on the respective interests of a broad cross section of professions and disciplines. Further, the definition has evolved as our scientific understanding of the physiology and pathology of the disease has advanced. A consensus definition, however, was reached by an interdisciplinary workgroup convened by the National Heart, Lung, and Blood Institute (NHLBI) as part of a process to develop and disseminate treatment guidelines for asthma (National Institutes of Health [NIH], 1991). The following updated and revised working definition is based on current knowledge and was developed by the NHLBI in 1995 (NIH, 1999):

> Asthma is a chronic inflammatory disorder of the airways in which many cells and cellular elements play a role, in particular, mast cells, eosinophils, T lymphocytes, macrophages, neutrophils, and epithelial cells. In susceptible individuals, this inflammation causes recurrent episodes of wheezing, breathlessness, chest tightness, and coughing, particularly at night or in the early morning. These episodes are usually associated with widespread but variable airflow obstruction that is often reversible either spontaneously or with treatment. The inflammation also causes an associated increase in the existing bronchial hyperresponsiveness to a variety of stimuli [p. 2].

A variety of stimuli elicit the release of inflammatory mediators from the cells that line the passages of the pulmonary airways, with the results of (1) inducing contraction of the smooth muscles that line the walls of the airway passages, which results in spasm of the airway passages, and (2) causing leakage in vascular walls, which increases the production of mucous and hyperreactivity.

The frequency of symptoms varies from patient to patient and for any given patient from time to time. Symptoms, as described in the definition, may remit either spontaneously or with treatment. As a consequence, health care providers use a functional definition that is based on an assessment of symptoms occurring over an extended period of time and on categories of disease derived from the severity of symptoms and the status of lung function. The more commonly used functional definitions describe four levels of the disease: mild intermittent, mild persistent, moderate persistent, and severe persistent. A stepwise treatment strategy employing these levels is incorporated in the NIH disease management and treatment guidelines for asthma (NIH, 1991, 1997).

In lay terms, the disease is manifested by difficulty in breathing resulting from a narrowing of the airways in the lung. During an asthma episode, the airways become narrow as the muscles around the airways tighten, the inner lining of the airways becomes edematous (swollen), and increased amounts of mucous are produced that clog the smaller airways. Breathing becomes difficult, and a wheezing or whistling sound is heard as attempts to inhale force air through the narrowed airways.

The Epidemiology of Asthma

Epidemiologists have been primarily concerned with investigating the factors that cause a healthy person to develop asthma and the factors that then affect the course of the disease and its outcomes. The conducting of studies to elucidate causal factors and associations has been made difficult by the lack of consensus on diagnostic criteria and classification, the lack of standardization of measurement techniques, and the uncertainties in determining whether the events that are monitored and measured to assess disease morbidity reflect morbidities that are true consequences of the disease process or morbidities that are a consequence of conditions and situations related to access to care or to disease management (Pearce et al., 1998).

Asthma is the most common chronic disease of children in the United States and other industrialized countries (von Mutius, 2000). In 1990, asthma was the leading cause of school absenteeism in the United States, with more than ten million school days missed by children between the ages of five and seventeen. Children in this age group also had an estimated 860,000 emergency room visits and 160,000 hospitalizations (Weiss, Gergen, & Hodgson, 1992) for asthma. A two- to threefold increase in morbidity is reported in African American children compared to other groups of children (Hayman, Mahon, & Turner, in press), and the prevalence of disability due to asthma is reported as higher for adolescents, African American children, and children from low-income and single-parent families (Newacheck & Halfon, 2000).

Creer and Bender (1995) describe the following risk factors as contributing to asthma in minority children, particularly African American children who live in the inner city: (1) poverty; (2) environmental factors such as maternal smoking, air pollution, and dust mites; (3) psychological factors; (4) familial factors, particularly family dysfunction, large family size, and small homes; and (5) physical factors, particularly low birthweight and a maternal age younger than twenty years at the child's birth (Evans, 1992; Weitzman, Gortmaker, & Sobol, 1990). Other precipitating or aggravating factors that have been cited include viral respiratory infections, cockroach antigens and animal dander, exercise, changes in weather and exposure to cold air, food, food additives, and preservatives (NIH, 1999).

Prevalence

The prevalence of asthma is increasing. In 1993 and 1994, an estimated 13.7 million people in the United States were reported to have asthma. From 1980 to 1994, the age-adjusted prevalence rose from 30.7 per 1,000 population in 1980 to a two-year average of 53.8 per 1,000 in 1993 and 1994. In 1998, a state-specific estimate of asthma reported that the disorder affected an estimated 17,299,000 people in the United States, or 6.4 percent of the U.S. population (Centers for Disease Control and Prevention [CDC], 1998).

The prevalence of asthma is higher among children than among adults and higher among African Americans than among whites. Among the general population the prevalence of asthma is higher among females; however, among children the prevalence is higher among males.

The prevalence among children ages five to fourteen increased 74 percent from 1980 to 1993 and 1994, from 42.8 to 74.4 per 1,000. Among children up to four years of age, asthma prevalence increased 160 percent, from 22.2 per 1,000 in 1980 to 57.9 per 1,000 in 1993 and 1994 (Mannino et al., 1998).

Mortality

In spite of the therapeutic advances in drug treatment and the availability of disease management guidelines, rates of death from asthma in the United States sharply increased from 0.8 per 100,000 in the general population in 1977 and 1978 to 2.0 per 100,000 in 1989 and 2.1 per 100,000 in 1994 (Sly & O'Donnell, 1997). The number of deaths from asthma was reported as 1,674 in 1977, 5,487 in 1994, and 5,637 in 1995. Death from asthma is two to six times more likely to occur among African Americans and Hispanics than among whites (U.S. Department of Health and Human Services, 2000).

Costs and Expenditures

This increasing prevalence accounts for the escalating costs associated with asthma. Weiss, Gergen, and Hodgson (1992) found the estimated economic cost of asthma in the United States was $6.2 billion in 1990. This figure included $3.64 billion for direct costs of asthma care (for example, costs for physicians, medications, laboratory procedures, hospitalizations, and emergency room care). More than half of the direct costs of asthma were due to hospitalizations and emergency room care, and 10 percent went for physician services. Approximately 35 percent of hospital costs were for persons under eighteen years of age. Finally, Weiss and his colleagues found that 30 percent of direct medical costs were associated with the 7.5 million prescriptions dispensed for asthma management and prevention. Recent estimates by others (for example, Smith et al., 1997; Stempel, Sturm, Hedblom, & Durcanin-Robbins, 1995) report similar findings.

Lozano, Sullivan, Smith, and Weiss (1999) analyzed data from the National Medical Expenditure Survey conducted in 1987. Among the major findings were the following:

- Forty-one percent of families with an asthmatic child had no health insurance.
- Children with asthma used substantially more services in all categories of care than children without asthma did: 3.1 times as many prescriptions, 1.9 times as many ambulatory provider visits, 2.2 times as many emergency room visits, and 3.5 times as many hospitalizations.
- Children with asthma incurred an average expenditure of $1,129 per child annually in total health care expenditures compared with $468 for children without asthma.

Treatment of Acute Asthma

With the role of inflammatory processes now characterized as a critical determinant in the pathogenesis of asthma, the advances in drug therapy have been targeted and dramatic. Current practices incorporate quick-relief medications to control acute symptoms in combination with longer-acting drugs designed for long-term control and maintenance. Bronchodilators are prescribed for acute attacks, and inhaled steroids and cromolyn sodium preparations are employed for maintenance and prophylaxis.

There is a continuing and expanding effort to ensure access to quality care and continuity of care for those children who are at highest risk for preventable morbidity and mortality from asthma. The Third International Pediatric Consensus Statement on the Management of Childhood Asthma describes these aims for therapeutic management (Warner, Naspitz, & Cropp, 1998, p. 3):

- To achieve rapid resolution of acute symptoms
- To employ environmental control where indicated by history and allergy test results
- To use prophylactic drugs when morbidity of asthma is sufficient to justify their use, taking into account their potential side effects
- To optimize quality of life with no sleep disturbance and prevent exercise-induced asthma
- To use delivery devices that are appropriate to the drug and the patient's age

With the continuing advances in drug therapy and medication to control asthma symptoms, the broad dissemination and implementation of asthma guidelines for medication usage (NIH, 1999), and patients' adherence to individualized asthma management and action plans, the goals for asthma treatment should be attainable for all children with asthma.

Many associated factors are critical to the achievement of these therapeutic goals. A written and individualized management and action plan should be prepared to guide self-management of disease episodes when appropriate and to direct the patient and family to seek care when appropriate. This plan must be written in a manner that the family can understand and can implement within their usual daily activities. (Words the family members cannot comprehend must be avoided, for example.) The family members involved in care provision and supervision, and, to the extent feasible, the child as well, must be taught the plan.

Equally critical to the optimal and effective use of prescribed medications is access to the appropriate inhalation devices (spacers and nebulizers) and the knowledge, skills, and ability to use these devices effectively. Access to appropriate drugs and inhalation devices remains a critical barrier for significant numbers of African American children with asthma.

An unacceptably high number of children lack health insurance and other financial resources necessary to ensure the availability and usage of appropriate control and maintenance therapy, placing these children at unnecessarily high risk. Adherence to appropriate therapeutic management is further complicated by the low numbers of children at high risk who have a primary source of care and who have a management plan to guide their use of medications and health services. Even when the necessary resources are in place, however, all too often adherence with ongoing therapy remains inconsistent or absent (Celano, Geller, Phillips, & Ziman, 1998).

The Role of Self-Management and Self-Efficacy

Almost three decades ago a number of trends and forces converged, catalyzing the development of effective self-management intervention programs for individuals with asthma, particularly pediatric asthma (Creer, Bender, & Lucas, in press). A major trend was the increasing prevalence of asthma and its associated morbidity, which resulted in pressure to encourage patients to become partners with health care providers in the management of their disease. The self-management concept was further advanced by recognition and acknowledgment of the health management process as a shared responsibility and by experiences in the previous decade during the time self-management techniques were being developed and tested (Creer, 1979; Creer & Christian, 1976). When resources became available to support collaboration between behavioral scientists and clinicians, a wide array of self-management programs were designed, implemented, and incorporated in care management plans for pediatric asthma. These practices were further promoted by the 1991 NIH treatment guidelines that underscored the role patients should play in the treatment and control of asthma. By the time the revised asthma treatment guidelines were issued (NIH, 1997), the partnership roles to be played by health care providers and patients were clearly spelled out. As we look to the future, it can be expected that asthma medications will become more specific and more potent and that the value of having a common blueprint that is shared by all members of an interdisciplinary team, including patients and their families, will increase.

Creer and Holroyd (1997) clearly and precisely describe the processes that promote self-management and self-efficacy. These processes include the following sequential and iterative steps:

- Goal setting, a process jointly shared by patients and their health care providers
- Information collection, particularly data gathered through the use of peak flow meters, asthma diaries, and records of acute symptomatic episodes
- Information processing and evaluation
- Decision making
- Action
- Self-reaction

These processes support the current treatment guidelines for asthma that specify the role to be played by patients. Key recommendations include the following (NIH, 1997):

- Patient education beginning at the time of diagnosis and integrated into every step of asthma care
- Patient education provided by all members of the team, including behavioral scientists
- An information and treatment approach that teaches asthma self-management skills and is tailored to fit the needs of each patient
- Patient education that teaches and reinforces behavioral skills (inhaler use, self-monitoring, and environmental control)
- Joint development of treatment plans by team members and patients
- Encouragement of an active partnership by providing written agreements and individualized action plans for patients
- Encouragement of adherence to the treatment jointly developed by the interdisciplinary team that includes the patient

It is within this framework and set of expectations that a number of community-based asthma intervention models and programs have designed strategies for high-risk families that give community health workers a role in the self-management process. As an example, community health workers employed by the Zap Asthma initiative employ a needs assessment instrument to tailor individualized support, teaching, and assistance during the acquisition of self-management competencies, and they intervene at the family and community level to eliminate barriers to the achievement of the goals and objectives of the self-management process.

Psychological and Behavioral Aspects of Childhood Asthma

As noted, epidemiological data fails to convey the potential influence of asthma on the psychological, social, and cognitive development of children. Conclusions about the psychological consequences of pediatric asthma are inconsistent; conclusions about childhood asthma, in particular, reflect both variations in research methodologies and differences in patient populations. The following section, based on research summarized by Bender and Creer (in press), Creer and Bender (1995), and Creer, Bender, and Lucas (in press), will review and critique findings on the psychological consequences of pediatric asthma, as well as explore important mediating variables regarding psychology and asthma.

Asthma and Psychological Development

Childhood asthma has often been associated with psychological disorders (Bender & Creer, in press; Creer & Bender, 1995; Creer, Bender, & Lucas, in press). Anxiety and depression in children with asthma, as well as distress these disorders induce in families, are the most frequently documented disorders. There are studies in the literature that imply that a large portion of children with asthma have been psychologically compromised by their illness and therefore are in need of mental health services (for example, Bussing, Halfon, Benjamin, & Wells, 1995). Inconsistency in the findings, however, limits the conclusions that can be drawn from the studies (Creer, Bender, & Lucas, in press). For example, while some experimenters reported a relationship between disease severity and psychological distress, others did not. Variations in sampling of subjects and different methodology used in the studies likely contributed to the inconsistencies and confusion about the relationship between asthma and psychological adaptation in children.

Two methodological shortcomings are found in many of these investigations (Annett & Bender, 1994; Bender & Klinnert, 1998). First, most relied on parental reports concerning asthma diagnosis, severity, medication use, and symptom control; these reports, however, were not corroborated by objective information, such as pulmonary test results, medical chart review, or physician verification of findings. Second, many investigators recruited what are referred to as samples of convenience. In particular, the tendency was to recruit as potential subjects single-site samples whose demographic and illness characteristics may have produced unique outcomes not found with other samples. For example, as described throughout the chapter, conducting a study such as Zap Asthma with minority groups in the inner city is not representative of the overall population of children with asthma.

Some of the variability in findings on the relationship between disease severity and psychological adaptation are due to differences in definitions of asthma severity (Creer, Bender, & Lucas, in press). In some instances, inclusion in a study was based only upon a report of asthma by the parent, with no diagnostic or severity-related assessment procured from health care providers. In most cases where illness severity was assessed by pulmonary function measures, frequency of asthma attacks, or medication use, no direct illness or psychopathology relationship was found. Measures of functional control, such as days of asthma-related school absence (for example, Klinnert, 1997) or activity restriction (Bussing, Halfon, Benjamin, & Wells, 1995), however, were frequently associated with the child's psychological adaptation as measured by standardized parent-report questionnaires. In all cases, this illness-adaptation relationship was relatively weak. Creer, Bender, and Lucas (in press) note that all variables were less significant determinants of psychological adaptation than were characteristics of the family such as parental psychopathology, exposure to stressful life events, family conflict, and maternal social support.

The Child Asthma Management Program (CAMP) is the largest multicenter study ever conducted on pediatric asthma. One thousand children in eight cities in North America have been followed in this investigation. Findings gathered thus far indicate that mild to moderate asthma does not result in an increase in cognitive, emotional, or behavioral problems in children. Bender (1998) reported that baseline psychological testing conducted in CAMP found no increase in scores indicative of behavioral problems, as assessed by the Child Behavior Checklist; depression, as assessed by the Children's Depression Inventory; or anxiety, as assessed by the Revised Children's Manifest Anxiety Scale. Furthermore, results from intelligence and school achievement tests revealed a distribution of scores that was no different from those of a normative, age-matched population of children (Annett, 1996).

Psychological Distress in Children with Asthma. Pediatric asthma is distressing for children and their families. All one has to do is watch a child try to breathe and be unable to do so. The sense of helplessness experienced by the child and family members is an alarming and unforgettable experience. Data from the Childhood Asthma Management Program indicate most children with asthma do not have psychological disorders. Short of inducing a psychological disorder, however, asthma can be difficult and stressful. Asthma interferes with normal physical and social activity in that children with asthma are often restricted in play and participation in sport (Newacheck & Halfon, 2000). Peer interactions can be impeded, and the natural evolution of childhood friendships interrupted. Children with asthma are often unable to experience the same social experiences as peers who do not have asthma. The lack of this experience may not only deprive children with asthma of those social interactions needed for success in our society but, in turn, can produce a sense of loss, self-doubt, and withdrawal.

Families of Asthmatic Children and Distress. Earlier, activity limitations and school absenteeism among asthmatic children were described. Chronic illness and the continual need for medical care create financial burdens, force parents to miss work, and interfere with family activities. Marital conflict often increases, and siblings receive less attention because parents must devote more time and energy to caring for a child with asthma. Environmental control measures, including intense cleaning of the interior of houses, replacement of carpeting, and restricted access to pets, generate work and expense for families. And, even when dramatic alterations are made in a home, there is the never-ending task of keeping triggers of asthma, such as dust, allergens, mold, and cigarette smoke, from the child's environment.

These circumstances indicate that asthma induces stress for patients, their families, and everyone having regular contact with an asthmatic child, such as a baby-sitter, grandparents, and so on. The constant stress, in turn, has a direct impact on the quality of life of all concerned with the child. Although difficult to measure, the concept of quality of life captures the notion that chronic illness interferes with daily life and the sense of satisfaction and enjoyment that it can produce. Quality of life questionnaires capture a degree of stress brought on by the illness, but have little or no demonstrable capacity to assess significant psychological change or disorder (Bender, 1996).

Poverty and Urban Minority Groups. As we've noted, asthma mortality and hospitalization rates are greater among nonwhite and low-income patients. Reasons cited for this data include lack of access to health care, failure to use asthma medications appropriately, inadequate recognition of illness severity, poor treatment adherence, and greater exposure to respiratory infections and environmental conditions that tend to trigger and exacerbate asthma. The latter would include environmental factors often found in the inner city, including air pollution, dust mites, indoor molds, and cigarette smoke.

Mediators of the Relationship Between Asthma and Psychological Disorder

Without question, some children with asthma develop psychological disorders. The prevailing problem is determining what circumstances or situations propel a child with asthma towards psychopathology. Variables suggested as potential mediators of the relationship between asthma and psychological disorder include asthma severity and other illnesses, presence of stressful life events, school absenteeism, allergies, and medication side effects. Bender and Creer (in press) and Creer, Bender, and Lucas (in press) recently summarized data on these factors; this information will be briefly examined in the following sections.

Disease Severity and Other Illness. Severe asthma can bring a heightened level of distress that significantly adds to the psychological burden for children and their families. With increased severity of asthma, the level of debilitation and activity restriction is often heightened, financial burdens grow, and interruption of the families' lives dramatically increases. There are many days when discomfort, pain, suffering, and a gnawing anxiety about the possibility of death from asthma intrude on the entire family's sense of well being. Most of the evidence supports the conclusion that a psychological disorder is increased in children only when their asthma is severe, although investigators have reported no severity-mediated relationship between the disorder and psychological adaptation. Inaccuracy in the assessment of asthma severity may occur in such studies because they rely solely upon parent-report measures, include no objective disease measures, and fail to represent severe asthma. Absence of an observed severity-psychopathology relationship, on the other hand, may reflect the absence of patients with severe asthma.

Another important factor is the degree of control established over asthma. If asthma is uncontrolled, it can be a major source of distress to families no matter the severity of the disorder. When it is controlled, however, even patients with severe asthma and their families may experience no more disruption of their lives than is found in youngsters with a milder form of the condition.

The occurrence of other illnesses in addition to asthma may further compromise the psychological adaptation of the children and their families. Results from the U.S. National Health Interview Survey on Child Health in 1988 found that the most common pediatric chronic illnesses were respiratory disorders, including asthma and allergies (Newacheck & Stoddard, 1994). Approximately 20 percent of the sampled children had one chronic condition. For the five percent of children who had two or more chronic health conditions, a three-fold increase for risk of learning difficulties and school absenteeism was reported (Creer, Bender, & Lucas, in press). Children with more than one physical illness or physical disability are more likely to develop psychopathology than are children with only one such condition. In a study of 551 asthmatic children, children with asthma and another chronic medical condition demonstrated more behavioral or psychological problems than children with asthma alone (Bussing, Halfon, Benjamin, & Wells, 1995).

Stressful Life Events. Stressful life events, such as moving frequently, parental job loss, and death or absence of a family member increase the psychological duress for a child with asthma. A study of behavior problems and social competence in eighty-one children between the ages of six and fourteen with a chronic disorder found that negative life events predicted increased behavioral problems as found on the Internalizing score from the Child Behavior Checklist. Negative life events suggested increased withdrawal and depression, while illness severity did not (MacLean, Perrin, Gortmaker, & Pierre, 1992). "Undesirable life events" were also predictive of psychopathology in a study of thirty-six asthmatic children; they played a greater role in predicting psychopathology than did other factors including illness severity (Steinhausen, Schindler, & Stephan, 1983).

Asthmatic children with irritable temperament, an outcome that frequently occurs as a consequence of the illness itself, may induce a greater degree of parental irritability than occurs with a healthy child. Temperament profiles of children with asthma have been compared both to children with other chronic illnesses and to normal youngsters. Creer, Bender, and Lucas (in press) pointed out that such investigations have found that asthmatic children were characterized by significantly lower adaptability, lower intensity of reaction, more negative mood, and less persistence. Parents of children with asthma have been found to be more critical of their children than parents of healthy children. Illness improvement is often greater when children or adolescents with asthma are removed from critical or overprotective parents for treatment of the disorder, although stated reasons for these findings were questioned by Renne and Creer (1985).

School Absenteeism. Children with asthma miss school more often than do children without a chronic illness. Parcel and his colleagues (1979) revealed that children with asthma in one school district were absent from school 7 percent of the time, in comparison with 2 percent absence for the remaining children. Frequent school absenteeism interrupts the process of learning and interferes with children's social interactions and participation in extracurricular activities (Creer & Yoches, 1971). Surprisingly, however, increased school absenteeism is associated neither with decreased achievement nor increased asthma severity. A study of ninety-nine children with moderately severe to severe asthma found no statistical correlation between academic performance and school absenteeism; it was further noted that the mean achievement of the asthmatic group was average to above average despite the fact that the children were absent from school 20 percent of the days in the semester prior to testing (Gutstadt et al., 1989). These findings indicate that school absence may temporarily interrupt the acquisition of new skills and knowledge without permanently impeding academic progress.

A survey of parents of inner-city children found that 40 percent reported that their children with asthma were having difficulty at school due to frequent absenteeism (Freudenburg et al., 1980). The findings suggest that for inner-city children with asthma, school absence may be a greater problem than for other children. A subsequent study, however, reported that low socioeconomic status did not predict school absenteeism among children with chronic illness, including asthma (Fowler, Johnson, & Atkinson, 1985).

Allergy-Mediated Neuropsychological Changes. Some investigators have raised the possibility that the presence of childhood asthma or allergies may result in, or be associated with, specific changes in the brain. If this is so, then academic difficulties should be increased, and specific associated learning disabilities identified in children with asthma and allergies. Bender and Creer (in press) and Creer, Bender, and Lucas (in press) noted that research examining these questions has been plagued by methodological problems that, at times, have resulted in erroneous or conflicting conclusions. For instance, one study reported results of a parent questionnaire that indicated almost 40 percent of children with asthma had difficulty in school, particularly with reading; surveys of other select groups of parents, however, do not yield objective information about the incidence of learning problems in children with asthma. Studies that employed larger groups of asthmatic children and that used standardized tests of educational achievement have generally not found decreased academic skills relative to children without asthma. In the largest study of children with asthma, including 1,041 patients in eight cities, mean IQ, cognitive, and achievement test scores were normally distributed (Annett, 1996). Even among children with more severe asthma, there is no clear evidence of increased risk for learning disability or lagging academic skills. In a study of ninety-nine children who have been hospitalized with moderate persistent to severe persistent asthma, average scores on the Slosson Intelligence Test, Woodcock Reading Mastery Test, Woodcock-Johnson Psychoeducational Battery, and Key Math Diagnostic Arithmetic Test were well above the 50th percentile relative to age-based norms (Gutstadt et al., 1989).

Theories proposing a direct link between allergic disorder, brain function, and learning disabilities have not been validated in subsequent research. When samples of hyperactive children were evaluated, an increased incidence of allergic disorders was not found (for example, Creer, Bender, & Lucas, in press). In addition, these authors reported that achievement levels among allergic children were no lower than those of nonallergic children. Furthermore, an association between reading disability, immune disorder, and left-handedness proposed by Geschwind and Galaburda (1987) has not, for the most part, been supported in subsequent research.

Medication Side Effects. Medication side effects may serve as yet another perturbation to the psychological adaptation of asthmatic children. Because children with severe, poorly controlled asthma are likely to receive more medications at larger doses, risk factors increase to the greatest degree in this segment of the asthmatic population. While the psychological effects of theophylline are not as severe as once believed, the caffeine-like effects of theophylline have been well documented. These include a slight trend towards more anxiety and hand tremor in treated versus untreated children; these behaviors are often accompanied by slightly increased attention and verbal memory (Bender, Lerner, & Poland, 1991; Bender & Milgrom, 1992). Classic antihistamines, such as diphenhydramine, have been found to cause drowsiness in some children (Vuurman, Veggel, Uiterwijk, Leutner, & O'Hanlon, 1993), although a recent study demonstrated no difference in effect upon learning of children treated with classic or nonsedating antihistamines (Bender, Milgrom, & McCormick, submitted for publication). Individual case studies have reported an association between sympathomimetics and a variety of unusual behaviors in children, including aggressiveness and visual hallucinations (Bender & Milgrom, 1995). Asthmatic children stabilized on high doses of oral corticosteroids (40 to 80 mg per day) can experience significant depression, anxiety, and impairment of long-term memory compared to children on low maintenance doses of corticosteroids (2 to 20 mg per day) (Bender, Lerner, & Kollasch, 1988). The steroid-induced psychosis reported in adults, however, has not been documented in children. Of particular interest is the finding that children with a preexisting history of emotional difficulties were more likely to become anxious and depressed while receiving high doses of prednisone than were children without such histories (Bender, Lerner, & Poland, 1991). This further supports the conclusion that a combination of risk factors heightens the potential for mal-adaptation. Inhaled steroids have not been associated with cognitive or behavioral changes in children with asthma (Bender, Ikle, DuHamel, & Tinkelman, 1998).

In summary, available evidence indicates that while asthma is a stressful and disruptive chronic illness, psychological development is not significantly altered for most children with mild-to-moderate asthma. The risk of psychological disorder is increased where children have severe asthma or are exposed to height-ened stress, live in poverty, or belong to a minority group. Other factors hypoth-esized to alter the developmental course for children with asthma—school absence, hypoxia, allergy-mediated changes in brain functions, and medication side effects—appear to have little impact.

Comprehensive Strategies to Reduce Preventable Morbidity and Optimize Health and Quality of Life

Erika von Mutius (1997) notes that the heterogeneity of the disease and the inad-equacy of our science and methods suggest that a discussion of primary pre-vention remains premature. She further observes that "apart from primary prevention strategies that have the potential to reduce rates of acquisition of asthma and atopic sensitization, secondary prevention is needed once asthma is established to reduce morbidity and mortality" (p. 14). The opportunities and strategies for secondary prevention are mentioned throughout this chapter and include allergen avoidance, reduction in exposure to air pollutants (such as envi-ronmental tobacco smoke), and the use of drugs that reduce the severity of the disease.

Studies have repeatedly concluded that preventable morbidity and mortality associated with asthma in high-risk populations can be attributed to a complex interaction of factors that include high levels of exposure to environmental aller-gens and irritants, lack of access to quality medical care and lack of financial re-sources, insufficient self-management skills, and inadequate social support (Creer & Bender, 1995; Kattan et al., 1997; Clark, Jones, Keller, & Vermeire, 1999). Successful efforts to improve the health and quality of life of African American children with asthma who live in urban settings will therefore require the coordi-nation of clinical, preventive, and social interventions to overcome the complex array of barriers to health.

Information obtained from data collected by quality-of-life instruments, needs assessment surveys, and focus groups among participants in programs im-plemented by the Zap Asthma initiative in Atlanta have identified an array of specific barriers and opportunities at multiple levels, which have been described by practitioners and researchers working in inner-city and high-risk communi-ties. These include but are not limited to

- The reliance on episodic care through the use of emergency rooms
- The absence of an asthma management plan and lack of knowledge about the proper use of medications
- Caregivers and school personnel who lack knowledge about the disease and lack the skills to take appropriate actions
- School policies that impede the ability of children to obtain medications in a timely fashion during school hours
- The lack of linguistically appropriate and culturally competent health education and health promotion resources

For the purpose of developing specifications for a comprehensive approach to ensuring conditions that will sustain improvements in the health and quality of life of asthmatic children at high risk, it may be helpful to examine health factors and barriers with the aid of an ecological health model. Such a model offers the opportunity to identify and examine explicit institutional factors, intrapersonal factors, interpersonal factors, community factors, and public policies that should be considered.

Institutional and health care system factors include (1) health care professionals that lack adequate training for diagnosing the disease and delivering quality care in compliance with current treatment and disease management guidelines, (2) health care systems that fail to employ case management strategies that would optimize care through individualized medication and management plans and through enhanced coordination and continuity of care, (3) inflexible policies and practices that do not accommodate the needs of families for extended hours and weekend availability of primary care services, and (4) resources and programs that are inadequate to ensure access to care and the availability of medications for children who are uninsured. Rust et al. (1996), in a study to assess the capacity of federally funded community health centers in the Southeast to meet the needs of low-income asthmatic patients, found that 29 percent had no mechanism to provide services for the uninsured and only 17 percent could provide peak flow meters to asthmatic patients.

Intrapersonal factors include patient and caregiver literacy, lifestyle, myths and personal beliefs, and self-management skills (Creer & Holroyd, 1997).

Interpersonal factors include the relationship and level of communication with health care providers and other caregivers including family members, teachers, and friends, and involvement in formal and informal networks and support groups.

Community factors include air quality and availability of affordable and safe housing, transportation, social support, and child care.

Public policy factors involve significant policies that affect health outcomes for asthmatic children living in both urban and isolated settings. They include school policies related to truancy and those that impede children's access to medication and treatment. They also include antipoverty policies such as welfare policy and the Personal Responsibility and Work Opportunity Reconciliation Act of 1996, which can make caregiving more difficult for the parent of a child with a chronic illness (Leviton, Snell, & McGinnis, 2000).

In spite of all these overwhelming and complex challenges, Leviton, Snell, and McGinnis (2000) express optimism about the potential for implementing new models for health promotion that engage urban inner-city residents as assets and partners in developing sustainable solutions to the growing disparity in chronic disease outcomes. These models are all based on collaborative and multisector approaches to capacity building in community systems as outlined in the recent CDC publication *Principles of Community Engagement* (1997). Among the growing numbers of collaborative partnerships and demonstrations that have been established to improve health outcomes for asthmatic children at highest risk, the contributions of community health workers are often cited as critical assets in the implementation of comprehensive community-based interventions (Butz et al., 1994; ORC Macro, 2000).

The core values and program elements that appear to be common to successful asthma collaborations include broad participation in planning and implementation from a diverse array of stakeholders associated with the direct and indirect contributing factors, grassroots leadership, self-organizing and transformative processes that build new capacities at the community level (individual skills and competencies, community systems, multisector collaborations, and so forth), enhanced communication vehicles and learning venues for all stakeholders and participants, and the availability of a wide range of opportunities for participation and contribution (Fisher et al., 1996; ORC Macro, 2000).

The aims and purposes are usually comprehensive in scope, mobilizing the collective assets of the partnership. They are designed to (1) remove the barriers to quality care that reside at the community, health system, and policy levels; (2) implement asthma education for patients, caregivers, and health professionals and asthma awareness in the general population as a critical component of a comprehensive strategy to improve clinical care, self-management, and efficacy; (3) influence policies that will reduce exposures to environmental triggers; and (4) address the broad range of social and environmental determinants that are critical to reductions in preventable morbidity and mortality.

Conclusion: Future Directions in Asthma Management

Lara (1999) presented a *four-point strategy* for asthma control in a recent invited conference to discuss future directions in the management of pediatric asthma. These four points and her additional strategies also summarize many of the concepts touched on in this chapter.

- *Educate* the public, providers, patients, and caregivers.
- *Simplify* treatment modalities, patient and physician education, and monitoring of patient progress.

- *Motivate* patients and providers through financial and other incentives.
- *Regulate* through public health vehicles and health care quality standards.

Lara identifies similar levers and strategies for children and their caregivers:

- *Educate* utilizing simple and multilingual messages.
- *Simplify* medication and equipment regimens (for example, provide "asthma tool kits").
- *Motivate* by offering free comprehensive care as an incentive to adhere to "well asthma care" programs.

She identifies specific opportunities and levers for health care providers:

- *Educate* through the dissemination of guidelines and interactive education.
- *Simplify* and automate systems for patient tracking, reminders, and prescriptions.
- *Motivate* by offering incentives and rewards for appropriate prescribing practices, primary care follow-up, and decreased tertiary care.
- *Regulate* through certification systems and health care process and performance standards.

In closing, Lara offers the following levers for intervention at the community and policy levels:

- *Educate* widely through the use of media campaigns.
- *Simplify* the ability to support continuity of care by coordinating health care and community-based efforts at the policy level.
- *Motivate* by assisting schools with asthma education and surveillance.
- *Regulate* by legislating comprehensive health insurance for children, school-based screening and referral, and tracking and monitoring of high-risk children and families.

Despite all of the efforts made to date, we still do not understand the underlying causes of the asthma epidemic in which we are currently trapped. Theories currently in vogue blame such disparate factors as outdoor air quality, increasingly energy-efficient homes that reduce the entry of fresh air and simultaneously trap air pollutants generated in the home inside it, and an increasingly sedentary lifestyle. Further study is needed to identify the true causes of the asthma epidemic and then to design, test, and implement appropriate strategies to mitigate the causative factors.

New and creative approaches need to be developed to address the heavy impact of asthma on inner city residents, as many remain afflicted by the effects of poorly controlled asthma despite our current efforts.

Appendix: Resources

Allergy and Asthma Network
Mothers of Asthmatics, Inc.
2751 Prosperity Avenue, Suite 150
Fairfax, VA 22031
(800) 878-4403; (703) 641-9595
Web site: www.aanma.org

American Academy of Allergy, Asthma & Immunology
611 East Wells Street
Milwaukee, WI 53202
(800) 822-ASMA (2762); (414) 272-6071
Web site: www.aaaai.org

American College of Allergy, Asthma & Immunology
Allergy, Asthma & Immunology Online
(800) 842-7777
Web site: www.allergy.mcg.edu

American Lung Association
1740 Broadway
New York, NY 10019
(800) LUNG-USA (586-4872); or call your local Lung Association
Web site: www.lungusa.com

Asthma and Allergy Foundation of America (AAFA)
1233 20th Street NW, Suite 402
Washington, DC 20036
(800) 7-ASTHMA (727-8462); (202) 466-7643
E-mail: info@aafa.org
Web site: www.aafa.org

Asthma Information Center, Journal of the American Medical Association
515 North State St.
Chicago, IL 60610
(312) 464-2402
Web site: www.ama-assn.org/special/asthma/asthma.htm

Breath of Life
United States National Library of Medicine
History of Medicine Department
Building 38, Room B1E21D

8600 Rockville Pike
Bethesda, MD 20892
(888) FIND-NLM (346-3656); (301) 594-5983
Web site: www.nlm.nih.gov/hmd/breath/breathhome.html

Foundation for Better Health Care
6 East 32nd Street
New York, NY 10016
(212) 835-2146
Web site: http://fbhc.org/modules/asthma.cfm

Healthy Lives
Glaxo Wellcome Inc.
Five Moore Drive
P.O.Box 13398
Research Triangle Park, NC 27709
(888) TALK2GW (825-5249); (919) 483-2100
Web site: www.healthylives.com

My Life Path
National Heart, Lung, and Blood Institute
National Institutes of Health
Bethesda, MD 20892
(800) 424-6521
Web site: www.mylifepath.com

National Asthma Education and Prevention Program (NAEPP)
National Heart, Lung, and Blood Institute
Health Information Center
P.O. Box 30105
Bethesda, MD 20824-0105
(301) 592-8573
E-mail: NHLBIinfo@rover.nhlbi.nih.gov
Web site: www.nhlbisupport.com/asthma.coalitioncorner/index.htm

National Institute of Allergy and Infectious Diseases, National Institutes of
Health
NIAID Office of Communications and Public Liaison
Building 31, Room 7A-50
31 Center Drive MSC 2520
Bethesda, MD 20892-2520
(301) 496-5717
Web site: www.niaid.nih.gov

National Institute of Environmental Health Sciences, Asthma Research
Office of Communications
P.O. Box 12233
Research Triangle Park, NC 27709
(919) 541-3345
E-mail: webcenter@niehs.nih.gov
Web site: www.niehs.nih.gov/airborne/home.htm

References

Annett, R. D. (1996, May). *Psychological growth and development studies and characteristics of the Childhood Asthma Management Program (CAMP) participants.* Paper presented at the annual meeting of the American Thoracic Society, New Orleans, LA.

Annett, R. D., & Bender, B. G. (1994). Neuropsychological dysfunction in asthmatic children. *Neuropsychological Review, 4,* 91–115.

Bender, B. (1996). Measurement of quality of life in pediatric asthma clinical trials. *Annals of Allergy, Asthma, and Immunology, 77,* 438–447.

Bender, B. (1998, April). *Is there a relationship between psychological dysfunction and disease severity in children with mild-to-moderate asthma?* Presented at the annual meeting of the American Thoracic Society, Chicago, IL.

Bender, B. G., & Creer, T. L. (in press). Asthma. In A. Christensen & M. Antoni (Eds.), *Chronic medical disorders: Behavioural medicine's perspective.* Oxford: Blackwell.

Bender, B. G., Ikle, D., DuHamel, T., & Tinkelman, D. (1998). Neuropsychological and behavioral changes in asthmatic children treated with beclomethasone dipropionate versus theophylline. *Pediatrics, 101,* 355–360.

Bender, B. G. & Klinnert, M. D. (1998). Psychological correlates of asthma severity and treatment outcome in children. In H. Kotses & A. Harver (Eds.). *Self-management of asthma* (pp. 63–88). New York, NY: Marcel Decker.

Bender, B., Lerner, J., & Kollasch, E. (1988). Mood and memory changes in asthmatic children receiving corticosteroids. *Journal of the American Academy of Child and Adolescent Psychiatry, 27,* 720–725.

Bender, B., Lerner, J, & Poland, J. (1991). Association between corticosteroids and psychological change in hospitalized asthmatic children. *Annals of Allergy, 66,* 414–419.

Bender, B., & Milgrom, H. (1992). Theophylline-induced behavior change in children: An objective evaluation of parents' perceptions. *Journal of the American Medical Association, 267,* 2621–2624.

Bender, B., & Milgrom, H. (1995). Neuropsychiatric effects of medications for allergic diseases. *Journal of Allergy and Clinical Immunology, 95,* 523–528.

Bender, B. G., Milgrom, H., & McCormick, D. *Lack of effect of diphenhydramine and loratadine on school performance.* Manuscript submitted for publication.

Busse, W. W., & Reed, C. E. (1988). Asthma: Definitions and pathogenesis. In E. Middleton Jr., C. E. Reed, E. F. Ellis, N. F. Adkinson Jr., & J. W. Yunginger (Eds.), *Allergy: Principles and practice* (3rd ed., pp. 969–989). St. Louis, MO: Mosby.

Bussing, R., Halfon, N., Benjamin, B., & Wells, K. B. (1995). Prevalence of behavior problems in U.S. children with asthma. *Archives of Pediatric and Adolescent Medicine, 149,* 565–572.

Butz, A. M., Malveaux, F. J., Eggleston, P., Thompson, L., Schneider, S., Weeks, K., Huss, K., Murigande, C., & Rand, C. S. (1994). Use of community health workers with inner-city children who have asthma. *Clinical Pediatrics, 33,* 135–141.

Celano, M., Geller, R. J., Phillips, K. M., & Ziman, R. (1998). Treatment adherence among low-income children with asthma. *Journal of Pediatric Psychology, 6,* 345–349.

Centers for Disease Control and Prevention. (1997). *Principles of community engagement.* Atlanta, GA: Author.

Centers for Disease Control and Prevention. (1998). Forecasted state-specific estimates of self-reported asthma prevalence: United States, 1998. *Morbidity and Mortality Weekly Report, 47,* 1022–1025.

Clark, N., Jones, P., Keller, S., & Vermeire, P. (1999). Patient factors and compliance with asthma therapy. *Respiratory Medicine, 93,* 856–862.

Creer, T. L. (1979). *Asthma therapy: A behavioral health-care system for respiratory disorders.* New York: Springer.

Creer, T. L., & Bender, B. G. (1995). Pediatric asthma. In M. C. Roberts (Ed.), *Handbook of pediatric psychology* (2nd ed., pp. 219–240). New York: Guilford Press.

Creer, T. L., Bender, B. G., & Lucas, D. (in press). Respiratory diseases. In *Health / behavioral handbook: Vol. 2.* Washington, DC: American Psychological Association.

Creer, T. L., & Christian, W. P. (1976). *Chronically-ill and handicapped children: Their management and rehabilitation.* Champaign, IL: Research Press.

Creer, T. L., & Holroyd, K. A. (1997). Self-management. In A. Baum, C. McManus, S. Newman, J. Weinman, & R. West (Eds.), *Cambridge handbook of psychology, health, and medicine* (pp. 255–257). New York: Cambridge University Press.

Creer, T. L., & Yoches, C. (1971). The modification of an inappropriate behavioral pattern in asthmatic children. *Journal of Chronic Diseases, 24,* 507–513.

Evans, R., III. (1992). Asthma among minority children: A growing problem. *Chest, 101,* [supplement], 368S–371S.

Fisher, E. B., Strunk, R. C., Sussman, L. K., Arfken, C., Sykes, R. K., Munro, J. M., Haywood, S., Harrison, D., & Bascom, S. (1996). Acceptability and feasibility of a community approach to asthma management: The Neighborhood Asthma Coalition (NAC). *Journal of Asthma, 33,* 367–383.

Fowler, M. G., Johnson, M. P., & Atkinson, S. S. (1985, April). School achievement and absence in children with chronic health problems. *Journal of Pediatrics, 106*(4), 683–687.

Freudenburg, N., Feldman, C. H., Clark, N. M., Millman, E. J., Valle, I., Wasilewski, Y. (1980). The impact of bronchial asthma on school attendance and performance. *Journal of School Health, 50,* 522-526.

Geschwind, N., & Galaburda, A. (1987). Cerebral lateralization: Biological mechanisms, associations and pathology: II. A hypothesis and program for research. *Archives of Neurology, 42,* 521–552.

Gutstadt, L. B., Gillette, J. W., Mrazek, D. A., Fukuhara, J. T., LaBrecque, J. F., Strunk, R. C. (1989). Determinants of school performance in children with chronic asthma. *American Journal of Diseases of Children, 143,* 471–475.

Hayman, L., Mahon, M., & Turner, R. (Eds.). (In press). *Health and behavior in childhood and adolescence: Cross disciplinary perspectives.* Mahwah, NJ: Erlbaum.

Kattan, M., Mitchell, H., Eggleston, P., Gergen, P., Crain, E., Redline, S., Weiss, K., Evans, R., III., Kaslow, R., Kercsmar, C., Leickly, F., Malveaux, F., & Wedner, H. J. (1997). Characteristics of inner-city children with asthma: The National Cooperative Inner-City Asthma Study. *Pediatric Pulmonology, 24,* 253–262.

Keeney, E. L. (1964). The history of asthma from Hippocrates to Meltzer. *Journal of Allergy, 35,* 215–226.

Klinnert, M. D. (1997). Guest editorial: Psychosocial influences on asthma among inner-city children. *Pediatric Pulmonology, 24,* 234–236.

Lara, M. (1999, January). *Barriers to effective management of pediatric asthma.* Paper presented at the Robert Wood Johnson Foundation conference *Future Directions in the Management of Pediatric Asthma,* Princeton, NJ.

Leviton, L., Snell, E., & McGinnis, M. (2000). Urban issues in health promotion strategies. *American Journal of Public Health, 90*(6), 863–866.

Lozano, P., Sullivan, S. D., Smith, D. H., & Weiss, K. B. (1999). The economic burden of asthma in U.S. children: Estimates from the National Medical Expenditure Survey. *Journal of Allergy and Clinical Immunology, 104,* 957–963.

MacLean, W. E., Perrin, J. M., Gortmaker, S., Pierre, C. B. (1992). Psychological adjustment of children with asthma: Effects of illness severity and recent stressful life events. *Journal of Pediatric Psychology, 17,* 159–171.

Mannino, D., Homa, D., Pertowski, C., Ashizawa, A., Nixon, L., Johnson, C., Ball, L., Jack, E., & Kang, D. S. (1998). Surveillance for asthma: United States, 1960–1995. *Morbidity and Monthly Weekly Report, 47*(SS-1), 1–27.

McFadden, E. R., Jr., & Stevens, J. B. (1983). A history of asthma. In E. Middleton Jr., C. E. Reed, & E. F. Ellis (Eds.), *Allergy: Principles and Practice* (2nd ed., pp. 805–809). St. Louis, MO: Mosby.

National Institutes of Health. (1991). *Executive summary: Guidelines for the diagnosis and management of asthma* (NIH Publication No. 91-3042A). Washington, DC: U.S. Department of Health and Human Services.

National Institutes of Health. (1997). *Expert panel report 2: Guidelines for the diagnosis and management of asthma* (NIH Publication No. 97-4051A). Washington, DC: U.S. Department of Health and Human Services.

National Institutes of Health. (1999). *Expert panel report 2: Guidelines for the diagnosis and management of asthma* (NIH Publication No. 98-4051). Washington, DC: U.S. Department of Health and Human Services.

Newacheck, P. W., & Halfon, N. (2000). Prevalence, impact, and trends in childhood disability due to asthma. *Archives of Pediatric and Adolescent Medicine, 154,* 287–293.

Newacheck, P. W., & Stoddard, J. J. (1994). Prevalence and impact of multiple childhood chronic illnesses. *Journal of Pediatrics, 124,* 40–48.

ORC Macro. (2000, May). *Evaluation of the Zap Asthma Project* (Contract No. 200-96-0598, Task 14). Atlanta, GA: Centers for Disease Control and Prevention, National Center for Environmental Health.

Parcel, G. S., Gilman, S. C., Nader, P. R., & Bunce, H. (1979). A comparison of absentee rates of elementary schoolchildren with asthma and nonasthmatic schoolmates. *Pediatrics, 64,* 878–881.

Pearce, N., Beasley, R., Burgess, C., & Crane, J. (1998). *Asthma epidemiology: Principles and methods.* New York: Oxford University Press.

Renne, C. M., & Creer, T. L. (1985). Asthmatic children and their families. In M. L. Walraich & D. K. Routh (Eds.), *Advances in developmental and behavioral pediatrics* (Vol. 6, pp. 41–81). Greenwich, CT: JAI Press.

Rust, G. S., Murray, V., Octaviani, H., Schmidt, E. D., Howard, J. P., Grant-Anderson, V., & Willard-Jelks, K. (1996). Asthma care in community health centers: A study by the Southeast Regional Clinicians' Network (Abstract). *Journal of the National Medical Association, 91,* 398–403.

Sly, R. M., & O'Donnell, R. (1997). Stabilization of asthma mortality. *Annals of Allergy, Asthma, and Immunology, 78,* 347–354.

Smith, D. H., Malone, D. C., Lawson, K. A., Okamoto, L. J., Battista, C., & Saunders, W. B. (1997). A national estimate of the economic costs of asthma. *American Journal of Respiratory and Critical Care Medicine, 156,* 787–893.

Steinhausen, H., Schindler, H., Stephan, H. (1983). Correlates of psychopathology in sick children: An empirical model. *Journal of the American Academy of Child Psychiatry, 22,* 559–564.

Stempel, D. A., Sturm, L. L., Hedblom, E. C., & Durcanin-Robbins, J. F. (1995). Total costs of asthma care. *Journal of Allergy and Clinical Immunology, 95,* 217.

U.S. Department of Health and Human Services. (2000). *Healthy people 2010: Understanding and improving health* (DHHS Publication No. 017–001–00543–6). Hyattsville, MD: Author.

von Mutius, E. (1997). Toward prevention. *Lancet, 350*(Suppl. 2), 14–17.

von Mutius, E. (2000). The burden of childhood asthma. *Archives of Disease in Childhood, 82,* [supplement 2], 2–5.

Vuurman, E. F., Veggel, F. L., Uiterwijk, M. M., Leutner, D., & O'Hanlon, J. F. (1993). Seasonal allergic rhinitis and antihistamine effects on children's learning. *Annals of Allergy, 71,* 121–126.

Warner, J. O., Naspitz, C. K., & Cropp, G.J.A. (1998). The Third Annual Pediatric Consensus Statement on the Management of Childhood Asthma. *Pediatric Immunology, 25,* 1–17.

Weiss, K. B., Gergen, P. J., & Hodgson, T. A. (1992). An economic evaluation of asthma in the United States. *New England Journal of Medicine, 326,* 862–866.

Weitzman, M., Gortmaker, S. L., & Sobol, A. M. (1990). Racial, social and environmental risks for childhood asthma. *American Journal of Diseases of Children, 144,* 1189–1194.

Williams, S., Sehgal, M., Falter, K., Dennis, R., Jones, D., Boudreaux, J., Homa, D., Raskin-Hood, C., Brown, C., Griffith, M., Redd, S. (2000). Effect of asthma on the quality of life among children and their caregivers in the Atlanta Empowerment Zone. *Journal of Urban Health. 77* (2), 268–279.

PART FOUR

LIFESTYLE BEHAVIORS

CHAPTER SIXTEEN

HIV/AIDS

Loretta Sweet Jemmott, John B. Jemmott III,
M. Katherine Hutchinson

The HIV/AIDS epidemic has seriously challenged our nation, calling into question many of our approaches to understanding disease—its prevention, treatment, and management (Kaiser Family Foundation, 1998). Despite tremendous advances in public health, biomedical science, and social science, human immunodeficiency virus/acquired immune deficiency syndrome continues to spread in the African American community, eluding both a cure and a preventive vaccine. Surveillance reports indicate that HIV and AIDS disproportionately affect African Americans. Because infection with HIV is associated with behaviors that facilitate the exchange of blood, semen, and vaginal secretions, behavioral interventions to teach ways of avoiding HIV infection are our most promising methods to prevent the spread of AIDS among African Americans. Unfortunately, research on HIV risk-reduction interventions in the African American community has been extremely limited (Jemmott & Jemmott, 1992a). The purpose of this chapter is to explore the impact of HIV/AIDS on African American communities and to describe innovative research-based approaches for reducing HIV risk-related behaviors.

Background and Significance of the Problem

In the earliest years of the U.S. epidemic, HIV/AIDS was thought to be a disease of white, gay men. However, since the early 1980s, African Americans have been disproportionately affected by HIV/AIDS. Although African Americans comprised only 12 percent of the population in 1982, they accounted for 23 percent of the AIDS cases at that time (Centers for Disease Control and Prevention [CDC], 1982). Since then, African Americans have been almost two times more likely than whites to be diagnosed with AIDS, and this disparity appears to be increasing (CDC, 1998).

Overall, 37 percent of the more than 733,000 AIDS cases reported through 1999 occurred among African Americans (CDC, 1999a). African American men accounted for 33 percent of all AIDS cases among adolescent and adult males, and African American women represented 57 percent of the cumulative AIDS cases reported among females. Rates among children mirrored those for women—African American children made up 58.5 percent of all pediatric AIDS cases reported through December 1999 (CDC, 1999a). As disturbing as these numbers are, they may be only the tip of the iceberg. Cumulative numbers of AIDS cases may actually underrepresent the extent of the current HIV/AIDS threat in the African American community. Cumulative or total numbers of AIDS cases include all individuals diagnosed with AIDS from the earliest years of the epidemic through December 1999. Newer trends in infection patterns may be difficult to discern when viewed in combination with the large number of cases reported over two decades.

Numbers of newly reported HIV and AIDS cases may more accurately reflect recent patterns in the transmission and epidemiology of HIV/AIDS among African Americans. Because many years may elapse between the time of infection with HIV and the development of an AIDS-defining condition, new HIV case numbers may be the most sensitive to recent trends in infection, although these data are limited to thirty-four areas with confidential HIV reporting (CDC, 1999a). For example, although African American males account for 33 percent of the cumulative AIDS cases among men, they account for 42.3 percent of the new AIDS cases and 47 percent of the new HIV cases reported among men in the past year (CDC, 1999a).

Data for HIV/AIDS among African American women paint an even more dramatic picture of escalating risk. Cumulative incidence rates for AIDS are more than fifteen times higher among African American women than among white women (CDC, 1995; Smith & Moore, 1996), and as already noted, more than half (57 percent) of all AIDS cases in women have occurred in African American women. Newer statistics are even more frightening, as more than two-thirds (69 percent) of new HIV cases among adolescent and adult females occurred among African Americans (CDC, 1999a). African American women represent one of the fastest growing subgroups of new HIV/AIDS cases. Women made up approximately 26 percent of new AIDS cases among adolescent and adult African Americans in 1994 (CDC, 1994). This proportion increased to 29.4 percent by 1997 and 31 percent by 1999 (CDC, 1997, 1999a).

Although there are nonsexual means of contracting HIV, including injection drug use (IDU) and blood transfusions, the worldwide AIDS pandemic has been largely fueled by sexual transmission. Among African Americans in the United States, sexual transmission is one of the most common routes of HIV transmission, particularly among women and adolescents. According to the most recent CDC data (1999a), 11 to 14 percent of new HIV cases among African American men and 9 percent of cases among African American women were associated with IDU. Sexual behaviors accounted for a much larger proportion of cases in both men and women. The risk category men who have sex with men (MSM) was associated with 26 percent of HIV cases among African American men. An additional 3 percent of cases occurred in men with both IDU and MSM risk (CDC, 1999a). Further, African American men represent an increasing proportion of AIDS cases among gay and bisexual men, rising from 31 percent in 1989 to 52 percent in 1998 (CDC, 2000).

Among women, the significance of heterosexual transmission of HIV may be underestimated by reporting practices (Smith & Moore, 1996). Nonetheless, heterosexual contact has surpassed IDU as the most common transmission route for new HIV infections among African American women. Thirty-five percent of new HIV cases among African American women were attributed to heterosexual transmission, with an additional 55 percent attributed to "no identifiable risk (NIR)" (CDC, 1999a). After further investigation, the CDC reclassified many of these NIR cases from 1998 and issued a revised report (1999b). Following these revisions, 63.5 percent of new AIDS cases among twenty-five- to thirty-nine-year-old African American women were attributed to heterosexual transmission, as were 54.7 percent of cases among forty- to sixty-four-year-old women.

African American adolescents and youths are also at high risk for HIV/AIDS, particularly from sexual transmission. Because of the long latency period between infection with HIV and the development of AIDS-defining conditions, it is likely that many of the young adults who are diagnosed with AIDS were infected during adolescence (Smith & Moore, 1996). HIV seroprevalence data validate that adolescents and young adults, particularly women, continue to be at great risk for HIV/AIDS. Fifteen percent of all HIV infections among African American males and 24 percent of cases among African American females occurred in thirteen- to twenty-four-year-olds (CDC, 1999a). Further, adolescent women appear to be at even greater risk than adolescent males. The number of HIV infections among adolescent African American females (aged thirteen to nineteen), exceeds that for adolescent African American males (1,965 versus 1,242) (CDC, 1999a).

Heterosexual transmission appears to be the primary route of infection among these young women. Of the thirteen- to nineteen-year-old females who were diagnosed with HIV during 1999, only 4 percent reported any history of injection drug use. Among twenty- to twenty-four-year-old women, this IDU proportion was slightly higher although still quite small (7 percent) (CDC, 1999a). Following risk reclassification of 1998 data, the CDC reported that 78.5 percent of new AIDS cases among African American women aged thirteen to twenty-four were due to heterosexual contact (CDC, 1999b).

Although it seems well documented that African Americans are at high risk of HIV/AIDS, several questions remain unanswered. How do we assist African Americans to reduce their risk? What are the most effective risk-reduction messages? How do we design effective culturally sensitive interventions to meet the needs of African American communities? Who are the most effective interveners? What are the long-term effects of such interventions? What are the effects of the interventions on the incidence of sexually transmitted diseases other than HIV? The next major section of this chapter will focus on prevention research. It considers results of studies testing the effectiveness of behavioral interventions for African Americans that have been implemented in community and clinical settings by the first two authors of this chapter, John B. Jemmott and Loretta Sweet Jemmott.

Effective Strategies for Reducing HIV Risk-Related Sexual Behavior

At present there is no cure for AIDS nor is there a vaccine against HIV. Because the risk of HIV infection is strongly tied to personal behavior, changing behavior is necessary to reduce risk. Hence culturally appropriate and creative HIV education and prevention programs are needed to assist African Americans to postpone the initiation of sexual intercourse, reduce numbers of sexual partners, reduce the frequency of unprotected intercourse, and change drug use behaviors that facilitate the spread of HIV/AIDS.

Several well-controlled studies have documented that HIV prevention interventions are most likely to be effective when they are (1) based on formative research with members of the study population, (2) tailored to the specific needs of the target population, and (3) grounded on a solid theoretical framework. By developing theoretically based prevention interventions and measuring the theoretical mediators of behavioral change, a better conceptual understanding of risk behavior has emerged. Interventionists and researchers are better able to understand not just whether behavioral change occurred but why and how it occurred. The theory of planned behavior, the theory of reasoned action, social cognitive theory, and the health belief model are the most commonly used theoretical frameworks employed in studies of HIV-related risk behavior and HIV prevention programs. These theories share a number of similarities. Several highlight the importance among individuals of beliefs, outcome expectancies, perceived norms, skills, self-efficacy, and intentions as determinants of HIV risk-associated behavior. We have based most of our own research and HIV risk-reduction intervention programs with African Americans on the theory of planned behavior. In this section we describe the theory of planned behavior and how it applies to a specific HIV risk-associated sexual behavior, condom use.

The theory of planned behavior (Ajzen, 1991; Ajzen & Fishbein, 1980) provides a particularly useful way of organizing much of the literature on determinants of HIV risk-associated behavior. According to the theory of planned behavior, specific behavioral intentions are the determinants of behaviors (see Figure 16.1). Several studies provide evidence that intentions are strong predictors of behavior, including condom use (Ajzen, 1991; Jemmott, Jemmott, &

FIGURE 16.1. THE THEORY OF PLANNED BEHAVIOR.

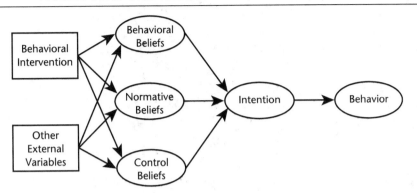

Hacker, 1992). Thus, for instance, people's use of a condom whenever they have sexual intercourse is a function of their intention to use a condom on all occasions of sexual intercourse.

The theory further holds that a behavioral intention is determined by attitudinal or behavioral beliefs about the consequences of the behavior, normative beliefs about whether important people approve of the behavior, and control beliefs about the ease or difficulty of performing the behavior. Thus people intend to perform a behavior when they evaluate that behavior positively, when they believe significant others think they should perform it, and when they feel confident of their ability to do the behavior.

Three types of behavioral beliefs have received considerable attention (Jemmott & Jemmott, 1994): (1) prevention belief—in the case of condom use, the belief that the use of condoms can prevent pregnancy, sexually transmitted disease (STD), and HIV infection (Jemmott & Jemmott, 1991, 1992a; Jemmott, Jemmott, Spears, Hewitt, & Cruz-Collins, 1992); (2) hedonistic belief—the belief about the consequences of condom use for sexual enjoyment (Jemmott & Jemmott, 1992a; Jemmott, Jemmott, Spears et al., 1992; NIMH Multisite HIV Prevention Trial Group, 1998); and (3) partner reaction belief—the belief that partners would react favorably to efforts to use condoms (Jemmott & Jemmott, 1992a).

Subjective norms are determined by normative beliefs (whether specific significant referents approve or disapprove of the behavior). In the case of condom use, the key referents would certainly include sexual partners (Jemmott & Jemmott, 1991; 1992a). Other referents that are sources of normative influence for adolescents' sexual behavior include peers, parents, and other family members (DiClemente, 1991; Fisher, Misovich, & Fisher, 1992; Fox & Inazu, 1980; Jemmott, Jemmott & Hacker, 1992; Hofferth & Hayes, 1987; Milan & Kilmann, 1987).

Finally, control beliefs, the beliefs about the ease or difficulty of performing the behavior, reflect past experience as well as anticipated impediments, resources, and opportunities. Thus, to the extent that people believe that they have the requisite skills and resources to use condoms, they should be more likely to plan to use condoms. Control beliefs have affinity with the social cognitive theory construct of perceived self-efficacy, that is, individuals' conviction that they can perform a specific behavior. Jemmott, Jemmott, and Fong (1992), Jemmott, Jemmott, & Hacker, 1992; Jemmott, Jemmott, Spears et al., 1992; Jemmott, Jemmott, and Fong (1998), and Jemmott and Fry (in press) have distinguished four types of control beliefs: (1) availability beliefs, which concern individuals' confidence that they can have condoms available when needed; (2) impulse control beliefs, which concern individuals' confidence that they can control themselves enough to use condoms when sexually excited; (3) negotiation beliefs, which concern individuals' confidence that they can persuade sexual partners to use condoms; and (4) technical skill beliefs, which concern individuals' abilities to use condoms with facility and without ruining the mood.

According to the theory of planned behavior, HIV prevention interventions that seek to reduce HIV risk-associated behavior should affect such behavior by affecting the variables that determine such behavior. Application of the theory of planned behavior has been successful in our HIV prevention research. We have used this theory in randomized, controlled HIV prevention trials with African American males attending a weekend community program (Jemmott, Jemmott, & Fong, 1992), middle school–aged African American youths (Jemmott, Jemmott, Fong, & McCaffree, 1999), and very young African American adolescents attending a special community weekend program (Jemmott, Jemmott, & Fong, 1998). These interventions were found to be effective in reducing sexual risk behaviors, including the frequency of unprotected sex, multiple sexual partners, frequency of sexual intercourse, and early age of sexual initiation.

Critical Questions

During the past ten years, our intervention research studies have addressed several critical questions about HIV behavioral interventions with African Americans, particularly adolescents: Can the behavior of high-risk populations be changed? Can culture-sensitive interventions be effective when implemented by facilitators who do not share the ethnic group membership or gender of participants? Can abstinence-based interventions be effective? How effective are peer educators? Can behavioral interventions influence health outcomes? Can research findings be translated into community-based programs? This section describes five studies that address these questions.

Can the Behavior of High-Risk Populations Be Changed?

To answer the first question, we focused on African American male adolescents. We conducted a randomized controlled trial to test the efficacy of an HIV risk-reduction intervention designed to reduce HIV risk-associated sexual behavior among inner-city African American male adolescents—a population at high risk for STDs (Jemmott, Jemmott, & Fong, 1992). For the most part, research on adolescents' sexual behavior has focused on female adolescents. Typically left out of the picture have been male adolescents, especially African American male adolescents. What makes the absence of intervention data on African American male adolescents especially troublesome is that (1) males are the ones who use condoms and (2) African American males are thought to be especially resistant to using them.

We randomly assigned 157 African American male adolescents to an HIV risk-reduction condition or a control condition. Each condition was delivered to small groups of about six boys each, led by a male or female African American facilitator. Those in the HIV risk-reduction condition received an intensive five-hour intervention. To develop the intervention, we conducted elicitation surveys and focus groups with members of the study population to identify potential mediators of behavioral change and drew on social cognitive theory, the theory of reasoned action, and its extension the theory of planned behavior. This culturally sensitive intervention involved small-group discussions, videos, games and interactive exercises, skill-building activities, and role-playing designed to influence (1) HIV risk-reduction knowledge; (2) behavioral beliefs about the consequences of condom use for sexual enjoyment; and (3) behavioral skills and self-efficacy regarding refusal, negotiation, and condom use. In addition, this intervention encouraged the adolescents to make proud and responsible decisions to protect themselves and their community from health risks.

To diminish the plausibility of alternative explanations involving Hawthorne effects or nonspecific features, including group interaction and special attention, we also implemented a five-hour intervention with the adolescents in the control condition. Structurally similar to the HIV intervention, it involved culturally and developmentally appropriate videotapes, exercises, and games, but the topic was career opportunities.

Although the mean age of the study participants was only 14.6 years, 83 percent reported engaging in coitus at least once. Of the 58 percent who reported coitus in the previous three months, 21 percent reported never using condoms during those experiences, and only 30 percent reported always using condoms. Analyses of covariance (ANCOVAs), controlling for preintervention measures, revealed that immediately after the intervention the adolescents who received the HIV risk-reduction intervention scored higher in AIDS knowledge, lower in attitudes toward HIV risk-associated sexual behaviors, lower in intentions to engage in such behaviors, and higher in hedonistic beliefs and self-efficacy than did the adolescents in the control condition. Three-month follow-up data collected on 96 percent of the 157 original participants indicated that those who had received the HIV risk-reduction intervention scored lower on an HIV risk-associated behavior index than did those in the control condition. Analyses on specific self-reported behaviors revealed that the HIV intervention participants had coitus less often, had fewer partners, used condoms more consistently, had unprotected sex on fewer occasions, and had a lower incidence of anal intercourse than did the control group.

Surprisingly, there was no evidence that male facilitators were more effective at changing the male adolescent participants' sexual risk behavior. In addition, social desirability bias, as indexed by the Marlowe-Crowne Social Desirability Scale, was unrelated to self-reported HIV risk-associated sexual behavior at preintervention and the three-month follow-up or to change in such behavior. There was no evidence of *contamination* effects due to cross-talk between conditions. About 18 percent of participants said they discussed the group activities with someone from another group in the study. ANCOVAs on AIDS knowledge, attitudes, intentions, and risky sexual behavior at the three-month follow-up revealed no significant interaction between the intervention and whether participants reported discussing group activities with someone from another group.

This study demonstrated that HIV risk-associated sexual behavior can be reduced in a key population—inner-city African American male adolescents—and that the intervention did not encourage sexual intercourse but decreased it. Those adolescents who did have sex were more likely to protect themselves by using condoms.

Can Culture-Sensitive Interventions Be Effective When Implemented by Facilitators Who Do Not Share the Ethnic Group Membership or Gender of Participants?

The second critical question addresses whether it is possible for a theory-based, culture-sensitive HIV intervention to be effective when the race and gender of participants and facilitators are not matched or when group members are of mixed gender.

To answer this question, Jemmott, Jemmott, Fong, and McCaffree (1999) conducted a randomized controlled trial to test the effects of our intervention among younger adolescents and examine practical questions about the best way to intervene with African American adolescents. Although many writers have pointed out the value of matching the gender and race or ethnicity of participants and facilitators and of conducting groups that are homogeneous in gender, little empirical research has tested the generality of intervention effects across such parameters. Practically speaking, sometimes HIV education may be implemented in situations where it is not possible to match all involved by gender or race and ethnicity. Unfortunately, little is known about the likely outcomes under such circumstances. Is it possible for an HIV intervention to be effective when race and ethnicity and gender are not matched or when the groups are not homogeneous in gender? The Jemmott, Jemmott, and Fong (1992) study suggested that African American female facilitators can be effective with African American male adolescents.

To pursue these questions further, 496 African American adolescents (mean age 13.2 years) were recruited from public schools in Trenton, New Jersey, via announcements made by project staff during seventh and eighth grade assemblies or lunch periods. About 54 percent of the recruits were female. Preintervention self-reports indicated that 55 percent of respondents had experienced coitus at least once, and 30 percent of respondents had had coitus in the previous three months. About 18 percent reported ever having anal intercourse, and 8.3 percent reported such involvement in the previous three months. Few reported ever sharing needles (1.2 percent) or having a sexual relationship with a person of their own gender (1.4 percent).

We randomly assigned the adolescents to a five-hour HIV risk-reduction intervention or a five-hour general health promotion intervention and also to a small group that was either homogeneous or heterogeneous in gender and led by a male or female facilitator who was African American or white. A total of forty-one adults served as facilitators: twenty implemented the HIV risk-reduction intervention, and twenty-one implemented the health promotion intervention.

We found that immediately after the intervention, the adolescents who received the HIV risk-reduction intervention expressed stronger intentions to use condoms, had more favorable hedonistic beliefs, and greater self-efficacy to use condoms than did those who received the control intervention. The return rate was high at the three-month (97 percent) and six-month follow-ups (93 percent) and did not differ by intervention condition. Analyses on the three-month follow-up HIV risk-associated sexual behavior index revealed that although the means were in the right direction, the difference between adolescents in the HIV intervention and those in the health intervention was nonsignificant. At the six-month follow-up, however, the difference was significant. The HIV risk-reduction intervention participants reported less HIV risk-associated sexual behavior than did their counterparts who had received the health promotion intervention. In addition, adolescents who received the HIV intervention reported less unprotected sexual intercourse and a lower incidence of anal intercourse than did the control group.

We conducted additional analyses to empirically test the matching hypothesis: that is, whether effects of the intervention were enhanced when the characteristics of the participants and facilitators were matched. These analyses centered on the race and gender of the facilitator, the gender of the participants, and the gender composition of the intervention groups. No such effects were found. The effects of the HIV intervention did not vary depending on the race of the facilitator, the gender of the facilitator, the gender of the participants, or the gender composition of the intervention group.

This study demonstrates that risk behavior can be reduced among young adolescents and that the effects of a theory-based, culturally sensitive intervention can generalize across implementation by facilitators of diverse race and gender. It also suggests that the influence of the race and gender of facilitators may be more complex than previously assumed. At first blush the lack of empirical support for the matching hypothesis may seem puzzling. After all, both the social psychological literature on the importance of similarity in attitude change and persuasion and real-world casual observations on the nature of social interaction and trust among individuals of different as opposed to the same gender and ethnicity can be marshaled to support the matching hypothesis. So why did we find no support for such an intuitively obvious notion?

One possible explanation revolves around the nature of our intervention. First, the intervention itself was designed to be culturally sensitive. Second, the activities were highly structured, and the training of the facilitators emphasized the importance of implementing the interventions according to the protocol. This would have minimized the importance of differences between facilitators. Third, the fact that all facilitators trained together might have helped them to calibrate their facilitation styles so that they were more similar to each other than they might have been otherwise. Thus, if such training had been absent, if culturally inappropriate materials had been used, and if the intervention had been less highly structured, differences in facilitator behavior by race and gender might have emerged. Under such circumstances the results might have been different from those we observed. Whether similar results would have been obtained with participants of other ethnic groups, including Latinos, is unknown.

Can Abstinence-Based Interventions Be Effective? How Effective Are Peer Educators?

To answer questions about the effectiveness of interventions that promote abstinence and the effectiveness of peer educators, a study was designed to test the effects of two types of HIV risk-reduction messages, abstinence and safer sex, delivered by two types of interveners, adult facilitators and peer cofacilitators.

A central issue for HIV behavioral interventions is determining the risk-reduction message that is most appropriate and effective. Sexual transmission of HIV is tied to unprotected sexual intercourse—that is, sexual intercourse without the use of a latex condom. To decrease the risk of sexually transmitted HIV infection, behavioral interventions must reduce the frequency of unprotected sexual intercourse. There are two ways to achieve this objective: the abstinence strategy, which focuses on reducing the frequency of sexual intercourse, and the safer sex strategy, which focuses on increasing the frequency of condom use. Whether abstinence or safer sex should be the focus of intervention efforts for adolescents has been vigorously debated among public health experts, educators, parents, and other advocates for youth.

The abstinence approach has appeal because adolescents, particularly young adolescents, may not have the knowledge and judgment to make informed choices about methods to protect themselves from pregnancy and STDs or to grapple with the adverse consequences of unprotected sexual intercourse. Consistent with this sentiment, the U.S. Congress, as part of the welfare reform act of 1996, allocated $50 million annually from 1998 to 2002 for educational programs that teach the social, psychological, and health benefits of abstaining from sexual activity. Supporters of the safer-sex strategy assert that the abstinence message is ineffective; that it is unrealistic to believe that an intervention can prevent, eliminate, or reduce sexual intercourse among adolescents; and that prevention programs should instead focus on increasing condom use. The debate has shed more heat than light. Despite the fact that both safer sex and abstinence approaches have the potential to decrease unprotected intercourse, no randomized controlled trial has considered the efficacy of both intervention approaches. Our study was a first step in addressing this important issue.

In addition to addressing the effectiveness of abstinence and safer sex messages, we examined the relative effectiveness in delivering HIV risk-reduction messages of two types of interveners or messengers—peers and adults. On one hand, it is often asserted that interventions for adolescents may be especially efficacious if peers implement them. Peer educators are likely to share the same experiences as the adolescents and may have a good appreciation of adolescents' issues and concerns. Peer educators may be better at establishing rapport. On the other hand, adult facilitators may also be efficacious. Adults have more life experience and a broader perspective that they can bring to bear during interventions. Adults may generate more respect and may be perceived as more credible sources of information because of their experience and maturity. In previous HIV prevention intervention studies, we have successfully employed adult facilitators.

In our randomized controlled trial (Jemmott, Jemmott, & Fong, 1998), the participants were 659 inner-city sixth and seventh grade African American adolescents (with a mean age of 11.8 years), recruited from three middle schools serving low-income African American communities in Philadelphia, Pennsylvania, via announcements by project staff in assemblies, classrooms, and lunchrooms, and letters to parents or guardians. About 53 percent were female. Preintervention self-reports indicated that 25 percent of the respondents had had coitus at least once, and 15 percent of respondents had had coitus in the previous three months. Few (1.6 percent) reported having sexual relationships with a person of their own gender.

Intervention Conditions. Participants were stratified by gender and age and, on the basis of computer-generated random number sequences, were randomly assigned to one of three interventions: an abstinence HIV intervention, a safer-sex HIV intervention, or a health promotion intervention that served as the control condition. They were also randomized to a group of six to eight adolescents led by one male or one female adult facilitator or by two male, two female, or one male and one female peer cofacilitators. The study was conducted in three cycles or replications, one at each of the three schools. The abstinence intervention acknowledged that condoms can reduce risks but emphasized abstinence to eliminate the risk of pregnancy and STDs, including HIV. The safer-sex intervention indicated that abstinence is the best choice but emphasized the importance of using condoms to reduce the risk of pregnancy and STDs, including HIV, if participants were to have sex. The control condition received a health promotion intervention designed to be as valuable and enjoyable as the HIV interventions.

It focused not on AIDS or sexual behavior but on behaviors associated with risk of cardiovascular disease, stroke, and certain cancers—health problems that are among the seven leading causes of premature death among African Americans.

Each intervention was highly structured and was implemented by facilitators who used intervention manuals. Designed to be educational but also entertaining and culturally sensitive, each intervention involved group discussions, videos, games, brainstorming, experiential exercises, and skill-building activities. Each intervention incorporated the "Be Proud! Be Responsible!" theme (Jemmott, Jemmott, & McCaffree, 1995) that encouraged the participants to be proud of themselves and their community, to behave responsibly for the sake of themselves and their community, and to consider their goals for the future and how unhealthful behavior might thwart attainment of those goals.

Facilitators and Facilitator Training. The adult facilitators were twenty-five African American men and women. We began with a pool of people who had the skills to implement any of the interventions. After stratifying them by age and gender, we randomly assigned them to be trained to implement one of the three interventions. In this way we randomized facilitator characteristics across interventions; hence the effects of the interventions cannot be attributed to the facilitators' preexisting characteristics. The peer facilitators were 45 African American adolescents (with a mean age of 15.6). About 56 percent were female. We also stratified them by age and gender and assigned them randomly to be trained in one of the three interventions.

Effects on Conceptual Variables Related to Abstinence. Immediately after the intervention the adolescents in the abstinence condition believed more strongly that practicing abstinence would prevent pregnancy and AIDS, expressed less favorable attitudes toward sexual intercourse, and reported weaker intentions to have sexual intercourse in the next three months than did those in the control condition or the safer sex condition. Adolescents in the abstinence condition also believed more strongly than did the control group that practicing abstinence would help them achieve their career goals, but did not differ in this belief from those in the safer sex condition.

Effects on Conceptual Variables Related to Condom Use. Immediately after the intervention the adolescents in the safer sex condition scored significantly higher in condom-use knowledge, believed more strongly that condoms can prevent pregnancy, STDs, and HIV, believed more strongly that using condoms would not interfere with sexual enjoyment, and expressed greater confidence that they could have condoms available when they needed them than did those in the control condition or the abstinence condition. Adolescents in the safer sex condition reported greater confidence that they could exercise sufficient impulse control to use condoms and greater self-efficacy for using condoms than did those in the control condition, but not more than those in the abstinence condition. Adolescents in the safer sex condition did not differ from those in the other two conditions in technical skills belief, negotiation skills belief, or condom use intentions.

Effects of Behavioral Interventions on Sexual Behavior. About 97 percent of the participants attended the three-month follow-up, 94 percent attended the six-month follow-up, and 93 percent attended the twelve-month follow-up. Adolescents in the abstinence group were significantly less likely to report having sexual intercourse in the three months after the intervention than were those in the control group and marginally less likely to report such behavior than were those in the safer sex group. Safer sex intervention participants were more likely to report consistent condom use at the three-month follow-up than were those in the control group or the abstinence group. Self-reported frequency of condom use was also significantly higher in the safer sex condition than in the control condition. Adolescents in the safer sex condition were less likely to report having unprotected sexual intercourse in the previous three months than were those in the control condition. Adolescents in the safer sex condition also reported less unprotected sexual intercourse than did those in the control condition. The interaction between intervention condition and preintervention sexual experience on self-reported unprotected sexual intercourse at three-month follow-up was significant. Among sexually inexperienced adolescents, there were no significant effects of the interventions on unprotected sexual intercourse. In contrast, among sexually experienced adolescents, those who received the safer-sex intervention reported less unprotected sexual intercourse than did those in the control condition or the abstinence condition.

At the six-month follow-up, the abstinence intervention did not reduce self-reported sexual behavior compared with the other interventions. However, safer sex intervention participants reported less frequent sexual intercourse and more frequent condom use than did the control group. At the twelve-month follow-up, those in the abstinence intervention did not reduce self-reported sexual behavior compared with those in the other interventions. However, adolescents in the safer sex and abstinence interventions reported more frequent condom use than did those in the control condition.

The intervention effects did not differ depending on whether the groups were implemented by an adult or by peer cofacilitators. Consistent with Jemmott, Jemmott, Fong, & McCaffree (1999), we found that the results also did not differ as a function of facilitator gender or of matching facilitator gender with participant gender.

Importance of Findings. The results demonstrate that culturally sensitive cognitive-behavioral interventions stressing abstinence or condom use can reduce HIV risk-associated sexual behavior among young African American adolescents. The abstinence intervention caused positive changes in theory-based mediators of abstinence at the immediate postintervention assessment and increased self-reported abstinence at the three-month follow-up. The safer sex intervention increased mediators of condom use postintervention and self-reported condom use at the three-month follow-up. Each intervention had the predicted positive impact on its targeted outcome, but only the safer sex intervention significantly reduced unprotected sexual intercourse—the outcome most closely linked to the risk of exposure to HIV and other STDs. The safer sex intervention's effects on condom use were sustained six and twelve months postintervention. Although the abstinence intervention was effective in the short term, its effects diminished with longer-term follow-up. Future research must seek to increase the longevity of these promising effects.

Can Behavioral Interventions Influence Health Outcomes?

To answer the question of whether behavioral interventions affected health outcomes we tested the effectiveness of four theory-based interventions on African American women's self-reports of sexual risk behaviors and incidence of clinically documented STDs. Although considerable evidence exists to indicate that behavioral interventions are effective in reducing self-reported HIV sexual risk behavior, relatively few randomized controlled trials have tested the long-term effects of such interventions on inner-city African American women. Even fewer have incorporated objective measures of sexual risk behaviors, such as STD incidence.

Moreover, there is a need to develop behavioral interventions that are appropriate and can be implemented in primary health care settings, where it is possible to reach a wide range of women, including those who may or may not proactively seek HIV prevention services. In this study, we tested the effectiveness of four theory-based interventions that contrasted two methods of intervention delivery—group and individual—and two types of intervention content—information and skill building. The objective was to identify effective interventions that are appropriate for clinics and other primary health care facilities.

The participants were 564 black women (mean age 27.2 years) seeking care at the outpatient Women's Health Clinic of a large hospital in Newark, New Jersey. About 70 percent were unemployed, and 20 percent tested positive for STDs at baseline. All participants reported having had sexual intercourse, and 90 percent reported sexual intercourse in the three months prior to study enrollment. Only 24 percent of those who had had sexual intercourse in the previous three months reported always using condoms.

Interventions. Participants were randomly assigned to one of five single-session interventions: a 20-minute one-on-one HIV information intervention, a 20-minute one-on-one HIV behavioral skill training intervention, a 3.33 hour group HIV information intervention, a 3.33 hour group behavioral skill training HIV intervention, or a 3.33 hour group control intervention on health issues unrelated to sexual behavior. In designing the interventions, we gathered information by conducting elicitation research and focus groups with women from the study population, and we drew on social cognitive theory and the theory of planned behavior. Although the interventions focused on sexual risk reduction, they also provided information about reducing the risk associated with injection drug use.

In both one-on-one interventions, the facilitator tailored the twenty-minute module to the specific needs of each participant. The one-on-one HIV information intervention included a sexual risk assessment interview, a review of a specially designed "Sister to Sister" HIV prevention information brochure, and a discussion of basic HIV information. In contrast, the one-on-one HIV skill training intervention included the assessment interview, a review of a specially designed "Sister to Sister" HIV prevention behavioral skill brochure, video clips, a condom demonstration, and role-playing.

The three group interventions were highly structured. Each one consisted of four fifty-minute modules involving group discussions, videos, games, and brainstorming. The group HIV information intervention was designed to increase participants' knowledge about HIV sexual risk and risk-reducing behaviors. The group HIV behavioral skill training intervention was designed to increase participants' knowledge about correct condom use, enhance their hedonistic beliefs regarding effects of condom use on sexual enjoyment, and increase their skills and self-efficacy beliefs regarding their ability to use condoms. Unlike the information intervention, it included skill-building activities such as condom demonstrations and role-playing.

Participants in the control group received a group health promotion intervention designed to be as valuable and enjoyable as the HIV interventions. It focused not on HIV but on behaviors associated with the risk of heart disease, stroke, and certain cancers.

The facilitators were twenty-eight African American female nurses. We began with a pool of nurses who had the skills to implement any of the five interventions. After stratifying them by age, we randomly assigned them to receive eight hours of training to implement one of the five interventions. The facilitator training stressed the importance of implementation fidelity. Implementation fidelity was also emphasized before each intervention session when the facilitators met with their trainers for one hour to review intervention.

Measures. Participants completed questionnaires before and immediately after the intervention and at three-, six-, and twelve-month follow-ups. The primary outcomes measured were self-reported sexual behaviors in the previous three months, including consistent condom use, condom use at most recent sexual intercourse, frequency of unprotected sexual intercourse, and sexual intercourse associated with alcohol and drug use. Secondary outcomes measured were STDs and potential mediators of the effects of interventions on HIV risk-associated sexual behavior. We examined *Neisseria gonorrhoeae, Chlamydia trachomatis,* and *Trichomonas vaginalis,* as clinically documented by physical exams and laboratory tests, preintervention and at the six-month and twelve-month follow-ups.

Effects of Behavioral Interventions on Sexual Behaviors. The return rates were 92 percent, 90 percent, and 87 percent for the three-, six-, and twelve-month follow-ups, respectively. The return rates did not differ by intervention condition and were unrelated to preintervention measures of self-reported behavior. The effects of the interventions on sexual behavior outcomes were tested using generalized estimating equations (GEE) and controlling for baseline measures. Considering the three follow-up periods together, the women who received the skill training interventions, as compared to the control group, were more likely to report using a condom the last time they had sexual intercourse. Considering the follow-up periods individually, the proportion of women reporting condom use the last time they had sex was significantly higher among those who had the skill interventions than among those in the control group at the three-month and the twelve-month follow-up. Over the three follow-up periods, women in the skill training interventions were more likely to report consistent condom use compared to those in the control group. Similarly, over the entire follow-up period and at the three-month follow-up specifically, the skill training intervention participants reported fewer days on which they had unprotected sexual intercourse than did the members of the control group.

Although the interventions did not have significant effects on the self-reported number of sexual partners, they did cause significant reductions in the frequency of unprotected sexual intercourse and unprotected sexual intercourse in conjunction with alcohol or drug use. As compared with the frequencies self-reported by the control group, the self-reported frequency of sexual intercourse and the frequency of unprotected sexual intercourse while high on alcohol or drugs were significantly lower among women in the skill training interventions and those in the information interventions at each follow-up and considering the follow-ups together. For the most part the group skill intervention and the one-on-one skill intervention did not significantly differ in effects on self-reported behavior. The only exception was that compared to the group skill intervention, the one-on-one skill intervention was more effective in reducing the frequency of intercourse while high on alcohol or drugs reported at the twelve-month follow-up. Marlowe-Crowne Social Desirability Scale scores did not interact with intervention conditions to affect self-reported sexual behaviors at any of the follow-ups.

Effects of Behavioral Interventions on Clinical STDs. GEE analyses controlling for baseline measures revealed that, considering the two STD follow-up periods together, the interventions did not reduce STD incidence. However, there was a significant interaction between the skill training intervention and the follow-up time. Although the interventions did not reduce STD incidence at the six-month follow-up, the women in the skill training interventions were less likely to have an STD at twelve-month follow-up than were those in the control group.

Effects of Behavioral Intervention on Conceptual Variables. ANCOVAs controlling for baseline measures revealed that immediately after the interventions the women in the skill training interventions as well as those in the information interventions scored higher in condom use knowledge, intention to use condoms, and attitude toward using condoms than did those in the control condition. In addition, the group skill intervention caused significantly greater increases in condom use knowledge than did the one-on-one skill intervention. Women who received the skill training intervention believed more strongly that using condoms would not interfere with sexual enjoyment and expressed greater confidence that they could exercise sufficient impulse control to use condoms than did women in the control group. The skill training intervention participants expressed marginally greater confidence that they could have condoms available when they needed them than did those in the control group. Those in the group skill training intervention scored higher in these condom availability beliefs than did those in the one-on-one skill intervention.

Participants' evaluations of the interventions were very favorable (means > 4.4 on 5-point scales). There were no significant differences in evaluations among participants in the skill training intervention, the information intervention, and the control groups. However, women in group interventions indicated they liked the interventions more, participated more actively, and learned more than did women in the one-on-one intervention, and they also indicated they were more likely to recommend the program.

Importance of Findings. The results demonstrate that culturally sensitive, skill-based, theory-based interventions can reduce HIV risk-associated sexual behavior and STD incidence among African American women. The skill interventions caused positive changes on mediators of condom use (hedonistic beliefs, perceptions of self-efficacy, and impulse control). Further, compared with the control group, the skills intervention group increased self-reported consistent condom use and condom use at most recent sexual intercourse and reduced reported days on which women had unprotected sex over the entire follow-up period. In addition, women in the skill training interventions were less likely to have an STD at twelve-month follow-up as compared with the control group. Surprisingly, the lengthier skills interventions delivered in the skill-based groups did not produce outcomes superior to the twenty-minute individual skills sessions.

Skill building in a group context has the potential to benefit from modeling and feedback from other group members. However, it is likely that the individually delivered intervention was able to elicit more personal disclosure and skill-building practice and hence greater tailoring of the training to the individual woman's life situation. We also found that the HIV interventions were especially effective in reducing sexual behavior in conjunction with alcohol and drug use. Women in both the skill-building and the knowledge interventions reported fewer days on which they had sex while high and fewer days of unprotected sex while high compared to the control group over the entire follow-up period.

In conclusion, then, skill-building interventions reduced HIV sexual risk behaviors and STDs among African American women in an outpatient women's health setting. Clearly, many women have the potential to be helped by intensive small-group and individual interventions that provide opportunities for practicing condom use and sexual negotiation skills. This study, with a twelve-month follow-up period and excellent retention rates, also showed that nurses can be effective in changing sexual risk-associated behavior.

Can Research Findings Be Translated into Community-Based Programs?

Often the results of intervention research remain buried in the pages of scientific journals where they are unlikely to come to the attention of the community people who could make the best use of them. Unfortunately, the ideal of translating research results into practical community-based programs is seldom realized. Recently, we attempted to address this issue by adapting our HIV risk-reduction interventions for use in a program implemented by a community-based organization, the Urban League of Metropolitan Trenton (Jemmott & Jemmott, 1992a).

This HIV/AIDS prevention program drew upon our experiences with the Jemmott, Jemmott, and Fong (1992) study and the Jemmott, Jemmott, Spears, et al. (1992) study and used many of the same activities. It was designed to be meaningful and culturally appropriate for the specific population of inner-city African-American adolescent women who would receive it. Prior to program implementation, individual and focus group interviews were conducted with adolescents from Trenton. These interviews suggested that many of the adolescents had a strong sense of identification with Africa. Thus posters used to advertise the program were colored red, black, and green (the black liberation colors) and bore a map of Africa and the motto "Respect Yourself, Protect Yourself—Because You Are Worth It." When the adolescents completed the program they were given T-shirts with the phrase "Respect Yourself, Protect Yourself" and a map of Africa colored in red, black, and green on the front and the phrase "Because I am worth it" on the back.

The program was six hours long and designed to be implemented in three two-hour sessions. The first session focused on factual information about the cause, transmission, and prevention of AIDS and the risks faced by black women of childbearing age in New Jersey. The second session focused on beliefs regarding partner reactions and hedonistic beliefs. The third session focused on skill building and self-efficacy to use condoms. Videotapes, games, and exercises were used to reinforce learning and to encourage active participation. The participants received the intervention in small groups of six to ten, each group led by a specially trained African American female health educator who was a native Trenton resident.

The program participants included 109 sexually experienced African American female adolescents (with a mean age of 16.8 years). About 72 percent reported that they had had coitus in the past three months. As in previous research on inner-city African American adolescents, the chief risky sexual behavior reported by participants was the failure to use condoms. About 19 percent of those who had had coitus in the past three months reported that condoms were never used on those occasions, and only 29 percent reported that condoms were always used on those occasions. Analyses revealed that the adolescents scored higher in intentions to use condoms, AIDS knowledge, hedonistic beliefs, prevention beliefs, and self-efficacy to use condoms after the intervention than they did before it (Jemmott & Jemmott, 1992a). In addition, increased perceptions of self-efficacy and more favorable hedonistic beliefs and beliefs regarding a sexual partner's support for condom use were significantly related to increased condom use intentions, but increases in general AIDS knowledge and specific prevention-related beliefs were not.

One potential weakness of the study was that the changes in intentions might reflect history rather than true intervention effects. Jemmott and Jemmott (1992a) reasoned that history is an unlikely explanation, however, because the women participated in intervention groups that were run sequentially over a six-month period. In this view, it is unlikely that events in addition to the intervention activities could have occurred between preintervention and postintervention and increased scores for these multiple intervention groups. Although history cannot account for the differential predictive power of perceived self-efficacy and hedonistic beliefs as compared with AIDS knowledge and prevention beliefs, the fact that the study did not include a control group that did not receive HIV risk-reduction interventions limits our ability to draw causal inferences about intervention effects.

In summary, our research suggests that intensive theory-based interventions can reduce HIV sexual-risk behaviors among inner-city African American adolescents and women. This body of research supports the view that effective behavioral HIV risk-reduction interventions (1) have an explicit theoretical basis and (2) are tailored to the study population or culture on the basis of formative research with members of the study population. A strength of this research is that it considers not only the effectiveness of the interventions in changing behavior but also the functioning of the theoretical mechanisms—the variables hypothesized to mediate intervention effects.

Lessons Learned

What have we learned from our research? How does what we have learned affect the ways African American communities might design and implement HIV prevention interventions? This section describes some of the lessons we have learned about the social context of HIV/AIDS risk in the African American community and the common barriers to prevention and also lessons about substance abuse issues, women's issues, adolescents' issues, intervention design issues, and the building of bridges between communities and researchers.

Social Context of HIV/AIDS Risk in the African American Community

Among the many cultural factors that may function as obstacles to effectively addressing and reducing HIV/AIDS risk among African Americans are racism, distrust of researchers, religious beliefs, homophobia, economic variables, and diversity within the community. For example, strong negative attitudes held by many African Americans about homosexuality and perceptions of AIDS as a "gay disease" may hinder efforts to engage African Americans in AIDS prevention programs (Butts, 1988; Icard, Schilling, El-Bassel, & Young, 1992). Beliefs that illness is a form of punishment by God (Taylor, 1998) and attitudes that AIDS is a consequence of sinful behavior (Butts, 1988; Mays & Cochran, 1987) also affect ways in which African Americans respond to AIDS prevention efforts. Commonly held views that AIDS is a form of racial warfare against African American people (DeParle, 1991; Jemmott & Jones, 1993; Madhubti, 1990) also may significantly impede prevention efforts in African American communities. Given such attitudes, HIV/AIDS prevention programs must be innovative, anticipate the myriad social and historical influences that may act as barriers to effective intervention efforts, and involve African American community members and leaders in program development from the earliest planning stages.

Racism, Trust, and Suspicion. The issues of racism and of lack of trust in the programs and efforts of the white majority continue to play major roles in the HIV epidemic. Like other communities of color in the United States, the African American community deals with both the legacy and the current reality of racism. These realities find their way into health care systems at all levels. One infamous incident is the Tuskegee Syphilis Study during the early 1900s. A sample of African American men took part in an experiment, sponsored by the federal government, in which their diagnosed syphilis was observed over time without treatment being offered, although a treatment was available. With this historical fact in the African American communal memory, there is little wonder that African Americans would be wary of health education programs (Jemmott & Jones, 1993), doubt medical research, distrust researchers who seek to recruit them for studies, and disbelieve government officials and health authorities who offer recommendations to reduce the risk of AIDS. Because of this past incident, African Americans may believe that they are being used as guinea pigs in experiments to try out procedures that would not be tried on whites. Distrust and feelings of being exploited may discourage participation in AIDS-related studies and negatively affect the quality of the data that are collected (Marin & Marin, 1991).

Suspicion contributes to the various beliefs some African Americans have about HIV infection and the AIDS crisis. Many African Americans believe that the linkage of HIV to Africa and the explosive penetration of the virus in the black community are consistent with a racist, genocidal origin in white America. This belief can be understood in part as a consequence of feelings of alienation and distrust and of an escalation of racially motivated hate acts perpetrated by whites against blacks. Such distrust may also be based on a belief that researchers will draw interpretations that disparage African Americans. There has been great concern that psychological testing and research has been used inappropriately to label African Americans as pathological or intellectually inferior (Jemmott & Jones, 1993; Marin & Marin, 1992; Williams, 1980).

Ironically, rejecting messages and programs designed to modify behavior in a safer, protective direction may be one way of resisting what is perceived as manipulation by whites. The reactions to centuries of racism cannot be ignored if one is to attempt to understand cultural responses to the AIDS crisis.

Religion and the Church. Many believe that religion is the backbone of the African American community. Religion influences attitudes and behaviors concerning sex; specific sexual practices; contraceptive use; and premarital, extramarital, homosexual, and other intimate relationships. It is important to understand the nature of African American religious affiliations because they provide an insight into sources of support, social networks, and potential organizing structures for prevention activities. Religious affiliations also provide points of reference for understanding the values and norms in African American communities. Hence it is important that researchers and intervention planners understand something about the different religions most prevalent in the African American communities in which they work.

Homophobia. One of the most important barriers to HIV prevention efforts is the homophobia in the African American community. Traditional black families and black churches frequently have negative attitudes toward men who have sex with men. There may be an overwhelming lack of compassion from the African American community in which gay men live. Community institutions, including churches, may be less supportive of gay men than of other community residents. Therefore African American men who have sex with men may be more closeted about sexuality and HIV status and may be reluctant to seek out and participate in HIV risk-reduction programs.

Poverty. The disproportionate representation of African Americans among those living in poverty is equally important to consider when designing prevention programs and evaluating the abilities of program participants and residents to accept HIV/AIDS prevention messages and adhere to safer sex and other HIV risk-reduction behaviors. For lower-income African Americans, day-to-day struggles such as paying the rent, providing for children, and obtaining and maintaining employment may reduce the perceived importance of HIV/AIDS (de la Cancela, 1989). When entire communities are economically disenfranchised, they may have little or no capital to provide residents with adequate health care or HIV prevention programs. Individual and community-level poverty are realities in many African American communities that must be incorporated into the design of prevention programming. For example, are the costs associated with child care and transportation potential barriers to participation in an HIV risk-reduction program? Are program sessions scheduled during work hours, requiring participants to miss work and putting them at risk for losing their jobs?

Diversity Within the Community. The African American community is by no means monolithic. With regional as well as class variations, this community continues to struggle for citizenship. From the outside, the African American community is too often viewed as homogeneous. However, this community's social values and norms include conservative and liberal points of view and diverse religious orientations including Christian sects, Islamic communities, Catholic communities, and traditional African religious practices. By not anticipating such diversity and incorporating it into programs, researchers and interventionists court disaster.

Moreover, blacks may differ not only in their degree of identification with African Americans in general but also in their ethnicity within the black community. Thus there are Afro-Caribbean Americans as well as African Americans who trace their roots to the Southern United States. Research programs have yet to grasp fully the behavioral implications of within-ethnic-group variation, yet without this knowledge, change efforts may miss key features of a subgroup's responses to behavioral change messages (Jemmott & Jones, 1993).

Substance Abuse Issues

Substance abuse is directly and indirectly fueling the spread of HIV in the United States and in African American communities.

Injection Drug Use. The association between injection drug use and the seroprevalence of HIV is well documented (Turner, Miller, & Moses, 1990). As the relationship between injection drug use and HIV infection was elucidated by the scientific community (Jaffe, Bregman, & Selik, 1983), several institutionally supported HIV risk-reduction models began to emerge. Foremost among these was the street-oriented community outreach approach, which usually employed recovering drug users to teach risk-reduction techniques and distribute materials to active injection drug users (Des Jarlais & Friedman, 1987; Newmeyer, 1988). Effective outreach programs address a number of issues, including the recruitment of outreach workers, building lost trust, the language and demeanor of workers, and the risk of relapse among participants. Outreach workers disseminate information, distribute tangible goods and materials, and serve as role models for current injection drug users.

Dramatic increases in the adoption of safer injection practices have been reported among injection drug users as a result of outreach interventions and a variety of other approaches, including HIV antibody screening and counseling, office-based education, needle exchange programs, and drug treatment or some combination of these general strategies (Becker & Joseph, 1988; Booth & Weibel, 1992; Calsyn, Saxon, Wells, & Greenberg, 1992; Chitwood, Comerford, & Trapido, 1991; Des Jarlais, Friedman, & Casriel, 1990; Friedman et al., 1989; Guydish, Temoshok, Dilley, & Rinaldi, 1990; Stephens, Feucht, & Roman, 1991). Although strategies for decreasing IDU and promoting safer injection practices have met with moderate success, modifying high-risk sexual behaviors among drug users has received less attention. Programs that have attempted to reduce sexual risk behaviors among drug users have frequently been less than effective.

Women who inject drugs are at particularly high risk of HIV infection due to their drug-using risk behaviors and their sexual relationships with male partners who inject (Brown, 1998; Cohen, Navaline, & Metzger, 1994; Tortu, Beardsley, Deren, & Davis, 1994). Female drug users are the fastest growing segment of the HIV-infected population. Approximately 80 percent of all female injection drug users with AIDS are African American or Latina (CDC, 1991). Studies reveal that female injectors report multiple HIV risks, including male sexual partners who are injectors (Allen, Battjes, Slododa, & Grace, 1991; Brown & Primm, 1988; Leigh, 1990; Watkins, Metzger, Woody, & McLellan, 1992, 1993), infrequent condom use, multiple sexual partners, and the exchange of sex for money or drugs. Despite evidence of widespread high-risk sexual practices among injection drug users, high-risk injection behavior has dominated the attention of researchers, with sexual transmission of HIV among drug users receiving far less attention.

Noninjection Drug Use. Although most attention has been directed to HIV risk among injecting drug users, HIV infection is also increasing at alarming rates among noninjecting drug users (Des Jarlais et al., 1991). Studies have tied alcohol and marijuana use to inconsistent condom use and multiple sexual partners among black women (Wingood & DiClemente, 1998). Crack cocaine use has been associated with sexual transmission of HIV and other STDs (Kral, Bluthenthal, Booth, & Watters, 1998) and with high-risk sexual behaviors in women (Booth, Watters, & Chitwood, 1993; Coyle, 1998; Tortu, Beardsley, Deren, & Davis, 1994) that include exchanging sex for money or drugs, multiple partners (Balshem, Oxman, van Rooyen, & Girod, 1992; Edlin et al., 1992; Hudgins, McCusker, & Stoddard, 1995; Weatherby et al., 1992), and infrequent condom use (Cohen et al., 1994; Coyle, 1998; Fullilove, Fullilove, Haynes, & Gross, 1990; Jones et al., 1998). Due to both high numbers of sexual encounters and frequent high-risk sexual behaviors, crack users have rates of HIV infection as high as the rates among injection drug users (Booth et al., 1993; Coyle, 1998).

Comprehensive programs for drug users must provide the information, skills, and support necessary to reduce both injection-related and sexual risks. At the same time, HIV and STD prevention services and drug treatment services must be better integrated to take advantage of the multiple opportunities for intervention and to address the multiple stressors and risks in the lives of drug users.

Women's Issues

Perhaps the most critical feature of behavioral change necessary for preventing sexual transmission of HIV to women is that it requires the cooperation of another person, namely, the woman's sex partner. Unfortunately, many of the women at highest risk for HIV/AIDS are poor and dependent upon their male partners for economic security and survival (Airhihenbuwa, DiClemente, Wingood, & Lowe, 1992; Kane, 1991). Many of these women lack the sexual communication and negotiation skills necessary to persuade their male partners to use condoms. Some women fear that they will lose desired partners if they insist on condom use. Requesting condom use may be viewed as an insult to the male partner or as an indication that the woman has been unfaithful to her partner or has a sexually transmitted disease (de Bruyn, 1992; Fullilove, Fullilove, Haynes, & Gross, 1990; Kenan & Armstrong, 1992). It may be particularly difficult to implement condom use in a long-term relationship. Changing behavior during the relationship may be much more difficult than initiating condom use at the beginning of a new relationship. Clearly, HIV risk-reduction interventions for women have to address these relationship and partner issues.

Several controlled studies have shown that behavioral interventions with women can reduce HIV risk-associated behavior and influence theory-based determinants of such behavior (Jemmott, Jemmott, & O'Leary, 2000; O'Leary & Wingood, 2000; Wingood & DiClemente, 1996). Studies have demonstrated significant increases in condom use (Belcher et al., 1998; DiClemente & Wingood, 1995; El-Bassel & Schilling, 1992; Kelly et al., 1994; Schilling, El-Bassel, Schinke, Gordon, & Nichols, 1991) and reductions in unprotected sexual intercourse (Belcher et al., 1998; Kelly et al., 1994) among women who received HIV risk-reduction interventions as compared with those in control groups. A recent study found that an HIV intervention reduced the incidence of STD in both Mexican American women (70 percent) and African American women (30 percent) (Shain et al., 1999). Thus evidence suggests that interventions can reduce women's HIV sexual risk behaviors.

Nonetheless there is an urgent need for woman-controlled prevention methods (Gollub, 1995). The female condom, which has only recently become available in the United States but has been available for some time in some European countries, may confer superior protection because it is made of polyurethane, a material tougher than latex, and possibly also because it covers more tissue area (Nowak, 1993). However, as the presence of the female condom is obvious to the male, issues of cooperation and trust remain potentially problematic. It is of utmost importance that female-controlled and undetectable HIV prevention technologies be developed (Cates, Stewart, & Trussell, 1992; Gollub, 1995; Rosenberg & Gollub, 1992; Stein, 1992, 1993). Vaginal microbicides offer one such hope. At present, development and testing of these agents is under way, but no such products are yet commercially available.

Adolescents' Issues

Adolescents account for less than 1 percent of all reported AIDS cases in the United States (CDC, 1997); however, this statistic underestimates the potential for HIV infection among adolescents. Because HIV has an incubation period that spans many years, it is likely that many African American young adults became infected during adolescence. Increasing rates of STDs and unintended pregnancy suggest an elevated risk of HIV infection among African American adolescents compared to their white counterparts (Alan Guttmacher Institute, 1994; Kann et al., 1996). National surveys of adolescents have consistently indicated that compared with whites and Latinos, a greater proportion of African Americans report being sexually active (CDC, 1991; Hofferth & Hayes, 1987; Kann et al., 1996; Pratt, Mosher, Bachrach, & Horn, 1984; Sonenstein, Pleck, & Ku, 1989; Taylor, Kagay, & Leichenko, 1986); this is so even when socioeconomic background is statistically controlled (Hofferth, Kahn, & Baldwin, 1987). Although the use of latex condoms can reduce substantially the risk of STDs, including HIV (Cates & Stone, 1992; CDC, 1988; Stone, Grimes, & Magder, 1986), most sexually active adolescents do not consistently use condoms (Hingson, Strunin, Berlin, & Heeren, 1990; Jemmott & Jemmott, 1990; Keller et al., 1991; Mosher & Pratt, 1990; Sonenstein et al., 1989; Jemmott & Jones, 1993; Jemmott, Jemmott, & Fong, 1998).

Considerable evidence indicates that behavioral interventions can reduce HIV sexual risk behavior among adolescents (National Institutes of Health, 1997; Jemmott & Jemmott, 2000; Kim, Stanton, Li, Dickersin, & Galbraith, 1997). For instance, studies have demonstrated significant increases in condom use (Jemmott, Jemmott, & Fong, 1992, 1998; Main et al., 1994; Orr, Langefeld, Katz, & Caine, 1996; Rotheram-Borus, Koopman, Haignere, & Davies, 1991; Stanton et al., 1996; Walter & Vaughan, 1993), reductions in frequency of sexual intercourse (Jemmott, Jemmott, & Fong, 1992; St. Lawrence, Brasfield, Jefferson, Alleyne, & O'Brannon, 1995), and reductions in the frequency of unprotected sex (Jemmott, Jemmott, Fong, & McCaffree, 1999; St. Lawrence et al., 1995) among adolescents who received HIV risk-reduction interventions as compared with adolescents in control groups.

Most recently, studies have begun examining the influence of families, particularly parents, on adolescents' sexual risk attitudes and behaviors. Early evidence shows that parents are likely to have an impact on their adolescents' sexual practices. Direct communication is one means through which parents socialize adolescents about important family values, beliefs, and behaviors, including sexual behavior. Parent-child communication about sex has been linked to later initiation of sexual activity (DiIorio, Kelley, & Hockenberry-Eaton, 1999; Hutchinson, 2000a, 2000b; Whitaker & Miller, 2000), less sexual activity (DiIorio, Kelley, & Hockenberry-Eaton, 1999; Jaccard & Dittus, 2000; Kotchick, Dorsey, Miller, & Forehand, 1999; Mueller & Powers, 1990; Pick & Palos, 1995), and consistent condom use (Hutchinson, 2000a, 2000b; Shoop & Davidson, 1994; Whitaker & Miller, 2000). Parents may also serve as a buffer against peer pressure to have sex by providing continual reinforcement of norms and beliefs (Santelli, DiClemente, Miller, & Kirby, 1999; Whitaker & Miller, 2000). Female teens who talked with their parents about when they should have sex were less influenced by whether they thought their friends had initiated sexual activity than were those who had not talked to parents (Whitaker & Miller, 2000). Clear, open parent-teen sexual communication can provide adolescents with a sense of their family's "relevant moral context" (Jaccard & Dittus, 2000) and can prevent misperceptions about parents' attitude toward adolescent sexual activity. Adolescents' perceptions of mothers' disapproval of adolescent sex are associated with a lower probability of sexual intercourse and pregnancy (Jaccard & Dittus, 1991; Jaccard, Dittus, & Gordon, 1996, 1998; Dittus & Jaccard, 2000).

In order to serve as positive role models and communicate effectively with adolescents about sexual risk issues and HIV and STD prevention, parents must possess accurate, up-to-date information about the current sexual risk milieu and the parenting and communication skills necessary to communicate with their children and prepare them to protect themselves from HIV and other STDs. We are currently conducting prospective controlled trial studies on the effectiveness of family-based interventions in reducing the sexual risk behaviors and outcomes of African American adolescents.

HIV Prevention Program Design Issues

Among the issues for HIV prevention program designers to consider are the potential uses of theoretical models and the relative emphases to place on knowledge and skill building on the one hand and between safer sex and abstinence on the other.

Theoretical Models. Behavioral theories can be a helpful tool for HIV prevention program planners. Formal health behavior theories can help service providers understand the various components of behavior and the steps that commonly lead individuals to behavioral change. Basic behavioral science explores the social, behavioral, and cultural influences that help explain why people put themselves at risk and why people continue to get infected with HIV. Theoretical models do not dictate what service providers must do, but they can suggest new ways of thinking about program elements and provide a framework for organizing program content. Behavioral change theory is also useful in HIV prevention because it assists the interventionist in understanding why and how individuals change behaviors that put them at risk for HIV infection. Finally, theoretical models can help providers explore which components of programs are more effective and which programs work well in certain populations (Valdiserri, West, Moore, Darrow, & Hinman, 1992; Herlocher, Hoff, & DeCarlo, 1995). Incorporating theory into HIV prevention interventions can help improve the overall quality of those interventions and help planners to conserve limited resources (University of California, San Francisco, 1995). Many evaluations of HIV interventions demonstrate that programs based on sound theoretical models are the most effective at affecting behavioral change (Fisher & Fisher, 1992; Holtgrave et al., 1995; Valdiserri, West, Moore, Darrow, & Hinman, 1992).

A number of formal theories have proven useful in understanding HIV-related sexual risk behaviors and have been used extensively in HIV prevention programs.

Some of the most commonly employed theoretical models summarized in the literature include the health belief model (Becker, 1974), social cognitive theory (Bandura, 1977), the theory of reasoned action (Ajzen & Fishbein, 1980), the theory of planned behavior, and the transtheoretical model (Prochaska, Redding, Harlow, Rossi, & Velicer, 1994).

The Relationship Between Knowledge Content and Skill-Building Content. For

HIV prevention efforts to successfully modify risk behaviors requires more than the dissemination of information. Knowledge, in and of itself, is not a sufficient motivator of behavioral change (Becker & Joseph, 1988; Jemmott, Jemmott, Spears, et al., 1992). In addition to effective information transfer, individuals need to acquire the social and practical skills necessary to avoid risk-taking situations and behaviors. The inclusion of skill training is a critical component that cannot be overlooked for behavioral change programs. For example, the literature on HIV risk-reduction interventions with African American adolescents illustrates that a focus on increasing AIDS knowledge is an ineffective way of changing behavior. This was demonstrated, as discussed earlier, in the Jemmott, Jemmott, Spears, et al. (1992) study in which an intervention offering AIDS information alone had a weaker effect on intentions to use condoms than did an intervention focusing on perceived self-efficacy and hedonistic beliefs. Similarly, the Jemmott and Jemmott (1992a) study suggested that changes in intentions to use condoms were not associated with changes in knowledge.

Several studies have suggested that interventions that address safer sex skills and perceived self-efficacy are more likely to be effective than information-only programs. Although skills and perceived self-efficacy are likely to be correlated—people who have the skills to implement safer sex behaviors are also likely to feel efficacious—they are not identical, and it is unclear which of the two is more important to behavioral change.

A number of types of skills and efficacy have been highlighted in the literature. Perhaps the most widely recognized type of skill or perceived efficacy is negotiation or resistance skill—the ability of the individual to convince a sexual partner to practice protected sexual intercourse or to resist partner pressure to practice unprotected sexual intercourse. Much less attention has been paid to technical skill in condom use, particularly skill at using condoms without ruining the mood. However, this type of skill may be just as important as negotiation skill (Jemmott, Jemmott, & Hacker, 1992). HIV risk-reduction interventions must teach participants how to use condoms. It is not enough to simply tell them they should use condoms. Role-plays are one way to enhance negotiation skills, and condom exercises can be used to rehearse use of condoms. Because of the importance of negotiation and technical skills and perceived self-efficacy, it is important to employ well-trained facilitators who are comfortable with sexual matters. A facilitator who is uncomfortable with sexual matters may give the skills short shrift. Yet these skills are a critical feature of the intervention.

The Relationship Between Abstinence Content and Safer Sex Content. The goal of HIV risk-reduction interventions is to decrease unprotected sexual intercourse so as to reduce the risk of exposure to HIV. Empirical evidence does not clarify whether the best strategy to accomplish this goal is to stress decreases in sexual activity (for example, abstinence) or to stress the consistent use of condoms during sexual activity. Although interventions should emphasize that the decision to practice abstinence or to have sexual intercourse is one that the individual has to make, they should also make clear that abstinence is an acceptable choice that many people make and that abstinence is the only way to completely eliminate the risk for pregnancy and sexually transmitted diseases including HIV infection. In addition, interventions should emphasize that those who decide to have sexual intercourse should use condoms to reduce their risk of sexually transmitted infection and, ideally, employ another method of contraception in addition to condoms.

The issue of contraception frequently arises during such programs. Adolescents in particular are often far more concerned about pregnancy than about STDs. Also, they may believe that condoms are unnecessary if they are already using birth control pills or another hormonal contraceptive. It should be emphasized that both pregnancy prevention and STD prevention are important and that even if the female partner uses hormonal contraceptives it is still necessary to use a latex condom to prevent sexually transmitted infections.

Prevention Messages and Messengers. To be effective, messages should be (1) persuasive without producing message avoidance because of the fears they engender, (2) compatible with community group norms, (3) focused to address behaviors that can be implemented, (4) delivered by indigenous community members who are credible to the target community, and (5) disseminated wherever community members normally congregate—at workplaces, homes, hairdressers, churches, and bars and also through street outreach. Persuasive strategies will be considerably more effective if a concerted effort is made to include practices that facilitate the adoption and maintenance of HIV preventive behaviors.

Cultural Sensitivity. In order for HIV risk-reduction interventions to be effective they must be sensitive to the cultural values of the participants and based on a sound theoretical framework (Jemmott & Jemmott, 1992a, Fishbein & Middlestadt, 1989; Fisher & Fisher, 1992; Mays & Cochran, 1988). It is likely to be more effective to develop and implement HIV prevention programs that are adapted to a community's existing practices and beliefs than to try to change those practices and beliefs to fit the program (Hubley, 1986). Culturally inappropriate program frameworks account for the failure of many social and behavioral programs formulated in a dominant group construct for later implementation in minority communities (Airhihenbuwa, DiClemente, Wingood, & Lowe, 1992).

Developing culturally sensitive health intervention programs is a continuous process of adapting the program to the cultural characteristics of the ethnic group being targeted. Integrating cultural components and cultural awareness into HIV prevention education programs for ethnic groups should span the entire phase of program development: planning, implementation, and evaluation. Only those HIV/AIDS intervention strategies that respect culture will be effective in changing risk behaviors.

When designing HIV risk-reduction programs for the African American community, one needs to consider such social norms and values of the African American community as religiosity, caring, sensitivity, family, concern with the welfare of others, adaptability, responsibility, reciprocity, cooperativeness, mutual aid, inclusivity, and interdependence (Akbar, 1977). These social norms and values should be incorporated into HIV education and prevention efforts. For African Americans, ethnically based values of cooperation and unity may be more powerful motivators of behavioral change than appeals to individualist action (Mays & Cochran, 1988). HIV prevention efforts targeted toward African Americans therefore need to address the significance of the African American extended family as well as promote individual survival and well-being. Furthermore, effective HIV prevention programs require long-term interventions that focus on ensuring the general health of African American communities; this long-term approach will empower African Americans to adopt and maintain effective HIV risk-reduction strategies (Airhihenbuwa, DiClemente, Wingood, & Lowe, 1992). It is important that in designing prevention efforts for the African American community we recognize the richness and value of the support networks, culture, and tradition that have helped this community mount successful efforts against many other ills (Mays, 1989).

The AIDS epidemic calls for ways to develop outreach and educational programs that are sensitive to the particular dynamics of African American culture and that use the knowledge of the African American community and the institutions that play key roles in community development and stability, including African American churches, social organizations, informal networks of friends, and extended family ties. Some of these efforts have been called Afrocentric. An Afrocentric approach draws on the strengths of the culture and promotes cultural pride and community, family and individual empowerment. If these types of elements can be built into HIV prevention programming efforts, and if communication processes can be developed that relate to the unique strengths of African American culture, community members at risk and their families may become more receptive to HIV intervention strategies.

Building Bridges Between Communities and Researchers

Finally, to enlist support for behavioral change interventions, researchers must be aware of and sensitive to the values, beliefs, and concerns of the population of African Americans who will be the target of intervention efforts. This may mean seeking community input in the design, planning, and implementation of HIV risk-reduction studies. The use of individual and focus group interviews and meetings with community opinion leaders may be useful in this connection. In addition, there is a need for more African American scientists who are actively involved in HIV risk-reduction research in community settings.

Researchers and social scientists should also make themselves available to communities as consultants. African American community groups and community AIDS organizations have long been conducting innovative grassroots prevention programs, but they have rarely been carefully evaluated. It is now essential to integrate more closely community interventions with research evaluation methodologies so that ineffective approaches can be discarded and effective approaches widely disseminated.

As effective HIV interventions are identified, an important concern that arises is whether those interventions are being disseminated to likely end-users, those who work with African American adults and adolescents in various clinical, school, and community settings. There is always the possibility that successful interventions will remain buried in the pages of scientific and public health journals, unavailable to those who might be in the best position to apply them. However, there has been progress along these lines. A fine example is the curriculum dissemination project of the Division of Adolescent and School Health (DASH) of the Centers for Disease Control and Prevention. Entitled Research to Classrooms: Programs that Work, the project identifies HIV prevention curricula that have credible scientific evidence of their effectiveness in changing the behavior of youths and that are user friendly and then brings them to the attention of educators and others concerned with youths' welfare. We were honored when the CDC selected our Be Proud! Be Responsible! curriculum as one of five programs identified as effective and worthy of dissemination. More such efforts are needed to disseminate what works.

Directions For Future Research

The literature on HIV risk-reduction interventions for African Americans is relatively small. There are a number of important questions that remain to be addressed in future studies. Although it is important to use culturally appropriate educational materials, one question that is unanswered is whether there are limits to the gains that can be achieved through tailoring interventions to the target population's culture. For example, many of our interventions were culturally appropriate, but none of them were Afrocentric. If a culturally appropriate intervention is effective, would an Afrocentric intervention be measurably more effective? Studies are needed to develop, implement, and contrast the effects of Afrocentric interventions with those of culturally sensitive interventions.

More broadly, a series of studies is needed that contrasts different types of interventions to determine which interventions are most effective. At this point we in the research community know that it is possible to change HIV risk-associated behavior among African Americans. What we need is empirical evidence that tells us what types of intervention strategies will bring about the greatest changes in behavior. Studies are also needed to further clarify the circumstances that lead to the greatest changes in behavior.

Because people are becoming infected with HIV at younger ages, prevention efforts of the future must be targeted to young people and sustained over time, with emphasis on preventing the initiation of drug use and unprotected sexual behavior. Family-based interventions that promote parent-child communication about risk, transmission of values, and monitoring of behavior may be particularly well suited to these purposes.

Conclusion

Although HIV therapies are improving and are prolonging life, prevention remains a critical priority. HIV prevention is both more humane and more cost effective than treatment for HIV/AIDS. Even a vaccine will not halt the spread of HIV unless people have access to it. Thus we must continue to focus on preventing HIV infection

Research on HIV risk reduction among African Americans in community and clinical settings is in an early stage of development. Few intervention studies have been conducted, and accordingly, the inferences that can be drawn are limited. There is clearly a need for additional, methodologically rigorous studies in this area. However, there are also potential obstacles to such studies, including logistical problems and community distrust of researchers and skepticism about recommendations for behavioral change. The authors of this chapter are optimistic that through sensitivity to the values, beliefs, and concerns of the community, it may be possible to conduct the theory-based, culturally sensitive, methodologically sound studies that are necessary to inform HIV risk-reduction efforts for and with African Americans.

References

Airhihenbuwa, C. O., DiClemente, R. J., Wingood, G. M., & Lowe, A. (1992). HIV/AIDS education and prevention among African Americans: A focus on culture. *Journal of AIDS Education and Prevention, 4,* 267–276.

Ajzen, I. (1991). The theory of planned behavior. *Organizational Behavior and Human Decision Processes, 50,* 179–211.

Ajzen, I., & Fishbein, M. (1980). *Understanding attitudes and predicting social behavior.* Upper Saddle River, NJ: Prentice Hall.

Akbar, N. (1977). *Natural psychology and human transformation.* Chicago: World Community of Islam.

Alan Guttmacher Institute. (1994). *Sex and America's teenagers.* New York: Author.

Allen, K., Battjes, J. R., Slododa, J., & Grace, W. C. (Eds.). (1991). *The context of HIV risk among drug users and their sexual partners* (National Institute of Drug Abuse Research Monograph No. 143, pp. 48–63). Washington, DC: National Institute of Drug Abuse.

Balshem, M., Oxman, G., van Rooyen, D., & Girod, K. (1992). Syphilis, sex and crack cocaine: Images of risk and morality. *Social Science and Medicine, 35,* 147–160.

Bandura, A. (1977). *Social learning theory.* Upper Saddle River, NJ: Prentice Hall.

Becker, M. H. (1974). The Health Belief Model and personal health behaviors. *Health Education Monographs, 2,* 324–508.

Becker, M. H., & Joseph, J. (1988). AIDS and behavioral change to reduce risk: A review. *American Journal of Public Health, 78,* 394–410.

Belcher, L., Kalichman, S., Topping, M., Smith, S., Emshoff, J., Norris, F., & Nurss, J. (1998). A randomized trial of a brief HIV risk reduction counseling intervention for women. *Journal of Consulting and Clinical Psychology, 66,* 856–861.

Booth, R., Watters, J., & Chitwood, D. (1993). HIV risk-related sex behaviors among injection drug users, crack smokers, and injection drug users who smoke crack. *American Journal of Public Health, 83,* 1144–1148.

Booth, R., & Weibel, W. (1992). Effectiveness of reducing needle related risks for HIV through indigenous outreach to injection drug users. *American Journal of Addictions, 1,* 277–287.

Brown, E. (1998). Female injecting drug users: Human immunodeficiency virus risk behavior and intervention needs. *Journal of Professional Nursing, 14,* 361–369.

Brown, L., & Primm, B. (1988). Sexual contacts of intravenous drug users: Implications for the next spread of the AIDS epidemic. *Journal of the National Medical Association, 80,* 651–656.

Butts, J. (1988). Sex therapy, intimacy, and the role of the black physician in the AIDS era. *Journal of the National Medical Association, 80,* 919–922.

Calsyn, D.A., Saxon, A.J., Wells, E.A., & Greenberg, D.M. (1992). Longitudinal sexual behavior changes in injecting drug users. *AIDS, 6,* 1207–1211.

Cates, W., Stewart, F., & Trussell, J. (1992). The quest for women's prophylactic methods: Hope vs. science. *American Journal of Public Health, 82,* 1479–1482.

Cates, W., & Stone, K. M. (1992). Family planning, sexually transmitted diseases and contraceptive choice: A literature update: Pt. 1. *Family Planning Perspectives, 24,* 75–84.

Centers for Disease Control and Prevention. (1982). Kaposi's sarcoma (KS), pneumocystis carinii pneumonia (PCP), and other opportunistic infections (OI): Cases reported to CDC as of June 15, 1982. First report.

Centers for Disease Control and Prevention. (1988). Condoms for the prevention of sexually transmitted diseases. *Morbidity and Mortality Weekly Report, 37,* 133–137.

Centers for Disease Control and Prevention. (1991). Premarital sexual experience among adolescent women: United States, 1970–1988. *Morbidity and Mortality Weekly Report, 39,* 929–932.

Centers for Disease Control and Prevention. (1994). *HIV/AIDS Surveillance Report, 6*(2,entire issue).

Centers for Disease Control and Prevention. (1995). *HIV/AIDS Surveillance Report, 7*(2, entire issue).

Centers for Disease Control and Prevention. (1997). *HIV/AIDS Surveillance Report, 9*(2, entire issue).

Centers for Disease Control and Prevention. (1998). *HIV/AIDS Surveillance Report, 10*(2, entire issue).

Centers for Disease Control and Prevention. (1999a). *HIV/AIDS Surveillance Report, 11*(2, entire issue).

Centers for Disease Control and Prevention. (1999b). *HIV/AIDS Surveillance Supplemental Report, 5*(3, entire issue).

Centers for Disease Control and Prevention. (2000). HIV/AIDS 1989–1998. *Morbidity and Mortality Weekly Report, 49,* 4.

Chitwood, D.J., Comerford, M., & Trapido, E.J. (1991). Strategies for enhancing existing studies of the natural history of HIV-1 infection among drug users. *NIDA Research Monograph, 109,* 9–28.

Cohen, D., Navaline, H., & Metzger, D. (1994). High risk behaviors for HIV: A comparison between crack-abusing and opioid-abusing African American women. *Journal of Psychoactive Drugs, 26,* 233–240.

Coyle, S. (1998). Women's drug use and HIV risk: Findings from NIDA's cooperative agreement for community-based outreach/intervention research programs. *Women and Health, 27,* 1–18.

de Bruyn, M. (1992). Women and AIDS in developing countries. *Social Science & Medicine, 34,* 249–262.

de la Cancela, V. (1989). Minority AIDS prevention: Moving beyond cultural perspectives towards sociopolitical empowerment. *AIDS Education & Prevention, 1*(2), 141–153.

DeParle, J. (1991, August 11). For some blacks, social ills seem to follow white plans. *New York Times,* p. E5.

Des Jarlais, D., Abdul-Quader, A., Minkoff, H., Hoegsberg, B., Landesman, S., & Tross, S. (1991). Crack use and multiple AIDS risk behaviors. *Acquired Immune Deficiency Syndrome, 4,* 446–447.

Des Jarlais, D., & Friedman, S. (1987). HIV infection among intravenous drug users: Epidemiology and risk reduction. *AIDS, 1,* 67–76.

Des Jarlais, D., Friedman, S., & Casriel, C. (1990). Target groups for preventing AIDS among intravenous drug users: The "hard" line studies. *Journal of Consulting & Clinical Psychology, 58*(1), 50–56.

DiClemente, R. J. (1991). Predictors of HIV-preventive sexual behavior in a high-risk adolescent population: The influence of perceived peer norms and sexual communication on incarcerated adolescents' consistent use of condoms. *Journal of Adolescent Health, 12,* 385–390.

DiClemente, R. J., & Wingood, G. M. (1995). A randomized controlled trial of a community-based HIV sexual risk reduction intervention for young adult African-American females. *Journal of the American Medical Association, 274,* 1271–1276.

DiIorio, C., Kelley, M., & Hockenberry-Eaton, M. (1999). Communication about sexual issues: Mothers, fathers, and friends. *Journal of Adolescent Health, 24,* 181–189.

Dittus, P., & Jaccard, J. (2000). Adolescents' perceptions of maternal disapproval of sex: Relationship to sexual outcomes. *Journal of Adolescent Health, 26,* 268–278.

El-Bassel, N., & Schilling, R. F. (1992). 15-month follow-up of women methadone patients taught skills to reduce heterosexual HIV transmission. *Public Health Reports, 107,* 500–504.

Edlin, B., Irwin, K., Ludwig, D., McCoy, H., Serrano, Y., Word, C., Bowser, B., Faruque, S., McCoy, C., & Schilling, R. (1992). High-risk sex behavior among young street-recruited crack cocaine smokers in three American cities: An interim report (The Multicenter Crack Cocaine and HIV Infection Study Team). *Journal of Psychoactive Drugs, 24,* 363–371.

Fishbein, M., & Middlestadt, S. (1989). Using the theory of reasoned action as a framework for understanding and changing AIDS-related behaviors. In V. Mays, G. Albee, & S. Schneider (Eds.), *Primary prevention of AIDS: Psychological approaches* (pp. 93–110). Thousand Oaks, CA: Sage.

Fisher, J. D., & Fisher, W. A. (1992). Changing AIDS risk behavior. *Psychological Bulletin, 111,* 455–474.

Fisher, J. D., Misovich, S., & Fisher, W. A. (1992). Impact of perceived social norms on adolescents' AIDS-risk behavior and prevention. In R. DiClemente (Ed.), *Adolescents and AIDS: A generation in jeopardy* (pp. 117–136). Newbury Park, CA: Sage.

Fox, G. L., & Inazu, J. K. (1980). Patterns and outcomes of mother-daughter communication about sexuality. *Journal of Social Issues, 36,* 7–29.

Friedman, G. L., Des Jarlais, D. C., Neaigus, A., Abdul-Quader, A., Sotheran, J., Sufian, M., Tross, S., & Goldsmith, D. (1989). AIDS and the new drug injector. *Nature, 339* (6223), 333–334.

Fullilove, M. T., Fullilove, R. E., III, Haynes, K., & Gross, S. (1990). Black women and AIDS prevention: A view towards understanding the gender rules. *Journal of Sex Research, 27,* 47–64.

Gollub, E. (1995). Women-centered prevention techniques and technologies. In A. O'Leary & L. Jemmott (Eds.), *Women at risk: Issues in the primary prevention of AIDS* (pp. 43–82). New York: Plenum.

Guydish, J., Temoshok, L., Dilley, J., & Rinaldi, J. (1990). Evaluation of a hospital based substance abuse intervention and referral service for HIV-affected patients. *General Hospital Psychiatry, 12*(1), 1–7.

Herlocher, T., Hoff, C., & DeCarlo, P. (1995, August). *Can theory help in HIV prevention?* [Fact sheet]. San Francisco: University of California, San Francisco, Center for AIDS Prevention Studies.

Hingson, R. W., Strunin, L., Berlin, B., & Heeren, T. (1990). Beliefs about AIDS, use of alcohol and drugs, and unprotected sex among Massachusetts adolescents. *American Journal of Public Health, 80*, 295–299.

Hofferth, S., Kahn, J., & Baldwin, W. (1987). Premarital sexual activity among U.S. teenage women over the past three decades. *Family Planning Perspectives, 19*, 46–53.

Hofferth, S. L., & Hayes, C. D. (Eds.). (1987). *Risking the future: Adolescent sexuality, pregnancy, and childbearing* (Vol. 2). Washington, DC: National Academy Press.

Holtgrave, D. R., Qualls, N. L., Curran, J. W., Valdiserri, R. O., Guinan, M. E., & Parra, W. C. (1995). An overview of the effectiveness and efficiency of HIV prevention programs. *Public Health Reports, 110*, 134–146.

Hubley, J. H. (1986). Barriers to health education in developing countries. *Health Education Research: Theory and Practice, 1*(4), 233–245.

Hudgins, R., McCusker, J., & Stoddard, A. (1995). Cocaine use and risky injection and sexual behaviors. *Drug and Alcohol Dependency, 37*, 7–14.

Hutchinson, M. K. (2000a, July). *Influence of family structure and communication variables on the sexual risk behaviors of late adolescent females.* Paper presented at the NIMH Conference on the Role of Families in Preventing and Adapting to HIV/AIDS, Chicago.

Hutchinson, M. K. (2000b). *Sexual risk communication with mothers and fathers: Influence on the sexual risk behaviors of adolescent daughters.* Manuscript submitted for publication.

Icard, L., Schilling, R., El-Bassel, N., & Young, D. (1992). Preventing AIDS among black gay men and black gay and heterosexual male intravenous drug users. *Journal of Social Work, 37*, 440–445.

Jaccard, J., & Dittus, P. (1991). *Parent-teenager communication: Towards the prevention of unintended pregnancies.* New York: Springer-Verlag.

Jaccard, J., & Dittus, P. (2000). Adolescent perceptions of maternal approval of birth control and sexual risk behavior. *American Journal of Public Health.*

Jaccard, J., Dittus, P., & Gordon, V. (1996). Maternal correlates of adolescent sexual and contraceptive behavior. *Family Planning Perspectives, 28*, 159–165, 185.

Jaccard, J., Dittus, P., & Gordon, V. (1998). Parent-adolescent congruency in reports of adolescent sexual behavior and in communications about sexual behavior. *Child Development, 69*, 247–261.

Jaffe, H. W., Bregman, D. J., & Selik, R. M. (1983). Acquired immune deficiency syndrome in the United States: The first 1,000 cases. *Journal of Infectious Diseases, 148*, 339–345.

Jemmott, J. B., III, & Fry, D. (in press). The abstinence strategy for reducing sexual risk behavior. In A. O'Leary (Ed.), *Beyond condoms.* New York: Plenum.

Jemmott, J. B., III, & Jemmott, L. S. (1993). Alcohol and drug use during sex and HIV risk-associated sexual behavior among inner-city black male adolescents. *Journal of Adolescent Research, 8*, 41–57.

Jemmott, J. B., III, & Jemmott, L. S. (1994). Interventions for adolescents in community settings. In R. DiClemente & J. Peterson (Eds.), *Preventing AIDS: Theory and practice of behavioral interventions* (pp. 141–174). New York: Plenum.

Jemmott, J. B., III, & Jemmott, L. S. (2000). HIV behavioral interventions for adolescents in community settings. In J. L. Peterson & R. J. DiClemente (Eds.), *Handbook of HIV Prevention* (pp. 103–127). New York: Plenum.

Jemmott, J. B., III, & Jemmott, L. S. (2000). HIV risk reduction behavioral interventions with heterosexual adolescents. *AIDS. 14 Supplement 2,* s40–s52.

Jemmott, J. B., III, Jemmott, L. S., & Fong, G. T. (1992). Reductions in HIV risk-associated sexual behaviors among black male adolescents: Effects of an AIDS prevention intervention. *American Journal of Public Health, 82,* 372–377.

Jemmott, J. B., III, Jemmott, L. S., & Fong, G. T. (1994). *Reducing the risk of AIDS in black adolescents: Evidence for the generality of intervention effects.* Under review.

Jemmott, J. B., III, Jemmott, L. S., & Fong, G. T. (1998). Abstinence and safer sex HIV risk-reduction interventions for African American adolescents: A randomized controlled trial. *Journal of the American Medical Association, 279,* 1529–1536.

Jemmott, J. B., III, Jemmott, L. S., Fong, G. T., & McCaffree, K. (1999). Reducing HIV risk-associated sexual behavior among African American adolescents: Testing the generality of intervention effects. *American Journal of Community Psychology, 27,* 161–187.

Jemmott, J. B., III, Jemmott, L. S., & Hacker, C. I. (1992). Predicting intentions to use condoms among African American adolescents: The theory of planned behavior as a model of HIV risk-associated behavior. *Journal of Ethnicity and Disease, 2,* 371–380.

Jemmott, J. B., III, Jemmott, L. S., Spears, H., Hewitt, N., & Cruz-Collins, M. (1992). Self-efficacy, hedonistic expectancies, and condom-use intentions among inner-city black adolescent women: A social cognitive approach to AIDS risk behavior. *Journal of Adolescent Health, 13,* 512–519.

Jemmott, J. B., III, & Jones, J. M. (1993). Social psychology and AIDS among ethnic minority individuals: Risk behaviors and strategies for changing them. In J. B. Pryor & G. D. Reeder (Eds.), *The social psychology of HIV infection* (pp. 183–224). Hillsdale, NJ: Erlbaum.

Jemmott, L. S., & Jemmott, J. B., III. (1990). Sexual knowledge, attitudes, and risky sexual behavior among inner-city black male adolescents. *Journal of Adolescent Research, 5,* 346–369.

Jemmott, L. S., & Jemmott, J. B., III. (1991). Applying the theory of reasoned action to AIDS risk behavior: Condom use among black women. *Nursing Research, 40,* 228–234.

Jemmott, L. S., & Jemmott, J. B., III. (1992a). Increasing condom-use intentions among sexually active inner-city black adolescent women: Effects of an AIDS prevention program. *Nursing Research, 41,* 273–279.

Jemmott, L. S., & Jemmott, J. B., III. (1992b). Family structure, parental strictness, religiosity and sexual behavior among black male adolescents. *Journal of Adolescent Research, 7,* 192–207.

Jemmott, L. S., Jemmott, J. B., III, & McCaffree, K. (1995). *Be Proud! Be Responsible! Strategies to empower youth to reduce their risk for AIDS.* New York: Select Media Publications.

Jemmott, L. S., Jemmott, J. B., III, & O'Leary, A. (2000). *HIV prevention for African American women in primary care settings: a randomized controlled trial.* Manuscript submitted for publication.

Jones, D. L., Irwin, K. L., Inciardi, J., Bowser, B., Schilling, R., Word, C., Evans, P., Faruque, S., McCoy, V., & Edlin, B. R. (1998). The multicenter crack cocaine and HIV infection study team. *Sexually Transmitted Diseases, 25* 187–193.

Kaiser Family Foundation. (1998). *National survey of African Americans on HIV/AIDS.* Washington, DC: Kaiser Family Foundation.

Kane, S. (1991). HIV, heroin and heterosexual relations. *Social Science and Medicine, 32,* 1037–1050.

Kann, L., Warren, C., Harris, W., Collins, J., Williams, B., Ross, J., Kolbe, L., & State and Local YRBSS Coordinators. (1996). Youth risk behavior surveillance: United States, 1995 (CDC Surveillance Summaries). *Mortality and Mortality Weekly Report, 45*(SS-4), 1–84.

Keller, S. E., Barlett, J. A., Schleifer, S. J., Johnson, R. L., Pinner, E., & Delaney, B. (1991). HIV-relevant sexual behavior among a healthy inner-city heterosexual adolescent population in an endemic area of HIV. *Journal of Adolescent Health, 12,* 44–48.

Kelly, J. A., Murphy, D. A., Washington, C. D., Wilson, T. S., Koob, J. J., Davis, D. R., Ledezma, G., & Davantes, B. (1994). The effects of HIV/AIDS intervention groups for high-risk women in urban clinics. *American Journal of Public Health, 84,* 1918–1922.

Kenan, R.H., & Armstrong, K. (1992). The why, when, and whether of condom use among female and male drug users. *Journal of Community Health, 17,* 303–317.

Kim, N., Stanton, B., Li, X., Dickersin, K., & Galbraith, J. (1997). Effectiveness of the 40 adolescent AIDS risk-reduction interventions: A quantitative review. *Journal of Adolescent Health, 20,* 204–215.

Kotchick, B., Dorsey, S., Miller, K., & Forehand, R. (1999). Adolescent sexual risk-taking behavior in single-parent ethnic minority families. *Journal of Family Psychology, 13,* 93–102.

Kral, A., Bluthenthal, R., Booth, R., & Watters, J. (1998). HIV seroprevalence among street-recruited injection drug and crack cocaine users in 16 US municipalities. *American Journal of Public Health, 88,* 108–112.

Leigh, B. (1990). The relationship of substance use during sex to high-risk sexual behavior. *Journal of Sex Research, 27,* 199–233.

Madhubti, H. R. (1990). *Black men: Obsolete, single, dangerous?* Chicago: Third World Press.

Main, D. S., Iverson, D. C., McGloin, J., Banspach, S. W., Collins, J. L., Rugg, D. L., & Kolbe, L. J. (1994). Preventing HIV infection among adolescents: Evaluation of a school-based education program. *Preventive Medicine, 23,* 409–417.

Marin, B., & Marin, V. (1991). *Research with Hispanic populations* (Applied social research series, Vol. 23). Thousand Oaks, CA: Sage.

Marin, B., & Marin, V. (1992). Predictors of condom accessibility among Hispanics in San Francisco. *American Journal of Public Health, 82,* 592–595.

Mays, V. M. (1989). AIDS prevention in black populations: Methods of a safer kind. In V. M. Mays, G. W. Albee, & S. F. Schneider (Eds.), *Primary prevention of AIDS: Psychological approaches* (pp. 264–279). Newbury Park, CA: Sage.

Mays, V. M., & Cochran, S. D. (1987). Acquired immunodeficiency syndrome and black Americans: Special psychosocial issues. *Public Health Reports, 102,* 224–231.

Mays, V. M., & Cochran, S. D. (1988). Issues in the perception of AIDS risk and risk reduction activities by black and Hispanic/Latina Women. *American Psychologist, 43,* 949–957.

Milan, R. J., & Kilmann, P. R. (1987). Interpersonal factors in premarital contraception. *Journal of Sex Research, 23,* 289–321.

Mosher, W. D., & Pratt, W. F. (1990). *Contraceptive use in the United States: Advance data from Vital and Health Statistics, 1973–1988* (No. 182). Hyattsville, MD: National Center for Health Statistics.

Mueller, K., & Powers, W. (1990). Parent-child sexual discussion: Perceived communicator style and subsequent behavior. *Adolescence, 25,* 469–482.

National Institutes of Health. (1997, February 11–13). Interventions to prevent HIV risk behaviors. *NIH Consensus Statement, 15*(2), 1–41.

Newmeyer, J. A. (1988). Why bleach? Development of a strategy to combat HIV contagion among San Francisco intravenous drug users. *NIDA Research Monograph, 80,* 151–159.

NIMH Multisite HIV Prevention Trial Group. (1998). The National Institute of Mental Health Multisite HIV Prevention Trial: Reducing HIV sexual risk behavior. *Science, 280,* 1889–1894.

Nowak, R. (1993, January). Research reveals condom conundrums. *The Journal of NIH Research, 5,* 32–33.

O'Leary, A., & Wingood, G. (2000). Interventions for sexually active heterosexual women. In J. L. Peterson and R. J. DiClemente (Eds.), *Handbook of HIV prevention.* New York: Plenum.

Orr, D. P., Langefeld, C. D., Katz, B. P., & Caine, V. A. (1996). Behavioral intervention to increase condom use among high-risk female adolescents. *Journal of Pediatrics, 128,* 288–295.

Pick, S., & Palos, P. (1995). Impact of the family on the sex lives of adolescents. *Adolescence, 30,* 667–675.

Pratt, W., Mosher, W., Bachrach, C. & Horn, M. (1984). Understanding U.S. fertility: Findings from the National Survey of Family Growth, Cycle III. *Population Bulletin, 39,* 1–42.

Prochaska, J., Redding, C., Harlow, L., Rossi, J., & Velicer, W. (1994). The transtheoretical model of change and HIV prevention: A review. *Health Education Quarterly, 21,* 471–486.

Rosenberg, M., & Gollub, E. (1992). Methods women can use that may prevent sexually transmitted diseases including HIV. *American Journal of Public Health, 82*(11), 1432–1478.

Rotheram-Borus, M. J., Koopman, C., Haignere, C., & Davies, M. (1991). Reducing HIV sexual risk behaviors among runaway adolescents. *Journal of the American Medical Association, 266,* 1237–1241.

St. Lawrence, J., Brasfield, T., Jefferson, K., Alleyne, E., & O'Brannon, R. A., III. (1995). Cognitive-behavioral intervention to reduce African-American adolescents' risk for HIV infection. *Journal of Consulting and Clinical Psychology, 63,* 221–237.

Santelli, J., DiClemente, R., Miller, K., & Kirby, D. (1999). Sexually transmitted diseases, unintended pregnancy, and adolescent health promotion. In M. Fisher, L. Juszczak, and L. Klerman (Eds.). *Adolescent medicine: Prevention issues in adolescent health care,* 87–108.

Schilling, R. F., El-Bassel, N., Schinke, S. P., Gordon, K., & Nichols, S. (1991). Building skills of recovering women drug users to reduce heterosexual AIDS transmission. *Public Health Reports, 106,* 297–304.

Shain, R. N., Piper, J. M., Newton, E. R., Perdue, S. T., Ramos, R., Champion, J. D., & Guerra, F. A. (1999). A randomized, controlled trial of a behavioral intervention to prevent sexually transmitted disease among minority women. *New England Journal of Medicine, 340,* 93–100.

Shoop, D., & Davidson, P. (1994). AIDS and adolescents: The relation of parent and partner communication to adolescent condom use. *Journal of Adolescence, 17,* 137–148.

Smith, D., & Moore, J. (1996). Epidemiology, manifestations, and treatment of HIV infection in women. In A. O'Leary & L. Jemmott (Eds.), *Women and AIDS: Coping and caring* (pp. 1–24). New York: Plenum.

Sonenstein, F. L., Pleck, J. H., & Ku, L. C. (1989). Sexual activity, condom use and AIDS awareness among adolescent males. *Family Planning Perspectives, 21,* 152–158.

Stanton, B. F., Li, X., Ricardo, I., Galbraith, J., Feigelman, S., & Kaljee, L. (1996). A randomized, controlled effectiveness trial of an AIDS prevention program for low-income African-American youths. *Archives of Pediatric and Adolescent Medicine, 150,* 363–372.

Stein, Z. (1992). The double bind in science policy and the protection of women from HIV prevention. *American Journal of Public Health, 82,* 1471–1472.

Stein, Z. (1993). HIV prevention: An update on the status of methods women can use. *American Journal of Public Health, 83,* 1379–1382.

Stephens, R. C., Feucht, T. E., & Roman, S. W. (1991). Effects of an intervention program on AIDS-related drug and needle behavior among intravenous drug users. *American Journal of Public Health, 81,* 568–571.

Stone, K. M., Grimes, D. A., & Magder, L. S. (1986). Personal protection against sexually transmitted diseases. *American Journal of Obstetrics and Gynecology, 155,* 180–188.

Taylor, H., Kagay, M., & Leichenko, S. (1986). *American teens speak: Sex myths, TV, and birth control.* Washington, DC: Planned Parenthood Federation of America.

Taylor, R. J. (1998). Structural determinants of religious participation among black Americans. *Review of Religious Research, 30,* 114–125.

Tortu, S., Beardsley, M., Deren, S., & Davis, W. R. (1994). The risk of HIV infection in a national sample of women with injection drug-using partners. *American Journal of Public Health, 84,* 1243–1249.

Turner, C., Miller, H., & Moses, L. (1990). *AIDS: Sexual behavior and intravenous drug use.* Washington, DC: National Academy Press.

University of California San Francisco-Center for AIDS Prevention Studies (1995). Can theory help in HIV prevention? [on-line]. Available: www.caps.ucsf.edu/theorytext.html.

Valdiserri, R. O., West, G. R., Moore, M., Darrow, W. W., & Hinman, A. R. (1992). Structuring HIV prevention service delivery systems on the basis of social science theory. *Journal of Community Health, 17,* 259–269.

Walter, H. J., & Vaughan, R. D. (1993). AIDS risk reduction among a multiethnic sample of urban high school students. *Journal of the American Medical Association, 270,* 725–730.

Watkins, K., Metzger, D., Woody, G., & McLellan, A. (1992). High-risk sexual behaviors of intravenous drug-users in- and out-of-treatment: Implications for the spread of HIV infection. *American Journal of Drug and Alcohol Abuse, 18,* 389–398.

Watkins, K., Metzger, D., Woody, G., & McLellan. A. (1993). Determinants of condom use among intravenous drug users. *AIDS, 7,* 719–723.

Weatherby, N. L., Shultz, J. M., Chitwood, D. D., McCoy, H. V., McCoy, C. B., Ludwig, D. D., & Edlin, B. R. (1992). Crack cocaine use and sexual activity in Miami, Florida. *Journal of Psychoactive Drugs, 24,* 373–380.

Whitaker, D., & Miller, K. (2000). Parent-adolescent discussions about sex and condoms: Impact on peer influences of sexual risk behavior. *Journal of Adolescent Research, 15,* 251–273.

Williams, R. L. (1980). The death of white research in the black community. In R. L. Jones (Ed.), *Black psychology* (pp. 403–416). New York: Harper & Row.

Wingood, G. M., & DiClemente, R. J. (1996). HIV sexual risk reduction interventions for women: A review. *American Journal of Preventive Medicine, 12,* 209–217.

Wingood, G. M., & DiClemente, R. J. (1998). The influence of psychosocial factors, alcohol, and drug use on African-American women's high risk sexual behavior. *American Journal of Preventive Medicine, 15,* 54–60.

CHAPTER SEVENTEEN

TOBACCO

From Slavery to Addiction

Sandra W. Headen, Robert G. Robinson

Race, geography, culture, and economic context are themes that have shaped the history and experiences of African Americans with tobacco and tobacco use from the beginning of slavery to the present. The term African American encompasses individuals who trace their ancestry of origin to sub-Saharan Africa. Their fate in the new world is popularly associated with the cotton crop, but tobacco is the product that spawned the African slave trade that resulted in the unprecedented diaspora from the African continent. Greed and racial prejudice allowed white settlers to rationalize a system that lasted for almost four hundred years and created a set of beliefs and norms that influences American life today. For African Americans, tobacco has been a source of physical and emotional harm from the days when they were forced to grow it to their eventual addiction to it.

Tobacco has a unique status in contemporary American society, and its use creates a troubling dilemma for professionals charged with protecting the public's health. Tobacco products are legally sold to adults and easily accessible to children, yet scientific evidence shows that nicotine is both addictive and harmful to health. When used as directed, tobacco often leads to illness, disability, and death. In spite of this observation, tobacco is protected in many ways. It is exempt from the kind of scrutiny and government regulation required of many other substances. For example, the composition of each cigarette brand is considered to be a trade secret and there is no requirement to disclose ingredients to the public. Tobacco is also a cultural icon, a product from which individual citizens and the country as a whole have reaped economic benefits. However, the price that Americans have paid for these apparent benefits from tobacco has been enormous.

Tobacco use is the single most preventable cause of disability and death in the United States. Each year over 400,000 people, including over 45,000 African

Americans, die from smoking-related illnesses such as heart disease, cancer, stroke, and emphysema and other respiratory illnesses (U.S. Department of Health and Human Services [DHHS], 1998). Cigarettes contain over 600 different chemicals and additives that affect the taste of the cigarette or the burning qualities of the tobacco. Many of these additives are harmful to health individually, and their combined effects are unknown (U.S. Environmental Protection Agency [EPA], 1992). Sidestream, or secondhand, smoke from lighted cigarettes also contains chemicals that are harmful to anyone who inhales them. Approximately 3,000 adult nonsmokers die each year from exposure to secondhand smoke. Secondhand smoke is also associated with higher rates of colds, ear infections, and asthma attacks in children (EPA, 1992). In spite of these daunting statistics, 3,000 young people become regular smokers every day, replacing older smokers who become ill or die. At least a third of these youths will die prematurely from smoking-related causes (DHHS, 1994).

Recently, the tobacco industry was challenged in the courts by the attorneys general of four states (Mississippi, Texas, Minnesota, and Florida) that were seeking reimbursement for the costs of treating sick smokers. The lawsuits resulted in out-of-court settlements with the tobacco industry. The sums awarded ranged from $3.3 billion for Mississippi to $14.5 billion for Texas to be paid over the next twenty-five years. The tobacco companies also participated in negotiations that resulted in a settlement with the remaining thirty-seven states that had filed legal actions against them. According to the Master Settlement Agreement (MSA), the tobacco industry will pay the states a total of $206 billion over the next twenty-five years. The amount of the payments to individual states will be determined by selected criteria. These actions have provided states with funds that could be used to prevent young people from starting to smoke and to help current smokers to quit. However, states are free to decide how this money is to be spent. The MSA also sets restrictions on youths' exposure to tobacco advertising and youths' access to tobacco products. For example, cartoon characters, like Joe Camel, are banned from advertising and promotion campaigns; brand-name sponsorship of events with substantial youth attendance is restricted; distribution and sale of clothing and other products with brand-name logos is banned after July 1999; and free samples are prohibited, except in adult-only establishments. Other restrictions are also included in the MSA. The settlement has also created the American Legacy Foundation, a national foundation with $250 million to spend over the next ten years, and a public education fund ($1.45 billion to spend between 2000 and 2003) to reduce youth smoking (Wilson, 1999).

A significant consequence of the lawsuits against the tobacco companies was the release of millions of pages of previously secret tobacco company documents. Some of the documents were minutes from meetings held by tobacco company executives to discuss such topics as marketing cigarettes to teens, women, and African Americans and the research results from experiments conducted over the years on the health effects of cigarette smoking and nicotine. These documents, which revealed that tobacco industry executives and scientists knew of the health damaging effects of tobacco use as far back as the 1950s, strengthened the evidence against the industry and helped the states to obtain the MSA. The documents are now available to the public on the Internet (Wilson, 1999).

This introduction highlights just a few of the complex issues that shape the broader social, economic, and political context of tobacco use in America. In the last ten years, public health efforts to control tobacco use have been initiated in every state and in many territories of the United States through Project ASSIST (American Stop Smoking Intervention Study), funded by the National Cancer Institute, and the IMPACT program, funded by the Centers for Disease Control and Prevention. Massachusetts, Arizona, Oregon, and Minnesota have also raised excise taxes on tobacco and earmarked funds to support tobacco control. In all of these programs, efforts have been made to address disparities in health outcomes and resources devoted to tobacco control so that African Americans and other minorities will no longer bear a disproportionate burden of illness from tobacco-related causes compared with whites.

The remainder of the chapter summarizes the themes and critical issues that describe the African American experience with tobacco from the beginning of the African slave trade to the present. Behavioral aspects of smoking initiation, nicotine addiction, and quitting specific to African Americans is reviewed as well as the health effects of tobacco use, the public health response to the problem of tobacco use, and the African American response to tobacco and the national tobacco control movement. We also present an innovative model that represents a vision for African American action on tobacco control in the year 2000 and beyond.

Tobacco and Slavery

Tobacco played a pivotal role in the success of the early colonies in America. The first waves of settlers on the Chesapeake Bay in Virginia were concerned about immediate survival, but as time passed they looked for ways to ensure stability and comfort in life. Tobacco, and several other labor- and resource-intensive crops such as indigo and rice, provided solutions to their problem. The first shipment of tobacco reached Europe around 1592 from the West Indies. The first tobacco grown in the Americas was planted in Virginia in 1612. Tobacco became very popular in Europe, and the high demand for it meant that growers could command high prices when they sold it. Indeed, the profits earned from growing tobacco were many times higher than returns from other crops. For this reason, tobacco was called the *money crop* and became the backbone of the colonial economy in Maryland, Virginia, and northern Carolina. Over 20,000 pounds were produced in 1619, and 500,000 pounds in 1627. Peak production was in 1790, when 118,000 hogsheads (barrels) of tobacco were exported. By 1814, only 3,000 hogsheads were exported (Kulikoff, 1986; Christian, 1995).

Events that followed the completion of the war of independence from England changed the agricultural outlook for tobacco, rice, and indigo. Land for growing high-quality tobacco crops was difficult to find, and the cultivation of rice expanded beyond the traditional flood plains to a broader area. The loss of traditional markets in Europe also affected the production of tobacco and indigo. Farmers were looking for another cash crop. The opportunity came in 1793 with the invention of the cotton gin by Eli Whitney. Some farmers grew cotton before this period, but it was not profitable. When harvested, the cottonseed had to be separated from the usable cotton fiber by hand, a slow and labor-intensive process. The cotton gin increased the speed of this process and lowered production costs, allowing American farmers to meet the ever-increasing demand for cotton fiber that was now emerging from the newly mechanized textile factories in England (Kulikoff, 1986; Christian, 1995; Carnes, Schlesinger, & Fox, 1996).

At the height of its economic strength, tobacco helped to shape the history and lifestyles of colonial America. Growing tobacco was a labor-intensive process that involved cultivating the land, tending seedbeds, hoeing weeds, topping (breaking the flowers from the tops of young plants), picking worms and other insects from the leaves, harvesting, sorting, stripping, and curing the crop to prepare it for market and then packing the tobacco into hogsheads to be taken to market.

Tobacco was planted on both large and small farms, but the wealth was to be had on the larger farms, or plantations, which required a large and steady supply of labor to maintain production. Plantations were the logical extension of decisions that the colonists made about farming methods. Their Indian neighbors used the *crop rotation* method of farming, which meant planting a different crop on a plot of land every two to three years or allowing the land to lie fallow (unplanted) periodically. This process produced higher-quality plants and higher yields because nutrients lost in one year would be replenished in the next. The tremendous profitability of tobacco and the high demand for it from Europe encouraged the colonial farmers to plant as much tobacco as they could each year. They used a process called *land rotation*, which meant planting a crop on the same plot of land in consecutive years and abandoning the plot when it was no longer fertile. Land rotation depleted so many nutrients from the soil that a plot of land so treated would not support healthy crops or any crops at all for many years afterward. The decision to employ the land rotation method of farming explains why successful colonial planters lived on very large plantations. As time passed and more and more land was depleted, the population moved away from the coast seeking new land and richer soil to grow tobacco on (Kulikoff, 1986; Christian, 1995; Carnes, Schlesinger, & Fox, 1996).

Growing tobacco was very profitable, but prices fluctuated, and retaining labor at the right wage was a recurring problem. Indentured servants did much of the work in the beginning. Many Europeans who came to America were poor and paid for their passage by selling their labor for a set number of years. It is believed that the first Africans to arrive in Virginia, in 1619, were sold as indentured servants, not slaves; and for years black and white indentured servants worked side by side in the fields. However, this system did not solve the labor problem for tobacco farmers because indentured servants eventually earned their freedom. Sometimes they established a farm nearby and grew their own tobacco, affecting the amount of tobacco grown in the area and, perhaps, the price of tobacco in any given year (Christian, 1995).

Two events were responsible for solving the labor shortage problem, at least from the colonial farmer's perspective. The first was the mass importation of African slaves into the colonies. Slaves were ideal workers for several reasons. Physically they were strong enough to work long hours in the sun and hardy enough to survive the infectious diseases that often killed native Indians or white indentured servants. A second desirable quality of slaves was their permanence. They had been stolen from their homelands, brought thousands of miles over vast oceans, and subjected to physical and psychological trauma. Returning home was not an option, and they had little knowledge of the environment outside the plantation itself.

The second event that eased the labor shortage on tobacco farms was the enslavement of free Africans and African Americans. As more slaves were imported, the colonists felt an increasing need to control the black population. Enslavement of all black people formalized the status differences between blacks and whites and eliminated distinctions among blacks. These actions provided the tobacco farmers and the colonial economy as a whole with a supply of workers that was permanent and self-replenishing (Kulikoff, 1986; Christian, 1995; Carnes et al., 1996).

History shows that the slave-driven plantation system was a double-edged sword. It allowed farmers to grow a lot of tobacco, but the price of tobacco fluctuated greatly. Very low income from tobacco in some years made it difficult for farmers to meet the fixed costs of running a plantation, such costs for maintaining slaves and equipment and for the upkeep of the plantation. Tobacco also depleted land resources, making them less valuable. By 1814, agricultural markets were changing and the demand for tobacco grown in the Americas had declined. Farmers were looking for alternative crops to grow and agricultural activity was now moving further south where the soil was still rich. These events did not change the fates of African Americans who were firmly entrenched as slaves in the new world. Their racial identity and history had been irrevocably changed, and their relationship to tobacco would remain strong and complex. During the eighteenth and nineteenth centuries, even free men and women were most likely to be working in tobacco and slaves sometimes earned their freedom by hiring themselves out as tobacco laborers. After emancipation, some African Americans farmed tobacco, a practice that was most common in North Carolina, South Carolina, Georgia, and Virginia. In the twentieth century, however, the number of tobacco farms owned by African Americans has declined dramatically (Christian, 1995; Carnes, Schlesinger, & Fox, 1996).

Contemporary Themes and Experiences

In the twentieth century, African Americans continued to have a very complex relationship to tobacco and the tobacco industry that involved the following activities: (1) agricultural production of tobacco and manufacturing of tobacco products, (2) increased consumption of tobacco products and greater exposure to advertising messages encouraging smoking, and (3) increased reliance on the marginal benefits that flowed from philanthropy by the tobacco industry.

Work and Wages

Historically, most of the jobs that African Americans have held in the tobacco industry were menial and poorly paid. During the post-colonial period, African Americans and whites worked side-by-side in small tobacco factories that formed a cottage industry. However, the introduction of the cigarette-making machine in the mid-1800s created many changes in the industry. White women were hired as the primary work force because it was believed that they alone had the dexterity to handle the new machines. African Americans were not allowed to work beside white women and were relegated to more menial jobs in the factories, a practice which continued to the 1930s.

The large number of African Americans working in tobacco in the early twentieth century allowed them to benefit from union-organizing activities. For example, the United Tobacco Workers Local 22 encouraged members to exercise their right to vote and was credited with facilitating the election of an African American city council member in Winston-Salem, North Carolina, in 1947. This union continued to be the strongest in the South, having far more influence than its rival, the Food, Tobacco, Agriculture, and Allied Workers Union. The strength of African Americans in the unions likely contributed to two progressive actions, both taken by the R. J. Reynolds Tobacco Company in Winston-Salem. African Americans were allowed to work on cigarette-making machines after World War II, and in 1961 a factory was opened that included integrated production lines and desegregated facilities (DHHS, 1998).

Advertising and Promotion of Tobacco Products

Several events occurred between the early 1950s and mid-1970s that changed the relationship between African Americans and the tobacco industry in the second half of the twentieth century. First, African Americans became important consumers of tobacco products after World War II. More African American than white men smoked cigarettes during the 1950s, and tobacco advertising began to reflect this new market. Magazines read by African Americans increased tobacco advertising during the 1960s and featured African American models and themes perceived to be attractive to African Americans, such as status-seeking, high-quality products, and brand loyalty. African American athletes were also an early symbol of marketing targeted to African Americans. The activities of the Liggett and Myers Tobacco Company are indicative of some of the strategies that were used. For example, in the 1950s they marketed the Chesterfield brand of cigarette to African Americans, featuring popular African American athletes in ads and placing the ads in newspapers and magazines read by African Americans. This targeted advertising campaign also included six documentary films about African American achievements that were shown in movie theatres and on college campuses. The success of this effort led to thirteen additional films on African American celebrities. By 1971, Liggett and Myers employed an advertising agency that specialized in marketing to African Americans to sell its L & M cigarette to men and women and to market the Eve cigarette to African American women. Similar steps were taken by other tobacco companies in response to the ban on television advertising of tobacco in 1971 (DHHS, 1998).

Menthol cigarettes were very popular when they were introduced in the 1950s, constituting 5 percent of the market by 1957, an impressive showing for a new product. They were not originally targeted to African Americans, but received favorable ratings from test marketing in African American communities. African American smokers now prefer menthol cigarettes to brands without menthol, and these cigarettes are heavily advertised in magazines and other media targeted to African Americans. A 1987 analysis of cigarette advertisements in magazines with a predominantly African American readership found that 65.9 percent featured menthol cigarettes compared with only 15.4 percent of cigarette advertisements in magazines designed for the general population. Newport, a menthol cigarette, is the most popular brand among African American adults and youth (DHHS, 1998).

Television advertising of tobacco products was banned in 1971. The strategies that tobacco companies employed in response to this event involved targeted marketing in a variety of media including newspapers, magazines, point-of-sale advertising on storefronts and sales counters, and outdoor advertising on full-scale billboards and smaller displays called eight sheets. Studies that were conducted in selected communities in Los Angeles, San Francisco, and Columbia, South Carolina, have shown that advertising of tobacco products is higher in African American communities and in some Hispanic and Asian communities than in white communities in spite of the lower percentages of these groups in the population (DHHS, 1998). These findings suggest that tobacco companies have devoted large quantities of their advertising resources to encouraging tobacco use in ethnic communities.

In the past twenty years, tobacco companies have shifted an increasing percentage of their marketing budgets into promotional activities instead of direct advertising. Product promotion is a subtle way to sell a product by linking the product name to sponsorship of a variety of activities that divert attention away from commercial motives. Tobacco money has supported many cultural events important to the African American community. Examples include the Kool Jazz Festival (sponsored by Brown and Williamson until 1985) and the Parliament World Beat Concert Series.

One of the most visible events in the African American community, the Ebony Fashion Fair, was sponsored by R. J. Reynolds' More cigarettes. However, public pressure eventually forced the sponsor, Johnson Publications, to break the relationship between the fashion show and its most lucrative sponsor. Over the years, tobacco companies have also contributed to the political campaigns of African American elected officials at the local, state, and federal levels (Robinson, Pertschuk, & Sutton, 1992; Robinson, Barry, et al., 1992). This type of support may have contributed to the reluctance of many African American political leaders to speak out against the dangers that tobacco poses for the health of African Americans.

Tobacco companies have appeared to be generous to African Americans, but use of their products also robbed the African American community of valuable leaders who had many more contributions to make to their families, communities, and the nation. The African American response to these facts should be clear. African American leaders and organizations that receive tobacco money should divest themselves of these funds and find replacement dollars to support their missions and activities. It is not possible to build the African American community on the one hand and to support products that disable and kill its people on the other. Divestiture of tobacco money will not be easy. Replacing these dollars puts a tremendous burden on individuals and organizations that may be marginally staffed, but the effort must be made. In addition, other community leaders should step forward to design a plan to facilitate divestiture so that everyone shares the burden of finding alternative financial support.

Harold Freeman (an African American physician at Harlem Hospital, tobacco control advocate, and past president of the American Cancer Society) described the problem succinctly when he said that some African American leaders and organizations are as addicted to tobacco money as smokers are addicted to tobacco (Fiore, Novotny, et al., 1990). This fact only underscores the importance of shaping a long-term strategy that will allow organizations to wean themselves from tobacco industry largesse.

Philanthropy

In the twentieth century, the relationship between the African American community and the tobacco industry has been very complex. Tobacco is responsible for over forty-five thousand preventable deaths annually and for countless years of disability and lost wages in this community. These devastating health outcomes are discussed infrequently because the tobacco industry has positioned itself to distribute an objectively meager amount of resources over a wide range of individuals, organizations, and activities that are important to African Americans. Recipients of tobacco dollars have included notable civil rights organizations such as the National Association for the Advancement of Colored People, the Urban League, the Leadership Conference on Civil Rights, 100 Black Men of America, Inc., and the National Coalition of 100 Black Women, and professional organizations, such as the National Association of Black Social Workers, the National Association of Negro Business and Professional Women's Clubs, the National Conference of Black Lawyers, and the National Black Police Association. Tobacco companies have given money to support education through scholarships in specific professions, such as journalism, and by supporting black colleges and universities through the United Negro College Fund.

Tobacco companies also support the publication of resource guides, a service that benefits African American organizations by providing free publicity. For example, since 1981 Philip Morris has published the *Guide to Black Organizations* on a biennial basis. The guide lists national, regional, and local nonprofit organizations, as well as state and local caucuses. In communities where tobacco companies have factories and offices, there is even greater support for local organizations and activities such as funding of local chapters of the Young Men's Christian Association or support of Christmas tree lighting ceremonies.

Tobacco Use Among African Americans

Tobacco use in the U.S. population has been monitored annually since 1964, when the first surgeon general's report on smoking and health concluded that cigarette smoking is linked to lung cancer in men (U.S. Department of Health, Education, and Welfare, 1964). By the early 1990s, there was sufficient evidence to describe who is likely to smoke and why these individuals become addicted to tobacco. Contrary to the tobacco industry's assertion that smoking is an adult behavior and starting to smoke is an adult decision, cigarette smoking should be thought of as a pediatric health problem that begins in the teen years or earlier. In one national survey, over 80 percent of adults aged thirty to thirty-nine who had become regular smokers reported that they tried their first cigarette before the age of eighteen and over half (53 percent) reported that they were regular smokers before age eighteen. Adolescents and young children often try their first cigarette between the ages of twelve and fourteen, although recent surveys show that the age of first use may be declining (DHHS, 1994). Some studies also suggest that African Americans start smoking at somewhat older ages than whites; one year later for males and two years later for females (DHHS, 1998; Centers for Disease Control and Prevention [CDC], 1991).

Becoming a smoker occurs in several stages. The first stage, preparation, involves forming attitudes about the functional value of smoking as a means of coping with stress or as a tool in social interaction. In the trying stage, adolescents may take a puff from a cigarette that someone else is smoking, followed by smoking a whole cigarette or several cigarettes. Many youths report experiencing negative reactions such as dizziness, coughing, or nausea when they first smoke, but these symptoms are greatly reduced or disappear as smoking continues. The severity of these symptoms and the social reinforcement individuals get for smoking determines whether and how quickly they go on to the next stage. Being an experimenter means smoking repeatedly but not regularly. Smoking at this stage is often done in response to a specific situation like a party or social gathering with friends. Regular smoking is the fourth stage and means that smoking is a habit that occurs at least weekly and across many situations and acquaintances. In the final stage, addiction and nicotine dependence, a tolerance for nicotine develops, and smokers will experience withdrawal from nicotine if they quit. The process of becoming a smoker may take two or three years (DHHS, 1994; Leventhal, Fleming, & Glynn, 1988). One study of youths who were experimenting with cigarettes found that half were smoking daily just one year later (McNeil, 1991).

Smoking has been called a *gateway drug* because it precedes or accompanies many problem behaviors. Smokers and nonsmokers differ in important ways. Smokers are more likely than nonsmokers to have personal and social problems such as low school performance, disciplinary problems in school, or frequent absences from school. Smokers are also more likely to report emotional distress, anxiety, depression, or other mood disorders. Teen smokers more often live in households where one or both parents or some other family member is a smoker (Fleming, Leventhal, Glynn, & Ershler, 1989; Bachman et al., 1991).

Teens themselves perceive that smoking has some functional value—to reduce stress or to look and feel cool. Studies of adolescent smokers confirm these perceptions, reporting that teen smokers do so to cope with boredom or with difficult situations, to look mature, to be accepted by friends and peers, or to be rebellious. Results of a qualitative study of the functional value and imagery of smoking or not smoking for teens aged twelve to seventeen were even more specific. Smokers and nonsmokers held similar images of adolescents who smoked, perceiving them to be losers and misfits who did not do well in school and frequently got into trouble. Smoking itself was perceived as unattractive. Paradoxically, smokers said that they smoked to be cool and thought that they looked cool when they were smoking. Smoking also served a deeper functional value for smokers from diverse racial backgrounds; it defined their personal and social identities. Smoking was associated with a look, a set of attitudes and behaviors, and a lifestyle that set one group of adolescents apart from another. Interestingly, nonconformity was the only common factor associated with the different lifestyles that teen smokers from different backgrounds described (Mermelstein & Tobacco Control Network Writing Group, 1999).

African American Smoking and Quitting Patterns

Whites and African Americans differ significantly in smoking patterns and behavior. Most (75 percent) African American smokers prefer menthol brands of cigarettes and most white smokers prefer nonmenthol brands. Newport and Marlboro are the most popular brands for African Americans and whites respectively. African Americans are lighter or less intense smokers than whites. On average, white smokers consume twenty-five cigarettes per day compared with fifteen cigarettes per day for African American smokers (Robinson, Pertschuk, & Sutton, 1992; DHHS, 1998). Also, the percentage of African Americans who reported smoking fewer than fifteen cigarettes per day increased from 56.0 percent in the period from 1978 to 1980 to 63.9 percent in 1994 and 1995, indicating a trend toward even lighter cigarette smoking (DHHS, 1998). Two reasons have been offered to explain why African Americans smoke less than whites. First, the cigarette brands preferred by African Americans are higher in nicotine and may satisfy the addiction with fewer cigarettes. Second, the economic disparity that exists between blacks and whites may reduce African Americans' ability to smoke large numbers of cigarettes (DHHS, 1998).

Quitting smoking is a difficult process that often requires repeated attempts. Smokers must be psychologically ready to quit. The following stages of behavioral change provide a useful framework for assessing when smokers are likely to succeed in quitting: (1) in the precontemplation stage, smokers are not thinking about quitting and are not ready to try to quit; (2) in the contemplation stage, smokers have begun to think about the advantages of quitting and the disadvantages of continuing to smoke, and they may be encouraged to try to quit if presented with additional information about the benefits of quitting or the risks in remaining a smoker; (3) in preparing for the third stage, the action stage, smokers remove cigarettes, ashtrays, and other cues to smoke from their homes, cars, and workplaces and alert family and friends that they plan to quit and seek their support; they have a plan to change eating and exercise habits to avoid weight gain and reduce stress; and they set a quit date and stick to it; (4) in the maintenance stage of quitting, ex-smokers are successfully living a smoke-free life. Staying off cigarettes for twenty-four hours is considered a quit attempt, and being a nonsmoker twelve months later is a useful definition of successful quitting. However, most smokers experience one or more relapses (smoking a cigarette) before they become nonsmokers. When this occurs, the smoker should begin the action phase again and repeat it as often as necessary to achieve his or her goal, which is maintenance of the smoke-free lifestyle (Robinson, Orleans, James, & Sutton, 1992; Prochaska & DiClemente, 1983).

African Americans are less successful at quitting smoking than are whites. In one study, African Americans were strongly motivated to quit smoking and were more likely than whites or Hispanics to report quit attempts during the previous year. However, among smokers who stayed off cigarettes for at least twenty-four hours during the previous year, fewer African Americans were nonsmokers one month later, and more of them relapsed to daily smoking or became occasional smokers (Bachman et al., 1991). Findings from another study suggest an intriguing explanation of why African Americans have difficulty quitting smoking. In the study, African Americans were reported to retain cotinine (the major [urinary] metabolite of nicotine) in their blood at significantly higher levels than whites or Mexican Americans. These observed differences were not considered to be attributable to various alternative explanations such as exposure to environmental tobacco smoke; number of smokers living in the home; number of cigarettes smoked per day; or age, sex, or weight of the smokers. Although there are still many unknowns regarding the potential role of metabolites in tobacco addiction, these findings suggest that African Americans may have a stronger physical addiction to tobacco than other groups, which may account for the greater difficulty quitting smoking (Caraballo et al., 1998).

Tobacco Use Among African American Youths

African American youths are often portrayed as having risky health habits that lead to negative outcomes such as teenage parenthood or sexually transmitted diseases. Trends in tobacco use reflect a refreshing and different image. Since the late 1970s, when annual surveys were first taken, African American youths have had significantly lower smoking rates than white youths. These early surveys were conducted with high school seniors, and it was initially argued that the racial gap was the result of higher dropout rates among African American smokers compared with the rates for white smokers or of a later age of initiation to smoking. Statistics on dropout rates did not support this assertion. Household surveys of smoking and other drug use that included a wider segment of the youth population, twelve- to seventeen-year-olds with no regard to school enrollment, found similar results (DHHS, 1998). In 1992, annual surveys of high school students were expanded to include eighth and tenth graders as well as seniors. The size and magnitude of the gap in smoking between white and African American teens was shown for all three grades (see Table 17.1) (Johnston, O'Malley, & Bachman, 1999a).

The gap between African American and white teens is even greater when daily smoking is considered (see Table 17.2). For example, daily smoking rates averaged for the years 1996–1997 were similar among white (28.9 percent) and African American (24.9 percent) youths. By the years 1979–1980, daily smoking for white youths had declined to 23.9 percent and remained at approximately the same level until 1995–1996 when it began to increase. During this same period, daily smoking among African American high school seniors declined from 17.4 percent in 1979–1980 to 4.1 percent in 1992–1993, after which it began to rise. It is evident that the gap between whites and African Americans is narrowing. However, daily smoking rates remained extremely low for African American youths—only 7.7 percent in 1998–1999 compared with 26.9 percent for white youths in those years. The public health implications of the increase in tobacco use among African American youth are major and should not be ignored. If this trend continues into early adulthood, it could undermine the potential gains that African Americans may have achieved in reducing deaths from smoking-related illnesses.

The size and consistency of the racial gap in teen smoking focused considerable attention on African American youths and possible explanations of their success in resisting tobacco use. Quantitative measures of smoking behavior and attitudes shed little light on the subject. However, a recent qualitative study of the functional value of smoking or not smoking to teens from diverse racial and ethnic backgrounds produced some useful hypotheses. The multisite study was conducted by investigators at thirteen universities. Over 1,000 teens aged twelve to seventeen, smokers and nonsmokers, participated in focus group discussions that explored the reasons why the teens smoked or did not smoke cigarettes and their images of smokers and nonsmokers. The findings of this study were provocative; both race and ethnicity and gender were important factors in distinguishing

TABLE 17.1. SMOKING IN THE PAST 30 DAYS
BY 8TH, 10TH, AND 12TH GRADERS.

	Survey Year					
	1992 (%)	1993 (%)	1995 (%)	1997 (%)	1998 (%)	1999 (%)
8th grade						
African American	5.3	6.6	8.9	10.9	10.6	10.7
White	16.2	17.8	20.7	22.8	21.5	20.1
10th grade						
African American	6.6	7.5	11.5	12.8	13.7	12.5
White	24.1	26.0	29.7	34.4	33.2	30.8
12th grade						
African American	8.7	9.5	12.9	14.3	14.9	14.9
White	31.8	33.2	36.6	40.7	41.7	40.1

Smokers are those who reported smoking one or more cigarettes during the thirty days before the survey.

Source: Johnston, O'Malley, & Bachman, 1999a.

teens' explanations and motivations for their behavior. The present discussion is restricted to observations for white and African American youths.

African American teens reported that family members expressed very strong disapproval of smoking, would not allow them to smoke in their presence, and did not allow them to smoke at home. African American females expressed the strongest negative impressions of smokers, saying that cigarette smoking damaged personal and social images and led to illicit drug use or other undesirable behaviors. This impression of smokers by African American females was supported by the responses of their peers. When asked, "How do you spend your free time after school and on weekends?" African American smokers and nonsmokers said very different things. Nonsmokers reported that they participated in a variety of activities including watching television, playing video games, reading magazines, playing sports, and hanging out with friends at their homes or in a recreation center. Smokers reported that they engaged in a smaller range of activities that included hanging out with friends, attending parties, and socializing. In addition to smoking, other risky behaviors took place at these events. Thus the association of smoking with undesirable behaviors reflected what African American girls were observing in their environments. White youths reported that their parents did not want them to smoke, but accepted it as a "lesser evil" compared to sexual activity or illicit drug use. Among white smokers, many said that their parents gave them cigarettes and allowed them to smoke at home as a way to avoid the risky environments that they might encounter otherwise (Mermelstein & Tobacco Control Network Writing Group, 1999). The results of this study suggest that white and African American youths may receive very different messages about smoking—how dangerous it is and how acceptable it is—from the normative environment that includes parents, family members, and other adults.

TABLE 17.2. DAILY SMOKING BY HIGH SCHOOL SENIORS.

Survey Year	African American (%)	White (%)
1977	24.9	28.9
1980	17.4	23.9
1985	9.9	20.4
1991	5.1	21.5
1992	4.2	20.5
1993	4.1	21.4
1995	6.1	23.9
1996	7.0	25.4
1997	7.2	27.8
1999	7.7	26.9

Note: Daily smokers are those who reported smoking one or more cigarettes per day during the thirty days before the survey.
Percentages for each year represent combined data for that year and the previous year.

Source: Johnston, O'Malley, & Bachman, 1999b.

Racial differences in behavior may simply reflect the different messages that they receive.

Tobacco Use Among African American Adults

Prior to the 1950s, more white than African American adults smoked cigarettes. A crossover occurred during the 1950s, which left African American men with a 10 percent higher smoking rate than white men. Smoking prevalence among African American women surpassed that of white women during the 1970s, but only by about three percentage points on average. Trends in smoking among all adults and among younger adults show a more complex picture. For example, among adults eighteen years and older (Table 17.3), white (34.3 percent) and African American (32.1 percent) women had similar smoking rates in 1965, but African American men (59.2 percent) smoked more than white men (50.8 percent). Among women, smoking rates have remained similar except for a period in the mid-1970s. However, African American men continued to have slightly higher smoking rates than white men from the early 1960s to the mid-1990s, although the gap narrowed each year. More recent data show that approximately a quarter of white and African American men in the United States smoke cigarettes. Reductions in smoking among African American adults ages eighteen and older were partly attributable to dramatic declines in smoking among younger adults ages eighteen to twenty-four (Table 17.4). These differences began to appear in the late 1970s and the 1980s, occurring slightly earlier for women than for men and resulting in a larger gap in smoking rates between African American and white women.

Declines in smoking among young African American adults may be related to a cohort effect in which low smoking prevalence among African American

TABLE 17.3. CURRENT SMOKING AMONG ADULTS 18 YEARS AND OLDER.

Group	1965 (%)	1974 (%)	1979 (%)	1983 (%)	1987 (%)	1991 (%)	1993 (%)	1995 (%)
				Survey Year				
African American								
Male	59.2	54.0	44.1	41.3	39.0	34.7	33.2	28.5
Female	32.1	35.9	30.8	31.8	27.2	23.1	19.8	22.0
White								
Male	50.8	41.7	36.5	34.1	30.4	27.0	27.0	26.4
Female	34.3	32.3	30.6	30.1	27.2	24.2	23.7	23.6

Source: National Center for Health Statistics. (1998). *Health United States, 1998* (DHHS Publication No. 98-1232). Hyattsville, MD: Public Health Service.

TABLE 17.4. CURRENT SMOKING AMONG ADULTS 18 TO 24 YEARS OLD.

Group	1965 (%)	1974 (%)	1979 (%)	1983 (%)	1987 (%)	1991 (%)	1993 (%)	1995 (%)
				Survey Year				
African American								
Male	62.8	54.9	40.2	34.2	24.9	15.0	19.9	14.6
Female	37.1	35.6	31.8	32.0	20.4	11.8	8.2	8.8
White								
Male	53.0	40.8	34.3	32.5	29.7	25.1	30.4	28.4
Female	38.4	34.0	34.5	36.5	27.8	25.1	26.8	24.9

Source: National Center for Health Statistics. (1998). *Health United States, 1998* (DHHS Publication No. 98-1232). Hyattsville, MD: Public Health Service.

youths is carried over to early adulthood. If this trend continues over the next several decades, it will result in further declines in overall adult smoking and will finally reduce the disproportionate burden in illness and death from smoking-related diseases that African Americans have borne for so long.

Health Consequences of Tobacco Use

More than 400,000 Americans die prematurely each year from heart disease, cancer, emphysema, and other diseases as a result of tobacco use. African Americans, who are second to American Indians and Alaskan Natives in cigarette smoking prevalence, currently bear the greatest health burden in terms of incidence and mortality rates. Approximately 45,000 African Americans die each year from tobacco-related diseases, representing a greater magnitude of disease risk relative to whites. An explanation of this racial disparity is complex and involves other factors besides tobacco use. Smoking is an important contributor to the difference, however (DHHS, 1998).

Cancer. African American men have high rates of tobacco-related cancers in comparison to males in other population groups in the United States. Death rates for African American men from respiratory cancers surpassed the rates for white men between 1950 and 1960 and have continued to be higher—a fact that may be related to the increased smoking rates of African Americans that occurred in the 1950s and the higher quit rates of white males after the 1950s. The respiratory cancer death rates of black women and white women have been similarly patterned. Since the 1990s, death rates from malignant neoplasms of the respiratory system decreased for African American males but remain significantly higher than death rates for white and African American women or for white males (see Table 17.5) (DHHS, 1998).

Chronic Obstructive Pulmonary Disease. The morbidity and mortality rates for chronic obstructive pulmonary disease (COPD) are lower for African Americans than for whites. The prevalence of self-reported chronic bronchitis and emphysema for African Americans and whites is shown in Table 17.6. African Americans and whites report similar experiences with bronchitis among the forty-five- to sixty-four-year-old age group, but there are clearly more cases of bronchitis reported among whites than African Americans in the sixty-five and older age group. The prevalence of self-reported emphysema shows a different pattern. There are fewer cases reported among younger (forty-five- to sixty-four-year-old) age groups, but whites have a significantly higher prevalence than African Americans. This racial gap virtually disappears among the older age group, with African Americans and whites reporting similar experiences with emphysema. African Americans are also less likely than whites to die of COPD. One strong hypothesis explaining this (unexpected) difference is the possible relationship of COPD to rates of *ever smokers*

TABLE 17.5. DEATHS FROM MALIGNANT NEOPLASMS (PER 100,000).

Group	Survey Year 1990	Survey Year 1995
African American		
Men	91.0	80.5
Women	27.5	27.8
White		
Men	59.0	53.7
Women	26.5	27.9

Source: DHHS, 1998.

TABLE 17.6. PREVALENCE OF SELF-REPORTED ILLNESS (PER 1,000).

	Age	
Group	45–64	65+
Chronic bronchitis		
African American	55.2	42.7
White	59.7	73.8
Emphysema		
African American	3.6	41.5
White	13.8	46.1

Source: DHHS, 1998.

(Mannino, Brown, & Giovino, 1997). For example, the aggregated percentage for the years 1987, 1988, 1990, and 1991 of African Americans who were ever smokers was 45.5 percent compared with 53.3 percent of whites (DHHS, 1998). Among former smokers, whites are also more likely than African Americans to have a longer lifetime duration of smoking, which may increase adverse health effects.

Coronary Heart Disease. Studies that examined differences between African Americans and whites in coronary heart disease (CHD) have shown conflicting results. In one study, a cohort of men was followed in Evans County from 1960 through 1980. African Americans had an overall lower rate of death from CHD than whites, with a ratio of 0.86 (Tyroler et al., 1984). Other studies have reported lower death rates for African American men than for white men, but slightly higher rates for African American women than for white women (DHHS, 1998). Cumulative incidence rates of fatal CHD were observed to be higher for African American men and women than for white men and women, but cumulative incidence rates of nonfatal CHD were higher among whites. The epidemiological profile is further complicated by the higher mortality rates for African Americans than for whites among middle-aged adults but lower mortality rates for elderly African Americans compared to elderly whites (National Center for Health Statistics [NCHS], 1996). A clearer understanding of differences in CHD incidence and mortality between African Americans and whites and the associated factors of age, gender, tobacco use, and comorbidity, requires additional research.

Cerebrovascular Disease. African Americans are more likely than whites to die from cerebrovascular disease (DHHS, 1998). For example, from 1992 to 1994, the rate of death per 100,000 was 53.1 for African American men and 40.6 for African American women but only 26.3 per 100,000 for white men and 22.6 per 100,000 for white women.

The Public Health Response to Tobacco

The public health effort to curb tobacco use and the unnecessary deaths and disability associated with tobacco is taking place on the national, state, and community levels.

National and State Initiatives

The unique qualities of tobacco—its deep historical roots in the life and economy of America, its devastating impact on the health and well-being of Americans—called for an aggressive response from the professionals charged to protect the public's health. They have embraced the environmental model for tobacco prevention and control as a conceptual framework that promotes a comprehensive, dynamic, and multifaceted approach to social change. The model employs diverse strategies including public education, media advocacy, and policy interventions targeting excise taxes, youth access to tobacco, restrictions on environmental tobacco smoke, and industry marketing of tobacco products in order to change the behavior of individuals as well as the broader environment in which they live. These strategies have been implemented through several national programs (DHHS, 1991).

The National Cancer Institute's Project ASSIST (American Stop Smoking Intervention Study) provided funding to seventeen states for the purpose of promoting statewide tobacco control coalitions, developing comprehensive tobacco control initiatives, and refocusing tobacco control program activities toward environmental policy approaches. In the first four years of this program, majority communities in the seventeen states funded developed capacity and infrastructure to carry out activities that would reduce the burden of tobacco on the health of their citizens. It was assumed that these broad-based activities would be sufficient to mobilize African American communities to become fully involved in the tobacco control movement. However, African Americans and members of other communities of color perceived that they were poorly integrated into tobacco control activities in many states and at the national level and expressed their dissatisfaction with this situation. Consequently, new strategies were adopted that allowed greater input and leadership from people of color to develop approaches that fit the needs of their cultures and environments (Robinson & Headen, 1999).

The Robert Wood Johnson Foundation and American Medical Association also launched broad-based initiatives to reduce the burden of tobacco use. The Smokeless States Program was a statewide effort that focused on policy initiatives and related education and media advocacy activities. In addition, the Centers for Disease Control and Prevention (CDC), Office on Smoking and Health, funded thirty-three states and U.S. territories to initiate tobacco control activities. However, we assert that these programs had many of the same limitations as the NCI's Project ASSIST. African Americans benefited from the activities that were carried out, but did not build capacity and infrastructure within their communities to carry out their own initiatives. This capacity and infrastructure are defined by the presence of the following elements: (1) targeted tobacco control research studies on African Americans, conducted by African American researchers, (2) targeted tobacco control programs and materials, (3) dedicated leadership, (4) organizations able to carry out tobacco prevention and control initiatives, and (5) networks of leaders and organizations experienced in tobacco control issues. Examples of states where African American communities have made progress in capacity building and infrastructure development are North Carolina and South Carolina, funded under the ASSIST program, and California, which provides substantial ongoing support to all communities of color (Robinson, Shelton, et al., 1995; Robinson & Headen, 1999).

A national initiative funded by the Centers for Disease Control and Prevention under the auspices of the Office on Smoking and Health was explicitly designed to build capacity and infrastructure in national organizations representing communities of color, youths, women, and agricultural workers. The results have been credible. African American leadership and organizations have participated in the elimination of the X cigarette, organized the successful Say No to Menthol Joe Community Campaign, partnered with the Office on Smoking and Health in a national communication campaign targeting African American smokers and making available via an 800 number the *Pathways to Freedom Smoking Cessation Guide,* and joined with the Summit Health Coalition in educating Congressional Minority Caucus members on the principles in legislation that would meet the specific needs of the African American community. One weakness in this program was the limited development of community-based organizations with related missions. However, the resources created by this national organizations initiative have facilitated the emergence of African American leaders who have national standing and who contribute to a dialogue concerning strategic next steps in the ongoing tobacco control struggle. These individuals, along with the handful of leaders who have emerged from state initiatives, have also produced programs that provide lessons to guide efforts in other states. The success of such tobacco control initiatives is a validation of the critical need for such efforts to ensure that capacity and infrastructure development are prioritized and supported (Robinson, Shelton, et al., 1995; Robinson & Headen, 1999).

Community-Based Initiatives

The inclusion of African Americans and other communities of color in the tobacco control movement as an explicit policy objective is very recent, and community-level initiatives have been woefully underfunded. In spite of this obstacle, African Americans have achieved notable accomplishments on the community level.

The Uptown Coalition. Black communities have carried out successful community-based campaigns to counter targeted advertising and marketing of tobacco products to African Americans. The first initiative was in Detroit in the mid-1980s, but a more crucial one occurred in Philadelphia in 1990. R. J. Reynolds developed a cigarette brand called Uptown, which was specifically designed for African American smokers. It was second only to the company's unfiltered Camel brand in nicotine content. Uptown was presented in a handsome black and gold pack with the cigarettes packaged upside down. It was believed that this practice favored the preference of working-class African Americans, who frequently held manual labor jobs, for having a borrower take a cigarette from the bottom to avoid soiling the others in the pack. The theme of the Reynolds campaign was "Uptown, the taste, the place." Philadelphia was one of two cities where the brand was to be test marketed (Robinson, Shelton, et al., 1995; Robinson & Headen, 1999).

The African American community in Philadelphia organized to protest against the Uptown campaign. It was a historic event, as this was the first time that the African American community had unified and launched a serious effort against the tobacco industry. The Uptown coalition was broad based, and its leaders included a public health researcher, a member of the clergy, a communications specialist, and a medical doctor. The primary theme of the protest was the right of African Americans to choose the products that would enter their community. Other themes included the excessive tobacco advertising in the community, the lack of empowerment, the threat to African American youths, the lethal nature of cigarettes in terms of tar and nicotine content, and the appropriation of community symbols, such as the name Uptown, which was a popular theatre frequented by African Americans in Philadelphia.

The Uptown coalition was historic because it was a movement by and for African Americans and led by African American leaders. In addition, the protest produced several important outcomes. First, it highlighted the importance of developing community-based tobacco control initiatives that are tailored to fit the social contexts of diverse cultural settings. It also emphasized the importance of diversifying the leadership of the tobacco control movement and the unexpected benefits obtained when communities of color choose their own leaders and methods for addressing tobacco control issues (Robinson, Shelton, et al., 1995).

The 'X' Cigarette. The tobacco industry suffered a second defeat in marketing another cigarette especially targeted to African Americans. In 1995 in Boston, a small independent distributor, Stowecraft Distributors, began marketing a cigarette called 'X' in a red, black, and green pack. The company claimed to be unaware that this 'X' could make people think of Malcolm X, an African American activist for social justice, or that the colors had significance as symbols of liberation for some African Americans. Leaders of a local organization, Churches Organized to Stop Tobacco (COST), became aware of the sale of the 'X' cigarette and contacted tobacco control activists in Philadelphia and California to plan a response. They launched a national campaign and were successful in stopping the sale of 'X' cigarettes. An important outgrowth of this effort was the establishment of a national communications network and the demonstrated capacity of African Americans in tobacco control to coordinate and implement successful media and advocacy campaigns (Robinson & Headen, 1999).

The Say No to Menthol Joe Community Crusade. A third demonstration of the impact that community action by African Americans can have on the tobacco industry occurred in 1996. New menthol brands were developed specifically for African American smokers. Philip Morris developed Marlboro menthols and R. J. Reynolds developed Camel menthols. However, the Reynolds Company decided to introduce its product with fanfare, and it attracted the attention of NAAAPI (the National Association of African Americans for Positive Imagery), an organization that emerged shortly after the Uptown victory in Philadelphia. This organization began tracking the activity of the Camel menthol brand to determine whether it was being targeted specifically to African Americans. It soon became apparent that Camel menthols were being advertised separately from the non-menthol brand and in predominantly black communities and in black media. In January 1997, R. J. Reynolds rolled out a national advertising campaign for Camel menthols, and NAAAPI alerted colleagues in several major cities to launch a response. Walgreen's stores were a major outlet for Camel menthols in Chicago, and a campaign to boycott these stores led to the withdrawal of the product from the shelves not only in Chicago but in the 2,256 stores across the nation. R. J. Reynolds subsequently recalled all advertising featuring the Joe Camel character from U.S. markets. Camel menthols continue to be sold, but without the Joe Camel logo (Robinson & Headen, 1999).

Prevention Strategies Targeted to African Americans: Ujima!

In the past the low prevalence of smoking among African American youths was sometimes interpreted to mean that prevention programs were not needed in African American communities. The alarming rise in smoking among African American males in the 1990s has dispelled this idea and emphasized the need for a better understanding of African American teen smoking patterns and for prevention programs tailored to these youths' history, culture, and lifestyles. As a consequence of the underfunding of programs for communities of color in general, few resources have been devoted to this effort. The Ujima! African American Youth Initiative in North Carolina is one exception. This program is designed to be a first step in mobilizing the African American community by empowering youth organizations as tobacco control advocates and community activists. Their charge is to educate their peers about the dangers of tobacco and the benefits of being a nonsmoker, to educate their parents and other adults, to conduct community projects on tobacco control, to receive training in tobacco use prevention and reduction, and to serve as trainers or teen representatives at various statewide tobacco control events. A strength of the Ujima! initiative is that youths are trained in groups that return intact to their local communities and have sufficient numbers to actually implement projects. Adult leaders also participate in training workshops, sometimes joining the youths and at other times concentrating on topics tailored to their own needs and broader responsibilities. An important benefit of this approach is that many of the behavioral challenges of working with youths—maintaining discipline, sustaining motivation, reinforcing lessons learned, supervising community projects—are the responsibility of adult group leaders who view these activities as complementing their organizational mission.

Ujima is a Swahili word that means "collective work and responsibility." The term is one of the seven Nguzo Saba, or principles, associated with Kwanzaa, an African American cultural holiday that is celebrated from December 26 to January 1 (Karenga, 1998). The initiative itself was designed and implemented by the African American Action Team of North Carolina Project ASSIST for the purposes of creating capacity and infrastructure in the African American community and of encouraging independent action to initiate tobacco control programs in the future. Members of this coalition included public health professionals, community volunteers, and adult leaders of community-based youth groups. A researcher trained in social and community psychology and public health served as a consultant to the Action Team. The foundation of the Ujima! African American Youth Initiative is the skill-building training that youths and their adult leaders receive during summer retreats and follow-up midyear retreats in late winter. The retreat curriculum, titled Ujima! African American Youths Collectively Working for a Smoke Free Community, incorporates four other principles associated with Kwanzaa to describe components of the training model. Plenary sessions attended by youths and their adult leaders are called *Umoja,* which means "to strive for and maintain harmony." Skill-building workshops are called *Kujichagulia,* which means self-determination, "to define ourselves" or "to speak for ourselves." Culturally based entertainment and expression is referred to as *Kuumba,* meaning "creativity." *Imani,* or "faith," is an implicit component of the training model that allows participants to acknowledge the importance of religion in African American life. The curriculum also includes training modules on the topics of media literacy, addressing policy through media advocacy, leadership development, the epidemiology of tobacco use among African Americans and other communities of color, preventing tobacco use, slavery and tobacco, American Indians and tobacco, and communication and presentation skills. Youths also present outcomes of ongoing or recently completed community projects and develop action plans for future projects. Activities in the curriculum that encourage positive personal, cultural, and group identity include formal and informal participation in sports and performances by African American storytellers, dancers, and musicians.

The significance of the Ujima! African American Youth Initiative is that it includes many of the elements for building capacity and infrastructure that will allow African Americans in North Carolina to develop independent programs in tobacco control well into the future. The African American Action Team represented a core of experts in tobacco control who in turn formed a network of advocates and organizations that could conduct tobacco control initiatives. With the assistance of researchers and expert consultants, the action team developed training modules that were culturally appropriate to African American youths. The Ujima! youth initiative is an excellent example of how a community development approach to tobacco control can empower communities of color to actualize their potential to mobilize their organizations and people.

The Ujima! African American Youth Initiative achieved the following outcomes over a four-year period: (1) institutionalized the inclusion of African Americans as key stakeholders in tobacco control efforts in North Carolina, and increased the number of individuals available to serve in this role; (2) promoted national goals for diversity and inclusiveness by encouraging action team members, youths, and their adult leaders to participate in national tobacco control conferences and events; (3) developed and pilot tested a unique, culturally appropriate tobacco use prevention model that mobilizes African American youths as tobacco control advocates, trainers, and activists; (4) developed a core of experts in tobacco control among action team members, youths, and their adult leaders; and (5) assisted youths to organize an African American Action Team Youth Advisory Council, which receives in-depth training and has greater responsibilities in the areas of media advocacy, training other youths in the state, and participating in national tobacco-use prevention activities.

The Ujima! African American Youth Initiative has greatly enriched North Carolina Project ASSIST and has established a blueprint for implementing prevention programs with African American youths in other states. The Ujima! initiative also served as an inspiration for a statewide summit on teen smoking prevention and a grant from the Robert Wood Johnson Foundation to establish four media centers throughout the state to train youths as media advocates for tobacco-use prevention and reduction. Ujima! was further recognized by the Robert Wood Johnson Foundation as a recipient of an award under the Innovators in Substance Abuse Prevention program which included funds to support its national dissemination. Innovative programs like the Ujima! African American Youth Initiative, which produce substantial outcomes and benefits with minimal resources, highlight the critical need for dedicated funding for tobacco control in communities of color and showcase the enormous talent waiting to use those resources in creative ways.

Community-Based Smoking Cessation Strategies

Educating the public about the dangers of smoking and tobacco use was one of the initial steps that launched a national tobacco control movement. The first surgeon general's report on smoking linked smoking to lung cancer in men (U.S. Department of Health, Education and Welfare, 1964). The Office of the Surgeon General has since released new reports annually documenting population trends in tobacco use, morbidity and mortality from smoking-related illnesses, and new scientific evidence about the harmful effects of tobacco on health. These reports have been effective in convincing many smokers to quit, but most of these individuals have been members of the majority population. Large-scale efforts to promote quitting in communities of color have not been conducted. However, African American researchers and tobacco control activists have made significant strides in developing comprehensive and culturally appropriate programs and interventions in the area of smoking cessation. One important example is the Pathways to Freedom program.

The Pathways to Freedom Program

The Pathways to Freedom (PTF) Smoking Cessation Program was developed at Fox Chase Cancer Center in Philadelphia, Pennsylvania, and it was the first effort that employed the components of a comprehensive tobacco control initiative to target the African American community (Robinson, Orleans, James, & Sutton, 1992). Participants in PTF receive a self-help guide and video. The primary focus of the guide is to help people quit smoking by using methods proven to be effective for African Americans and all smokers. The guide also analyzes the advertising and promotion tactics of the tobacco industry and emphasizes the social need to support a smoke-free lifestyle by changing environmental norms and promoting policies that help accomplish this goal. The PTF program has been very effective in mobilizing African American leaders and residents in many local communities across the United States to become involved in tobacco control issues. Church-based programs have also adopted Pathways to Freedom, and efforts to tailor PTF by incorporating Bible-based prompts are being carried out to enhance its relevance for smokers who participate in quitting programs in church settings. The Congress of National Black Churches and the National Medical Association also support the use of PTF in their tobacco control initiatives (Robinson & Headen, 1999).

One study that evaluated the outcome of participating in the PTF program reported a twelve-month quit rate of 15 percent for African American smokers using the PTF guide compared with a quit rate of 8.8 percent for smokers who received usual care (a self-help smoking cessation guide, *Clearing the Air,* that was not designed for African American smokers). The attainment of such high quit rates for a self-help program may have resulted from the methods used to recruit smokers. Studies have shown that radio is an effective medium for disseminating information to African Americans. In this study, paid radio ads with culturally appropriate content were aired in targeted communities during a broad range of time slots, including early morning hours. This process was designed to attract African American listeners and may have resulted in a larger audience for the ads including more smokers. The high quit rates with the Pathways program also may have been a response to a reservoir of need in the African American community where cessation services may not be widely available and culturally appropriate services of any kind are absent. The PTF program has been so successful that the American Cancer Society adopted it as its cessation materials of choice for African Americans and collaborated with the Office on Smoking and Health to disseminate PTF (Robinson & Headen, 1999).

Comprehensive Tobacco Control Initiatives That Incorporate PTF

The PTF program has received additional research support from the Office on Smoking and Health and the National Cancer Institute for the development of cessation programs tailored to health care settings (provider counseling protocol) and to community environments (grassroots cessation initiatives) (Headen & Berman, 1996). These programs are a part of an emerging smoking cessation program called Uhuru-No Smoke, a toolbox of smoking cessation strategies for African Americans. The provider counseling protocol enhances opportunities for physicians and other health care providers to counsel African American smokers to quit. Its design is informed by research on cessation and features of previous effective clinic-based cessation interventions (Braithwaite et al., 1997). A unique feature of the protocol is its dual function as both a passive and an active intervention for smokers. Studies show that 90 percent of smokers who quit do so on their own without the help of programs (Fiore, Novotny, et al., 1990; DHHS, 1998). The provider counseling protocol is designed to facilitate self-quitting by exposing smokers to messages and materials that help them to progress along the continuum of behavioral change from precontemplation (not thinking about smoking), through contemplation, action, and on to maintenance of nonsmoker status. As an active intervention, the protocol provides a comprehensive training manual that is based on Agency for Health Care Policy and Research (AHCPR) guidelines and supporting materials that serve as cues to stimulate providers to counsel their patients (Fiore, Bailey, et al., 1996). The protocol also contains additional elements that incorporate the PTF smoking cessation program: (1) a poster that displays counseling tips from the PTF guide, matched to the stages of readiness to quit smoking; (2) a calendar of African American family portraits framed by messages on the benefits of quitting to the smoker and his or her loved ones; and (3) a behavioral prescription pad that offers PTF stage-matched tips on quitting and relapse prevention. The behavioral prescription is designed to add potency to the counseling session by reinforcing the verbal message. The provider signs the behavioral prescription tip sheet, tears it off, and hands it to the patient in a manner similar to that used for medical prescriptions (Robinson & Headen, 1999).

The materials for the provider counseling protocol have now been extended to include a smoking cessation counseling protocol for pregnant women, also based on the PTF guide. This component allows the patient and her provider to examine myths about pregnancy and smoking that the patient may hold, examine the reality of these myths, and identify strategies for eliminating the myths as barriers to behavioral change. On her own the patient is expected to set a quit date, to quit smoking, and to engage in the behaviors that will allow her to remain smoke free. Materials for this protocol include a tabletop flip chart for the provider, an identical take-home companion brochure for the patient, and a take-home brochure for a significant other with tips for supporting the quitting process (Robinson & Headen, 1999).

Churches and other community-based organizations frequently become involved in smoking cessation activities to help their members and loved ones to quit smoking. There are few guidelines, however, to assist them in identifying specific roles and activities that fit their organizational objectives and available resources. The PTF Community-Based Smoking Cessation Protocol was developed for this purpose. It provides a blueprint for implementing smoking cessation activities by community volunteers that help individual smokers to quit and support tobacco-free lifestyles. Specifically, the protocol achieves the following: (1) identifies goals and objectives related to smoking cessation that are achievable by community organizations, and (2) outlines the steps involved in accomplishing specific outcome objectives. More important, the protocol supports a multistage approach to program implementation and seeks to improve on the train-the-trainer model by tailoring the curriculum content to a workforce of community volunteers. The smoking cessation content of the program may be used alone or in conjunction with a broader program of lifestyle change that includes nutrition and physical activity. Distinctive features of the smoking cessation toolbox for African American communities include the following: (1) a three-part train-the-trainer curriculum that reflects a staged program implementation process that encourages reassessment and redesign at various intervals, (2) a brief smoking cessation counseling protocol tailored to nonprofessionals that facilitates understanding of the process of quitting, (3) case studies of hypothetical smokers whose circumstances reflect themes found in African American smoking patterns and barriers to quitting, (4) small-group exercises that allow participants to identify stages of readiness to quit smoking and to practice counseling smokers to quit, and (5) a resource manual that describes case studies of cessation activities conducted in community settings and methods of evaluating outcomes.

The PTF Community-Based Smoking Cessation Program promotes a comprehensive approach to tobacco-use prevention and reduction and encourages community organizations to view their specific cessation activities within a broader framework that may include the following activities: (1) educating the community on the causes of cigarette smoking, its health consequences, and the unique behaviors of African American smokers, (2) recruiting smokers to quit and identifying resources in the community that can facilitate this process, (3) distributing smoking cessation materials to smokers who want to quit including the PTF guide for African American smokers, (4) developing mass-media campaigns that support community norms for a smoke-free lifestyle, (5) designing activities that facilitate cessation by individual smokers and reward them for success, (6) encouraging clinics and health care providers to counsel their patients who smoke to quit, and (7) expanding the availability of cessation services by using the PTF Community-Based Smoking Cessation Protocol to train individuals and organizations to implement smoking cessation activities and programs. These activities help communities accomplish the overall program goal of providing ongoing opportunities for smokers to quit or to progress along the continuum of behavioral change that leads to quitting. Additionally, community norms supporting smoke-free lifestyles will be strengthened, and the gap in access to cessation services for African American smokers will be reduced (Robinson & Headen, 1999).

The smoking cessation initiatives included in the Uhuru-No Smoke program incorporate the PTF program and offer a unique model for the design of comprehensive smoking cessation programs targeted to the African American community. The foundation is culturally competent materials that incorporate the cultural, historical, contextual, and geographic themes that shape community attitudes about tobacco and smoking. Only such truly comprehensive programs will provide training for counselors in smoking cessation techniques, inform them about the special needs of smokers in the African American community (and about responding to that community's heterogeneity), and provide strategies for designing activities that support a nonsmoking lifestyle in both the home and the community.

Pathways to Freedom has served as a critical component in designing and implementing capacity- and infrastructure-building initiatives in the African American community. It has reinforced the work of young researchers in tobacco control and stimulated funding agencies to target resources to developing PTF beyond its initial stage. It has proven effective in enabling African American leaders, organizations, and churches across a broad spectrum to use PTF in their initiatives. Most important, PTF has evolved as an identifiable product that is now broadly recognized and is a source of pride for African Americans involved in tobacco control.

A New Paradigm for the New Millennium: The Community Development Model for Public Health Applications

The critical issues in smoking and health facing the African American community relate to its readiness to respond to the emergent tobacco control environment of the twenty-first century. The tobacco control settlement is the most critical factor in the equation. The next five years will witness a flurry of activity and priority setting as decisions are made about policies, programs, and resource allocations that will impact tobacco control for the next quarter century or more. African Americans will be best served if they are able to engage the important players in their state tobacco control environments with statements of need and proposed programs and budgets that will allow them to implement comprehensive programs in their communities. Unfortunately, minimal work has been done to develop such a plan, either for the national community of African Americans or for communities of African Americans within their respective states.

We offer a solution to this problem by introducing a novel approach that can be used as a blueprint for program planning and implementation, resource allocation, and process and outcome evaluation to reduce disparities between majority populations and communities of color. The Community Development Model for Public Health Applications offers an approach that is different from the traditional way that public health professionals have thought about resource allocation and the role of race or ethnic group membership or the role of community as a defining category for allocation purposes (Robinson, 2000). The Community Development Model reflects the philosophy of the World Health Organization, which states that the concept of health involves more than just the presence or absence of illness. Health should be considered holistically, viewing individuals within the social contexts in which they live and incorporating the life experiences that are so important to shaping health outcomes and behaviors. These ideas have been described as the health promotion approach to pubic health that emphasizes strengthening communities, building supportive environments, and promoting political action and policies that improve health. Health promotion is a "people-centered" approach (Raeburn & Rootman, 1997; Raphael & Bryant, 2000). The concepts, relationships, and proposed action steps associated with this model, and also the barriers that must be overcome in adopting it, are outlined in the following discussion.

The population approach to health originates from epidemiological methods of analysis and the values that accompany a research approach that is often devoid of social or political context (Raeburn & Rootman, 1997). From a philosophical perspective, it contrasts sharply with the health promotion approach. Health is viewed as the absence of illness and is measured in terms of collections of individuals and not in terms of the social systems that they live in. The often-unstated values underlying the population approach are conservative in nature and support the status quo. Social policy is not perceived to be an appropriate strategy for enhancing the health of the public. The thinking that accompanies the population approach to public health presents significant barriers to adopting the ideas supported by the Community Development Model that must be overcome.

Barriers to Adopting the Model in the Public Health Environment

The first barrier to adopting the model is represented by issues involving the epidemiological methods used to analyze key questions in public health and the assumptions and cognitive biases that influence how answers to these questions are framed. First, statistical modeling in epidemiology, as in other fields, is limited in its ability to reflect what happens in the real world. Scientists who develop these models go to great lengths to include all the variables relevant to predicting or explaining the behavior or outcome of interest, but this method allows them to make only approximations and estimates. When public health professionals apply the findings from these models too literally, errors in conclusions and subsequent policy and program objectives may occur. One excellent example of this appears in the debate over the cause of racial gaps in various health indicators. Efforts to explain these gaps employ statistical models that often include race and socioeconomic status in the same equation. In this context, the variable race is sometimes nonsignificant, leading many to conclude that race can be ignored and that socioeconomic status can be used as the relevant category in designing and implementing public health applications and programs. Yet the personal and community experiences of many Americans suggest that race is a very important factor that influences a broad spectrum of issues either directly or indirectly. A health promotion perspective would highlight these often qualitative community-level variables and incorporate them as central elements of problem definition, analysis, and solutions in public health.

The nonsignificance of race as a variable in epidemiological analyses may simply reflect profound differences in our ability to measure the critical components of the concept of race and our ability to measure class or status, especially when the latter is measured by income or education. The latter are quite tangible; race is not. In addition, relying on socioeconomic indicators reflects a certain tunnel vision that encourages drawing conclusions based on assessment of statistical results rather than making a more complex evaluation that relates the importance of race to the communities in which people live. It is simpler to rely on statistics, but decisions and resulting intervention strategies based solely on statistical outcomes ignore the reality that people with low socioeconomic status continue to live in geographic areas that are defined by race. Segregated living patterns continue to be the norm in American society, with estimates of 70 percent of the population residing in de facto segregated geographic areas. In essence, prevention strategies must consider the communities or locations in which people live in addition to the particular educational or economic strata that categorize individuals living within these communities.

Comprehensive prevention strategies will need to target community and race and build racial and ethnic communities' capacity and infrastructure. These efforts, if carried out systematically, will eliminate population gaps, especially when they are employed as additions to intervention efforts that target population strata. The goal is not *either/or* but *both/and*, with the important principle asserting that individuals require "people-centered" interventions that recognize their race and community membership as well as their characteristics associated with socioeconomic status. In essence, the significance of race is only partially dependent on multivariate statistical analysis. Ultimately, the final decision must address the type of intervention deemed appropriate to address the defined problem. Eliminating population disparities depends on comprehensive efforts to build capacity and infrastructure, and these strategies specifically address the needs of racial or ethnic groups and the communities in which they reside. These interventions and strategies must therefore be culturally competent and based on the underlying determinants of history, culture, context, and geography.

The second barrier to addressing this community development model is the way that problems and solutions in public health are framed. Researchers, policymakers, and practitioners exhibit a limited ability to think about public health problems holistically, even though that is often the goal. For example, it is easier to conceptualize socioeconomic status than race and community because the former can be transformed into concrete indicators of education and income. This fits well with the reductionism inherent in epidemiological methods. However, from our perspectives, race and community are best viewed as whole entities, and we posit that they are determined by the history, culture, social context, and geography associated with a particular group of people living in a given location. Lacking holistic models of conceptualization and analysis, researchers tend to frame both the problem and the solution in disaggregated or fragmented constructs. This fragmentation robs problem and solution statements of contextual meaning and threatens the validity of epidemiological analyses and of behavioral research and programs based on them.

A third barrier to adopting this community development model is the propensity for public health professionals to think about problems in a simplistic, one-dimensional way that fails to take into account the complexity that is necessary to understanding and prediction. This complexity is especially problematic because it involves understanding the history, culture, context, and geography related to race and ethnicity and that understanding rests largely on qualitative measures. Political systems as well as scientific methodologies tend to ignore the consciousness inherent in collectivities such as race and community and prefer to frame social reality as a manifestation of individual life experience that can be measured and quantified. It is then easy to evolve laws and regulations that ignore society's responsibility for the well-being of communities and races and to emphasize instead society's responsibility to individuals. Consistent with the population approach to public health, the social context of health and illness is ignored. To summarize, current thinking and methods of analyzing problems in public health reflect a population-focused approach that emphasizes individual characteristics and behaviors and may oversimplify reality by ignoring the social context of health and illness. These ideas represent significant barriers to the adoption of our community development model that represents a more "people-centered" approach (Raeburn & Rootman, 1997; Raphael & Bryant, 2000).

Concepts, Relationships, and Action Steps in the Community Development Model

Race and community are key elements of self-definition for many groups in America, and they also define the way in which members of the majority population relate to other groups. Therefore, allocating funds to communities of color should be a high priority in the tobacco control movement for the explicit purpose of empowering these communities to develop capacity and infrastructure to implement comprehensive tobacco control initiatives in each state and to coordinate activities at the national level. These ideas can be summarized with the following four activities that reflect the philosophy of the Community Development Model: (1) promoting communities rather than individuals as a unit of analysis in public health, (2) including race as a concept in statistical analyses, decision making, and all activities that must reflect accurate representations of the real world, (3) assessing community capacity and infrastructure in making decisions about resources needed to achieve objectives for comprehensive tobacco control programs, and (4) explicitly incorporating the goal of eliminating disparities between majority communities and communities of color in decisions regarding resource allocation. A more detailed discussion of each of these concepts follows.

The appropriate unit of analysis in public health is the community environment, which is both complex and unique from one setting to the next. In the community development model, community is viewed as having elements that are homogeneous and elements that are heterogeneous in terms of racial or ethnic composition or other characteristics of people in groups. The heterogeneity of communities is evident when a more holistic view is taken. For example, communities that are homogeneous with respect to race or ethnicity may be heterogeneous with respect to income or education. An appreciation of the ways in which heterogeneity can influence communities suggests that different programs and interventions would be designed for Asians of Japanese descent and Asians of Vietnamese descent. Thus considering these multiple dimensions of community can enhance the effectiveness of programs implemented and may be essential to achieving the long-term goal of eliminating disparities among population groups.

Concepts that influence how community is defined include history, geography, culture, and context. Communities and racial and ethnic groups differ from one another in the way in which these four components interact. The result in each case is a unique environment that shapes behaviors and outcomes of the particular racial or ethnic groups or communities and the multiplicity of groups that are a part of it. One's perception of community is culturally competent when race is considered to be a key element of community and is addressed at this aggregate level. Public health professionals must broaden their thinking and allow themselves to design programs that begin to take these complex factors into account. The success of this effort will define the extent to which these programs will be culturally competent, that is, congruent with the history, geography, culture, and context of specific groups. When a community is viewed holistically and its heterogeneity is considered, the criteria for achieving cultural competence is more complex. However, the value of these programs may be difficult to assess using epidemiological methods that underestimate the significance of race. The solution to this problem is to use the results of epidemiological analyses as a guide rather than as a blueprint for designing and redesigning programs, to recognize the inherent limits of reductionism, and to use creativity and findings from qualitative research to design programs and interventions that more appropriately reflect the complex environments that people live in.

Regardless of the outcomes of epidemiological analyses, race is always a significant concept in the real world. For many Americans, race is a central feature of their personal and social identity and greatly influences how they behave and how they organize their environments. Homogeneity of racial and ethnic groups is still a feature of both physical and psychological communities. Race, defined as a discrete category (black, white, and so on), is an operational concept in public health that may satisfy the needs of researchers to analyze problems with methods that rely on quantification, but may not reflect what "race" means to many people nor capture how it might be measured. At a minimum, history, culture, context, and geography influence the meaning of race. These factors also affect what it means to categorize people into specific races, and how doing so has an impact on problem definition, analysis, and the development of public health applications.

Reducing health disparities between majority communities and communities of color must take into account the resources available in community settings to stimulate the changes necessary to achieve these outcomes. The objective of tobacco control is to design comprehensive programs that result in environmental and behavioral changes that reduce smoking and lower morbidity and mortality from smoking-related illnesses. An intermediate goal on the way to accomplishing this is to provide subgroups and communities with the capacity and infrastructure that is needed to achieve this goal—that is, the resources required to implement programs, sustain them over time, and expand them for greater coverage and improved results. Communities with high capacity have the following characteristics: (1) a body of research that identifies the factors critical to behavioral change and program success, (2) programs and models that can be implemented, (3) leaders in a variety of fields including science, public health, and medicine who are also involved in tobacco control, (4) organizations that can provide the necessary services, and (5) networks of trained public health professionals who can design and implement tobacco control programs.

In order to eliminate disparities between majority populations and communities of color in factors important to tobacco control, the allocation of resources to communities and ethnic groups must take this policy explicitly into account. That is, communities should be assessed along the five dimensions of capacity and infrastructure just listed. Communities judged to have low capacity and infrastructure should receive an infusion of resources that would allow them to improve on all dimensions. Communities that are high in infrastructure and capacity need fewer resources to maintain existing programs and to develop new ones. Groups that have disparities in resources, health outcomes, or other dimensions, such as low income in comparison to majority groups, but do not function as communities in a geographic or psychological sense will require less-comprehensive efforts related to building capacity and infrastructure. The basic point is that the lion's share of the resources for tobacco control should not continue to go into communities that already have high capacity and infrastructure at the expense of other communities, usually those of color, that have considerably lower capacity and infrastructure. In addition, policymakers should not be confused by the array of multicultural groups demonstrating disparities but should be guided by assumptions that help to define communities more coherently and by assessments that make explicit existing levels of capacity and infrastructure related to tobacco prevention and control.

Finally, the process of reducing disparities between the majority population and communities of color should take place in an atmosphere of trust and with a philosophical commitment to multiculturalism, inclusiveness, and cultural competence. Indeed, cultural competence is best viewed as protocols, materials, or images that reflect and resonate with the history, geography, culture, and context of the community that is being targeted. Given the abundance of resources now available for tobacco control, eliminating population disparities in services, resource allocation, and health outcomes is entirely feasible. The Community Development Model for Public Health Applications is a useful conceptual framework for achieving this objective. Communities of color will be the immediate beneficiaries, but the public health community and the nation will share the victory.

Conclusion

Tobacco has played a complex role in the lives of African Americans. It was the cash crop that served as the incentive for Europeans to kidnap Africans from their homelands and transport them to the Americas, a deed that altered the racial identity of African people as well as the history of the Americas. Until the 1800s, when it was replaced by cotton, tobacco consumed the labor of African Americans on plantations, in small factories where cigarettes were first manufactured, and in larger factories where production of tobacco products became the backbone of the American economy.

African Americans benefited little from this prosperity, being paid nothing during four-hundred years of slavery and receiving only minimal pay for menial work throughout most of the twentieth century. After World War II, African Americans who worked in the tobacco industry benefited from some of the changes wrought by the union movement. For example, more comparable treatment compared with white workers within the unions may have influenced the R. J. Reynolds Tobacco Company to become the first company to desegregate the workplace. Union membership encouraged political participation among African Americans, which contributed to the election of an African American to the city council in Winston-Salem, North Carolina.

Following World War II, more African Americans began to smoke, a factor that again changed their relationship to the tobacco industry. As consumers of tobacco products, African Americans were now the targets of advertising and product promotions campaigns that were designed to increase the attractiveness of tobacco to African American smokers and potential smokers. The success of these campaigns led to higher smoking rates among African Americans (especially men), with peak rates occurring in the 1950s for men and in the 1970s for women. Smoking rates among African Americans and whites were comparable in the 1990s; about one-quarter of each group was classified as a current smoker. Selective contributions to organizations and causes that were important to African Americans also improved the image of the tobacco industry in the African American community. As science would predict, African Americans experienced the expected health consequences of tobacco use: higher rates of respiratory cancer than whites (especially among men), lower rates of nonfatal coronary heart disease but higher rates of fatal CHD, and serious illness from chronic obstructive lung disease (although fewer deaths than whites). All of these influences created the need for tobacco-use prevention efforts that would be tailored to African American historical experiences with tobacco, to the unique smoking patterns that they would eventually develop, and to the complex relationship that the African American community would have with the tobacco industry in the twentieth century.

It has been evident to the public health community for decades that the health of Americans cannot be enhanced until national rates of tobacco use have been greatly reduced. Since 1964, the Office of the Surgeon General has released annual reports documenting the impact of tobacco on the health of Americans, and in the 1990s a campaign was launched to address this problem on a national scale.

Three separate initiatives provided states with funding to reduce tobacco use among adults and to prevent young people from starting to smoke. These programs were Project ASSIST (American Stop Smoking Intervention Study) (the National Cancer Institute), the Smokeless States Initiative (the Robert Wood Johnson Foundation), and the IMPACT Initiative (Centers for Disease Control and Prevention, Office on Smoking and Health). A unique feature of the programs is that they used a common model, a comprehensive, environmental approach to tobacco-use prevention and reduction and common strategies to address the problem. Over a ten-year period, these programs made enormous strides in mobilizing communities to take action to reduce tobacco use, to convince many smokers to quit, and to make teens and adults aware of the influence of tobacco advertising and promotional activities on smoking initiation among youth. African Americans benefited in many ways from these efforts, but few of them addressed tobacco use in ways that were specific to their experiences. In addition, very few resources were devoted to developing African American leaders in tobacco control who could do this for their own communities. Despite this barrier, African American leaders did emerge and their influence on the tobacco control movement has been significant. In several community-based initiatives they responded to tobacco industry actions in unique and unexpected ways that altered history for themselves and for the nation as a whole. For example, the R. J. Reynolds tobacco company test marketed a new cigarette called Uptown in Philadelphia. The cigarette was designed to attract African American smokers and was named after a popular theatre in the area. Using diverse strategies that included grassroots organizing, coalition building, and media campaigns, African Americans were successful in influencing the company to remove the cigarette from the market. This campaign occurred in the 1980s, and in the 1990s, they were able to discourage the rapid distribution of a menthol brand of the Camel cigarette distributed by the R. J. Reynolds Company. Similarly, grassroots efforts in Boston were successful in preventing the mass distribution of the X cigarette.

In the past decade, African American leaders have contributed to their own communities and to the larger movement by developing tobacco prevention and control programs that are tailored to the unique history, culture, geography, and social context of African American life and experience. One program that has made a lasting impact on tobacco control activity among African Americans is the Pathways to Freedom (PTF) smoking cessation program. At least one study has demonstrated the effectiveness of this culturally appropriate program in helping African American smokers to quit. The PTF has also inspired the development of programs that encourage cessation activities targeted to African Americans in specific settings such as health facilities and community settings. For example, the Uhuru-No Smoke program is a toolbox for smoking cessation strategies targeted to African Americans that includes the Provider's Smoking Cessation Counseling Protocol and the Grassroots Smoking Cessation Initiative. The prevention of tobacco use among youth has been addressed by the innovative, nationally recognized Ujima! African American Youth Initiative. This program is also culturally appropriate, building upon the Nguzo Saba or the seven principles of Kwanzaa, an African American cultural holiday. It develops advocacy skills, leadership, and cultural appreciation among preadolescents and young adults.

The tobacco control movement has operated under a conceptual framework that promotes a comprehensive, environmental approach to social and behavioral change in reducing tobacco use. This model is indeed appropriate in addressing tobacco control issues in African American and other communities of color. However, the Community Development Model for Public Health Applications goes one step further in offering a conceptual framework that is more specific to the unique ways in which history, geography, culture, and social context have influenced the lives of people of color and their relationships to tobacco and the tobacco industry. Using this model will allow public health professionals to derive appropriate strategies for allocating resources that will achieve the dual purposes of reducing tobacco use in communities of greatest need and enhancing the overall health of Americans.

References

Bachman, J. G., Wallace, J. M., Jr., O'Malley, P. M., Johnston, L. D., Kurth, C. L., & Neighbors, H. W. (1991). Racial/ethnic differences in smoking, drinking, and illicit drug use among American high school seniors, 1976–1989. *American Journal of Public Health, 81,* 372–377.

Braithwaite, R. L., Hill, H. A., Stephens, T. T., Resnicow, K., Headen, S. W., & Hansen, A. (1997). African American physicians' and dentists' perceptions of smoking cessation: Solo versus HMO practices. *Ethnicity and Disease, 7,* 114–120.

Caraballo, R. S., Giovino, G. A., Pechacek, T. F., Mowery, P. D., Richter, P. A., Strauss, W. J., Sharp, D. J., Eriksen, M. P., Pirkle, J. L., Maurer, K. R., & Kurt, R. (1998). Racial and ethnic differences in serum cotinine levels of cigarette medicine. Smokers: Third National Health and Nutrition Examination Survey, 1988–1991. *Journal of the American Medical Association, 280,* 135–139.

Carnes, M. C., Schlesinger, A. M., & Fox, D. R. (1996). *A history of American life* (rev. ed.). New York: Simon & Schuster.

Centers for Disease Control and Prevention. (1991). Differences in the age of smoking initiation between blacks and whites: United States. *Morbidity and Mortality Weekly Report, 40,* 757–777.

Centers for Disease Control and Prevention. (1997). Cigarette smoking among adults: United States, 1995. *Morbidity and Mortality Weekly Report, 46,* 1217–1220.

Christian, C. M. (1995). *Black saga: The African American experience.* Boston: Houghton Mifflin.

Fiore, M. C., Bailey, W. C., Cohen, S. J., Dorfman, S. F., Goldstein, M. G., & Gritz, E. R. (1996). *Smoking cessation: Clinical Practice Guideline No. 18* (AHCPR Publication No. 96-0692). Rockville, MD: U.S. Department of Health and Human Services, Public Health Service, Agency for Health Care Policy and Research.

Fiore, M. C., Novotny, T. E., Pierce, J. P., Giovino, G. A., Hatziandreu, E. J., Newcomb, P. A., Surawicz, T. S., & Davis, R. M. (1990). Methods used to quit smoking in the United States: Do cessation programs help? *Journal of the American Medical Association, 263,* 2760–2765.

Fleming, R., Leventhal, H., Glynn, K., & Ershler, J. (1989). The role of cigarettes in the initiation and progression of early substance use. *Addictive Behaviors, 14,* 261–272.

Giovino, G. A., Schooley, M. W., Zhu, P. B., Chrismon, J. H., Tomar, S. L., Peddicord, J. P., Merritt, R. K., Husten, C. G., & Eriksen, M. P. (1994). Surveillance for selected tobacco-use behaviors: United States, 1900–1994. *Morbidity and Mortality Weekly Report, 43,* 1–36.

Headen, S. W., & Berman, B. (1996). *Strategies for counseling xmokers to quit: Targeted messages for African Americans and members of other minority groups* [Brochure]. Chapel Hill: University of North Carolina at Chapel Hill.

Johnston, L. D., O'Malley, P. M., & Bachman, J. G. (1999a, December 17). *The Monitoring the Future Study* (Press release). Ann Arbor: University of Michigan [On-line]. Available: www.monitoringthefuture.org/pressreleases/99drugpr.html

Johnston, L. D., O'Malley, P. M., & Bachman, J. G. (1999b). *The Monitoring the Future Study* [unpublished data]. Ann Arbor: University of Michigan.

Karenga, M. (1998). *Kwanzaa: A celebration of family, community, and culture.* Los Angeles: University of Sankore Press.

Kulikoff, A. (1986). *Tobacco and slaves.* Chapel Hill: University of North Carolina Press.

Leventhal, H., Fleming, R., & Glynn, K. (1988). A cognitive developmental approach to smoking intervention. In S. Maes, C. D. Spielberger, P. B. Defares, & I. G. Sarason (Eds.), *Topics in health psychology: Proceedings of the First Annual Expert Conference in Health Psychology.* New York: Wiley.

Mannino, D. M., Brown, C., & Giovino, G. A. (1997). Obstructive lung disease deaths in the United States from 1979 through 1992: An analysis using multiple-cause mortality data. *American Journal of Respiratory and Critical Care Medicine, 156,* 814–818.

McNeil, A. D. (1991). The development of dependence on smoking in children. *British Journal of Addiction, 86,* 589–592.

Mermelstein, R., & Tobacco Control Network Writing Group. (1999). Explanations of ethnic and gender differences in youth smoking: A multi-site, qualitative investigation. *Nicotine and Tobacco Research, 1,* S91–S98.

Mitchell, O., & Greenberg, M. (1991). Outdoor advertising of addictive products. *New Jersey Medicine, 88*(5), 331–333.

National Center for Health Statistics. (1996). *Health, United States, 1995* (DHHS Publication No. PHS 96-1232). Hyattsville, MD: Author.

National Center for Health Statistics. (1998). *Health, United States, 1998, with socioeconomic status and health chartbook* (DHHS Publication No. PHS 98-1232). Hyattsville, MD: Author.

Prochaska, J. O., & DiClemente, C. C. (1983). Stages and processes of self-change of smoking: Toward an integrative model of change. *Journal of Consulting and Clinical Psychology, 51,* 390–395.

Raeburn, J., & Rootman, I. (1997). *People-centered health promotion.* Ontario, CA: John Wiley & Sons.

Raphael, D., & Bryant, T. (2000, January-February). Putting the population into population health (editorial). *Canadian Journal of Public Health, 91*(9), 9–12.

Robinson, R. G. (2000, Spring). Eliminating population disparities in tobacco control (editorial). *Smokeless States Nobacco News, 6*(1), 5.

Robinson, R. G., Barry, M., Bloch, M., Glantz, S., Jordan, J., Murray, K. B., Popper, E., Sutton, C., Tarr-Whelan, K., Themba, M., & Younger, S. (1992). Report of the Tobacco Policy Research Group on marketing and promotions targeted at African Americans, Latinos, and women. *Tobacco Control: An International Journal, 1*(Suppl.), S24–S30.

Robinson, R. G., & Headen, S. W. (1999). Tobacco use and the African American community: A conceptual framework for the year 2000 and beyond. In M. L. Forst (Ed.), *Successful tobacco education programs* (pp. 83–112). Springfield, IL: Thomas.

Robinson, R. G., Orleans, C. T., James, D. A., & Sutton, C. D. (1992). *Pathways to freedom: Winning the fight against tobacco.* Philadelphia: Fox Chase Cancer Center.

Robinson, R. G., Pertschuk, M., & Sutton, C. (1992). Smoking and African Americans: Spotlighting the effects of smoking and tobacco promotion in the African American community. In S. E. Samuels & M. D. Smith (Eds.), *Improving the health of the poor* (pp. 124–185). Menlo Park, CA: Kaiser Family Foundation.

Robinson, R. G., Shelton, D. M., Hodge, F., Lew, R., Lopez, E., Toy, P., Merritt, R., & Yack, D. (1995). Tobacco control capacity index for communities of color in the United States. In K. Slama (Ed.), *Tobacco and health* (pp. 359–365). New York: Plenum.

Tuckson, R. V. (1989). Race, sex, economics, and tobacco advertising. *Journal of the National Medical Association, 81,* 1119–1124.

Tyroler, H. A., Knowles, M. G., Wing, S. B., Lougue, E. E., Davis, C. E., Heiss, G., Heyden, S., & Hames, C. G. (1984). Ischemic heart disease risk factors and twenty-year mortality in middle-age Evans County black males. *American Heart Journal, 108*(3, Pt. 2), 738–746 .

U.S. Department of Health, Education, and Welfare. (1964). *Smoking and health: Report of the Advisory Committee to the Surgeon General of the Public Health Service* (DHHS Publication No. PHS 1103). Washington, DC: U.S. Department of Health and Human Services, Public Health Service.

U.S. Department of Health and Human Services. (1991). *Strategies to control tobacco use in the United States: A blueprint for public health action in the 1990s.* (NIH Publication No. 92-3316). Public Health Service, National Institutes of Health, National Cancer Institute.

U.S. Department of Health and Human Services. (1994). *Preventing tobacco use among young people: A report of the surgeon general.* (DHHS Publication No. S/N 017-001-00491-0). Atlanta, GA: U.S. Department of Health and Human Services, Centers for Disease Control and Prevention, Office on Smoking and Health.

U.S. Department of Health and Human Services. (1996). *Physical activity and health: A report of the surgeon general.* (DHHS Publication No. S/N 017-023-00196-5). Atlanta, GA: U.S. Department of Health and Human Services, Centers for Disease Control and Prevention, National Center for Chronic Disease Prevention and Health Promotion.

U.S. Department of Health and Human Services. (1998). *Tobacco use among U.S. racial/ethnic minority groups: African Americans, American Indians and Alaska Natives, Asian Americans and Pacific Islanders, and Hispanic Americans: A report of the surgeon general.* (Publication No. S/N 017-001-00527-4). Atlanta, GA: Centers for Disease Control and Prevention, Office on Smoking and Health.

U.S. Environmental Protection Agency. (1992). *Respiratory health effects of passive smoking: Lung cancer and other disorders.* (EPA Publication No. 600/6-90/006F). U.S. Environmental Protection Agency, Office of Research and Development, Office of Air and Radiation.

Wilson, J. J. (1999, March). *Summary of the Attorneys General Master Tobacco Settlement Agreement.* Washington, DC: National Conference of State Legislatures. [On-line]. Available: www.ncsl.org/statefed/tmsasumm.htm.

CHAPTER EIGHTEEN

SUBSTANCE ABUSE

Tony L. Strickland

Due to the dramatic surge in use of drugs of abuse and their pernicious consequences, there is a pressing need to study the associated psychosocial and neurobehavioral consequences. Because the abuse of cocaine and related substances has been a long-standing problem for African American communities, the primary focus of the discussion of drug abuse in this chapter will be on stimulant abuse. Frequently abused stimulants such as methamphetamine and cocaine are extremely potent cerebral vasoconstrictors that continue to be used at escalating rates (*Pulse Check*, 1998). It is now well established that abuse of stimulants like cocaine and methamphetamine can lead to hypertensive encephalopathy and ischemic brain hemorrhage (Caplan, Hier, & Banks, 1982). Despite the evidence that indicates these drugs of abuse can induce significant cerebral pathology, little is known about any differences that might exist in the magnitude of brain impairment or the specific region(s) adversely affected. Moreover, although methamphetamine is similar to cocaine in pharmacological action, we do not know if the extent of cerebral dysfunction observed in cocaine abusers is also to be found in methamphetamine abusers. Still to be determined is whether methamphetamine has an affinity for the same brain regions affected by cocaine or induces a similar pattern(s) of psychosocial and neurobehavioral dysfunction. It is also unclear whether there are differential ethnic or gender effects secondary to methamphetamine abuse, or how long any observed deficits might persist. Increased knowledge in these areas will almost certainly improve the quality of substance abuse treatment for stimulant abusers.

Treatments of addictive disorders are typically standardized and are initiated with little regard for interindividual or intergroup variation. The further development of technologies in the fields of neuroimaging, pharmacokinetics, neuropsychometrics, and molecular biology will permit more advanced assessment of potential drug-induced neurobiological and psychosocial similarities and differences among and between groups (that is, by gender, socioeconomic status, ethnicity, and so on). For example, some researchers suggest greater preservation of brain blood flow secondary to cocaine abuse among women despite significantly greater drug use (Gur et al., 1982; Kosten, Malison, & Wallace, 1996; Rodriguez, Warkentin, Risberg, & Rosadini, 1988; Strickland et al., 1993). This observation illustrates the complexity of drug abuse and clearly highlights the need for more research related to individual differences. Unfortunately, current assessment practices are ill equipped to most effectively assess and treat African Americans. There is a limited understanding of the impact of culture, race, and socioeconomic status (SES) on assessment in general and on test development and test performance in particular (Heaton, Grant, & Matthews, 1996; Helms, 1997). Furthermore, the effects of learning styles, test-taking attitudes, and information-processing strategies on test performance and test interpretation are also not well known. The lack of test norms specific to African Americans often leads to a tendency to overdiagnose psychopathology in African Americans (Manly, Jacobs, Sano, Bell, & Merchant, 1998). These issues have significant implications for diagnosis and treatment. This chapter will address important issues we need to focus on for more culturally sensitive assessment and intervention, and it will present specific guidelines for working with addicted African Americans.

The significance of research aimed at clarifying ethnic, gender, and SES differences in the use and effects of drugs and also the differential effects of drugs within a class extends beyond the immediate practical application of clinical findings, that is, beyond developing better treatments for the respective groups. Such work also has very important theoretical implications. For example, if a particular response were evident in all groups, that finding would strongly support the existence of comparable (universal) neuropathological underpinnings for the disorder. In turn, these comparable neuropathological underpinnings would argue for generic psychobiological approaches to the treatment of that given substance abuse disorder. If group differences were noted, however, then group-specific treatment approaches might be justified. In addition, such a finding would point to possible differences in neuropathological mechanisms within the different groups. Currently, of course, there is a very large gap in our understanding of potentially differential neuropathological outcomes resulting from drugs of abuse that share similar pharmacological actions, of whether deficits observed at a given assessment point persist over time, and of the role of gender and ethnicity as possible influences on individuals' responses to specific drugs of abuse.

Epidemiological Trends in Stimulant Use

In addition to the often-cited National Household Survey on Drug Abuse, there are several other indicators of drug abuse trends that provide information on the prevalence and consequences of cocaine and methamphetamine use. First is *Pulse Check: National Trends in Drug Abuse,* a publication distributed by the Office of National Drug Control Policy, which tracks drug use through the impressions of ethnographers, law enforcement officials, and treatment providers across the country. Second is the information about emergency room admissions for California and other states generated by the Public Statistics Institute (PSI). These two sources provide timely assessment of trends—across the country in the case of *Pulse Check,* and in states such as California and other states in the case of the PSI emergency room admissions data.

Methamphetamine Use

A recent *Pulse Check* (Summer, 1998) included a special report on methamphetamine use in five Western states. This report reinforces the identification of methamphetamine as an emerging drug, according to ethnographers and law enforcement. Methamphetamine has been gaining popularity especially among individuals switching from cocaine. For example, analysis of emergency room admissions in California from 1984 to 1993 reveals a dramatic upward trend in its use (Cunningham, Thielmeir, & Micks, 1995). Amphetamine-related emergency admissions increased by 366 percent over this ten-year period.

In 1993, this trend produced a state average of 22 admissions per 100,000 population. Among the total number of persons admitted to emergency departments (EDs) in Los Angeles County, methamphetamines were mentioned as a factor in admission by 1.3 percent in the first half of 1992 and 3.5 percent in the second half of 1993 (U.S. Department of Health and Human Services [DHHS], 1995). In California in 1993, Los Angeles County experienced the most admissions (1,161), followed by San Diego County (996).

Except for a small decline between the fourth quarter of 1994 and the first quarter of 1995, the trend in the 1990s has been toward increased methamphetamine-related ED admissions. Amphetamine morbidity has been concentrated primarily among non-Hispanic Euro-Americans (hereinafter Euro-Americans). In Los Angeles County, 41 percent of the population and 75 percent of ED admissions involving methamphetamines were Euro-Americans. Hispanics, Asians, and African Americans were all underrepresented in amphetamine-related ED admissions relative to their proportion of the general population. (In the case of Hispanics, emergency department visits may be a substantial underestimation of amphetamine-related problems relative to other groups if immigration status is deterring people from seeking ED care.) The median age of these admissions rose slightly over the period, from twenty-eight to thirty-one years. Sixty-one percent of these patients were between eighteen and thirty-four years old. Following this trend, as of the first quarter of 1995, methamphetamine was reported to be their primary drug of abuse by 5 percent of the total sample of patients admitted to treatment programs. Seventy percent of these persons were Euro-Americans, but Hispanics were increasingly being admitted. Almost 50 percent of those admitted for methamphetamine abuse are male and between twenty-six to thirty-four years of age.

Cocaine Use

Although the most recent comprehensive estimates of drug abuse show declines in occasional use of cocaine, frequent (weekly) use shows no change (DHHS, 1995). In 1995, an estimated 1.4 million Americans aged twelve and older were current (past month) cocaine users, with crack being used by 0.5 million individuals. Higher proportional rates of cocaine use were found among African Americans (1.3 percent) and Hispanics (1.1 percent) compared to Euro-Americans. Yet, 62 percent of current cocaine users were Euro-American (due to their larger numbers in the total population) compared to 22 percent and 16 percent for African Americans and Hispanics, respectively. Police and treatment providers report similar impressions. Reports for the Los Angeles area suggest 60 percent of users are African American and most are twenty-six years old or older.

Cocaine-related emergency admissions from 1985 to 1994 appear to show an uneven pattern. In California, for example, rates surged from 14.0 per 100,000 population in 1985 to their first peak in 1988, at 37.5 per 100,000, then temporarily dropped before a making recent surge in 1994 to 41.5 per 100,000, a 22.4 percent increase over the previous year. There was an even greater surge (32 percent) in Los Angeles County to 60.8 per 100,000. Indeed, Los Angeles County accounted for 5,691 or 42 percent of the 13,496 cocaine-related admissions in California in 1994.

African Americans, constituting 45.9 percent of all cocaine-related admissions, dominated the admission rates although they constitute only 7 percent of the California population. Euro-Americans, Hispanics, and Asians were all underrepresented relative to their proportion in the population. The aging of cocaine users identified by *Pulse Check* is also well supported by emergency admission data, with median ages rising from twenty-nine years in 1985 and 1986 to thirty-six years in 1993 and 1994. Males predominate the population admitted, with 65.3 percent of admissions in 1994 and no significant change since 1985. The financial burden generated by cocaine-related admissions rose from a non-inflation-adjusted $24 million in 1985 to $178 million in 1994, which is a 642 percent increase, with the median hospital charge also nearly doubling to $13,354.

In conclusion, there has been a recent and dramatic upsurge in cocaine-related admissions, which, combined with other recent survey data, suggests the number of heavy users is increasing or the average heavy user is consuming more cocaine. These epidemiological trends pose a unique problem for treatment researchers and treatment providers. We anticipate that practically all the methamphetamine abusers will be Euro-Americans and Hispanics, and that African Americans, Hispanics, and Euro-Americans will be represented among the cocaine abusers. This ethnicity by drug type effectively precludes testing for potentially very interesting gender by ethnicity by drug type interactions and, by implication, unraveling the mystery of drug by ethnicity effects on substance abuse treatment. As a result, current research and practice can only partly address this issue by testing for gender differences within each drug use group. This is clearly a compromise solution to a problem that is inherent in the distribution of drugs of choice across ethnic populations.

Neurobiology and Neuropathology of Methamphetamine Use

It has been estimated that at least 4 million individuals in the United States have tried methamphetamine at least once (Substance Abuse and Mental Health Services Administration, 1994). According to the Drug Abuse Warning Network (DAWN), the number abusing methamphetamine has recently risen dramatically, with emergency department episodes up 237 percent from 1990 to 1994 (NIDA, 1998).

Much of what is known about methamphetamine is derived from a long line of research on the amphetamines in general. These drugs are indirect catecholamine agonists that release newly synthesized norepinephrine and dopamine (Carlsson, 1970; Carlsson, Lindqvist, Dahlstroem, Fuxe, & Masuoka, 1965; Carlsson & Waldeck, 1966; Chiueh & Moore, 1974; Javoy, Hamon, & Glowinski, 1970; Von Voigtlander & Moore, 1973). In contrast, cocaine acts through storage pools, not only through newly synthesized catecholamines (King & Ellinwood, 1992). The amphetamines are powerful sympathomimetics. Both diastolic and systolic blood pressure is elevated (Weiner, 1985). Tachycardia and cardiac arrhythmias have been observed (Ellinwood & Rockwell, 1988). These responses can combine to produce serious cerebrovascular pathology. Chronic high-dose abuse of amphetamines results in numerous pathophysiological changes, with central nervous system consequences among the most serious. Generalized depression of norepinephrine levels is found after acute withdrawal in monkeys, with persisting low levels in the midbrain and frontal cortex even after three to six months of abstinence (Seiden, Fischman, & Schuster, 1977).

Similar findings were reported for dopamine in the basal ganglia up to six months after the last amphetamine injection. These results combined with the findings of neuronal degeneration (Duarte-Escalante & Ellinwood, 1970; Ricaurte, Seiden, & Schuster, 1984; Ricaurte, Guillery, Seiden, Schuster, & Moore, 1982), a reduced number of dopamine transporters and uptake sites (Ricaurte, Schuster, & Seiden, 1980; Ricaurte, Guillery, et al., 1982), and reduced volume of tyrosine-beta-hydroxylase (Ricaurte, Schuster, & Seiden, 1980; Hotchkiss, Morgan, & Gibb, 1979) indicate that amphetamines are neurotoxic to the catecholamine system.

The study of drug-induced neuropathology is rich in studies that use amphetamine models. Cocaine and amphetamine have similar mechanisms of action on cerebral perfusion. The catecholamine release associated with both compounds leads to cerebral vasoconstriction. As early as 1977, Rumbaugh et al. showed that cocaine could lead to stroke in humans and in an experimental model of stroke showed that even a single oral dose of amphetamine could lead to severe cerebral vasospasm and stroke in monkeys. Interestingly, in this monkey model, oral use of amphetamine led to microinfarcts and small hemorrhages. This early literature on amphetamine-induced stroke (for example, Edwards, Russo, & Harwood-Nuss, 1987) mirrors the more recent experience with cocaine in which patients taking crack for the first time can suffer infarcts or hemorrhages in the spinal cord, brainstem, basal ganglia, subcortical white matter, or cortex (Mody, Miller, McIntyre, Cobb, & Goldberg, 1988). The sudden death of the basketball star Len Bias at the University of Maryland-College Park some years ago was a dramatic example that youth was no barrier to the potentially negative neurological consequences of cocaine.

Animal research on cerebrovascular changes following chronic amphetamine administration is notable for the clear-cut findings of neuropathology. Both three months and one year of methamphetamine administration to monkeys produced extensive pathology in small arterioles and capillary beds seen as beading, vascular filling or nonfilling, and fragmentation of the vessels (Rumbaugh, 1977). Associated with the vascular pathology was neuronal loss, proliferation of glial cells, and microhemorrhages in the cerebellum and hypothalamus. These findings are congruent with clinical reports of cerebral hemorrhage (Kalant & Kalant, 1979). Thus even short periods of use can have devastating consequences for the brain.

Research on single-dose amphetamine effects on blood flow is suggestive of decreased cerebral blood flow (CBF) (Kahn, Prohovnik, Lucas, & Sackeim, 1989). Single-dose methylphenidate (0.5 mg/kg IV), an amphetamine analog commonly used for attention deficit disorder, in normal males produced a whole-brain CBF decrement of 25 ± 11 percent after five to ten minutes and a persisting 20 ± 10 percent decrement after thirty minutes. An intriguing finding was the relative uniformity in regional decrements of 23 to 30 percent, which the study authors attributed to the drug's vasoconstrictive properties. At least one study of the cerebral metabolic effects of amphetamine has been reported (Wolkin et al., 1987). The authors administered d-amphetamine (0.5 mg/kg PO) or a placebo to chronic schizophrenics and normal controls. The amphetamine resulted in decreased glucose metabolism in all regions studied (frontal, temporal, and striatal). Psychiatric status did not influence the results, and in addition, metabolic effects were significantly associated with plasma drug levels.

An exhaustive search of the literature yielded only one study to date on the cerebral blood flow status among amphetamine abusers. Kao, Wang, and Yeh (1994) conducted HMPAO SPECT scans on twenty-one amphetamine abusers whose use ranged from one month to several years. Nearly all had at least small defects (95 percent), and most had multiple defects spanning both hemispheres (71 percent). Although there was no association between the degree of abnormality revealed by SPECT and the dose or duration of drug use or neuropsychiatric symptoms, statistical power was low due to the small number of subjects and the likely limited reliability of dose and duration estimates. It is possible that a replication of this research study, with a significantly larger sample size and more reliable dose and duration estimates, would yield significant associations between the abnormalities and the extent of neuropsychiatric symptoms.

Amphetamines, including methamphetamine, are known largely for their anorectant, autonomic, and potential psychotomimetic effects. However, the cerebrovascular pathology and neurochemical dysregulation are strongly suggestive of adverse neuropsychological effects as well. In contrast, single mild to moderate doses of these drugs in drug-naive individuals may produce positive effects on attention and psychomotor speed and are known to be helpful for many suffering from attention deficit hyperactivity disorder (Barkley, 1977). Unfortunately, very little is known about chronic abuse of methamphetamine relative to long-term neurobehavioral functioning, and even less is known about the potential influences of ethnicity and gender on these parameters.

Neurobiology and Neuropathology of Cocaine Use

The literature on the human neurobiology of cocaine use continues to develop at an impressive pace. Existing research indicates that there are serious medical and neuropsychological complications similar to those of methamphetamine use that can occur even in first-time users. These include acute myocardial infarction, cardiac arrhythmia, intestinal ischemia, brain hemorrhage, ischemic stroke, and cerebral vasculitis (Caplan et al., 1982; Chynn, 1975; Green, Kelly, Gabrielson, Levine, & Vandersant, 1990; Kaku & Lowenstein, 1989; Kaye & Fainstat, 1987; Klonoff, Andres, & Obana, 1989; Krendel, Ditter, Frankel, & Ross, 1990; Lehman, 1987; Lichtenfeld, Rubin, & Feldman, 1984; Mody et al., 1988; Moore & Peterson, 1989; Nalls, Disher, Dariabagi, Zant, & Eisenman, 1989; Notel & Gelman, 1989; Rogers, Henry, Jones, Froede, & Byers, 1986; Schwartz & Cohen, 1984; Wojak & Flamm, 1987). Noted complications in the neurocognitive domain include decreased attention and concentration, impaired memory, compromised abstraction and problem-solving ability, and episodic dyscontrol (Brandt, Butters, Ryan, & Bayog, 1983; Manschreck et al., 1990; Meek, Clark, & Solana, 1989; Miller, 1985). The more severe medical and neuropsychiatric complications are more prevalent among crack and freebase users.

Cocaine has been observed to induce cerebral hypertension, and the ensuing brain perfusion anomalies observed in chronic cocaine abusers may be related to cocaine-induced microvascular ischemia (Strickland, Mena, et al., 1993). Of interest is that in patients who suffer stroke from cocaine, routine cerebral angiography often is normal (Mody et al., 1988). The probable explanation is that cocaine causes ischemia in small vessels that are below the image resolution of this technique. With cocaine, occlusion of major vessels is uncommon and small white matter infarcts and lacunar infarcts are more typical sequelae. For example, Rowley, Lowenstein, Rowbotham, and Simon (1989) described three patients with a mean age of thirty-three who had small infarcts in the rostral midbrain and thalamus. Strokes in this area more typically occur in individuals over the age of fifty after their chronic hypertension leads to changes in medium-sized and small vessels.

More recently, Kaufman et al. (1997) used magnetic resonance angiography to demonstrate cerebral vasoconstriction following intravenous administration of cocaine in volunteers. Interestingly, greater lifetime cocaine use was associated with a greater likelihood of vasoconstriction.

Gender-Related Variations in Consequences of Cocaine Abuse

Researchers and clinicians have increasingly explored drug use patterns and consequences among substance-abusing women. However, knowledge concerning the factors that promote or maintain cocaine, alcohol, and other drug abuse patterns in women has lagged considerably behind the massive literature of such information on men. There is comparatively little information about gender variation among cocaine abusers in general, and even less is known about the neurobehavioral sequelae of cocaine abuse in women. Women who do not seek treatment in publicly supported programs or who do not come to the attention of public agencies, moreover, are rarely included in research studies, so most of what we know about the nature and extent of drug abuse among women has been derived almost completely from investigations involving women from the lower socioeconomic classes.

The limited information on gender differences in substance abuse has been gathered largely as a result of alcohol research. Because alcohol is frequently ingested in concert with cocaine, and chronic alcohol ingestion results in a global decrease in brain perfusion (Mathew & Wilson, 1991), and because cocaine is a significantly greater cerebral vasoconstrictor than alcohol, it is reasonable to hypothesize more adverse neurobehavioral complications from cocaine use in women, given the known differences in the absorption, distribution, and metabolism of drugs in women compared to men. For example, the rate of absorption distribution and metabolism of a range of compounds is more variable in women than in men and is affected by a number of neurohormonal factors such as progesterone levels that fluctuate during the menstrual cycle (Lex, 1991).

A gender-based CBF differential has been proposed by several other researchers (Esposito, Van Horn, Weinberger, & Berman, 1996; Gur et al., 1982; Rodriguez et al., 1988). Several studies using either PET or SPECT scans have found higher global CBF and glucose metabolism in women (Andreason, Zametkin, Guo, Baldwin, & Cohen, 1994; Baxter et al., 1987; Devous, Stokely, Chehabi, & Bonte, 1986; Gur et al., 1982; Rodriguez et al., 1988; Shaw et al., 1984), whereas others have not (Azari et al., 1992; Matsuda, Maeda, Yamada, Gui, & Hisada, 1984; Melamed, Lavy, Bentin, Cooper, & Rinot, 1980; Miura et al., 1990). Esposito and colleagues (1996) observed that most of those studies that found no effect were conducted with subjects at rest (Azari et al., 1992; Hannay, Leli, Falgout, Katholi, & Halsey, 1983; Matsuda et al., 1984; Melamed et al., 1980; Miura et al., 1990). Specific findings of differences included a higher rate of blood flow per unit of brain weight (Gur et al., 1982), greater difference in the frontal lobes than in the temporal, parietal, and occipital lobes (Mathew, Wilson, & Tant, 1986), and a diminished effect after young adulthood (Davis et al., 1983; Devous et al., 1986; Shaw et al., 1984). Of particular relevance to the current proposed study is a finding by Levin et al. (1994) of *fewer* cerebral perfusion anomalies among women cocaine abusers in their sample compared to men.

A significant base of research has been devoted to gender differences in neuropsychological functioning (for example, Burstein, Bank, & Jarvik, 1980; Kimura & Harshman, 1984; Kosten et al., 1996; Piazza, 1980), and these differences would likely be reflected in CBF and metabolism. These findings collectively illustrate the importance of employing a very well-matched control group to compare CBF and cerebral metabolism between clinical groups. We have recently observed evidence of gender differences in cerebral perfusion (Strickland, Miller, Stein, & Kowell, 2000) and in brain choline levels among cocaine abusers (Chang, Ernst, & Strickland, 1996).

Consistent with the findings of Levin and his colleagues (1994), findings from recent research on the neurobehavioral effects of cocaine strongly indicate gender differences (Chang et al., 1996; Strickland, Miller, Stein, & Kowell, 2000). Specifically, women cocaine abusers abstinent for at least five months exhibited better cerebral blood flow on SPECT scanning than men did. This is in striking contrast to the finding that the women in the study had an estimated lifetime cocaine intake *more than 2.5 times* that of men. We are currently exploring several explanations for these findings. Although we are analyzing gender difference in peak use and number of binges, one intriguing possibility is that women in general exhibit greater cerebral blood flow. Our current data show that female controls have greater CBF than male controls but also that the CBF for female cocaine abusers exceeds the CBF found for female controls.

Apolipoprotein Polymorphism and Stimulant Abuse

Recently, the use of apolipoprotein E genotyping has shown promise in identifying individuals with enhanced risk for developing neurocognitive deficits. In a number of studies of Euro-American populations, the frequency of the e4 allele of apolipoprotein E (APO-E) has been found to be approximately 25 percent and to increase late-onset Alzheimer's disease (AD) compared to control subjects (Saunders et al., 1993; Strittmatter et al., 1993; Pericak-Vance et al., 1991). The human APO-E gene encodes a cholesterol carrier lipoprotein (apolipoprotein E) produced in the liver and brain. APO-E is important in lipid transport and thought to be involved in postinjury repair in the central nervous system. Its exact role in dementia is unclear but may relate to formation of free radicals as well as amyloid deposition (Lethem & Orrell, 1997). It is polymorphic and occurs in three common allelic forms designated APO-E e2, e3, and e4, giving rise to six possible genotype combinations because everyone inherits two APO-E alleles, one from each parent.

Saunders et al. (1996) noted that it is not necessary to inherit an e4 allele to develop AD. The inheritance of the e4/e4 genotype (about 2 percent of the general population) is associated with a mean age of onset of AD of sixty to seventy years in most clinic populations. Few homozygous e4/e4 persons reach the age of ninety years without developing AD (Rebeck et al., 1994). Additionally, there is some indication that possession of APO-E e2 is underrepresented in AD populations and may protect against AD (Corder et al., 1994). In some families with early onset of AD before age sixty, particularly in those with a positive family history of AD, the presence of the e4 allele also may be increased in patients with multi-infarct dementia, and it is suggested that e4 is a marker of both AD and vascular dementia (Noguchi, Murakami, & Yamada, 1993).

The literature examining the relationship between APO-E frequencies, substance abuse, and neurobehavioral outcomes has been strikingly absent, and data for African Americans and Hispanics have been even more limited.

Maestre et al. (1995) studied 145 dementia patients and 206 healthy elderly controls who were divided among African Americans, Hispanics, and Euro-Americans. The results revealed a fivefold increase in the risk of Alzheimer's type dementia among all groups homozygous for APO e4, however, the risk was weaker for African Americans than for Hispanics and Euro-Americans. Conversely, the APO e2/e3 genotype was associated with an increased risk of dementia in African Americans but with reduced risk in Euro-Americans. These results suggest a potential differential risk pattern for genotype status and raise a question about the strength of the association between cognitive impairment and genotype frequencies among African Americans as compared to other racial and ethnic groups. As a consequence, future research should examine allele frequencies among substance-abusing cohorts. Significantly, we expect possible neuropsychological test findings among the differing ethnic and allele genotype groups in the future study samples.

Socioeconomic Status and Substance Abuse

There is substantial evidence and general consensus that socioeconomic status is a major contributor to differential morbidity and mortality resulting from a variety of physical and psychiatric disorders. In their excellent report, Williams and Collins (1995) review the evidence for the SES gradient in health and the basis for the consistent racial differences in health noted in most epidemiological reports. They note that there is unequivocal evidence of disproportionate risk for morbidity and mortality among the lower SES groups, and that race and ethnicity condition this relationship so that low-SES African Americans suffer a greater burden of morbidity and mortality than Americans of all other races and ethnic groups do. Several factors have been implicated in this inverse SES-health relationship, including a greater exposure to pathogenic social and environmental conditions, a greater life stress burden, more negative health behavior profiles, and less access to and utilization of quality health care (Blendon, Aiken, Freeman, & Corey, 1989).

Of even greater relevance to this chapter is the evidence that low SES is associated with earlier substance use initiation, a shorter transition from recreational drug use to regular use and abuse, and a greater prevalence of use of the more neurotoxic drugs such as crack cocaine (Lillie-Blanton, Anthony, & Schuster, 1994). There is also suggestive evidence of more severe negative consequences from the use of abusable substances such as tobacco (Sterling & Weinkam, 1989) and alcohol (Lex, 1991). All this evidence underscores the need to pay careful attention to the potential role that socioeconomic status might play in differences in substance abuse histories overall and the need to consider the possible differential functions of gender and ethnicity. Preliminary data from research conducted by members of our team also suggest that there may be SES-related differences in the neurobehavioral effects of heavy cocaine use and abuse, at least among African Americans, with the less affluent abusers evidencing more significant reductions in brain blood flow than their more affluent peers.

Neuropsychological Assessment of African Americans

Neuropsychology is "the scientific study of brain-behavioral relationships" (Meier, 1974). The value of neuropsychological assessment has been clearly demonstrated through the work of neuropsychologists such as Ralph M. Reitan (Reitan & Wolfson, 1992), Charles J. Golden (Golden, 1987; Golden, Hammeke, & Purish, 1978, 1980), and A. R. Luria (Luria, 1963, 1966, 1973), among others, over several decades (Horton, 1994). Neuropsychological test batteries such as the Halstead-Reitan Neuropsychological Test Battery (Reitan & Wolfson, 1992) and The Luria-Nebraska Neuropsychological Battery were developed by these researchers for research and clinical use (Golden et al., 1980). Descriptions of these batteries (too extensive to be included here) may be found in Horton and Wedding (1984), or Horton (1994) for the child versions. Suffice it to say that these batteries encompass many hours of complicated behavioral measurements including measures of intelligence, sensory perceptual functioning, motor skill, language, visuospatial ability, academic skill, memory, executive functioning, and emotional functioning (Horton & Wedding, 1984).

Interest in neuropsychology has increased at a tremendous rate in recent years. There have been multiple examples of successful applications of neuropsychological assessment methods (Horton, 1994; Horton & Wedding, 1984; Reitan & Davison, 1974; Reitan & Wolfson, 1992). At the same time, concern has been expressed regarding possible cultural and racial biases that may skew neuropsychological test findings (Adams, Boake, & Crain, 1982; Amante, VanHouten, Grieve, Bader, & Margules, 1977; Sue, Fujino, Hu, Takeuchi, & Zane, 1991). This concern includes great interest in the extent to which neuropsychological results for African Americans may be influenced by ethnic status. A significant issue for neuropsychological testing has been the limited normative data on minority groups such as African Americans (Strickland, D'Elia, James, & Stein, 1997). The lack of adequate neuropsychological data sets to evaluate the influences of race and culture prevents the development of firm conclusions regarding ethnic effects on neuropsychological assessment of African Americans. Without this information, there is the potential for errors to occur in diagnosis and treatment planning decision making as well as in placement for special services and in compensation decisions for acquired disabilities.

African Americans and Neuropsychological Research Findings

A number of studies are selectively reviewed in this section to present an overview of current research on the neuropsychological assessment of African Americans. The most frequently used design in this research seeks to compare the performance of African Americans with normative performance data for Euro-Americans. For example, Knuckle and Campbell (1984) used published norms to judge the neuropsychological test performances of one hundred nonreferred seventh- and eighth-grade African Americans. In this reportedly normal subject pool, about two-thirds were impaired on a measure of motor skill, and over a third were impaired on a measure of visuomemory ability. The overdiagnosis of impairment calls into question the relevance of the published norms for African American youths. Similarly, Harvey, Isaac, and Hynd (1986) found nonreferred five- to nine-year-old Euro-American subjects to perform better than African American children on a neuropsychological test measure that tapped the left tertiary region in the parietal lobes. Additionally, Campbell et al. (1996) examined the accuracy of several neuropsychological tests with normal African American adults. Again, published norms derived from nonminority populations by a number of conventional neuropsychological tests clearly overdiagnosed neuropsychological impairment in this normal African American sample. The failure of such studies to adequately control for SES, motivation, and cultural factors limits the degree to which these studies can be relied upon.

Finding spurious neuropsychological impairments in nonreferred normal children undercuts the value of neuropsychological testing for clinical decision making. These results argue strongly for the development of separate sets of neuropsychological test norms based on cultural and racial populations. So far, only one study could be identified (Strickland, D'Elia, et al., 1997) that has specifically addressed the urgent need for more normative data on neuropsychological tests in the African American population. Interestingly, however, Bernard (1989) failed to demonstrate spurious rates of neuropsychological impairment in a study of African American, Euro-American, and Hispanic American male youths when a full standardized neuropsychological test battery, the Halstead-Reitan Neuropsychological Test Battery (Reitan & Wolfson, 1992), was used. This study suggests that although spurious results may be found on a single neuropsychological test or a small number of neuropsychological tests, nonetheless, a full standardized neuropsychological battery, interpreted competently, may provide accurate results.

In summary, the scientific literature on the neuropsychological assessment of African Americans is minimal at best and potentially very misleading at worst. Only a handful of studies have compared African Americans with other groups. Also, the existing studies suffer from multiple methodological flaws and theoretical shortcomings. The greatest need is for large culturally and racially specific normative databases derived from normal African Americans of all ages to assist in neuropsychological assessment (Strickland, D'Elia, et al., 1997). After these normative databases are available, then the influences of drugs of abuse on the brain-behavior relationships of African Americans can be better understood. Until such time as these normative databases are available, the most reasonable approach to neuropsychological assessment with African Americans will be to use a full standardized neuropsychological test battery and to interpret the battery as a whole rather than to rely on single or small groups of neuropsychological tests.

Conclusion

Our hope and expectation is that this chapter will have highlighted for the reader the important problems related to substance abuse disorders among African Americans.

References

Adams, R., Boake, C., & Crain, C. (1982). Bias in a neuropsychological test classification related to education, age, and ethnicity. *Journal of Consulting and Clinical Psychology, 50,* 143–145.

Amante, D., VanHouten, V., Grieve, J., Bader, C., & Margules, P. (1977). Neuropsychological deficit, ethnicity, and socioeconomic status. *Journal of Consulting and Clinical Psychology, 45,* 524–535.

Andreason, P. J., Zametkin, A. J., Guo, A. C., Baldwin, P., & Cohen, R. M. (1994). Gender-related differences in regional cerebral glucose metabolism in normal volunteers. *Psychiatry Research, 51,* 175–183.

Azari, N. P., Rapoport, S. I., Grady, C. L., Gonzales-Aviles, A., Shapiro, M. B., & Horowitz, B. (1992). Gender differences in correlations of cerebral glucose metabolic rates in young normal adults. *Brain Research, 574,* 198–208.

Barkley, R. A. (1977). The effects of methylphenidate on various types of activity level and attention in hyperkinetic children. *Journal of Abnormal Child Psychology, 5*(4), 351–369.

Baxter, L. R., Jr., Mazziotta, J. C., Phelps, M. E., Selin, C. E., Guze, B. H., & Fairbanks, L. (1987). Cerebral glucose metabolic rates in normal human females versus normal males. *Psychiatry Research, 21,* 237–245.

Bernard, L. C. (1989). Halstead-Reitan Neuropsychological Test performance of black, Hispanic, and white young adult males from poor academic backgrounds. *Archives of Clinical Neuropsychology, 4,* 267–274.

Blendon, R. J., Aiken, L. H., Freeman, H. E., & Corey, C. R. (1989). Access to medical care for black and white Americans. A matter of continuing concern. *Journal of the American Medical Association, 261,* 278–281.

Brandt, J., Butters, N., Ryan, C., & Bayog, R. (1983). Cognitive loss and recovery in long-term alcohol abusers. *Archives of General Psychiatry, 40,* 435–442.

Burstein, B., Bank, L., & Jarvik, L. F. (1980). Sex differences in cognitive functioning: Evidence, determinants, implications. *Human Development, 23,* 289–313.

Caplan, L. R., Hier, D. B., & Banks, G. (1982). Current concepts of cerebrovascular disease-stroke: Stroke and drug abuse. *Stroke, 13,* 869–872.

Carlsson, A. (1970). Amphetamine and brain catecholamines. In E. Costa & S. Garattini (Eds.), *Amphetamines and related compounds* (pp. 289–299). New York: Raven Press.

Carlsson, A., Lindqvist, M., Dahlstroem, A., Fuxe, K., & Masuoka, D. (1965). Effects of the amphetamine group on intraneuronal brain amines in vivo and in vitro. *Journal of Pharmacy and Pharmacology, 17,* 521–524.

Carlsson, A., & Waldeck, B. (1966). Effects of amphetamine, tyramine, and protriptyline on reserpine resistant amine-concentrating mechanisms of adrenergic nerves. *Journal of Pharmacy and Pharmacology, 18,* 252–253.

Chang, L., Ernst, T., & Strickland, T. L. (1996). *Neurochemical abnormalities and gender effects in abstinent asymptomatic cocaine users* (Abstract). New York: International Society for Magnetic Resonance in Medicine.

Chiueh, C. C., & Moore, K. E. (1974). In vivo evoked release of endogenously synthesized catecholamines from the cat brain evoked by electrical stimulation and d-amphetamine. *Journal of Neurochemistry, 23,* 159–168.

Chynn, K. Y. (1975). Acute subarachnoid hemorrhage. *Journal of the American Medical Association, 233,* 55–56.

Corder, E. H., Saunders, E. M., Risch, N. J., Strittmatter, W. J., Schmechel, D. E., Gaskell, P. C., Jr., Rimmler, J. B., Locke, P. A., Conneally, P. M., & Schmader, K. E. (1994). Protective effect of apolipoprotein E type Z allele for late onset Alzheimer disease. *Nature Genetics, 7*(2), 180–184.

Cunningham, J., Thielmeir, M. A., & Micks, D. A. (1995). *Cocaine-related emergency admissions trends and regional variations in California (1985–1994).* Irvine, CA: Public Statistics Institute.

Davis, S. M., Ackerman, R. H., Correia, J. A., Alpert, N. M., Chang, J., Buonanno, R. E., Rosner, B., & Taveras, J. M. (1983). Cerebral blood flow and cerebrovascular CO_2 reactivity in stroke-age normal controls. *Neurology, 33,* 391–399.

Devous, M. D., Stokely, E. M., Chehabi, H. H., & Bonte, F. J. (1986). Normal distribution of regional blood flow measured by dynamic single-photon emission tomography. *Journal of Cerebral Blood Flow and Metabolism, 6,* 95–104.

Duarte-Escalante, O., & Ellinwood, E. H., Jr. (1970). Central nervous system cytopathological changes in cases with chronic methedrine intoxication. *Brain Research, 21,* 151–155.

Edwards, M., Russo, L., & Harwood-Nuss, A. (1987). Cerebral infarction with a single oral dose of phenylpropanolamine. *American Journal of Emergency Medicine, 5,* 163–164.

Ellinwood, E. H., & Rockwell, W.J.K. (1988). Central nervous system stimulants and anorectic agents. In B. Blackwell (Ed.), *Mewler's side effects of drugs* (pp. 1–26). New York: Elsevier.

Esposito, G., Van Horn, J. D., Weinberger, D. R., & Berman, K. F. (1996). Gender differences in cerebral blood flow as a function of cognitive state with PET. *Journal of Nuclear Medicine, 37,* 559–564.

Golden, C. J. (1987). *The Luria-Nebraska Neuropsychological Battery: Children's revision manual.* Los Angeles: Western Psychological Services.

Golden, C. J., Hammeke, T., & Purish, A. D. (1978). Diagnostic validity of a standardized neuropsychological battery derived from Luria's neuropsychological tests. *Journal of Consulting and Clinical Psychology, 49,* 410–417.

Golden, C. J., Hammeke, T., & Purish, A. D. (1980). *The Luria-Nebraska Neuropsychological Battery: Test manual (Revised).* Los Angeles: Western Psychological Services.

Green, R., Kelly, K. M., Gabrielson, T., Levine, S. R., & Vandersant, C. (1990). Multiple intracerebral hemorrhages after smoking "crack" cocaine. *Stroke, 21,* 957–962.

Gur, R. C., Gur, R. E., Obrist, W. D., Hungerbuhlez, J. P., Younkin, D., Rose, A. D., Skolnick, B. E., & Revich, M. (1982). Sex and handedness differences in cerebral blood flow during rest and cognitive activity. *Science, 217,* 659–661.

Hannay, J. H., Leli, D. A., Falgout, J. C., Katholi, C. R., & Halsey, J. H. (1983). rCBF for middle-aged males and females during right-left discrimination. *Cortex, 19,* 465–474.

Harvey, L., Isaac, W., & Hynd, G. (1986). Neurodevelopmental and racial differences in tactile-visual (cross-modal) discrimination in normal black and white children. *Archives of Clinical Neuropsychology, 1,* 139–145.

Heaton, K. K., Grant, L., & Matthews, C. G. (1996). Demographic influences on neuropsychological test performance. In I. Grant & K. M. Adams (Eds.), *Neuropsychological Assessment of Neuropsychiatric Disorders* (2nd ed.) (pp. 141–163). New York: Oxford University Press.

Helms, J. E. (1997). The triple quandary of race, culture, and social class in standardized cognitive ability testing. In D. P. Flanagan, J. L. Genshaft, & P. L. Harrison (Eds.), *Contemporary Intellectual Assessment* (pp. 517–532). New York: Guilford.

Horton, A. M., Jr., (1994). *Behavioral interventions with brain injured children.* New York: Plenum.

Horton, A. M., Jr., & Wedding, D. (1984). *Clinical and behavioral neuropsychology.* New York: Praeger.

Hotchkiss, A. J., Morgan, M. E., & Gibb, J. W. (1979). The long-term effects of multiple doses of methamphetamine on neostriatal tryptophan hydroxylase, tyrosine hydroxylase, choline acetyltransferase and glutamate decarboxylase activities. *Life Sciences, 25,* 1373–1378.

Javoy, F., Hamon, H., & Glowinski, J. (1970). Disposition of newly synthesized amines in cell bodies and terminals of central catecholaminergic neurons: 1. Effect of amphetamine and thioproperazine on the metabolism of CA in the caudate nucleus, the substantia nigra and the ventromedial nucleus of the hypothalamus. *European Journal of Pharmacology, 10,* 178–188.

Kahn, D. A., Prohovnik, I., Lucas, L. R., & Sackeim, H. A. (1989). Dissociated effects of amphetamine on arousal and cortical blood flow in humans. *Biological Psychiatry, 25,* 755–767.

Kaku, D. A., & Lowenstein, D. H. (1989). Recreational drug use: A growing risk factor for stroke in young people. *Neurology, 39*(Suppl. 1), 161–162, (Abstract).

Kalant, H., & Kalant, O. (1979). Death in amphetamine users: Causes and rates. In D. E. Smith (Ed.), *Amphetamine use, misuse, and abuse* (pp. 169–188). New York: G. K. Hall.

Kao, C. H., Wang, S. J., & Yeh, S. H. (1994). Presentation of regional cerebral blood flow in amphetamine abusers by 99Tcm-HMPAO brain SPECT. *Nuclear Medicine Communications, 15*(2), 94–98.

Kaufman, M. J., Levin, J. M., Ross, M. H., Lange, N., Rose, S. L., Kukes, T. J., Mendelson, J. H., Lukas, S. E., Cohen, B. M., & Renshaw, P. F. (1997). Cocaine-induced cerebral vasoconstriction detected in humans with magnetic resonance angiography. *Journal of the American Medical Association, 279,* 376–380.

Kaye, B. R., & Fainstat, M. (1987). Cerebral vasculitis associated with cocaine abuse. *Journal of the American Medical Association, 258,* 2104–2106.

Kimura, D., & Harshman, R. A. (1984). Sex differences in brain organization for verbal and non-verbal functions. *Progress in Brain Research, 61,* 423–441.

King, G. R., & Ellinwood, E. H. (1992). Amphetamines and other stimulants. In J. H. Lowinson, P. Ruiz, & R. B. Millman (Eds.), *Substance abuse: A comprehensive textbook* (pp. 247–270). Baltimore, MD: Williams & Wilkins.

Klonoff, D. C., Andres, B. T., & Obana, W. G. (1989). Stroke associated with cocaine use. *Archives of Neurology, 46,* 989–993.

Knuckle, E., & Campbell, A. (1984). *Suitability of neuropsychological test norms with black adolescents.* Paper presented at the International Neuropsychological Society meeting, Houston, TX.

Kosten, T. R., Malison, R., & Wallace, E. (1996). Neuropsychological abnormalities of cocaine abusers: Possible correlates in SPECT neuroimaging. In National Institute on Drug Abuse, *Neurotoxicity and neuropathology associated with cocaine/stimulant abuse* (NIDA Research Monograph No. 163, pp. 175–191). Bethesda, MD: National Institutes of Health, National Institute on Drug Abuse.

Krendel, D. A., Ditter, S. M., Frankel, M. R., & Ross, W. K. (1990). Biopsy-proven cerebral vasculitis associated with cocaine abuse. *Neurology, 40,* 1092–1094.

Lehman, L. B. (1987). Intracerebral hemorrhage after intranasal cocaine use. *Hospital Physician, 7,* 69–70.

Lethem, R., & Orrell, M. (1997). Antioxidants and dementia. *Lancet, 349,* 1189–1190.

Levin, J. B., Holman, L., Mendelson, J. H., Siew, K. T., Garada, B., Johnson, K. A., & Springer, S. (1994). Gender differences in cerebral perfusion in cocaine abuse: Technetium-99m-HMPAO SPECT study of drug abusing. *Journal of Nuclear Medicine, 35,* 1902–1909.

Lex, B. W. (1991). Some gender differences in alcohol and polysubstance abusers. *Health Psychology, 10,* 121–132.

Lichtenfeld, P. J., Rubin, D. B., & Feldman, R. S. (1984). Subarachnoid hemorrhage precipitated by cocaine snorting. *Archives of Neurology, 41,* 223–224.

Lillie-Blanton, M., Anthony, J. C., & Schuster, C. R. (1994). Probing the meaning of racial/ethnic group comparisons in crack cocaine smoking. *Journal of the American Medical Association, 269,* 993–997.

Luria, A. R. (1963). *Restoration of function after brain injury.* New York: Macmillan.

Luria, A. R. (1966). *Higher cortical functioning in man.* New York: Basic Books.

Luria, A. R. (1973). *The working brain.* New York: Basic Books.

Maestre, G., Ottoman, R., Gurland, B., Chun, M., Tang, M. X., Shelanski, M., Tycho, B., & Mayeux, R. (1995). Apolipoprotein E and Alzheimer's disease: Ethnic variation in genotypic risks. *Annals of Neurology, 37*(2), 254–259.

Manly, J., Jacobs, D., Sano, M., Bell, K., & Merchant, C. (1998). Cognitive test performance among nondemented elderly African Americans and whites. *Neurology, 50,* 1238–1245.

Manschreck, T. C., Schneyer, M. L., Weisstein, C. C., Laughery, J., Rosenthal, J., Celada, T., & Berne, J. (1990). Freebase cocaine and memory. *Comprehensive Psychiatry, 31,* 369–375.

Mathew, R. J., & Wilson, W. H. (1991). Substance abuse and cerebral blood flow. *American Journal of Psychiatry, 148,* 292–305.

Mathew, R. J., Wilson, W. H., & Tant, S. R. (1986). Determinants of resting regional cerebral blood flow in normal subjects. *Biological Psychiatry, 21,* 907–914.

Matsuda, H., Maeda, T., Yamada, M., Gui, L. X., & Hisada, K. (1984). Age-matched normal values and topographic maps for regional cerebral blood flow measurements by ^{133}Xe inhalation. *Stroke, 15,* 336–342.

Meek, P. S., Clark, H. W., & Solana, V. (1989). Neurocognitive impairment: The unrecognized component of dual diagnosis in substance abuse treatment. *Journal of Psychoactive Drugs, 21,* 153–160.

Meier, M. J. (1974). Some challenges for clinical neuropsychology. In R. M. Reitan & L. A. Davison (Eds.), *Clinical neuropsychology: Current status and applications* (pp. 289–324). New York: Wiley.

Melamed, E., Lavy, S., Bentin, S., Cooper, G., & Rinot, Y. (1980). Reduction in regional cerebral blood flow during normal aging in man. *Stroke, 11,* 31–35.

Miller, L. (1985). Neuropsychological assessment of substance abusers: Review and recommendations. *Journal of Substance Abuse Treatment, 2,* 5–17.

Miura, S. A., Shapiro, M. B., Grady, C. L., Kumar, A., Salerno, J. A., Kozachuck, W. E., Wagner, E., Rapoport, S. I., & Horowitz, B. (1990). Effect of gender on glucose utilization rates in healthy humans: A positron emission tomography study. *Journal of Neuroscience Research, 27,* 500–504.

Mody, C. K., Miller, B. L., McIntyre, H. B., Cobb, S. K., & Goldberg, M. A. (1988). Neurologic complications of cocaine abuse. *Neurology, 38,* 1189–1193.

Moore, P. M., & Peterson, P. I. (1989). Nonhemorrhagic cerebrovascular complications of cocaine abuse. *Neurology, 39*(Suppl. 1), 302.

Nalls, G., Disher, A., Dariabagi, J., Zant, Z., & Eisenman, J. (1989). Subcortical cerebral hemorrhages associated with cocaine abuse: CT and MR findings. *Journal of Computer Assisted Tomography, 13,* 1–5.

National Institute on Drug Abuse (NIDA). (1998, April). Methamphetamine: Abuse and addiction. (NIH publication No. 98-4210). *NIDA Research Report Series, 2.* On-line at: http://165.112.78.61/research reports/methamp/methamp.html

Noguchi, S., Murakami, K., & Yamada, N. (1993). Apolipoprotein-E genotype and Alzheimer's disease. *Lancet 342,* 737.

Notel, K. B., & Gelman, B. B. (1989). Intracerebral hemorrhage associated with cocaine abuse. *Archives of Pathology and Laboratory Medicine, 113,* 812–813.

Pericak-Vance, M. A., Bebout, J. L., Gaskell, P. C., Jr., Yamaoka, L. H., Hung, W. Y., Alberts, M. J., Walker, A. P., Bartlett, R. J., Haynes, C. A., & Welsh, K. A. (1991). Linkage studies in familial Alzheimer's disease: Evidence for chromosome 19 linkage. *American Journal of Human Genetics, 48*(6), 1034–1050.

Piazza, D. M. (1980). The influence of sex and handedness in the hemispheric specialization of verbal and nonverbal tasks. *Neuropsychologia, 18,* 163–175.

Pulse Check: National Trends in Drug Control Policy. (1998, summer).

Rebeck, G. W., Perls, T. T., & West, H. L. (1994). Reduced apolipoprotein epsilon 4 allele frequency in the oldest old Alzheimer's patient and cognitively normal individuals. *Neurology, 44,* 1513–1516.

Reitan, R. M., & Davison, L. A. (Eds.). (1974). *Clinical neuropsychology: Current status and applications.* New York: Wiley.

Reitan, R. M., & Wolfson, D. (1992). *The Halstead-Reitan Neuropsychological Test Battery: Theory and clinical interpretation* (2nd ed.). Tucson, AZ: Neuropsychology Press.

Ricaurte, G. A., Guillery, R. W., Seiden, L. S., Schuster, C. R., & Moore, R. Y. (1982). Dopamine nerve terminal degeneration produced by high doses of methylamphetamine in the rat brain. *Brain Research, 235,* 93–103.

Ricaurte, G. A., Schuster, C. R., & Seiden, L. S. (1980). Long-term effects of repeated methyl-amphetamine administration on dopamine and serotonin neurons in the rat brain: A regional study. *Brain Research, 193,* 153–163.

Ricaurte, G. A., Seiden, L. S., & Schuster, C. R. (1984). Further evidence that amphetamines produce long-lasting dopaminergic neurochemical deficits by destroying dopamine nerve fibers. *Brain Research, 303,* 359–364.

Rodriguez, G., Warkentin, S., Risberg, J., & Rosadini, G. (1988). Sex differences in regional cerebral blood flow. *Journal of Cerebral Blood Flow and Metabolism, 8,* 783–789.

Rogers, J. N., Henry, T. E., Jones, A. M., Froede, R. C., & Byers, J. M., III. (1986). Cocaine-related deaths in Pima County, AZ, 1982–1984. *Journal of Forensic Sciences, 31,* 1404–1408.

Rowley, H. A., Lowenstein, D. H., Rowbotham, M. C., & Simon, R. P. (1989). Thalamo-mesencephalic strokes after cocaine abuse. *Neurology, 39,* 428–430.

Rumbaugh, C. L. (1977). Small vessel cerebral vascular changes following chronic amphetamine intoxication. In E. H. Ellinwood & M. Kilbey (Eds.), *Cocaine and other stimulants* (pp. 241–251). New York: Plenum.

Saunders, A. M., Holette, C., Welsh-Bohmer, K. A., Schmechel, D. E., Crain, B., Burke, J. R., Alberts, M. J., Strittmatter, W. J., Breitner, J.C.S., Rosenberg, C., Scott, S. V., Gaskell, P. C., Pericak-Vance, M. A., & Roses, A. D. (1996). Specificity, sensitivity, and predictive value of apolipoprotein-E genotyping for sporadic Alzheimer's disease. *Lancet, 348,* 90–93.

Saunders, A. M., Strittmatter, W. J., Schmechel, D., George-Hyslop, P. H., Pericak-Vance, M. A., Joo, S. H., Rosi, B. L., Gusella, J. F., Crapper-Maclachlan, D. R., & Alberts, M. J. (1993). Association of apolipoprotein E allele epsilon 4 with late-onset familial and sporadic Alzheimer's disease. *Neurology, 43*(8), 1467–1472.

Schwartz, K. A., & Cohen, J. A. (1984). Subarachnoid hemorrhage precipitated by cocaine snorting. *Archives of Neurology, 41,* 705.

Seiden, L. S., Fischman, M. W., & Schuster, C. R. (1977). Changes in brain catecholamines induced by long-term methamphetamine administration in rhesus monkeys. In E. H. Ellinwood & M. Kilbey (Eds.), *Cocaine and other stimulants* (pp. 179–185). New York: Plenum.

Shaw, T. G., Mortel, K. F., Meyer, J. S., Rogers, R. L., Hardenberg, J., & Cutaia, M. M. (1984). Cerebral blood flow changes in benign aging and cerebrovascular disease. *Neurology, 34,* 855–862.

Sterling, T. D., & Weinkam, J. J. (1989). Comparison of smoking-related risk factors among black and white males. *American Journal of Industrial Medicine, 15*(3), 319–333.

Strickland, T. L., D'Elia, L. F., James, R., & Stein, R. (1997). Stroop color-word performance of African Americans. *The Clinical Neuropsychologist, 11,* 87–90.

Strickland, T. L., Mena, I., Villanueva-Meyer, J., Miller, B. L., Cummings, J., Mehringer, C. M., Satz, P., & Meyers, H. (1993). Cerebral perfusion and neuropsychological consequences of chronic cocaine use. *Journal of Neuropsychiatry and Clinical Neuroscience, 5,* 419–427.

Strickland, T. L., Miller, B. L., Stein, R. A., & Kowell, A. (2000). Neuropsychological aspects of cocaine abuse: Contributions from functional neuroimaging. *Neuropsychology Review.*

Strittmatter, W. J., Saunders, A. M., Schmechel, D., Pericak-Vance, M. A., Enghild, J., Salvenson, G. S., & Roses, A. D. (1993). Apolipoprotein E: High-avidity in late-onset familial Alzheimer's disease. *Proceedings of the National Academy of Science USA, 90*(5), 1977–1981.

Substance Abuse and Mental Health Services Administration. (1994). *Preliminary estimates from the 1993 national household survey on drug abuse.* Washington, DC: U.S. Department of Health and Human Services.

Sue, S., Fujino, D. C., Hu, L., Takeuchi, D., & Zane, N. W. (1991). Community mental health services for ethnic minority groups. A test of the cultural responsiveness hypothesis. *Journal of Consulting and Clinical Psychology, 59,* 533–540.

U.S. Department of Health and Human Services. (1995). *Preliminary estimates from the 1994 National Household Survey on Drug Abuse* (Advance Report No. 10). Hyattsville, MD: Author.

Von Voigtlander, P. F., & Moore, K. E. (1973). Involvement of nigro-striatal neurons in the in vivo release of dopamine by amphetamine, amantadine and tyramine. *Journal of Pharmacology and Experimental Therapeutics, 184,* 542–552.

Weiner, N. (1985). Norepinephrine, epinephrine and the sympathomimetic amines. In A. G. Gilman, L. S. Goodman, T. W. Rall, & F. Murad (Eds.), *The pharmacological basis of therapeutics* (pp. 145–180). New York: Macmillan.

Williams, D. R., & Collins, C. (1995). U.S. socioeconomic and racial differences in health: Patterns and explanations. *Annual Review of Sociology, 21,* 349–386.

Wojak, J. C., & Flamm, E. S. (1987). Intracranial hemorrhage and cocaine abuse. *Stroke, 18,* 712–715.

Wolkin, A., Angrist, B., Wolf, A., Brodie, J., Wolkin, B., Jaeger, J., Camero, R., & Rotrosen, J. (1987). Effects of amphetamine on local cerebral metabolism in normal and schizophrenic subjects as determined by positron emission tomography. *Psychopharmacology, 92,* 241–246.

CHAPTER NINETEEN

ALCOHOL USE AND MISUSE

Frederick D. Harper

This chapter explores alcohol drinking behaviors, consequences, and problems; research on alcohol, alcohol abuse, and blacks; culture-specific treatment, intervention, and counseling; and models and strategies for the prevention of alcohol-related problems. It also examines the implications of this information and presents recommendations. An appendix offers program resources and sources of information.

Drinking Behaviors, Consequences, and Problems

On the one hand, African American drinking patterns and behaviors are similar to those of the general U.S. population: that is, (1) males are more likely than females to drink alcohol and to be heavy drinkers and problem drinkers, (2) young adults in their twenties are more likely to drink and drink heavily than are adolescents and adults in their mid-thirties and older, (3) single and newly divorced persons drink more heavily than married persons do, and (4) persons residing in the western United States and large metropolitan areas drink more than those in the eastern and rural areas, respectively (National Institute on Alcohol Abuse and Alcoholism [NIAAA], 1997). On the other hand, a national survey of drinking behaviors by ethnicity indicates that African American adolescents and adults tend to have a slightly lower rate of alcohol use in the past year and a lower rate of heavy alcohol use in the past month when compared to the general U.S. population (Substance Abuse and Mental Health Services Administration [SAMHSA], 1998). Moreover, as compared to specific ethnic groups, in national survey results reported by the National Institute on Alcohol Abuse and

Alcoholism (NIAAA, 1997), African Americans presented lower rates of current drinkers and weekly drinkers when compared to whites and Hispanics, a lower rate of heavier drinkers when compared to Hispanics, and a similar rate of heavier drinkers when compared to whites. (Asian Americans have the lowest rate of drinkers and heavier drinkers when compared to African Americans, Hispanic Americans, Native Americans, and white Americans.)

However, when consequences are considered, African Americans seem to have a significantly higher percentage of problems associated with alcohol use than other U.S. populations do (NIAAA, 1990; Caetano & Clark, 1998; Herd, 1994). For example, Caetano's survey (1997) of drinking problems among subsamples of 723 blacks, 703 Hispanics, and 788 whites ($N = 2,214$) revealed that African Americans and Hispanics, regardless of gender, were more at risk for alcohol-related health and social problems. However, it must be kept in mind that Caetano's 1997 publication was based on data collected in 1992. Looking at more recent survey data, collected in 1995, Caetano and Clark (1998) found that although black men had a higher rate than white men of alcohol-related problems (11 percent versus 13 percent), between the years 1984 and 1995, black men showed a larger decrease in alcohol-related problems (a 16 to 13 percent decrease for black males versus a 12 to 11 percent drop for white males).

In contrast to Caetano's findings, Herd's analysis (1997) of national survey data indicated that African American women presented a lower rate than white women of risk for alcohol problems. Nevertheless, like Caetano (1997) and Caetano and Clark (1998), Herd (1994) found that African American men seem to have a higher rate of alcohol-related health and social problems when compared to white men but a lower rate of heavier drinkers. Even when the alcohol-related health problem of cirrhosis is considered, black men tend to have a higher rate of alcohol-related cirrhosis (NIAAA, 1997).

African American Youths

Consistently over the last two to three decades, African American youths have demonstrated similar or lower rates of alcohol use when compared to white youths or the general population (Braucht, 1982; Dawkins, 1976; Epstein, Botvin, & Diaz, 1998; Globetti, 1970; Johnston, O'Malley, & Bachman, 1998a, 1998b). Furthermore, a number of recent studies have found African American youths to have lower rates of alcohol use and heavier drinking when compared to other nonwhite American ethnic groups, except for Asian American youths (Bass & Kane-Williams, 1993; Epstein, Botvin, Baker, & Diaz, 1998; Epstein, Botvin, & Diaz, 1998; National Clearinghouse for Alcohol and Drug Information, 1995).

A national survey by the National Clearinghouse for Alcohol and Drug Information (1995) indicates that black youths fare favorably on alcohol use patterns and behaviors when compared to most other major American ethnic groups. For example, when compared to white youths and Hispanic youths, African American youths presented the lowest rates of lifetime alcohol use, current alcohol use, and episodic heavier drinking. In the same survey, African American female and male high school students had the lowest percentages of reported use of alcohol or other drugs during their last sexual intercourse experience as compared to their white and Hispanic counterparts.

Even when urban youths are surveyed alone, there appears to be a lower rate of risk for alcohol use among African American youths as compared to some of the other youth subsamples. For example, in a three-year self-report study of patterns of alcohol use involving a sample of 2,312 African American, Asian, Hispanic, and white youths in twenty-two urban schools in New York, Epstein, Botvin, and Diaz (1998) found that African American and Asian American youths demonstrated lower rates of alcohol use and fewer episodes of drunkenness when compared to Hispanic and white youths. (For external generalizability purposes the research participants were all urban youths in grades 6 and 7 who were primarily [67 percent] from two-parent homes.)

College Students

Studies are beginning to emerge that report a high level of binge drinking (five or more drinks per occasion) by white college students (Johnston, O'Malley, & Bachman, 1998b; Wechsler, Davenport, Dowdall, Moeykens, & Castillo, 1994). This binge drinking very often involves a period of heavy drinking over an extended weekend from Thursday through Sunday. Nevertheless, recent surveys (NIAAA, 1997) suggest that African American students are less involved in binge drinking than their white counterparts. For example, Meilman, Stone, Gaylor, and Turco (1990) carried out a study on 400 undergraduate students and found that 91.8 percent drank at least once a month and that a larger proportion of white students than minority students binge drank (8.6 percent versus 5.4 percent).

In a survey of 590 African American students from a traditionally black university in the south, Grenier, Gorskey, and Folse (1998) found 75.5 percent had taken at least one drink in the previous month; however, a very small percentage reported drinking daily (3 percent). Moreover, 85 percent of the African American college students reported that they would be willing to attend a nonalcoholic party.

The Research on Alcohol and Blacks

The research studies involving African Americans in general and African Americans and alcohol in particular are often based on Western-biased research questions, research variables and terms, measurements or instrumentation, and procedures (Butcher, 1982; Harper, 1996). For example, research variables are often based on such western concepts and values as an emphasis on self, a deficit orientation (which appears for example in deficit-oriented terminology), a focus on levels of performance on instruments, and a concern with deviance as dysfunction (as opposed to difference) and with health as the norm (as opposed to health as positive exceptionality or as a positive striving toward survival and growth).

Self-report data collection instrumentation is often Western oriented in content, Western defined (in an operational sense), and white-Western normed. Psychological diagnostic criteria and psychological assessment tools are often Western oriented (as are, for example, the *Diagnostic and Statistical Manual of Mental Disorders* [*DSM-IV*], the Rorschach assessment, personality inventories, and alcohol-drug self-report assessment instruments). Often African Americans are misdiagnosed due to Anglocentric or Americentric language and terms employed in printed, standardized instruments, language and terms that may differ from black English terms or may embody concepts different from ebonic concepts, resulting in the miscommunication of test or instrument items (Harper, Braithwaite, & LaGrange, 1999). Moreover, a significant number of tests and self-report instruments are normed primarily on white American samples and thus may be biased against African Americans or persons of African descent when it comes to interpretation of test or instrument results.

Also, the treatment modalities on which outcome research is often predicated are usually Western oriented (involving, for example, a medical model of diagnosis and treatment, medical detoxification of alcohol addicts, traditional group psychotherapy, individual psychotherapy, and Western theoretical or clinical approaches to counseling).

With regard to statistical procedures, there is an overemphasis on inferring and predicting, on associating rather than observing, on averaging (determining statistical means, for example), and in general on analyzing rather than understanding phenomena. In surveys on the use of alcohol and other drugs, there is also an overemphasis or sole emphasis on intergroup comparisons at the expense of intragroup comparisons. Nevertheless, the survey *Prevalence of Substance Use Among Racial and Ethnic Subgroups in the United States, 1991–1993,* by the Substance Abuse and Mental Health Services Administration (1998), is one good example of a broad-scale survey that examines a variety of intragroup differences for ethnic groups with regard to Hispanics (offering, for example, comparisons among Central Americans, Cuban Americans, Hispanics from South America, Mexican Americans, and Puerto Rican Americans).

Although various western statistical procedures are certainly useful, they should not be overemphasized and overvalued in deriving research results for the purpose of policy decision making, planning, and development. Along with collecting self-reported data on alcohol-related measures, researchers must also be able to observe and record behavioral events via direct observation methods (that is, without ethnocentrically biased and predetermined assumptions). Moreover, researchers should examine the characteristics of samples and statistical distributions as well as analyze mean and median differences on alcohol-related measures, especially when there are questions about the sample size and distribution. Certainly, there are nonparametric statistical procedures that have been overlooked in cases of analysis of small samples of black research participants or in cases where the data may not have been drawn from normally distributed populations.

In addition, researchers must raise realistic questions, ones that are based on sound ethnic-centered theory and initial pilot observations of an African American sociodemographic group, rather than raising biased research questions, ones that are based on their Western-biased training, and thus coming up with biased outcomes and interpretations.

In the area of research design and methods, there is a need for more longitudinal studies on blacks' use of alcohol and a need for time-series studies in order to ascertain patterns of drinking behaviors and alcohol-related problems across a specific period of time and among different sociodemographic groups of blacks. These time-series studies would allow for intermittent measures or observations over an extended period of time such as a month or year, whereas a longitudinal study is likely to measure trends over a number of years. Other research methods appropriate for understanding African American drinking behaviors are naturalistic studies (studies in a natural setting involving direct observation of African American drinking behaviors), content analysis studies (studies that analyze alcohol-related parameters in black literature such as black magazines, autobiographies, novels, and so on), qualitative studies in general, and historical studies of alcohol use during various periods of African American history. For example, there are questions about how the drinking behaviors of blacks prior to the Civil Rights Act of 1964 compare to blacks' drinking behaviors during the decades since then.

There is also a dire need to study alcohol use and misuse behaviors among middle-class and upper-class African Americans. The great majority of studies on blacks' use of alcohol have been carried out on "captive" black participants, those who have had little or no control over their role as study participants (for example, alcoholics in treatment, alcoholics in counseling, hospital patients, prison inmates, criminal offenders, homicide victims, welfare recipients, college students, and school youths).

Treatment, Intervention, and Counseling

Treatment, intervention, and counseling for African Americans who are alcoholic or who have alcohol-related problems should address cultural orientation, family dynamics, family needs, employment needs, overall health needs, and lifestyle change. With regard to culture-specific treatment, it is preferable that alcoholism treatment efforts for African Americans consider or encourage (1) cultural competence among the helping practitioners, (2) an understanding of the cultural diversity within the African American population, (3) the involvement of African American counselors where possible, (4) intervention programs that are located in black communities, and (5) the establishment of accessible Alcoholics Anonymous (AA) groups in the black community or ethnic-centered AA groups with a predominantly African American membership (Brisbane, 1998; Center for Substance Abuse Prevention, 1993; Harper & Saifnoorian, 1991). Nevertheless, even though these conditions of treatment are preferred, that preference does not preclude the treatment of African American alcoholics in mainstream programs or hospitals or their involvement in predominantly non-black-oriented settings when the preferred conditions or options are not available.

With respect to family orientation, treatment should train and counsel the black family on how to be a support system rather than an enabling system. Family members can learn how to support and encourage responsibility and the motivation to be sober on the part of the African American alcoholic or problem drinker who is in treatment, rather than succumbing to a situation in which the family, as a system, enables problem drinking or alcoholism through its emotional reactions to and rejection of the problem-drinking member. Moreover, counselors need to assess the effect of alcoholism or problem drinking on the family and aim to eliminate dysfunctional family interactions, while also addressing African American familial needs for health services, social services, education, and even employment. It should be noted that in a number of sociodemographic groups of African Americans, a significant proportion of black alcoholics are unemployed, lack stable employment, or are homeless (NIAAA, 1990).

African American family problems that are associated to some degree with alcoholism or heavy drinking include spousal and partner abuse (especially male-to-female violence), child abuse (physical and sexual abuse), financial problems, certain health problems, child neglect, inappropriate sharing of alcoholic beverages with babies and youths, violence related to gambling and drinking, and marital discord. A warning here is that many of these family disrupting alcohol-related problems have been found in research on urban or low-income African Americans; there is little research in this area on middle-class or upper-class African American families (Harper & Saifnoorian, 1991; Herd, 1989; NIAAA, 1997).

The theoretical orientation of the counseling or intervention should be based on cognitive-behavioral and holistic perspectives and *not* the intrapsychic, interpretative, psychoanalytic perspective or the various passive, slow, and introspective therapies, which include client-centered therapy. Nevertheless, existential psychotherapy's concepts of meaning, choice, and loneliness are worth pursuing with some African American alcoholics, as appropriate to the individual, in terms of addressing life issues. Also, counselors may find useful such Gestalt therapy techniques and concepts as unfinished business (resolving unfinished issues from the past), role-playing, homework (activities for outpatients to do between counseling sessions), confrontation (the counselor's confrontation of the client's resistance), role reversal (role-playing wherein the alcoholic exchanges roles with a family member or another significant person in his or her life), and empty chair (role-playing with an imaginary person in an empty chair, for example, someone who has died). For an excellent review of these techniques and concepts of counseling, see Nugent (1999).

Foremost and in general, the cognitive-behavioral counseling approaches and techniques are recommended because these are directive and action-oriented models that involve changing the illogical thoughts and irrational game playing of the alcoholic client. Illogical thoughts are perceived as driving the client's illogical or irrational alcohol-related actions and behaviors. Cognitive-behavioral techniques are also effective in dealing with resistive behavior, defense mechanisms, and the game playing that alcoholics frequently use to maintain their addiction and to arouse guilt, anger, and anxiety in their loved ones. Some examples of cognitive-behavioral approaches are rational behavior therapy (Maultsby, 1984), choice theory (Glasser, 1998), reality therapy (Glasser & Wubbolding, 1995), rational emotive behavior therapy (Dryden, 1995; Ellis, 1995), and transcendent counseling (Harper & Stone, 1999).

Counseling techniques and foci of cognitive-behavioral approaches often include (1) cognitive restructuring of illogical thoughts and beliefs, (2) persuading the client to think realistically and differently, (3) using stress management and relaxation techniques, and (4) teaching social learning or social skills development by inadvertent imitation of positive role models. These techniques all seem to be relevant and useful in counseling African American clients with alcohol problems and an *alcoholic personality*.

In the author's counseling, consulting, and research experiences, the following are some of the irrational or illogical thoughts that African American alcoholics verbalize in order to maintain or justify their continued heavy drinking:

> "Alcoholism is a white thing. I am not alcoholic, I just drink a lot of liquor."
>
> "I can quit tomorrow if I want to."
>
> "Everybody has a crutch, and mine is alcohol."
>
> "Lend me some money [to buy alcohol]. I'll pay you when my ship comes in."
>
> "If I can find me a good job, I'll stop drinking."
>
> "If it was not for my wife [or husband], I wouldn't have to drink."

The following treatment, intervention, and counseling strategies are also recommended.

• Treatment efforts should focus on *outreach counseling*, because black alcoholics and problem drinkers are not likely to self-refer or voluntarily come to treatment, and the family is not likely to refer a family member to treatment.

• Treatment programs and their counselors should focus on the *employment needs* of African Americans, because drinking may be related to unemployment, unstable employment, or even racial discrimination in employment à la the glass ceiling.

• Treatment activities and counseling efforts should focus on *holistic health*, regarding physical health, mental health, and spiritual health as being one and essential. This holistic orientation is very much a part of the African and Native American roots of black Americans and is also found in the religious and spiritual grounding of blacks in the church or through their religious family upbringing. Religion has been found to be an effective motivating force in the therapy and improvement of African American alcoholics and problem drinkers. Positive religious influences in the black community have mainly come from the Christian Protestant churches and the Nation of Islam, or black Muslims.

• Medical personnel or health care providers on both inpatient and outpatient staffs should interview, examine, and arrange to treat African American alcoholics for *diseases other than their alcoholism*, diseases or illnesses that may be compounded by heavy drinking (for example, diabetes, hypertension, lupus, HIV/AIDS, prostate conditions, kidney disease, cancer, cardiovascular and cerebrovascular diseases, and liver disease).

• Based on national input from counselors who work with African American alcoholics and problem drinkers, the following *treatment methods* are recommended, ranked in order of perceived importance: (1) outreach counseling; (2) individual, or one-to-one, counseling; (3) referrals to and from other agencies or programs; (4) participation in educational groups, including alcohol education groups; (5) job placement and employment counseling; (6) family counseling; (7) participation in AA groups; (8) aftercare, or follow-up, of the client after alcoholism treatment; (9) group counseling; (10) job training; (11) interpersonal skills development; (12) medical treatment; (13) public assistance and services as necessary; and (14) self-esteem development. Treatment methods that were mentioned by counselors but that ranked lowest included self-management skills, recreation, meditation or spiritual activity, and social modeling (Harper & Saifnoorian, 1991; also see Harper, 1979).

It is also important to consider some ongoing treatment issues related to black alcoholism, alcohol misuse, and problem drinking. For each issue presented here, an accompanying comment offers insights based on research, practice, and theory.

Issue. Can whites or nonblacks effectively counsel black alcoholics?

Comment. Black counselors who grow up in a black cultural milieu have an edge in cultural understanding; however, effective counseling also relies on the counselor's personal and professional experience with alcoholism, the counselor's personality, and the counselor's professional commitment to help the client as perceived by the client (Harper, 1983; Harper & Saifnoorian, 1991).

Issue. Isn't an alcoholic an alcoholic—that is, aren't all alcoholics the same regardless of ethnicity?

Comment. Biomedical research supports the contention that all alcoholics are subject to the same physiological mechanism of addiction due to sustained, heavy use of the drug alcohol, and all alcoholics tend to display similar physiological and psychological responses to alcohol addiction. Nonetheless, alcoholics differ in their language and their system of communication, their cognitive-perceptual styles, their drinking patterns (when, where, how, with whom, and what they drink), their cultural style, and their gender (NIAAA, 1990, 1997).

Issue. Should treatment programs or related agencies provide employment services and financial support for low-income alcoholics who are in treatment and who are often African Americans from urban communities?

Comment. Effective treatment surely requires a variety of supportive efforts for low-income African Americans. Many clients in treatment are in need of jobs, medical care, health insurance, and child care. For female alcoholics, child care is often a necessity during the several hours required for each outpatient visit (including both treatment and transportation time) or during the three weeks or more required for inpatient treatment. Therefore a holistic approach to alcoholism treatment should examine the comprehensive needs of each African American and seek to address those needs as appropriate.

Issue. Don't we have to recognize that alcohol is a means of black survival in the face of racism and racial discrimination?

Comment. Although alcohol, as a drug, offers a means of psychological escape from racial problems, daily stress, and painful misfortunes, its misuse cannot be justified as necessary for black survival and social adjustment because there are also positive solutions and positive mechanisms available for dealing with racism, daily stresses, and life's misfortunes—mechanisms such as counseling, family support, relaxation techniques, exercise, meditation, interpersonal effectiveness training, and self-management techniques. Alcohol misuse is actually a means of black self-destruction and the destruction of black families and communities.

Models and Strategies for the Prevention of Alcohol-Related Problems

Discussion of the prevention of alcoholism and alcohol-related problems is often couched in the context of three levels of prevention: primary prevention, secondary prevention, and tertiary prevention. Primary prevention efforts are designed to prevent alcohol misuse, inappropriate alcohol-related behaviors, and alcohol problems long before any drinking occurs. Secondary prevention is targeted at drinkers or probable drinkers who may be at risk for alcoholism or alcohol-related problems, that is, after drinking has started but before at-risk behaviors escalate to the level of manifested alcohol-related health or social problems. Tertiary prevention involves treating alcoholics or problem drinkers so that their disease or problem drinking is arrested or so that the likelihood of their becoming involved in alcohol-related problems in the future diminishes substantially (Maisto, Galizio, & Connors, 1999).

In terms of African Americans' use and misuse of alcohol, it seems we should have a primary focus on the prevention of alcoholism and heavy drinking and thus also a focus on the prevention of alcohol-related health and social problems, considering the evidence that compared to others in the general population, African Americans are likely to have a higher rate of alcohol-related health and social problems (NIAAA, 1990; Caetano, 1997). With regard to participants in prevention efforts, schools, community groups and leaders, families, and professionals should become involved, as well as any persons in a position to affect the alcohol industry and alcohol-related policy. In a broader sense, prevention efforts should involve a partnership among educational institutions at all levels, community organizations, businesses, government, and churches or religious groups. This collaborative ideology is tantamount to the nowadays trite but still highly meaningful African proverb "It takes a whole village to raise a child."

The Comer project is an example of a long-running, community-based, collaborative program that has focused on the primary prevention of school failure, violence, and alcohol and drug problems among urban African American youths. Formally referred to as the Yale Child Study Center's School Development Program (SDP), it was founded in 1968 at Yale University by James P. Comer, an African American professor. The Comer project is currently implemented in more than eighty-two school districts in twenty-one states and Washington, D.C. The project focuses on creating a cooperative and collaborative network of students, parents, teachers, administrators, and community leaders that works for the healthy development of youths, the prevention of violence and alcohol and drug abuse, and the improved academic achievement of students (Comer, 1993; Haynes, 1996). The Comer project has incorporated a number of significant protective factors associated with reducing the risk for alcohol and drug addiction, factors such as improved academic achievement (Rodney, Mupier, & O'Neal, 1997), positive self-esteem (Rodney, Mupier, & Crafter, 1996), and parental knowledge about alcohol as well as parents' involvement in the education of their children (Donnelly, Mowery, & McCarver, 1998).

Another school-centered alcohol and drug prevention program that emphasizes community involvement, organizational collaboration, and the use of positive role models is the Building Resiliency and Vocational Excellence (BRAVE) program in Atlanta. BRAVE is a federally funded program that employs violence and alcohol and drug abuse prevention strategies with African American teenage boys who have been intermittently expelled from public schools or identified by teachers or principals as threatening or difficult to manage (Harper & Griffin, 2000). BRAVE's prevention efforts emphasize alcohol and drug abuse prevention, anger management and violence prevention, job placement, assistance in academic schoolwork, and one-on-one, male role model mentoring. Again, all of these foci assist in developing the protective factors that act as buffers, reducing youths' risk for alcohol misuse and addiction.

Johnson and Johnson (1999) posit that although there are stressful conditions and events in urban living that influence heavier drinking and problem-drinking behaviors among some African Americans, there are also important cultural and familial factors that protect blacks from the risk of alcohol misuse and its related problems—factors such as the black church, some black parents' antismoking and antidrinking attitudes, and other black parents' values and beliefs about controlling drinking. With regard to additional psychological traits among African Americans that encourage black survival and discourage alcohol misuse, Na'm Akbar, at the Second National Conference on Preventing and Treating Alcohol and Other Drug Abuse, HIV Infection, and AIDS in Black Communities, postulated that "hope, will, love, and faith" are essential strengths of African Americans for addressing social and health problems (Center for Substance Abuse Prevention, 1993, p. 14).

Further protective factors in the African American family are suggested by research and theories on healthy families that are focusing more on the quality of family functioning than on the nature of family structure or on the traditional myth that the healthy family must have both biological parents present throughout a child's development. Certainly, two *nurturing* parents are as effective, if not more effective, than a single nurturing parent with regard to the healthy development of their offspring. Nevertheless, family therapists and family researchers are now giving increased attention to healthy and mature transactions between family members, that is, to the quality of functioning within the family as opposed to mainly the dysfunctional behaviors and dysfunctional transactions associated with the structure of family membership (Lewis, Dana, & Blevins, 1994). In documenting the importance of family functioning, a recent graduate from Howard University found in her doctoral dissertation research that family functioning was more important than family structure as a predictor of self-esteem, perceived parental nurturance, and healthy development in college youths (Terry-Leonard, 1999). Quality of family functioning may explain why black children from some single-parent families excel and why children from some two-parent families, regardless of race, can fail to achieve and fail to value themselves highly as human beings.

The following are additional culture-specific recommendations aimed at the prevention of alcoholism, heavy drinking, and alcohol-related problems among African Americans.

• Coordinated efforts should be made to eliminate alcohol billboard advertisements in urban African American neighborhoods.

• Communities should make an effort to eliminate or minimize the presence of alcohol outlets in black residential neighborhoods by altering city ordinances that allow the establishment and maintenance of liquor stores near homes and schools, a condition that offers easy access to alcohol and that influences the drinking behaviors of African Americans.

• Family members and helping professionals should discourage the practice of heavy drinking while gambling, especially among black males. The intoxicated gambler who loses money can become ego dejected, angry, and violence prone.

• Public alcohol education programs should focus on dispelling and eliminating such harmful intergenerational practices by some African Americans as (1) using alcohol to relieve chronic pain, (2) giving small amounts of alcohol to babies as a sedative to put them to sleep, and (3) practicing all-night house partying.

• Medical staff, health care professionals in general, educators, and alcohol abuse treatment professionals should encourage accurate knowledge and attitudinal changes about alcohol among African Americans who are at high risk due to drinking heavily while using prescribed medication. Moreover, heavy drinking should be discouraged for African Americans who have chronic diseases that are exacerbated by such heavy alcohol use and for African Americans who are at high risk for crises resulting from use of alcohol with illicit drugs.

Conclusion

According to national surveys, African Americans as a group have lower rates of drinkers and of heavier drinkers when compared to the general U.S. population; nevertheless, African Americans, especially males, have a higher rate of the health and social problems associated with alcohol use. Black women and black youths in particular tend to have lower rates of drinkers, heavier drinkers, and problem drinkers when compared to their counterparts (NIAAA, 1990, 1997; SAMHSA, 1998).

As African Americans increase in age, especially into the middle-age years, there is an increased possibility of social and health problems related to alcohol use. For example, white males record more alcohol-related problems in their twenties (ages eighteen to twenty-nine) than similarly aged black males, whereas black males in their thirties and older have more alcohol-related problems than their white male counterparts (Herd, 1989, 1997). An explanation here may be that black males have more social problems and fewer employment opportunities due to race when compared to white males. The stressful reactions to these types of racial conditions and barriers may very well influence incidents of alcohol misuse and their associated problems.

When the question arises about the rates of use of legal drugs (for example, tobacco and alcohol) as compared to the rates for illicit drugs among African Americans, recent national surveys indicate the following surprising patterns. In SAMHSA's national survey (1998) of U.S. substance abuse behaviors among various ethnic groups and subgroups ($N = 87,000$) from 1991 through 1993, African Americans presented lower rates of cigarette use than the rates for the general U.S. population in the past year and also lower rates of heavy cigarette use in the past month (a pack or more a day), alcohol use in the past year, alcohol dependence, and heavy alcohol use (five or more drinks per occasion); however, African Americans indicated higher rates of illicit drug use for marijuana use in the past year, cocaine use in the past year, and use of any illicit drug in the past year.

The overall interaction of alcohol use with predisposing diseases and health problems among African Americans is a concern that needs to be addressed by health care professionals and counseling or psychotherapeutic practitioners. Moreover, the interaction of stress and distress due to racism, racial discrimination, and poverty with alcohol use and misuse is another area of dire concern for helping professionals who work with black problem drinkers and alcoholics. As African Americans get older, the challenges of race coupled with the universal challenges of human development over the life span can result in overall life challenges greater than those faced by white America. Under the persistent stressful circumstances faced by black America, alcohol use and misuse can become an escape mechanism or an inadvertent means of addressing the challenges of survival and self-improvement in a racist world of inequality, racial rejection, and racial hostility.

Appendix: Resources

The following resources and agencies are presented for professionals and laypersons interested in additional knowledge and research on alcohol and the African American community or interested in information on grant funding opportunities for proposed research projects or community efforts.

National Clearinghouse for Alcohol and Drug Information
Web site: www.health.org/index.htm

The National Clearinghouse for Alcohol and Drug Information provides a list of free and low-cost materials such as survey reports, special populations reports, fact sheets, research abstracts and reports, educational brochures, prevention flyers, and videotapes that can be accessed on-line via the Internet or requested by telephone.

National Institute on Alcohol Abuse and Alcoholism
Web site: www.niaaa.nih.gov

The National Institute on Alcohol Abuse and Alcoholism is the federal agency designated by the U.S. Congress in 1970 to combat alcoholism and alcohol problems. It provides grant funds for biomedical and behavioral research, and it plays a role in policy development, in information distribution, and in the collaborative efforts of alcohol professionals, associations, and researchers.

National Council on Alcoholism and Drug Dependence
Web site: www.ncadd.org

The National Council on Alcoholism and Drug Dependence (formerly the National Council on Alcoholism) is the largest private organization that is aimed at alcohol and drug awareness and addiction prevention on both the national and local levels. It has local affiliates in many cities throughout the country that carry out its aims at the local and state levels.

All of these agencies and organizations have to some degree developed or distributed information on alcohol and blacks over the years and have coordinated various program efforts to serve nonwhite ethnic groups.

In addition, the U.S. Department of Education has funded projects related to the prevention of alcohol and other drug problems primarily among children and adolescents, and the U.S. Department of Transportation has focused on the problem of drinking and driving, working on efforts to prevent drunk driving and alcohol-related road accidents.

In the black community the effective efforts of the black Muslims, or Nation of Islam, to eliminate alcohol and drug use and addiction among black inmates in prisons as well as among African American converts to Islam in general cannot be overlooked. In addition, a number of black Christian churches have taken in persons with alcohol problems and have helped them to substitute a lifestyle of spirituality and church involvement for a lifestyle involving drinking friends and heavy drinking. Religious institutions and churches are definitely a valuable resource in the black community for addressing alcohol problems among African Americans.

References

Bass, L. E., & Kane-Williams, E. (1993). Stereotypes or reality: Another look at alcohol and drug use among African American children. *Public Health Reports, 108,* 78–84.

Braucht, G. N. (1982). Problem drinking among adolescents: A review and analysis of psychosocial research. In National Institute on Alcohol Abuse and Alcoholism, *Alcohol and health: Special populations issues.* (NIAAA Monograph No. 4, DHHS Publication No. ADM-82-1193, pp. 143–164). Rockville, MD: National Institute on Alcohol Abuse and Alcoholism.

Brisbane, F. L. (1998). *Cultural competence for health care professionals working with African American communities: Theory and practice* (CSAP Cultural Competence Series No. 7, DHHS Publication No. 98-3228). Rockville, MD: Center for Substance Abuse Prevention.

Butcher, J. N. (1982). Cross-cultural research methods in clinical psychology. In P. C. Kendall & J. N. Butcher (Eds.), *Handbook of research methods in clinical psychology* (pp. 273–308). New York: Wiley.

Caetano, R. (1997). Prevalence, incidence and stability of drinking problems among whites, blacks, and Hispanics, 1984–1992. *Journal of Studies on Alcohol, 58,* 565–572.

Caetano, R., & Clark, C. L. (1998). Trends in alcohol-related problems among whites, blacks, and Hispanics, 1984–1995. *Alcoholism: Clinical and Experimental Research, 22,* 534–538.

Center for Substance Abuse Prevention. (1993). *The second national conference on preventing and treating alcohol and other drug abuse, HIV infection, and AIDS in black communities: From advocacy to action* (Publication No. ADM-93-1969). Rockville, MD: Author.

Comer, J. P. (1993). *School power: Implications of an intervention project.* New York: Simon & Schuster.

Dawkins, M. P. (1976). Alcohol use among black and white adolescents. In F. D. Harper (Ed.), *Alcohol abuse and black America* (pp. 163–175). Alexandria, VA: Douglass.

Donnelly, F. M., Mowery, J. L., & McCarver, D. G. (1998). Knowledge and misconceptions among inner-city African American mothers regarding alcohol and drug use. *American Journal of Drug and Alcohol Abuse, 24,* 675–683.

Dryden, W. (Ed.). (1995). *Rational emotive behavior therapy.* Thousand Oaks, CA: Sage.

Ellis, A. (1995). *Rational emotive behavior therapy.* In R. J. Corsini & D. Wedding (Eds.), *Current psychotherapies* (5th ed., pp. 162–196). Itasca, IL: Peacock.

Epstein, J. A., Botvin, G. J., Baker, E., & Diaz, T. (1998). Patterns of alcohol use among ethnically diverse black and Hispanic urban youth. *Journal of Gender, Culture, and Health, 3,* 29–39.

Epstein, J. A., Botvin, G. J., & Diaz, T. (1998). Ethnic and gender differences in alcohol use among a longitudinal sample of inner-city adolescents. *Journal of Gender, Culture, and Health, 3,* 193–207.

Glasser, W. (1998). *Choice theory: A new psychology of personal freedom.* New York: HarperCollins.

Glasser, W., & Wubbolding, R. (1995). Reality therapy. In R. Corsini & D. Wedding (Eds.), *Current psychotherapies* (5th ed., pp. 293–321). Itasca, IL: Peacock.

Globetti, G. A. (1970). Drinking patterns of Negro and white high school students in two Mississippi communities. *Journal of Negro Education, 39,* 60–69.

Grenier, C. E., Gorskey, E. J., & Folse, D. W. (1998). A survey analysis of alcohol use at a black university in the deep south. *Journal of Child and Adolescent Substance Abuse, 7,* 79–92.

Harper, F. D. (1979). *Alcoholism treatment and black Americans* (Publication No. ADM 79-853). Washington, DC: U.S. Government Printing Office.

Harper, F. D. (1983). Alcoholism treatment and black Americans: A review and analysis. In T. D. Watts & R. Wright Jr. (Eds.), *Black alcoholism: Toward a comprehensive understanding* (pp. 71–84). Springfield, IL: Thomas.

Harper, F. D. (1996, November). Race, gender, and research as related to alcohol/drug use and Afrinesians. Paper presented at "Developing Research Collaborations Among Historically Black Colleges and Universities," a conference of the National Institute on Drug Abuse and the Center for Drug Abuse Research, Washington, DC.

Harper, F. D., Braithwaite, K., & LaGrange, R. D. (1999). Ebonics and academic achievement: Role of the counselor. *Journal of Negro Education, 67,* 25–34.

Harper, F. D., & Griffin, J. P., Jr. (2000). Creative and underused counseling strategies for the prevention of violence in schools. In D. S. Sandhu & C. B. Aspy (Eds.), *Violence in American schools: A practical guide for counselors* (pp. 185–200). Alexandria, VA: American Counseling Association.

Harper, F. D., & Saifnoorian, E. (1991). Drinking patterns among African Americans. In D. J. Pittman & H. R. White (Eds.), *Society, culture, and drinking patterns reexamined* (pp. 327–338). New Brunswick, NJ: Rutgers Center of Alcohol Studies.

Harper, F. D., & Stone, W. O. (1999). Transcendent counseling (TC): A theoretical approach for the year 2000 and beyond. In J. McFadden (Ed.), *Transcultural counseling: Bridging cultures* (2nd ed., pp. 83–108). Alexandria, VA: American Counseling Association Press.

Haynes, N. M. (1996). Creating safe and caring school communities: Comer School Development Program Schools. *Journal of Negro Education, 65,* 308–314.

Herd, D. (1989). The epidemiology of drinking patterns and alcohol-related problems among U.S. blacks. In National Institute on Alcohol Abuse and Alcoholism, *Epidemiology of alcohol use and abuse among U.S. minorities* (NIAAA Monograph No. 18, DHHS Publication No. ADM-89-1435, pp. 3–50). Washington, DC: U.S. Government Printing Office.

Herd, D. (1994). Predicting drinking problems among black and white men: Results from a national survey. *Journal of Studies on Alcohol, 55,* 61–71.

Herd, D. (1997). Sex ratios of drinking patterns and problems among blacks and whites: Results from a national survey. *Journal of Studies on Alcohol, 58,* 75–82.

Johnson, P. B., & Johnson, H. L. (1999). Cultural and familial influences that maintain the negative meaning of alcohol. *Journal of Studies on Alcohol, 13*(Suppl.), 79–83.

Johnston, L. D., O'Malley, P. M., & Bachman, J. G. (1998a). *National survey results on drug use from the Monitoring the Future Study, 1975–1997: Vol. 1: Secondary school students* (NIH Publication No. 98-4345). Rockville, MD: National Institute on Drug Abuse.

Johnston, L. D., O'Malley, P. M., & Bachman, J. G. (1998b). *National survey results on drug use from the Monitoring the Future Study, 1975–1997: Vol. 2: College students and young adults* (NIH Publication No. 98-4346). Rockville, MD: National Institute on Drug Abuse.

Lewis, J. A., Dana, R. Q., & Blevins, G. A. (1994). *Substance abuse counseling: An individualized approach* (2nd ed.). Pacific Grove, CA: Brooks/Cole.

Maisto, S. A., Galizio, M., & Connors, G. J. (1999). *Drug use and abuse* (3rd ed.). Ft. Worth, TX: Holt, Rinehart & Winston.

Maultsby, M. C., Jr. (1984). *Rational behavior therapy.* Upper Saddle River, NJ: Prentice Hall.

Meilman, P. W., Stone, J. E., Gaylor, M. S., & Turco, J. H. (1990). Alcohol consumption by college undergraduates: Current use and 10-year trends. *Journal of Studies on Alcohol, 51,* 389–395.

National Clearinghouse for Alcohol and Drug Information. (1995). *Youth risk behavior surveillance: United States, 1995.* Rockville, MD: Author.

National Institute on Alcohol Abuse and Alcoholism. (1990). *Seventh special report to the U.S. Congress on alcohol and health.* Rockville, MD: Author.

National Institute on Alcohol Abuse and Alcoholism. (1997). *Ninth special report to the U.S. Congress on alcohol and health.* Rockville, MD: Author.

Nugent, F. A. (1999). *An introduction to the profession of counseling* (3rd ed.). New York: Merrill.

Rodney, H. E., Mupier, R., & Crafter, B. (1996). Predictors of alcohol drinking among African American adolescents: Implications for violence prevention. *Journal of Negro Education, 65,* 434–444.

Rodney, H. E., Mupier, R., & O'Neal, S. (1997). African American youth in public housing showing low alcohol and drug use. *Journal of Child and Adolescent Substance Abuse, 6,* 55–73.

Substance Abuse and Mental Health Services Administration. (1998). *Prevalence of substance use among racial and ethnic subgroups in the United States, 1991–1993.* Rockville, MD: Author.

Terry-Leonard, B. L. (1999). *The relationship of self-esteem, perceived parental nurturance, and family functioning across three family structures in a sample of non-traditional undergraduate students.* Unpublished doctoral dissertation, Howard University, Washington, DC.

Wechsler, H., Davenport, A., Dowdall, G., Moeykens, B., & Castillo, S. (1994). Health and behavioral consequences of binge drinking in college: A national survey of students at 140 campuses. *Journal of the American Medical Association, 272,* 1672–1677.

CHAPTER TWENTY

NUTRITION

Shiriki K. Kumanyika, Angela Odoms

As we eat we not only survive corporally, we also express ourselves socially. . . .
Nutritional values are one thing, social values quite another.

ANNE MURCOTT, 1988 (p. 5)

Both dietary patterns and disease patterns have changed markedly during the twentieth century (Brewster & Jacobson, 1978; Friend, Page, & Marston, 1979; Federation of American Societies for Experimental Biology [FASEB], Life Sciences Research Office, 1995; Frazão, 1999). As a result the role of diet in the maintenance of good health has also changed. A large body of evidence has emphasized the role of nutrition and dietary intake not only in growth and development and in sustaining life but also in the prevention and management of chronic diseases (Committee on Diet and Health, 1989). Although nutrient deficiencies are still a concern in certain segments of the population, prevalent health conditions in the United States reflect problematic aspects of dietary patterns that may otherwise be adequate in the traditional sense (FASEB, 1995). Higher or lower than optimal intakes of certain dietary constituents are associated with cardiovascular diseases, obesity, diabetes, and cancer (Committee on Diet and Health, 1989; World Cancer Research Fund & American Institute for Cancer Research, 1997; Deckelbaum et al., 1999).

Disproportionately high rates of morbidity and mortality among black Americans due to chronic diseases have been clearly documented for more than a decade (U.S. Department of Health and Human Services [DHHS], 1985; National Center for Health Statistics [NCHS], 1999; Miller et al., 1996). Furthermore, problems associated with undernutrition are still present in the black community. Nutrition monitoring data (FASEB, 1995) indicate that the average intake of some essential nutrients are still below recommended levels in the African American population. Food insecurity (that is, the sense of not having enough to eat) is also more common in blacks than whites.

Several cross-cutting diet and health associations are summarized in Table 20.1. Factors associated with atherosclerosis, cancer, and diabetes include high intakes of calories, total fat, and saturated fat and salt and low intakes of fiber and complex carbohydrates. A high intake of foods containing antioxidant substances (for example, certain vitamins or minerals or other constituents of plant foods with antioxidant activity [*phytochemicals*]) has also been associated with protection from chronic diseases (Deckelbaum et al., 1999). High salt intake is associated with low potassium intake. The ratio of salt intake to potassium intake may be important as a predisposing factor to high blood pressure and stroke (Committee on Diet and Health, 1989). Other diet-disease associations of current public health interest include the relationship of calcium intake to osteoporosis and potentially to colon cancer, the association of cataracts with low intakes of antioxidants, and the association of folic acid and other nutrients with birth outcomes and immune function (Bendich & Deckelbaum, 1997). These associations have given rise to general recommendations to increase the proportion of caloric intake from plant foods in relation to animal foods (American Cancer Society, 1996; U.S. Department of Agriculture & U.S. Department of Health and Human Services [USDA & DHHS], 2000). Increased intakes of fruits, vegetables, whole grains, and legumes (such as dried beans and peas) are recommended as plant sources of dietary fiber and protein, with a commensurate decrease recommended in the consumption of meat and poultry (USDA & DHHS, 2000). Fish (other than fried fish) is recommended because it is lower in both total fat and saturated fat than a portion of meat with the equivalent amount of protein. Fish such as salmon, tuna,

TABLE 20.1. COMMON CLINICAL AND EPIDEMIOLOGICAL LINKS BETWEEN NUTRITIONAL FACTORS AND RISKS FOR CHRONIC DISEASES.

Dietary Intake	Disease Risk			
	Cancer	Arteriosclerosis	Obesity	Diabetes
High calories	↑[a]	↑	↑	↑
High total or saturated fat	↑[a]	↑	↑[b]	↑[b]
High salt	↑[c]	↑	. . .	↑
Low fiber and complex carbohydrates	↑	↑	. . .	↑
Low antioxidants	↑	↑	. . .	↑

Note: Arrows = increased risk; ellipses (. . .) = no definite association.

[a] High fat intake is associated with increased risk of certain cancers.

[b] Although some evidence indicates that higher proportions of total calorie intake from fat are associated with increased risk for obesity and type 2 diabetes, this point is still unresolved.

[c] Increased risk is associated with salts used in pickling or preserving meats and other foods.

Source: Reprinted by permission from R. J. Deckelbaum et al., 1999. Summary of a scientific conference on preventive nutrition: Pediatrics to geriatrics. *Circulation, 100*(4), p. 451.

and mackerel contain a type of fat (omega-3 fatty acids) that may have protective effects in relation to chronic disease development. The recommendations apply to the general population of children (over age two) and adults throughout life. An underlying rationale is that the genetic makeup of human beings is actually more attuned to the hunter-gatherer eating pattern of the past than to the current meat-based diets common in western countries (Davies, 1995).

In this chapter we describe the food habits and average dietary intakes of African American adults and discuss the implications for their health, illness, and quality of life. Relevant social and cultural factors and dietary change issues are described. See Kimm, Gergen, Malloy, Dresser, and Carroll (1990), Bronner (1996), and Deckelbaum et al. (1999) for detailed consideration of pediatric nutrition and health issues for children; see Kumanyika (1997a) for a review of nutrition issues for older African Americans.

What Do African Americans Eat?

Dietary patterns can be described both qualitatively (referred to here as *foodways* or *food habits*) and quantitatively (referred to as *food intakes* or *nutrient intakes* or *eating patterns*). Foodways are the historical, traditional aspects of food habits. Food habits are the general ways that people in a particular cultural group are predisposed to eat in relation to both historical and current sociocultural contexts. Food and nutrient intakes are what people actually consume on a day-to-day basis, and they reflect the choices that are made in relation to what is available and affordable. Assessments of food and nutrient intake reflect food habits but tend to understate their complexity.

As noted by Whitehead (1992), the difference or lack of difference between the particular foods one group eats and the foods another group eats is not necessarily a criterion for defining their food habits. Rather, factors such as the degree of identification with certain foods, the centrality of these foods to the culture or lifestyle, and the particular meanings attached to those foods define the food habits of a particular group. Food habits have many dimensions: the usual food choices, the foods considered core to the eating pattern, the typical ways foods are combined, the ways foods are cooked, the types of textures and flavors that are preferred, the size and timing of various meals, and the ways food is used in familial and social processes, for cultural expression, and for religious observance. Food habits tend to include certain foods and exclude other foods. They incorporate symbolic and connotative meanings (that is, the intangible social and emotional values that people attach to food). These symbolic meanings are perhaps the least likely aspects of food habits to be conveyed by quantitative assessments, but they may be the most important aspects to consider when attempting to change eating patterns to meet health outcomes.

Historical and Social Influences

Like all ethnic groups, African Americans have cultural food patterns that reflect their social and historical experiences. In fact, food may be a particularly salient ethnic symbol for people who have experienced severe forms of oppression such as slavery (Mintz, 1996). African American foodways are an amalgamation of African, European, and Native American food systems (Kittler & Sucher, 1998; Whitehead, 1992). African slaves brought traditional West African foods, such as black-eyed peas, okra, and watermelon, and cooking methods. Then West African food traditions were modified based on foods available to slaves in the South. As described by Poe (1999), plants indigenous to North America were substituted for traditional West African ingredients. However, for the most part, food availability was largely contingent on provisions from slave owners and as a result varied from plantation to plantation. Common foods included salt pork and corn with rice, salted fish, and molasses, the latter used to a lesser extent based on availability (Kittler & Sucher, 1998). Some slaves supplemented their diets with vegetables grown in "their" gardens. Slaves also caught and ate small animals (such as opossums, rabbits, and raccoons) and fish (such as catfish) in addition to the food they received. In the fall, hog slaughtering sometimes provided slaves with a variety of pork cuts including ham hocks and intestines (chitterlings).

Women were primarily responsible for food preparation on most plantations (Poe, 1999). Meal patterns were structured around plantation work schedules. Breakfast was the largest meal, to sustain slaves during work in the fields, with lunch or the afternoon meal consisting of leftovers or one-dish vegetable stews (Kittler & Sucher, 1998). Evening meals were also commonly one-pot dishes that were prepared in the morning and cooked throughout the day (Poe, 1999). Sundays and holidays were times during which extended family and friends came together to share larger meals. These gatherings reflected communal patterns and gatherings common in African societies (Poe, 1999).

These food patterns continued after emancipation from slavery and were shaped by the employment and economic situations of black Americans. For example, African American sharecroppers focused on cash crops and continued to acquire foods similar to those available during slavery (Whitehead, 1992). A significant amount of food was obtained from white landowners for cash or on credit. Northern migration brought new challenges as people had to adapt from agricultural to urban lifestyles. Although many dietary patterns continued, new work habits and food availability changed several aspects of the traditional meal patterns. Daily meals became lighter, whereas communal meals on Sunday and holidays continued to be large and to include extended kinship groups and traditional favorites (Jerome, 1969).

African American food habits are generally described as a U.S. *southern* diet (Veale-Jones & Darling, 1996; American Dietetic Association, 1998). This may reflect both the high proportion of African Americans who live or were raised in the South (Pollard & O'Hare, 1999) as well as the inability to label any other set of eating or food preparation patterns common to African Americans in general (see our later discussion of demographic diversity in the black American population). As shown in Table 20.2, typical African American core foods continue to reflect many of the foods and preparation methods brought from West Africa and foods available in the South. Characteristic preparation styles also continue to be popular, including frying meats in pork fat or other fat, stewing or boiling vegetables using pork as seasoning, and using excess sugars in desserts and drinks (Airhihenbuwa et al., 1996; Kittler & Sucher, 1998).

With respect to current dietary recommendations, African American food habits are a mixture of positives and negatives. Positives include the core position of certain plant foods such as legumes, dark green leafy vegetables, and yellow vegetables; these foods are inherently low in fat and salt and high in dietary fiber and are also good sources of several protective nutrients. At the same time, there is less habitual use of fresh fruits and vegetables, which are underconsumed by Americans in general. The traditional southern practice of cooking vegetables for long periods and of adding salted meat or fat as a seasoning for legumes or vegetables detracts from their potential positive health benefits. Similarly, the emphasis on rice, grits, and breads is consistent with the recommendation to eat several servings of grain products daily. However, if prepared in the traditional manner, high consumption of these foods may not be consistent with recommendations to decrease fat and salt intake. Whole grain foods, which are increasingly recommended for special emphasis in the grains category because of their high content of certain nutrients, are not cited as part of the core southern African American eating pattern. The traditional preference is for more refined "white" breads or corn bread (Kittler & Sucher, 1998).

Additionally, having meat as part of a meal is a core value in African American food habits that may be particularly problematic because meat is a major source of total and saturated fat. Placing a high value on meat might have been protective historically, when meat was relatively unavailable or expensive and could be obtained only in small quantities. However, because meat now is widely

TABLE 20.2. TYPICAL CHARACTER OF THE SOUTHERN AFRICAN AMERICAN DIET.

Core	Secondary	Infrequent
Rice	Bought (light) breads	
Corn bread	Spaghetti (meat)	
Biscuits	Macaroni and cheese	
Grits		
Meat (pork and chicken)	Fish	
Meat (variety cuts)		
Cooked green leafy vegetables	White potatoes	Fresh vegetables
Okra, tomatoes, legumes, corn, yams	Other vegetables	Fruits
	Desserts	Dairy

Source: Veale-Jones & Darling, 1996.

available and more affordable, African Americans may be predisposed to over-consumption of meat and poultry and disinclined to follow advice to consume fewer servings, to substitute plant-based protein sources, and to have some meat-less meals (Smit, Nieto, Crespo, & Mitchell, 1999).

Food and Nutrient Intakes and Dietary Quality

Cross-sectional national surveys such as the ongoing National Health and Nutrition Examination Survey (NHANES), conducted by the National Center for Health Statistics, and the Continuing Survey of Food Intakes by Individuals (CSFII), conducted by the U.S. Department of Agriculture (USDA), provide food and nutrient intake data for large, nationally representative samples of African Americans for both current and prior time periods (FASEB, 1995). In some large epidemiological studies (Willett, 1998), broadly representative dietary data have been gathered from participants who include African Americans. These sources provide quantitative estimates of food and nutrient intakes. Quantitative estimates are derived from interviews or records that ask people to recall or keep track of foods eaten over a specified time period (for example, several twenty-four-hour periods), with details of how much was eaten and how it was prepared (Thompson & Byers, 1994). Semiquantitative dietary assessment interviews or question-naires offer respondents a list of perhaps one hundred foods and ask them to indicate how often each food is usually eaten (for example, times per day, per week, or per month) and in what approximate quantity. Such measures are oriented to-ward collecting information that addresses the nutrient or chemical composition of food. Dietary quality indices are scoring systems that estimate the cumulative or simultaneous effects of food and nutrient intakes, expressed in terms of adher-ence to dietary guidelines.

Food Intake. The average daily servings of various food groups reported by black men and women, calculated according to the number and size of servings recommended on the Food Guide Pyramid (Figure 20.1), are shown in Table 20.3. These estimates, from Kumanyika and Krebs-Smith (in press), are based on the CSFII for 1994 to 1996. Data for whites are shown for reference. The data in Table 20.3 are reported without consideration of the effects of socioeconomic sta-tus, which will be discussed subsequently.

In general, food consumption patterns of Americans are not consistent with the Food Guide Pyramid recommendations (see Figure 20.1). Table 20.3 illus-trates the general finding that average consumption of grains, whole grains, and fruits tends to be lower than recommended and consumption of discretionary fats, added sugars, and meat higher than recommended. Table 20.3 also shows that, among both men and women, servings of grain products and whole grains, vegetables, fruits, and dairy products are lower for blacks than for whites and intakes of foods from the meat group and of added sugars are higher for blacks

FIGURE 20.1. FOOD GUIDE PYRAMID: A GUIDE TO DAILY CHOICES.

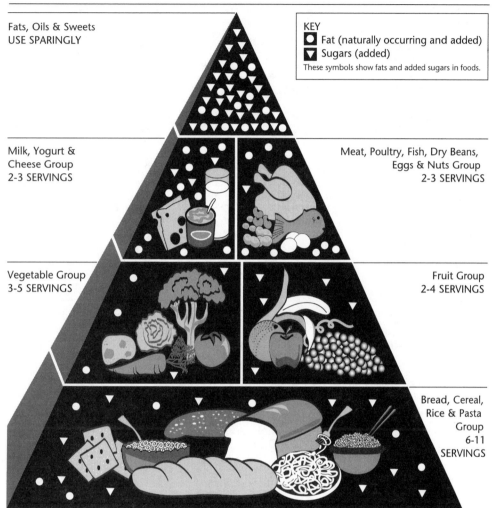

Note: A range of servings is given for each food group. The number of servings recommended depends on age, gender, and level of physical activity. The smaller number of servings applies to children ages two to six and to adults with lower energy needs (such as older women) and the largest number to adults with high energy needs (such as teenage boys and active men). Servings for others (such as older children, active women, and most men) are intermediate. Pyramid serving sizes are often smaller than those given on the Nutrition Facts Food Label.

Source: USDA & DHHS, 2000, pp. 14–15.

TABLE 20.3. FOOD GROUP INTAKES FOR BLACK AND WHITE NON-HISPANIC MEN AND WOMEN AGED 20 AND OVER, CSFII, 1994–1996.

Food Group	Men		Women	
	Black	White	Black	White
Total grain products	7.0 ± 0.4	8.1 ± 0.1	4.9 ± 0.1	5.7 ± 0.1
Whole grains	0.8 ± 0.1	1.3 ± 0.1	0.6 ± 0.1	1.0 ± 0.0
Total vegetables	3.9 ± 0.2	4.3 ± 0.1	2.9 ± 0.1	3.1 ± 0.0
Green/yellow	0.5 ± 0.1	0.4 ± 0.0	0.5 ± 0.0	0.4 ± 0.0
White potatoes	1.5 ± 0.2	1.5 ± 0.0	0.9 ± 0.1	0.8 ± 0.0
Dried beans/peas	0.3 ± 0.1	0.2 ± 0.0	0.1 ± 0.0	0.1 ± 0.0
Other starchy	0.3 ± 0.1	0.3 ± 0.0	0.2 ± 0.0	0.2 ± 0.0
Tomatoes	0.5 ± 0.0	0.6 ± 0.0	0.4 ± 0.0	0.4 ± 0.0
Other	0.9 ± 0.1	1.3 ± 0.0	0.8 ± 0.0	1.2 ± 0.0
Fruits	1.4 ± 0.1	1.5 ± 0.0	1.3 ± 0.1	1.5 ± 0.0
Milk/cheese/yogurt	1.0 ± 0.1	1.7 ± 0.0	0.8 ± 0.1	1.2 ± 0.0
Meat/meat alternatives	7.3 ± 0.2	6.2 ± 0.1	4.7 ± 0.2	3.7 ± 0.0
Meat/poultry/fish	6.6 ± 0.2	5.6 ± 0.1	4.3 ± 0.1	3.3 ± 0.0
Discretionary fat	25.3 ± 0.5	25.1 ± 0.2	25.4 ± 0.4	24.6 ± 0.2
Added sugars	16.4 ± 0.9	14.4 ± 0.2	17.9 ± 0.5	15.0 ± 0.3

Note: All serving values are mean ± SE per day; serving sizes are based on the Food Guide Pyramid.

Source: Adapted from Kumanyika & Krebs-Smith, in press.

than for whites. The finding of low dairy product consumption among blacks is associated directly or indirectly (that is, through related cultural practices) with the high prevalence of lactose intolerance found in several non-Caucasian populations; 50 percent of African Americans are lactose intolerant as compared to 10 percent of whites, with the highest prevalence (85 percent) of lactose intolerance found among Asians (Standing Committee on the Scientific Evaluation of Dietary Reference Intakes, 1999a).

Other CSFII tabulations for non-Hispanic black and white men and women aged twenty years and over (USDA, 1999) further refine the impression of ethnic differences suggested by the findings for the broad food categories shown on Table 20.3. For example, candy is a relatively greater source of sugar for whites than for blacks; black men and women who consume milk are more likely than whites to consume whole milk rather than low-fat or skim milk; black men and women consume more dark green leafy vegetables than whites do but fewer dark yellow vegetables and fewer lettuce or lettuce-based salads. Beverage consumption patterns also differ considerably. Coffee consumption is substantially lower among black men and women than among their white counterparts, and consumption of fruit drinks and ades is higher among blacks. Black women are more likely to consume regular carbonated drinks than white women and much less likely to consume low-calorie carbonated drinks: 45 percent of black versus 29 percent of white women reported consumption of regular soft drinks over a twenty-four-hour period; 5 percent of black versus 21 percent of white women reported consuming low-calorie soft drinks. The data in Table 20.3 suggest somewhat higher consumption of discretionary fat among black than white women. Fats added in cooking, frequent use of frying as a method of food preparation, use of mayonnaise in potato salad, and addition of sauces and gravies on meats have been mentioned as common sources of discretionary fat for African Americans (Dacosta & Wilson, 1996; Kittler & Sucher, 1998).

Although the ethnic differences in average daily servings are small, they reflect meaningful differences in food intake patterns, they trend in the same direction as qualitative descriptions of African American food habits, and they are relatively consistent across varied data sources (Borrud et al., 1989; Swanson et al., 1993; FASEB, 1995; Smit et al., 1999). For example, lower fruit intake in blacks was also reported in the 1989 to 1991 CSFII data; only 60 percent of black men and 69 percent of black women reported having consumed any fruit or fruit juice in a three-day period, compared to 69 percent of white men and 77 percent of white women (FASEB, 1995).

Nutrient Intake. All these descriptions and reports of food habits and food intakes of African Americans lead one to expect certain patterns of nutrient intake in comparison to patterns for whites. For example, one expects to observe higher consumption of total fat, saturated fat, and cholesterol (contained in animal products); lower consumption of fiber (contained in grains, fruits, and fresh vegetables), calcium (in dairy products), and potassium (in dairy products and fruits); and higher consumption of carotenes (vitamin A precursor substances found in dark green vegetables). The available nutrient intake data, presented in Table 20.4, are largely consistent with these expectations.

The nutrients listed in Table 20.4 address both meeting normal dietary needs and reducing chronic disease risks. In general, average intakes meet requirements for adequacy. Calcium intake is an exception. Average intake is below the recommended level of 1,000 to 1,200 mg per day (Standing Committee on the Scientific Evaluation of Dietary Reference Intakes, 1999a). With respect to fat intake and fiber, average intakes for both blacks and whites exceed current guidelines for fat ($<$ 30 percent of kilocalories as fat, $<$ 10 percent as saturated fat) and fail to meet requirements for fiber (20 to 25 g of fiber per day) (FASEB, 1995). The similar caloric intake of black and white women is inconsistent with the finding of a marked excess prevalence of obesity in African American women (Kumanyika, 1987; Flegal, Carroll, Kuczmarski, & Johnson, 1998). This may reflect underreporting of caloric intake by African American women but could also reflect the greater contribution to black female obesity of low levels of caloric expenditure associated with physical inactivity (Crespo, Smit, Andersen, Carter-Pokras, & Ainsworth, 2000). Average intakes of folate are also below current recommendations (Standing Committee on the Scientific Evaluation of Dietary Reference Intakes, 1999b). However, folate intake may be underestimated in these data, which were collected before the recent fortification of food with folic acid. The

TABLE 20.4. NUTRIENT INTAKES FOR BLACK AND WHITE NON-HISPANIC MEN AND WOMEN AGED 20 AND OVER, CSFII, 1994–1996.

Nutrient	Men		Women	
	Black	White	Black	White
Energy (kilocalories)	2,414 ± 138	2,472 ± 30	1,630 ± 29	1,649 ± 13
Protein (% of kcal)	16.3 ± 0.3	15.8 ± 0.1	15.8 ± 0.3	15.7 ± 0.1
Fat (% of kcal)	34.4 ± 0.5	33.5 ± 0.2	34.1 ± 0.5	32.3 ± 0.2
Saturated fat (% kcal)	11.3 ± 0.2	11.3 ± 0.1	11.1 ± 0.2	10.8 ± 0.1
Carbohydrate (% kcal)	48.4 ± 0.8	49.2 ± 0.2	50.3 ± 0.6	52.1 ± 0.2
Dietary fiber	15.8 ± 0.5	18.8 ± 0.3	11.3 ± 0.4	14.2 ± 0.2
Alcohol (% kcal)	1.9 ± 0.3	2.8 ± 0.2	0.9 ± 0.2	1.6 ± 0.1
Vitamin A (µg retinol equivalents)	1,263 ± 262	1,147 ± 25	867 ± 78	994 ± 23
Carotenes (µg retinol equivalents)	485 ± 30	552 ± 20	446 ± 30	508 ± 18
Folate (µg)	266 ± 11	307 ± 5	195 ± 9	229 ± 3
Vitamin B12 (µg)	9.82 ± 2.76	6.54 ± 0.32	4.53 ± 0.63	4.14 ± 0.14
Vitamin E (α-tocopherol equivalent)	9.1 ± 0.4	10.1 ± 0.2	6.3 ± 0.2	7.2 ± 0.1
Vitamin C (mg)	118 ± 12	106 ± 2	97 ± 6	87 ± 2
Thiamin (mg)	1.79 ± 0.09	1.92 ± 0.02	1.21 ± 0.03	1.34 ± 0.01
Riboflavin (mg)	2.06 ± 0.13	2.29 ± 0.03	1.39 ± 0.05	1.62 ± 0.02
Niacin (mg)	25.7 ± 0.8	28.3 ± 0.4	18.0 ± 0.4	18.9 ± 0.2
Vitamin B6 (mg)	2.03 ± 0.06	2.19 ± 0.03	1.42 ± 0.05	1.51 ± 0.02
Calcium (mg)	706 ± 59	924 ± 15	525 ± 20	668 ± 8
Phosphorus (mg)	1,345 ± 83	1,499 ± 19	904 ± 30	1,037 ± 8
Magnesium (mg)	274 ± 11	335 ± 5	194 ± 6	239 ± 2
Iron (mg)	18.1 ± 1.5	18.7 ± 0.3	11.4 ± 0.3	13.2 ± 0.1
Zinc (mg)	13.8 ± 1.0	14.0 ± 0.2	8.6 ± 0.2	9.2 ± 0.1
Copper (mg)	1.4 ± 0.1	1.5 ± 0.0	0.9 ± 0.0	1.1 ± 0.0
Sodium (mg)	3,889 ± 154	4,129 ± 57	2,667 ± 69	2,764 ± 29
Potassium (mg)	2,886 ± 151	3,262 ± 42	2,009 ± 51	2,371 ± 18
Cholesterol (mg)	395 ± 21	319 ± 5	246 ± 11	204 ± 3

Note: All intake values are mean ± SE.

Source: Adapted from Kumanyika & Krebs-Smith, in press.

average level of sodium intake is above the recommended upper limit of 2,400 mg per day.

Dietary Quality. The Healthy Eating Index (HEI) (Table 20.5) was developed by the USDA to help Americans evaluate their diets in relation to current dietary guidance (Bowman, Lino, Gerrior, & Basiotis, 1998). HEI data are calculated from the CSFII. The index has ten dietary components on which individuals are scored from 10 (the maximum score) to 0 (the minimum score). An HEI score of 81 or above indicates a good diet; a score of 51 to 80 indicates that the diet needs improvement and a score of less than 51 indicates a poor diet. Food group servings are based on the Food Guide Pyramid recommended levels, which vary ac-

TABLE 20.5. COMPONENTS OF THE HEALTHY EATING INDEX AND SCORING SYSTEM.

Component	Criteria for Maximum Score of 10[a]	Criteria for Minimum Score of 0[a]
Grain consumption	6–11 servings[b]	0 servings[b]
Vegetable consumption	3–5 servings[b]	0 servings[b]
Fruit consumption	2–4 servings[b]	0 servings[b]
Milk consumption	2–3 servings[b]	0 servings[b]
Meat consumption	2–3 servings[b]	0 servings[b]
Total fat intake	30% or less energy from fat	45% or more energy from fat
Saturated fat intake	Less than 10% energy from saturated fat	15% or more energy from saturated fat
Cholesterol intake	300 mg or less	450 mg or more
Sodium intake	2,400 mg or less	4,800 mg or more
Food variety	8 or more different items in a day	3 or fewer different items in a day

[a] People with consumption (intakes) between the maximum and minimum amounts are assigned scores proportionately.

[b] Number of servings depends on *recommended energy allowance*. All amounts are per day.

Source: Adapted from Bowman et al., 1998.

cording to the calorie levels specified for different age and gender groups. However, the HEI does not set limits on the overall calorie level.

The HEI scores for African Americans (Table 20.6) present a picture of African American dietary practices that suggests negative long-term health prospects. For the majority of the HEI components, less than 50 percent of African Americans meet recommended levels, except for cholesterol (data not shown). As Table 20.6 illustrates, African Americans score very low on the 10 to 0 HEI scale on intake of foods in the fruit and milk groups, consistent with the data presented earlier, and have a lower average score than whites on all components except meat and sodium. On the HEI scale, higher sodium scores mean lower sodium intake (see Table 20.5), indicating that scores for African Americans on this component are favorable relative to those of white Americans. The sodium intake of African Americans may be comparatively lower owing to blacks' lower consumption of grain products (Center for Nutrition Policy and Promotion, 1998). Processed grain products are major sources of sodium in the U.S. diet (USDA & DHHS, 2000). The score for meat consumption is based on achieving the recommended minimum number of Food Guide Pyramid servings, but does not address directly the possibility of overconsumption of meat or meat products, which may apply to some African Americans. In a breakdown by age group across the life span (Center for Nutrition Policy and Promotion, 1998), overall HEI scores were generally higher between the ages of two and ten years and after age fifty, but were lower for African Americans than whites in all age categories. The ethnic differences were smallest in children under age ten years.

TABLE 20.6. MEAN HEI SCORES FOR AFRICAN AMERICAN AND WHITE MEN AND WOMEN AGED 20 AND OVER, 1994–1996.

Healthy Eating Index Score Component	Black		White	
	Men	Women	Men	Women
Overall score	56.8	58.7	62.5	64.8
Grain consumption	5.9	5.4	6.8	6.2
Vegetable consumption	6.0	5.7	6.7	6.4
Fruit consumption	3.0	3.4	3.4	4.0
Milk consumption	3.9	3.2	5.8	4.9
Meat consumption	7.8	6.7	7.4	5.9
Total fat intake	6.0	6.3	6.6	6.9
Saturated fat intake	6.1	6.5	6.3	6.8
Cholesterol intake	6.0	8.0	7.0	8.7
Sodium intake	5.3	7.6	4.6	7.5
Food variety	6.7	6.0	8.0	7.5

Source: P. P. Basiotis (U.S. Department of Agriculture, Center for Nutrition Policy and Promotion) personal communication to S. K. Kumanyika, 2000.

Is it possible that these dietary data overstate or understate dietary problems among African Americans? Dietary data are inherently error prone because of the day-to-day variability in what people eat, because people have difficulty in remembering and describing what they eat, and because self-reports of eating behavior may be biased for psychosocial reasons. In addition, because of the considerable variation among individuals in nutrient requirements and because of variation in such other factors as consumption of fortified food, use of vitamin and mineral supplements, and physiological adaptability to varying levels of daily nutrient intakes, an individual with below average or below recommended intake might actually be meeting his or her nutrition needs. Moreover, in populations where diagnoses of diet-related conditions such as high blood pressure or diabetes are common, people might have modified their diets based on medical advice or might have reported their dietary intakes so as to make them closer to recommended levels. Many African Americans, for example, are aware of the relationship between high salt intake and high blood pressure (FASEB, 1995) and think their diets should be lower in salt.

Some findings of low dietary intake among African Americans (for folate and vitamin E, for example) (Ford & Bowman, 1999; Ford & Sowell, 1999), are corroborated by data from blood nutrient levels, suggesting that the impression obtained from the dietary data is indeed an accurate one. Such blood nutrient data would reflect added intakes from vitamin supplements. However, low intakes of certain nutrients among the African American population do not appear to be compensated for by supplement use. African Americans are less likely than whites to take vitamin and mineral supplements (FASEB, 1995; Ervin, Wright, & Kennedy-Stephenson, 1999), and the ethnic differences in blood nutrient levels are observed in both users and nonusers of vitamin supplements (Ford & Bowman, 1999; Ford & Sowell, 1999).

Demographic and Social Influences

Food and nutrient intakes vary according to numerous demographic factors, and it is important to consider how such variation relates to differences within the U.S. black population. For example, are there subgroups of African Americans for whom the impression given by national data could be misleading? The following sections consider this issue with respect to socioeconomic status, region of residence (considering both the area of the country and urban versus rural residence), country of birth, and religion.

Socioeconomic Influences

Socioeconomic status (SES) is a major predictor of dietary intake. African Americans are disproportionately represented among the low-income segment of the population, and low SES has been linked to a variety of dietary or nutrition problems (Levedahl & Oliveira, 1999; FASEB, 1995). In 1996, the majority of black persons (55 percent) lived in families that could be classified as poor or near poor (Pollard & O'Hare, 1999). The poverty rate for blacks (27 percent) was three times that for non-Hispanic whites (9 percent). Over two-thirds of black children live in poverty, particularly those in female-headed households. Families with limited financial resources are at great risk for food insecurity. From 1996 to 1998, approximately ten million households could be classified as food insecure (that is, not always having access to enough food to meet basic needs or experiencing hunger), with the greatest proportion affected being households with children (Nord, Jemison, & Bickel, 1999). Black households with children were about twice as likely as their white counterparts to be classified as experiencing hunger (Klein, 1998).

U.S. food assistance programs, including the Food Stamp Program (FSP) and Women, Infants, and Children (WIC), are intended to serve as a safety net to assist low-income families and individuals in meeting nutrition needs. As of 1998, about one-third of the low-income households participating in the Food Stamp Program were African American, whereas 23 percent overall of low-income households are African American (Basiotis, Kramer-Leblanc, & Kennedy, 1998). Participation in food assistance programs has the potential to improve nutritional status (Rush, Leighton, Sloan, Alvir, & Garbowski, 1988; Levedahl & Oliveira, 1999). However researchers predict that changes in welfare policy in the last decade will have long-term negative effects on food expenditure and consumption and, subsequently, on the nutritional adequacy of low-income households (Gundersen, LeBlanc, & Kuhn, 1999). By reducing per person benefits and restricting eligibility, the Personal Responsibility and Work Opportunity Reconciliation Act of 1996 (PRWORA) cut more funds from the Food Stamp Program than from any other social welfare program (Gundersen et al., 1999). PRWORA made the Food Stamp Program the only entitlement program remaining available to most low-income households, because it replaced the largest cash assistance entitlement program, Aid to Families with Dependent Children, with a nonentitlement program, Temporary Aid to Needy Families.

Dietary quality generally improves with increasing income or education. However, disparities in dietary quality and nutritional status between African Americans and whites appear to persist regardless of income. For example, HEI scores increase with income for both African Americans and whites but are lower for African Americans at every income level (P. P. Basiotis, personal communication to S. K. Kumanyika, 2000). Scores for persons with incomes between 0 and 185 percent of the poverty line versus scores for those with over 185 percent of the poverty line were, respectively, 55.5 and 57.7 for black men and 59.7 and 63.2 for white men. Comparable scores for women were 57.5 and 60.0 for blacks and 62.3 and 65.5 for whites. Multivariate analyses of HEI scores in models that included measures of nutrition knowledge and awareness suggest that these nutrition information variables may explain some of the residual race effect (Variyam, Blaylock, Smallwood, & Basiotis, 1998).

Geographic Region and Urban Versus Rural Residence Patterns

Food consumption in the United States varies by region and is greatly influenced by local food systems and food accessibility (Shortridge & Shortridge, 1998). For example, consumption of milk and milk products is generally higher in the Midwest and lowest in the South (Yadrick, Harris, & Idris, 1997). Dietary quality also shows regional variation as well. People who live in the Northeast have the best dietary quality, and those in the South have the lowest (Bowman et al., 1998). In a comparison of dietary intake in three areas of the United States, Swanson et al. (1993) reported that both blacks and whites in Detroit and New Jersey consumed fried foods and vitamin A–rich foods more frequently than blacks and whites in Atlanta. Several studies have reported that nutrient intakes are not significantly different for ethnic groups residing in the same region (Borrud et al., 1989; Harland, Smith, Ellis, O'Brien, & Morris, 1992; Ganguli et al., 1999). Based on data from a randomized clinical trial, Kristal, Shattuck, and Patterson (1999) noted similar total fat intake among black and white women living in two southern cities but cited differences in the sources of fat. Blacks consumed more fat from meats, and white women acquired more fat from dairy products.

Urbanization also influences food consumption. More than half of the black population lives in central cities, compared to fewer than one-quarter of non-Hispanic whites (Pollard & O'Hare, 1999). In central cities, African American neighborhoods in particular lack major supermarket chains, which can result in a greater dependence on smaller convenience stores for goods and services, higher prices, and often lower quality and less healthful foods (Brown, 1999). The availability of healthy food products in grocery stores influences the healthfulness of individual diets of community members (Cheadle et al., 1991). In addition to the lack of supermarkets, the wide availability of fast-food establishments further hinders inner-city residents' ability to obtain healthy foods (Freedman, 1990). Fast-food franchises pose a dilemma for many black communities. Although they often supply a type of food that is not considered healthful by current standards, they also serve as a vehicle for economic development and employment in areas with very limited resources.

Immigrant Population Patterns

Although individuals of African descent share a common origin, differences in historical and cultural patterns have resulted in variations in dietary practices throughout the diaspora. As we move into the twenty-first century, the level of heterogeneity within the African American population requires taking note of subgroups. Over the past three decades, the United States has seen an increasing number of immigrants of African descent. In 1980, about 3 percent of African Americans were foreign born. By 1998, that percentage had almost doubled (Pollard & O'Hare, 1999). Black immigrants come from Africa and the Caribbean, and most of them are clustered in a small number of large cities (Council of Economic Advisers for the President's Initiative on Race, 1998; Pollard & O'Hare, 1999). Caribbean Americans make up the majority of immigrants to the United States of African descent.

Like African Americans of U.S. southern heritage, Caribbean Americans have dietary habits influenced by their West African roots and by their experiences during slavery (Mintz, 1996; Kittler & Sucher, 1998). Staple foods such as cassava, yams, and plantains are a mainstay of the Caribbean diet. Caribbean Islanders developed some cooking methods comparable to those of black Americans. However, certain dietary practices that emerged among American blacks (for example, the consumption of collard greens and desserts) did not become prevalent in the Caribbean. Moreover, the availability of tropical fruits and vegetables allowed a wide array to be commonly eaten in the Caribbean.

Some evidence suggests that Caribbean Islanders maintain many aspects of their original dietary patterns after migration to the United States. In a study comparing dietary risk factors among blacks in central Harlem, Greenberg, Schneider, Northridge, and Ganz (1998) reported that Caribbean-born respondents generally had higher fruit and vegetable consumption compared to their Southern-born counterparts. Other studies suggest that Caribbean-born blacks also have lower rates of diet-related chronic diseases than black persons born in the United States (Greenberg & Schneider, 1991; Fang, Madhavan, & Alderman, 1996).

Although the dietary practices of Caribbean Americans have received some attention, few studies have explored the food consumption of African migrants. About 560,000 Americans were born in Africa (Pollard & O'Hare, 1999), and dietary practices of Africans are known to vary from country to country in Africa. Although we could not identify any studies of the dietary practices of African immigrants to the United States, it can be expected that the food habits of immigrant populations will have an influence on U.S.-born blacks.

Religious Influences

Religion has played a major role in the lives of African Americans. The majority of African Americans participate in Christianity, particularly in the Baptist and Methodist denominations, with a large percentage active in religious worship (Lincoln & Mamiya, 1990; Chatters, Taylor, & Lincoln, 1999). A significant number of African Americans are involved in religious faiths—such as Seventh-Day Adventist, Islam, Mormon, and Judaic or Hebrew Israelite—that advocate dietary practices that depart to various degrees from traditional African American food habits (Lincoln, 1999). For example, it has been estimated that as many as four million African Americans are Muslim (McCloud, 1995). Consumption of pork, one of the cornerstones of the traditional African American diet, is taboo for Muslims. However, many Muslims continue to use other traditional African American foods and preparation methods (Odoms, 1999). Members of the Nation of Islam, however, a predominately African American Muslim group, are required to abstain from eating most traditional foods including pork, cornbread, black-eyed peas, and sweet potatoes (McCloud, 1995; Muhammad, 1972). Traditional dietary habits are believed to be associated with slavery and thus a "fast road to death" (Muhammad, 1972). Other religious communities, including Seventh-Day Adventists and Hebrew Israelites, advocate vegetarian lifestyles (Murphy, Gwebu, Braithwaite, Green-Goodman, & Brown, 1997; Markowitz, 1996).

An increasing body of literature illustrates that dietary behaviors valued by these religious communities are consistent with lifestyle recommendations for reducing the risk of chronic disease (Phillips & Snowdon, 1985; Jarvis & Northcott, 1987; Levin & Vanderpool, 1989). Melby, Toohey, and Cebrick (1994) reported that African American Seventh-Day Adventists who adhered to religious recommendations of a vegetarian lifestyle had lower serum cholesterol and triglyceride levels than those who did not. The Adventist Health Study, a California-based prospective study, analyzed the association of food consumption in 1976 with mortality from all causes ascertained through 1985 in approximately 1,700 black men and women (Fraser, Sumbureru, Pribis, Neil, & Frankson, 1997). Even in highly educated populations (nearly half were college graduates) with lower than average meat consumption, a protective effect of certain dietary patterns was evident: frequent consumption of nuts, fruits, and green salads was significantly associated with a lower risk of death during the follow-up period.

Although the number of African Americans participating in religious communities with health-promoting dietary practices may be increasing, it is probably still too small to influence the data collected from national samples of African

Americans. Furthermore, the traditional black churches maintain a practice of providing highly favored, but not necessarily healthful meals during many of their functions. However, the Muslim communities and the Seventh-Day Adventists can provide insights into the issues of diversity in food choice and of health-related dietary habits in the African American community (Fraser et al., 1997; Odoms, 1999).

Diet-Related Health Issues

The observational epidemiological studies that have identified dietary factors associated with chronic diseases do not necessarily include African Americans, and when they are included in a study, data for them are not necessarily analyzed separately. Similarly, intervention studies in which regression of disease or risk factors is demonstrated in association with dietary changes may not include or present data for African Americans. Even when available, analyses for African American subgroups may not have sufficient numbers to be definitive, particularly when the question is whether apparent differences in the size of associations between blacks and whites are of clinical or only statistical significance. Thus inferences about the relevance of dietary practices to health for African Americans must be made indirectly.

In general the diet-health associations in Table 20.1 are thought to apply to African Americans. Some studies are available that specifically demonstrate that the risk factor–disease associations in blacks apply to whites (Hayes et al., 1999; Whittemore et al., 1995; Must et al., 1999; Giles, Croft, Greenlund, Ford, & Kittner, 2000), but such studies are relatively small in number. The circumstantial evidence—that is, high disease occurrence among African Americans in parallel with high prevalence of related dietary risk factors—is strong, however, and is accepted in the absence of any clear evidence or suspicion to the contrary. In addition, as with data from any race-based epidemiological studies, data for African Americans that do *not* show the expected associations between dietary factors and health outcomes require systematic evaluation before inferring that a particular dietary factor actually has a biological effect in African Americans that is different from what would be expected based on data for whites. Artifacts and unmeasured explanatory factors can lead to spurious inferences that there are genetically based "racial" differences (Kumanyika & Golden, 1991; Kumanyika, 1993). Moreover, diet-related health problems are generally impossible to attribute to diet alone. They are also influenced by many other factors, including many environmental and behavioral factors that also differ between blacks and whites such as access to and use of health services.

The clearest links between nutritional factors and health among African Americans relate to obesity. Although it is characteristically difficult to link dietary measures of calorie and fat intake to weight levels, the presence of obesity in a population is evidence of a chronic excess intake of calories in relation to caloric expenditure (from metabolic and physical activity). Obesity is as prevalent in African American men as in white men (that is, about one in five has a body mass index [BMI] of 30 or more) and nearly twice as prevalent in African American compared to white women. Approximately two in five African American women aged twenty and older are obese (with a BMI of 30 or more), and a substantial proportion of African American women are extremely obese (with a BMI of 40 or more) (Flegal et al., 1998). Obesity indices have been linked directly to the incidence or prevalence of diabetes, high blood pressure, and coronary heart disease and to precursors of these diseases in the African American population in national and population-based samples (Must et al., 1999). Obesity has also been linked to osteoarthritis of the knee and to functional disability in African Americans (Kumanyika, 1987, 1994). The International Collaborative Study of Hypertension in Blacks (Kaufman, Durazo-Arvizu, Rotimi, McGee, & Cooper, 1996) has demonstrated that the increasing gradients of obesity that are observed when comparing African-descent populations living in West Africa, the Caribbean, and the United States are directly correlated to a higher occurrence of hypertension in the Caribbean than in West Africa and in the United States than in the Caribbean. Moreover, a truly alarming trajectory of increased obesity has been observed in African American children (Troiano, Flegal, Kuczmarski, Campbell, & Johnson, 1995), with an increased incidence of pediatric Type 2 diabetes as one consequence (Rosenbloom, Joe, Young, & Winter, 1999).

Calcium intake is an aspect of African American dietary practices for which the health implications are not so clear. Direct application of data from white populations to black populations is contraindicated by the paradoxical finding of both lower calcium intakes and lower fracture rates in African Americans, when the expectation would be higher fracture rates (Kumanyika, 1993). Higher levels of obesity afford some protection from osteoporotic factors. However, other factors related to bone size and density and to vitamin D metabolism are also involved (Weinstein & Bell, 1988). The question of whether blacks and whites have different calcium requirements has been raised, and this has an intuitive appeal because of the higher prevalence of lactose intolerance in blacks than in whites. This issue remains unresolved at present. In any event, the possible role of calcium as a protective factor in colon cancer, currently under study by the Women's Health Initiative Study Group (1997), will be an additional consideration in establishing ethnicity-specific recommendations for calcium intake.

For any nutritional status variable, the issue of ethnicity-specific standards is very complex. Iron status (Perry, Byers, Yip, & Margen, 1992; Johnson-Spear & Yip, 1994; Berti & Leonard, 1995) and birthweight (Kleinman & Kessel, 1987) are other examples of phenomena that raise the possibility that current standards should be interpreted differently for blacks and whites. Such issues must be approached cautiously, however, for at least two reasons. One is that being African American can be viewed as more a social than a genetic variable, meaning that observed differences may be modifiable rather than inherent (LaVeist, 1996). Another is that the implementation of these different standards is likely to affect other standards as well (for example, for deciding eligibility for nutrition assistance programs such as WIC), which would pose both feasibility and policy issues.

Interventions

How much can be gained with respect to wellness, longevity, and reduction in health care costs by effecting dietary changes in the African American population? This question is not answerable at this time, partly because the means to effect permanent dietary changes have generally not been established (Kumanyika, Bowen, et al., 2000; Jeffery et al., 2000) and also because of the lack of research on dietary interventions in African American populations. For example, in spite of the high prevalence of obesity in black women, observed for several decades, an exhaustive evidence-based review of controlled weight reduction studies (National Heart, Lung, and Blood Institute, 1998) identified only one eligible randomized controlled trial of weight reduction in African Americans (Agurs-Collins, Kumanyika, Ten Have, & Adams-Campbell, 1997).

Achieving long-term dietary changes to meet health objectives is a daunting proposition (Kumanyika, Bowen, et al., 2000). To say, "lower your fat intake," or, "eat more dietary fiber," implies numerous specific behavioral changes to reach a specified level of reduction or consumption. These changes must be based on *knowledge* of which foods contain fat and fiber and which do not and also of how to prepare foods in ways that alter their fat and fiber content as well as on the *willingness* to make the indicated changes in food selections or food preparation. Lowering sodium intake can be especially complicated. Less use of the saltshaker is a relatively simple instruction, but most salt in the average person's diet comes from processed food or restaurant food and is not under the individual's direct control. Nutrition counselors attempt to simplify such changes with advice such as: "If you feel hungry between meals, try to eat a banana or an orange instead of chips or a candy bar," "Ask for whole-wheat bread instead of white bread when you order a sandwich," "Start buying skim milk instead of whole milk," and, "Rinse the salt off of canned vegetables before you cook them." To make a sufficient number of such changes to alter the dietary factor in question may require a willingness to reframe one's entire pattern of selecting and consuming foods and even one's food preferences.

The assumptions underlying nutrition counseling approaches are that health motivations can support the effort needed to learn the new behaviors, that the new behaviors will eventually become habitual (and therefore less onerous), and that the health benefits of the new eating pattern will help to sustain the behaviors. However, food preferences and eating patterns are strongly anchored by cultural, psychosocial, and lifestyle influences that do not necessarily yield to behavioral changes, even among highly motivated individuals. People attempting to make changes in the composition of their diet or the amount of food they eat may feel deprived of the pleasures of eating. The taste and cost of food are stronger influences on food choices than are nutrition or weight control issues, even among those for whom health is a primary lifestyle focus (Glanz, Basil, Maibach, Goldberg, & Snyder, 1998). Many tasty, low-cost foods are high in fat, low in fiber, and high in salt; and the need to make decisions about whether or not, or how often, to choose such foods must usually be made numerous times every day as these foods are aggressively advertised (sometimes in clever ways that are nutritionally misleading), prominently positioned on supermarket shelves or restaurant menus, offered by friends, and served at church functions. Situational factors such as limited income or limited choices (as when there is no supermarket in the neighborhood or when the neighborhood stores have limited options) may be additional constraints.

Some surveys indicate less knowledge and awareness of diet and health issues among African Americans than among white comparison populations (Frazão, 1999; Variyam et al., 1998), even within education or income strata. The reasons for this are not well established but might include differences in access to or use of the most effective sources of nutrition information or a lack of receptivity to certain current dietary advice because of preexisting beliefs that conflict with that advice. For example, African Americans' beliefs about what constitutes a healthful eating pattern may be influenced by nutritional adequacy considerations (for example, ideas that one has to eat substantial amounts of food to get enough protein, vitamins, and minerals). Folk beliefs and the role of food in traditional home remedies may also influence African Americans' beliefs and their responsiveness to nutrition information (Matthews, 1987). Nutritional adequacy was the primary focus of dietary guidance and nutrition policy in the United States and many other countries until the 1970s, and has continued to be the primary message in nutrition education in low-income communities and public nutrition programs such as school lunch and WIC until very recently (FASEB, 1995).

Based on the high prevalence of diet-related chronic conditions such as high blood pressure, obesity, and diabetes in the black community and related patterns of physician contact, one might expect African Americans to be more exposed to therapeutic dietary counseling than whites are. However, professional dietary advice may not be provided in many clinical settings where it would be relevant. For example, among 330 African men and women with high blood pressure or high cholesterol, including 15 percent who also had a diagnosis of diabetes, only 22 percent reported they had ever been counseled by a dietitian (Kumanyika, Adams-Campbell, et al., 1999).

A meaningful literature on dietary interventions for African American populations is only now emerging. The general clinical and research literature suggests that African Americans are less likely than whites to adhere to therapeutic or modified diets (Kumanyika, 1999). However, there is also some evidence that clinical benefits of dietary interventions are equivalent to or better than those observed in white populations from a dose-response perspective (Luft et al.,

1991; Brancati, Appel, Seidler, & Whelton, 1996; Kumanyika, 1997b; Svetky et al., 1999).

There has also been an increasing appreciation of the potential improvement in the effectiveness of behavioral change interventions when they are tailored to participant motivations and, with respect to minority populations, cultural contexts. For example, Agurs-Collins et al. (1997) reported promising results from a culturally adapted nutrition and exercise program for weight management and glycemic control among African Americans aged fifty-five and older. The program was offered at a hospital in the black community and with African American staff. Cultural adaptations included the use of program materials (for example, videos) depicting African American families, settings, language, and values; the use of recipes and cooking methods familiar to African Americans; and peer group discussions about social eating issues such as the content of church meals.

In another model oriented to dietary change in outpatient settings, Kumanyika, Adams-Campbell, et al. (1999) developed and evaluated an audiovisual nutrition education program suitable for African Americans with reading levels of fifth to eighth grade or above. The video depicted an intergenerational African American family in which a family member—the mother or grandmother—was faced with dietary change issues related to high blood pressure and high cholesterol. This motivational video was accompanied by a set of twelve audiocassette programs of vignettes in which family members confronted and resolved various dietary change tasks or issues. Core elements of the program included food picture cards and a booklet that employed a simplified color-coded scheme for recognition of foods that were low, medium, or high in fat, cholesterol, and sodium. In association with clinic monitoring and counseling every four months, these educational materials were effective in facilitating reductions in serum cholesterol and blood pressure among forty- to seventy-year-old African American men and women over a one-year period. Improvements in cholesterol and blood pressure at one year were greatest among those who reported more initial use of the printed materials.

Church-based programs may also be a very effective venue for nutrition interventions in African American communities. Advantages include the potential convenience and sustainability of such interventions as well as group support factors. In addition, as noted previously, meals served at church functions may be prime targets for modification in their calorie, fat, and salt content and in their perpetuation of traditional eating practices that are no longer considered healthful. Kumanyika and Charleston (1992) noted the feasibility of and receptivity of African American women to a weight control program sponsored by a black community hospital through state health department funding but offered in a church setting. Turner, Sutherland, Harris, and Barber (1995) reported some success with changing salt and meat consumption practices through a church-based health promotion program in an African American community in northern Florida. These authors articulated several inherent characteristics of churches that lend themselves naturally to health education initiatives and engaged church members in formulating and implementing the program.

A large-scale intervention that was effective in increasing fruit and vegetable consumption was conducted with fifty African American churches in ten rural counties in North Carolina (Campbell, Demark-Wahnefried, et al., 1999) as part of the National Cancer Institute's 5-a-Day research program. The intervention included providing bulletins tailored to individual church members and printed materials that could be used by Nutrition Action Teams established at the churches during the intervention component; arranging gardening activities, educational sessions, and cookbook sharing and recipe tasting; serving more fruits and vegetables at church functions; involving lay health advisors, community coalitions, and local grocers and vendors; providing information for pastors and involving them directly in health promotion activities; and offering other activities planned and implemented by the individual churches.

Campbell, Honess-Morreale, Farrell, Carbone, and Brasure (1999) also reported pilot test results that suggested the potential effectiveness of an innovative approach to providing nutrition education for a group of Food Stamp Program participants, of whom 85 percent were African American. Using computer technology and taking into account the results of formative research with the client population, the intervention used a soap opera video (with a courtroom drama and love triangle plot) to deliver nutrition information along with *infomercials* that were tailored to individual participants' interests and needs as revealed by their responses to a questionnaire. Participants watched the thirty-minute program in a kiosk at the food stamp office.

These types of studies have been slow in coming. However, the importance of conducting culture-specific studies in high-risk populations is increasingly recognized, and the groundwork is being laid for the development of a body of literature to clarify the most cost-effective and sustainable dietary change methods for African American communities.

Conclusion

Although the database on diet-related health issues for African Americans is relatively sparse and has many imperfections, the consistency of the evidence suggesting important, correctable nutrition problems in the black community is undeniable. These issues deserve much more attention and are to some extent unique to African Americans as opposed to minority populations in general, as reviewed elsewhere (Kumanyika & Krebs-Smith, in press). Current African American eating patterns reflect both historical factors, such as the evolution of dietary practices and traditions under conditions of slavery, and current societal conditions, such as the economics and ecology of food in inner-city communities.

The persistence of food insecurity and nutritional inadequacies in the African American population alongside an excess of "overnutrition"-related health problems means that the goals of nutrition interventions must be carefully formulated to address both these issues. Both clinical and community-based approaches are indicated as well as general communication strategies (for example, through the media) in order to facilitate the understanding and adoption of nutrition information. Several areas have been noted where a more complete picture is needed in order to understand the variations in nutrition-related attitudes and practices of black Americans. The formulation of such research and the translation of the resulting data into meaningful strategies and programs can benefit from the cultural knowledge that may be unique to African American researchers, and it will require collaboration among investigators trained in both social science and biomedical fields.

A complete review of nutrition issues in the black community would address many issues not covered here. As noted at the beginning of the chapter, specific considerations for children and the elderly have not been addressed here, partly to limit the scope of this chapter and partly because these life-stage groups have unique nutritional requirements. Obesity has also not been addressed here except to note that it is a critical issue, particularly for black women and children. Among the issues not adequately addressed due to the lack of data are nutrition issues for African Americans in rural areas. Current data sources are dominated by samples from urban areas, and findings for rural populations may differ from those described here. Similarly, issues for the higher socioeconomic status segment of the African American population differ from those of the segment living in poverty but cannot be fully explored with existing data sets. Finally, the increasing importance of studying separately subethnic groups in the African American community has been highlighted. For a variety of reasons, people of African descent whose core diet is African or Caribbean based have nutritional issues and potential risks different from those described here.

References

Agurs-Collins, T. D., Kumanyika, S. K., Ten Have, T. R., & Adams-Campbell, L. L. (1997). A randomized controlled trial of weight reduction and exercise for diabetes management in older African American subjects. *Diabetes Care, 20,* 1503–1511.

Airhihenbuwa, C. O., Kumanyika, S., Agurs, T. D., Lowe, A., Saunders, D., & Morssink, C. B. (1996). Cultural aspects of African American eating patterns. *Ethnicity and Health, 3,* 245–260.

American Cancer Society. Advisory Committee on Diet, Nutrition, and Cancer Prevention. (1996). Guidelines on diet, nutrition, and cancer prevention: Reducing the risk of cancer with healthy food choices and physical activity. *CA: A Cancer Journal for Clinicians, 46,* 325–341.

American Dietetic Association. (1998). *Food Guide Pyramid with popular southern fare* [On-line]. Available: www.eatright.org

Basiotis, P. P., Kramer-Leblanc, C. S., & Kennedy, E. T. (1998). Maintaining nutrition security and diet quality: The role of the Food Stamp Program and WIC. *Family Economics and Nutrition Review, 11,* 4–16.

Bendich, A., & Deckelbaum, R. (1997). *Preventive nutrition: The comprehensive guide for health professionals.* Totowa, NJ: Humana Press.

Berti, P., & Leonard, W. R. (1995). The merits of race-specific standards [Letter to the editor]. *American Journal of Clinical Nutrition, 61,* 616.

Borrud, L., Pillow, P., Allen, P., McPherson, R., Nichaman, M., & Newell, G. (1989). Food group contribution to nutrient intakes in whites, blacks and Mexican Americans in Texas. *Journal of the American Dietetic Association, 89,* 1061–1069.

Bowman, S., Lino, M., Gerrior, S., & Basiotis, P. (1998). The Healthy Eating Index, 1994–1996. *Family Economics and Nutrition Review, 11,* 2–14.

Brancati, F. L., Appel, L. J., Seidler, A. J., & Whelton, P. K. (1996). Effect of potassium supplementation on blood pressure in African Americans on a low-potassium diet. *Archives of Internal Medicine, 156,* 61–67.

Brewster, L., & Jacobson, M. F. (1978). *The changing American diet.* Washington, DC: Center for Science in the Public Interest.

Bronner, Y. L. (1996). Nutritional status outcomes for children: Ethnic, cultural, and environmental contexts. *Journal of the American Dietetic Association, 96,* 891–900, 903.

Brown, M. (1999). Supermarket blackout: There are few supermarkets in cities, meaning that blacks pay more for food, lose out on jobs, and go elsewhere for quality goods. *Black Enterprise, 29,* 81–92.

Campbell, M. K., Demark-Wahnefried, W., Symons, M., Kalsbeek, W. D., Dodds, J., Cowan, A., Jackson, B., Motsinger, B., Hoben, K., Lashley, J., Demissie, S., & McClelland, J. W. (1999). Fruit and vegetable consumption and prevention of cancer: The Black Churches United for Better Health project. *American Journal of Public Health, 89,* 1390–1396.

Campbell, M. K., Honess-Morreale, L., Farrell, D., Carbone, E., & Brasure, M. (1999). A tailored multimedia nutrition education pilot program for low-income women receiving food assistance. *Health Education Research, 14,* 257–267.

Center for Nutrition Policy and Promotion. (1998). *Report card on the dietary quality of African Americans: Insight 6. Nutrition Insights* [On-line]. Available: www.usda.gov/cnpp

Chatters, L., Taylor, R., & Lincoln, K. (1999). African American religious participation: A multi-sample comparison. *Journal for the Scientific Study of Religion, 38,* 132–145.

Cheadle, A., Psaty, B., Curry, S., Wagner, E., Diehr, P., Koepsell, T., & Kristal, A. (1991). Community-level comparisons between the grocery store environment and individual dietary practices. *Preventive Medicine, 20,* 250–261.

Committee on Diet and Health. Food and Nutrition Board. Commission on Life Sciences. National Research Council. (1989). *Diet and health: Implications for reducing chronic disease risk.* Washington, DC: National Academy Press.

Council of Economic Advisers for the President's Initiative on Race. (1998). *Changing America: Indicators of social and economic well-being by race and Hispanic origin* [On-line]. Available: www.access.gpo.gov/eop/ca/index.html

Crespo, C. J., Smit, E., Andersen, R. E., Carter-Pokras, O., & Ainsworth, B. E. (2000). Race/ethnicity, social class and their relation to physical inactivity during leisure time: Results from the Third National Health and Nutrition Examination Survey, 1988–1994. *American Journal of Preventive Medicine, 18,* 46–53.

Dacosta, K. O., & Wilson, J. F. (1996). Food preferences and attitudes in three generations of black and white women. *Appetite, 27,* 183–191.

Davies, S. (1995). Scientific and ethical foundations of nutritional and environmental medicine: Pt. 2. Further glimpses of "the higher medicine." *Journal of Nutritional and Environmental Medicine 5,* 5–11.

Deckelbaum, R. J., Fisher, E. A., Winston, M., Kumanyika, S., Lauer, R. M., Pi-Sunyer, F. X., St. Jeor, S., Schaefer, E. J., & Weinstein, I. B. (1999). Summary of a scientific conference on preventive nutrition: Pediatrics to geriatrics. *Circulation, 100*(4), 450–456.

Ervin R. B., Wright, J. D., & Kennedy-Stephenson, J. (1999). *Use of dietary supplements in the United States, 1988–1994* (Vital and Health Statistics, Series 11, No. 244, DHHS Publication No. PHS 99-1694). Hyattsville, MD: National Center for Health Statistics.

Fang, J., Madhavan, S., & Alderman, M. (1996). The association between birthplace and mortality from cardiovascular causes among black and white residents of New York City. *New England Journal of Medicine, 335,* 1545–1551.

Federation of American Societies for Experimental Biology. Life Sciences Research Office. (1995). *Third Report on Nutrition Monitoring in the United States* (Vol. 1, prepared for the Interagency Board for Nutrition Monitoring and Related Research). Washington, DC: U.S. Government Printing Office.

Flegal, K. M., Carroll, M. D., Kuczmarski, R. J., & Johnson, C. L. (1998). Overweight and obesity in the United States: Prevalence and trends, 1960–1994. *International Journal of Obesity, 22,* 39–47.

Ford, E. S., & Bowman, B. A. (1999). Serum and red blood cell folate concentrations, race, and education: Findings from the Third National Health and Nutrition Examination Survey. *American Journal of Clinical Nutrition, 69,* 476–481.

Ford, E. S., & Sowell, A. (1999). Serum alpha-tocopherol status in the United States population: Findings from the Third National Health and Nutrition Examination Survey. *American Journal of Epidemiology, 150,* 290–300.

Fraser, G. E., Sumbureru, D., Pribis, P., Neil, R. L., & Frankson, M.A.C. (1997). Association among health habits, risk factors, and all-cause mortality in a black California population. *Epidemiology, 8,* 168–174.

Frazão, E. (Ed.). (1999). *America's eating habits: Changes and consequences* (Agricultural Information Bulletin No. 750). Washington, DC: U.S. Department of Agriculture, Economic Research Service, Food and Rural Economics Division.

Freedman, A. M. (1990, December 19). Habit forming: Fast-food chains' central role in diet of the inner-city poor. *Wall Street Journal,* p. A6.

Friend, B., Page, L., & Marston, R. (1979). Food consumption patterns in the United States, 1909–1913 to 1976. In R. Levy, B. Rifkind, B. Dennis, & N. Ernst (Eds.), *Nutrition, Lipids, and Coronary Heart Disease* (pp. 489–522). New York: Raven Press.

Ganguli, M. C., Grimm, R. H., Svendsen, K. H., Flack, J. M., Grandits, G. A., & Elmer, P. J., for the TOMHS Research Group. (1999). Urinary sodium and potassium profile of blacks and whites in relation to education in two different geographic urban areas. *American Journal of Hypertension, 12,* 69–72.

Giles, W. H., Croft, J. B., Greenlund, K. J., Ford, E. S., & Kittner, S. J. (2000). Association between total homocyst(e)ine and the likelihood for a history of acute myocardial infarction by race and ethnicity: Results from the Third National Health and Nutrition Examination Survey. *American Heart Journal, 139,* 446–453.

Glanz, K., Basil, M., Maibach, E., Goldberg, J., & Snyder, D. (1998). Why Americans eat what they do: Taste, nutrition, cost, convenience, and weight control concerns as influences on food consumption. *Journal of the American Dietetic Association, 98,* 1118–1126.

Greenberg, M., & Schneider, D. (1991). Region of birth and mortality of blacks in the United States. *International Journal of Epidemiology, 21,* 324–328.

Greenberg, M., Schneider, D., Northridge, M., & Ganz, M. (1998). Region of birth and black diets: The Harlem Household Survey. *American Journal of Public Health, 88,* 1199–1202.

Gundersen, C., LeBlanc, M., & Kuhn, B. (1999). *The changing food assistance landscape: The Food Stamp Program in a post-welfare reform environment* (Agricultural Economic Report No. 773).

Washington, DC: U.S. Department of Agriculture, Economic Research Service, Food and Rural Economics Division.

Harland, B., Smith, S., Ellis, R., O'Brien, R., & Morris, E. (1992). Comparison of the nutrient intakes of blacks, Sioux Indians, and whites in Columbus County, North Carolina. *Journal of the American Dietetic Association, 92,* 348–350.

Hayes, R. B., Ziegler, R. G., Gridley, G., Swanson, C., Greenberg, R. S., Swanson, G. M., Schoenberg, J. B., Silverman, D. T., Brown, L. M., Pottern, L. M., Liff, J., Schwartz, A. G., Fraumeni, J. F., Jr., & Hoover, R. N. (1999). *Cancer Epidemiology, Biomarkers, and Prevention, 8,* 25–34.

Jarvis, G. K., & Northcott, H. C. (1987). Religion and differences in morbidity and mortality. *Social Science and Medicine, 25,* 813–824.

Jeffery, R. W., Drewnoswski, A., Epstein, L. H., Stunkard, A. J., Wilson, G. T., Wing, R. R., & Hill, D. R. (2000). Long-term maintenance of weight loss: Current status. *Health Psychology, 19,* 5–16.

Jerome, N. (1969). Northern urbanization and food consumption patterns of southern-born Negroes. *American Journal of Clinical Nutrition, 22,* 1667–1669.

Johnson-Spear, M. A., & Yip, R. (1994). Hemoglobin difference between black and white women with comparable iron status: Justification for race-specific standards. *American Journal of Clinical Nutrition, 60,* 117–121.

Kaufman, J. S., Durazo-Arvizu, R. A., Rotimi, C. N., McGee, D. L., & Cooper, R. S. (1996). Obesity and hypertension prevalence in populations of African origin (The investigators of the International Collaborative Study on Hypertension in Blacks). *Epidemiology, 7,* 398–405.

Kimm, S. Y., Gergen, P. J., Malloy, M., Dresser, C., & Carroll, M. (1990). Dietary patterns of U.S. children: Implications for disease prevention. *Preventive Medicine, 19,* 432–442.

Kittler, P. G., & Sucher, K. P. (1998). *Food and culture in America: A nutrition handbook* (2nd ed.). Washington, DC: West/Wadsworth.

Klein, B. (1998). Could there be hunger in America? *Family Economics and Nutrition Review, 11,* 52–54.

Kleinman, J. C., & Kessel, S. S. (1987). Racial differences in low birth weight: Trends and risk factors. *New England Journal of Medicine, 317*(12), 749–753.

Kristal, A., Shattuck, A., & Patterson, R. (1999). Differences in fat-related dietary patterns between black, Hispanic, and white women: Results from the Women's Health Trial Feasibility Study in Minority Populations. *Public Health Nutrition, 2,* 253–262.

Kumanyika, S. (1987). Obesity in black women. *Epidemiological Review, 9,* 31–50.

Kumanyika, S. K. (1993). Diet and nutrition as influences on the morbidity/mortality gap. *Annals of Epidemiology, 3,* 154–158.

Kumanyika, S. K. (1994). Obesity in minority populations: An epidemiologic assessment. *Obesity Research, 2,* 166–178.

Kumanyika, S. K. (1997a). Aging, diet and nutrition in African Americans. In K. S. Markides & M. R. Miranda (Eds.), *Minorities, aging and health* (pp. 205–235). Thousand Oaks, CA: Sage.

Kumanyika, S. K. (1997b). The impact of obesity on hypertension management in African Americans. *Journal of Health Care for the Poor and Underserved, 8,* 365–378.

Kumanyika, S. K. (1999, April). *Understanding adherence to dietary and lifestyle change in minority populations.* Presented at the American Heart Association conference on compliance in health care and research, Waltham, MA.

Kumanyika, S. K., Adams-Campbell, L., Van Horn, B., Ten Have, T., Treu, J., Askov, E., Williams, J., Achterberg, C., Zaghloul, S., Monsegu, D., Bright, M., Stoy, D. B., Malone-Jackson, M., Mooney, D., Deiling, S., & Caulfield, J. (1999). Outcomes of a cardiovascular nutrition counseling program in African Americans with elevated blood pressure or cholesterol. *Journal of the American Dietetic Association, 99,* 1380–1388.

Kumanyika, S. K., Bowen, D., Rolls, B. J., Van Horn, L., Perri, M. G., Czajkowski, S. M., & Schron, E. (2000). Maintenance of dietary behavior change. *Health Psychology, 19*(Suppl.), 42–56.

Kumanyika, S. K., & Charleston, J. B. (1992). Lose weight and win: A church-based weight loss program for blood pressure control among black women. *Patient Education and Counseling, 19,* 19–32.

Kumanyika, S. K., & Golden, P. M. (1991). Cross-sectional differences in health status in U.S. racial/ethnic minority groups: Potential influence of temporal changes, disease, and lifestyle transitions. *Ethnicity and Disease, 1,* 50–59.

Kumanyika, S. K., & Krebs-Smith, S. M. (in press). Preventive nutrition issues in ethnic and socioeconomic groups in the United States. In A. Bendich & R. J. Deckelbaum (Eds.), *Preventive Nutrition* (Vol. 2). Totowa, NJ: Humana Press.

LaVeist, T. A. (1996). Why we should continue to study race . . . but do a better job: An essay on race, racism, and health. *Ethnicity and Disease, 6,* 21–29.

Levedahl, J. W., & Oliveira, V. (1999). Dietary impacts of food assistance and programs. In E. Frazão (Ed.), *America's eating habits: Changes and consequences* (Agricultural Information Bulletin No. 750, pp. 307–330. Washington, DC: U.S. Department of Agriculture, Economic Research Service, Food and Rural Economics Division.

Levin, J., & Vanderpool, Y. (1989). Is religion therapeutically significant for hypertension? *Social Science and Medicine, 29,* 69–78.

Lincoln, C. E. (1999). *Race, religion, and the continuing American dilemma.* New York: Hill & Wang.

Lincoln, C. E., & Mamiya, L. H. (1990). *The black church in the African-American experience.* Durham, NC: Duke University Press.

Luft, F. C., Miller, J. Z., Grim, C. E., Fineberg, N. S., Christian, J. C., Daugherty, S. A., & Weinberger, M. H. (1991). Salt sensitivity and resistance of blood pressure: Age and race as factors in physiological responses. *Hypertension, 17*(Suppl.), I102–I108.

Markowitz, F. (1996). Israel as Africa, Africa as Israel: "Divine geography" in the personal narratives and community identity of the black Hebrew Israelites. *Anthropological Quarterly, 69,* 193–205.

Matthews, H. (1987). Rootwork: Description of an ethnomedical system in the American south. *Southern Medical Journal, 80,* 885–891.

McCloud, A. (1995). *African-American Islam.* New York: Routledge.

Melby, C., Toohey, M., & Cebrick, J. (1994). Blood pressure and blood lipids among vegetarian, semivegetarian, and nonvegetarian African Americans. *American Journal of Clinical Nutrition, 59,* 103–109.

Miller, B. A., Kolonel, L. N., Bernstein, L., Young, J. L., Jr., Swanson, G. M., West, D., Key, C. R., Liff, J. M., Glover, C. S., Alexander, G. A., Coyle, L., Hankey, B. F., Ries, L.A.G., Kosary, C. L., Harras, A., Percy, C., & Edwards, B. K. (Eds.). (1996). *Racial/ethnic patterns of cancer in the United States, 1988–1992* (NIH Publication No. 96-4104). Bethesda, MD: National Cancer Institute.

Mintz, S. W. (1996). *Tasting food, tasting freedom: Excursions into eating, culture and the past.* Boston: Beacon Press.

Muhammad, E. (1972). *How to eat to live* (Vol. 1). Chicago: Muhammad's Temple of Islam No. 2.

Murcott, A. (1988). Sociological and social anthropological approaches to food and eating. *World Review of Nutrition and Dietetics, 55,* 1–40.

Murphy, F., Gwebu, E., Braithwaite, R., Green-Goodman, D., & Brown, L. (1997). Health values and practices among Seventh-Day Adventists. *American Journal of Health Behavior, 21,* 43–50.

Must, A., Spandano, S., Coakley, E. H., Field, A., Colditz, G., & Dietz, W. (1999). The disease burden associated with overweight and obesity. *Journal of the American Medical Association, 282,* 1523–1529.

National Center for Health Statistics. (1999). *Health, United States, 1999 with health and aging chartbook* (DHHS Publication No. PHS 99-1232). Hyattsville, MD: Author.

National Heart, Lung, and Blood Institute. Expert Panel on the Identification, Evaluation, and Treatment of Overweight and Obesity in Adults. (1998). Clinical guidelines on the identification, evaluation, and treatment of obesity in adults: The evidence report. *Obesity Research, 6*(Suppl.), 51S–209S.

Nord, M., Jemison, K., & Bickel, G. (1999). *Measuring food security in the United States: Prevalence of food insecurity and hunger, by state, 1996–1998* (Food Assistance and Nutrition Research Report No. 2). Washington, DC: U.S. Department of Agriculture, Economic Research Service, Food and Rural Economic Division.

Odoms, A. (1999). *The role of religion in the dietary and food choice practices of African-American Muslim women.* Unpublished doctoral dissertation, Cornell University.

Perry, G. S., Byers, T., Yip, R., & Margen, S. (1992). Iron nutrition does not account for the hemoglobin differences between blacks and whites. *Journal of Nutrition, 122,* 1417–1424.

Phillips, R. L., & Snowdon, D. A. (1985). Dietary relationships with fatal colorectal cancer among Seventh-Day Adventists. *Journal of the National Cancer Institute, 74,* 307–317.

Poe, T. (1999). The origins of soul food in the black urban identity: Chicago, 1915–1947. *American Studies International, 37,* 4–33.

Pollard, K., & O'Hare, W. (1999). America's racial and ethnic minorities. *Population Bulletin, 54,* 1–34.

Rosenbloom, A. L., Joe, J. R., Young, R. S., & Winter, W. E. (1999). Emerging epidemic of type 2 diabetes in youth. *Diabetes Care, 22,* 345–354.

Rush, D., Leighton, J., Sloan, N. L., Alvir, J. M., & Garbowski, G. C. (1988). The national WIC evaluation: Evaluation of the Special Supplemental Food Program for Women, Infants, and Children: 2. Review of past studies of WIC. *American Journal of Clinical Nutrition, 48*(Suppl.), 394–411.

Shortridge, B., & Shortridge, J. (1998). Introduction: Food and American culture. In B. Shortridge & J. Shortridge (Eds.). *The taste of American place: A reader on regional and ethnic foods* (pp. 1–18). Lanham, MA: Rowman & Littlefield.

Smit, E., Nieto, F. J., Crespo, C. J., & Mitchell, P. (1999). Estimates of animal and plant protein intake in U.S. adults: Results from the Third National Health and Nutrition Examination Survey, 1988–1991. *Journal of the American Dietetic Association, 99,* 813–820.

Standing Committee on the Scientific Evaluation of Dietary Reference Intakes. Food and Nutrition Board. Institute of Medicine. (1999a). *Dietary reference intakes for calcium, phosphorus, magnesium, vitamin D, and fluoride.* Washington, DC: National Academy Press.

Standing Committee on the Scientific Evaluation of Dietary Reference Intakes. Food and Nutrition Board. Institute of Medicine. (1999b). *Dietary reference intakes for thiamin, riboflavin, niacin, vitamin B6, folate, vitamin B12, pantothenic acid, biotin, and choline.* Washington, DC: National Academy Press.

Svetky, L. P., Simons-Morton, D., Vollmer, W. M., Appel, L. J., Conlin, P. R., Ryan, D. H., Ard, J., & Kennedy, B. M. (1999). Effects of dietary patterns on blood pressure: Subgroup analysis of the Dietary Approaches to Stop Hypertension (DASH) randomized clinical trial. *Archives of Internal Medicine, 159,* 285–293.

Swanson, C., Gridley, G., Greenberg, R., Schoenberg, J., Swanson, M., Brown, L., Hayes, R., Silverman, D., & Pottern, L. (1993). A comparison of diets of blacks and whites in three areas of the United States. *Nutrition and Cancer, 20,* 153–165.

Thompson, F. E., & Byers, T. (1994). Dietary assessment resource manual. *Journal of Nutrition, 124*(11, Suppl.), 2245S–2317S.

Troiano, R. P., Flegal, K. M., Kuczmarski, R. J., Campbell, S. M., & Johnson, C. L. (1995). Overweight prevalence and trends for children and adolescents: The National Health and Nutrition Examination Surveys, 1963–1991. *Archives of Pediatric Adolescent Medicine, 149,* 1085–1091.

Turner, L. W., Sutherland, M., Harris, G. J., & Barber, M. (1995). Cardiovascular health promotion in north Florida African-American churches. *Health Values, 19,* 3–9.

U.S. Department of Agriculture. Agricultural Research Service. (1999). *Data tables: Food and nutrient intakes by Hispanic origin and race, 1994–1996* [On-line]. Available: www.barc.usda.gov/bhnrc/foodsurvey/home.htm

U.S. Department of Agriculture & U.S. Department of Health and Human Services. (2000). *Nutrition and your health: Dietary guidelines for Americans* (5th ed., Home and Garden Bulletin No. 232). Washington, DC: Author.

U.S. Department of Health and Human Services. Task Force on Black and Minority Health. (1985). *Report of the Secretary's Task Force on Black and Minority Health* (Vol. 1, Executive Summary). Washington, DC: U.S. Government Printing Office.

Variyam, J. N., Blaylock, J., Smallwood, D., & Basiotis, P. P. (1998). *USDA's Healthy Eating Index and nutrition information* (Technical Bulletin No. 1866). Washington, DC: U.S. Department of Agriculture, Economic Research Service, Food and Rural Economics Division.

Veale-Jones, D., & Darling, M. (1996). *Ethnic foodways in Minnesota: Handbook of food and wellness across cultures.* [On-line] Available: www.agricola.umn.edu/foodways

Weinstein, R. S., & Bell, N. H. (1988). Diminished rates of bone formation in normal black adults. *New England Journal of Medicine, 319,* 1698–1701.

Whitehead, T. L. (1992). In search of soul food and meaning: Culture, food, and health. In J. A. Baer & Y. Jones (Eds.), *African Americans in the south: Issues of race, class, and gender* (pp. 94–110). Athens: University of Georgia Press.

Whittemore, A. S., Kolonel, L. N., Wu, A. H., John, E. M., Gallagher, R. P., Howe, J. R., Burch, J. D., Hankin, J., Dreon, D. M., West, D. W., The, C. Z., & Paffenbarger, R. S., Jr. (1995). *Journal of the National Cancer Institute, 87,* 652–661.

Willett, W. (1998). *Nutritional Epidemiology* (2nd ed.). New York: Oxford University Press.

Women's Health Initiative Study Group. (1997). Design paper: The Women's Health Initiative Clinical Trial and Observational Study. *Controlled Clinical Trials, 19,* 61–109.

World Cancer Research Fund & American Institute for Cancer Research. (1997). *Food, nutrition and the prevention of cancer: A global perspective.* Washington, DC: American Institute for Cancer Research.

Yadrick, K., Harris, E., & Idris, R. (1997). *Food and nutrient intake of lower Mississippi delta residents: Nutrition and health status in the lower Mississippi delta of Arkansas, Louisiana, and Mississippi: A review of the existing data* (Lower Mississippi Delta Nutrition Intervention Research Consortium). Rockville, MD: Westat Delta NIRI Coordinating Center.

CHAPTER TWENTY-ONE

PHYSICAL ACTIVITY

Wendell C. Taylor, Antronette K. Yancey,
Deborah Rohm Young, William J. McCarthy

Physical activity improves physical and psychological health (U.S. Department of Health and Human Services [DHHS], 1996). Activity reduces the risk of heart disease, high blood pressure, diabetes, colon and other cancers, depression, anxiety, and dying prematurely. Regular physical activity promotes psychological well-being; helps control weight; and builds and maintains healthy bones, muscles, and joints (DHHS, 1996). Physical inactivity and dietary factors are second only to cigarette smoking as primary contributors to premature mortality in the United States (McGinnis & Foege, 1993) and are increasingly important contributors to premature mortality worldwide (Popkin & Doak, 1998). The black community can benefit immensely by increasing physical activity levels to improve quality of life and reduce health care costs. As a result, substantial public health gains can be achieved in the black community (Taylor, Baranowski, & Rohm Young, 1998).

Physical inactivity is associated with increased risk of premature morbidity and mortality (Blair et al., 1989) and is an independent predictor for coronary heart disease, the leading cause of death of all Americans (American Heart Association, 1997). The extrapolated cost of physical inactivity, based on 1986 mortality estimates, is $5.7 billion, which is higher than the cost of any other risk factors for coronary heart disease except elevated blood cholesterol levels (Hahn, Teutsch, Rothenberg, & Marks, 1990).

Regular physical activity is associated with reduced incidence of hypertension (American College of Sports Medicine, 1993), diabetes (Manson & Spelsberg, 1994) obesity (National Institutes of Health, 1998), and some types of cancers, such as colon cancer (Slattery, Edwards, Boucher, Anderson, & Caan, 1999; Thune & Lund, 1996; World Cancer Research Fund & American Institute for

Cancer Research, 1997) and breast cancer (Thune, Brenn, Lund, & Gaard, 1997; Carpenter, Ross, Paganini-Hill, & Bernstein, 1999). Given the disproportionate risk for these diseases among the black community, lack of participation in regular physical activity is of heightened concern. For example, blacks are at increased risk for hypertension and diabetes (American Heart Association, 1997) compared to whites, and black women are more likely to be overweight or obese compared to white women (Flegal, Carroll, Kuczmarski, & Johnson, 1998). Although most epidemiological investigations have not been conducted with sufficient sample sizes of blacks to allow ethnicity-specific analyses, regular physical activity is surely beneficial to persons of all ethnic origins. In summary, blacks are more likely than whites to have conditions (for example, obesity and hypertension) that can be prevented or managed with regular physical activity (Gillum, 1987; Rowland & Roberts, 1982). In this chapter, we present physical activity as a health enhancing behavior for the black community. We present definitions; we examine physical activity guidelines, levels, determinants, and interventions; and we discuss future directions and recommendations. Three appendices provide information about helpful Web sites, programs for youths, and national agencies and organizations.

Definitions

Physical activity, exercise, and *physical fitness* are terms with distinct meanings (Ainsworth & Macera, 1998; Caspersen, 1989). Physical activity is bodily movement produced by contracting skeletal muscles that substantially increases energy expenditure. Examples include such activities as participating in a sport, walking, dancing, gardening, vacuuming, stair walking, washing the car, and mowing the lawn (U.S. Department of Agriculture, 1995). Physical activity is a broad category; exercise is a subset of physical activity. Exercise is planned, structured, and repetitive bodily movement intended to maintain or improve physical fitness. Examples include jogging, swimming, aerobic classes, tennis, weight training, and other conditioning activities. Physical activity and exercise are behaviors involving repetitive, continual bodily movement.

In contrast, physical fitness is a set of attributes that people have or achieve that correspond to the ability to perform physical activity. Components of physical fitness include attributes related to health such as aerobic capacity, muscular endurance, muscular strength, body composition, and flexibility and attributes related to skill such as speed, balance, and agility. Fitness can be measured by a variety of tests: for example, aerobic capacity is measured by exercise testing on a treadmill or stationary cycle during which time oxygen utilization is directly measured or estimated. A physically fit person can carry out daily tasks and enjoy leisure time pursuits with vigor and energy. Further, a physically fit person can perform moderate to vigorous levels of physical activity without undue fatigue. (For a more complete description of terms, see Ainsworth & Macera, 1998; Caspersen, 1989; DHHS, 1996.)

Guidelines for Physical Activity

Physical activity is more challenging than many health enhancing behaviors (such as flossing one's teeth, using a seat belt, and so forth) because activity takes planning, consistency, time, effort, and exertion (Dishman, 1996). Only 22 percent of American adults engage in regular, sustained physical activity (DHHS, 1996). Most American adults are sedentary or irregularly active, and many youths are inactive (Centers for Disease Control and Prevention [CDC] & American College of Sports Medicine, 1993; DHHS, 1996; Pate, Long, & Heath, 1994).

A 1996 report of the surgeon general entitled "Physical Activity and Health" states that "all people over the age of 2 years should accumulate at least 30 minutes of endurance-type physical activity, of at least moderate intensity, on most—preferably all—days of the week" (p. 28).

Examples of moderate intensity activity range from stair walking, water aerobics, brisk walking, raking leaves, dancing, and gardening to washing windows or floors. The health benefits that can be achieved with regular physical activity include improvements in one's blood lipid profile, resting blood pressure, body composition, glucose tolerance, insulin sensitivity, bone density, immune function, and psychological function (Pate, Pratt, et al., 1995). Vigorous intensity activity, such as running or jogging, fast cycling, or playing basketball or racquetball, is associated with these same benefits to a greater degree and will improve cardiorespiratory fitness as well. Expending at least 200 calories per day in at least moderate intensity activity is sufficient to achieve significant health benefits (DHHS, 1996; Pate, Pratt, et al., 1995). Health benefits can be realized even if physical activity is accumulated in short bouts (for example, three ten-minute activity sessions per day). More physical activity, in terms of increased frequency, intensity, or duration, will accrue additional health benefits, although high levels of activity are also associated with increased risk of musculoskeletal injuries.

Levels of Physical Activity

Measures of physical activity include self-reports (for example, diaries, logs, recall surveys, global self-reports, and retrospective quantitative histories) and direct monitoring (behavioral observations, heart rate monitors, and motion sensors) (DHHS, 1996). Any measure is subject to bias, measurement error, inaccuracies, and incomplete assessment. Given these limitations, the existing literature documents ethnic differences in physical activity levels.

Several studies have compared levels of physical activity by ethnic group and gender. Consistent trends in the physical activity levels of black males have not been established. Nonetheless, there is evidence that compared to men from three other ethnic groups, black men have the highest levels of self-reported leisure time physical inactivity (DHHS, 1996). Further, black women report high levels of physical inactivity (Ainsworth, Keenan, Strogatz, Garrett, & James,

1991; Liu et al., 1989; Washburn, Kline, Lackland, & Wheeler, 1992; Wing et al., 1989). Data for 1992 from the Youth Risk Factor Surveillance System indicate that the prevalence of sedentary behavior is 1.6 times higher among black women than among white women (CDC, 1997). Only one study found no significant difference in energy expenditure in leisure time physical activity between black and white women, who in this study were thirty-five to seventy-four years old (Folsom et al., 1991). Among 189 college students, black women reported lower levels of physical activity than black men (Ainsworth, Berry, Schnyder, & Vickers, 1992). Physical activity levels decline dramatically during adolescence, particularly among girls, with the decline most apparent among black girls (Heath, Pratt, Warren, & Kann, 1994). Among high school students the rate of moderate to vigorous physical activity was lower in black girls (17.4 percent) than in white girls (27.5 percent) and Mexican American girls (20.9 percent) (CDC, 1992b). Overall, lack of participation by blacks in physical activity is a public health concern because of the array of health benefits that regular physical activity confers, particularly for diseases for which blacks are at increased risk.

Determinants of Physical Activity

Determinants of physical activity are factors, variables, or conditions associated with or predictive of that activity. Modifiable determinants are intrapersonal, interpersonal, and environmental factors that can be changed by physical activity interventions. Nonmodifiable determinants are factors such as gender and age. These nonmodifiable determinants define subgroups, and each subgroup may have unique modifiable determinants. There have been a number of reviews of determinants of physical activity in adults (King et al., 1992; Rohm Young & King, 1995) and youths (Sallis, Prochaska, & Taylor, 2000; Taylor, Beech, & Cummings, 1997; Taylor, Baranowski, & Sallis, 1994; Taylor & Sallis, 1997). Data are limited regarding physical activity determinants for blacks and other racial or ethnic minority groups.

Johnson, Corrigan, Dubbert, and Gramling (1990) interviewed black and white women in shopping malls in a southeastern city to determine barriers to physical activity. Most of the sample was under the age of forty years. In this study, there were no racial differences in physical activity participation; 37 percent of the women reported they currently engaged in a regular exercise program. There also were no racial differences in barriers to physical activity. Lack of time was the greatest barrier, most commonly lack of time due to work or school responsibilities. Another study assessed barriers to physical activity among older black women. Common barriers these women expressed were that places to exercise are far away, exercise is fatiguing, they might look funny in exercise clothes, and they were afraid to walk in their neighborhood (Jones & Nies, 1996).

Exercise knowledge and beliefs have been examined in older black and white women (Fitzgerald, Singleton, Neale, Prasad, & Hess, 1994). Racial differences were noted for exercise beliefs. For example, white women were less likely to believe that older people should avoid vigorous exercise. Also, white women had greater confidence for engaging in a regular schedule of physical activity compared to black women. However, black and white women had similar perceptions of obstacles related to being physically active, such as lack of time.

Airhihenbuwa, Kumanyika, Agurs, and Lowe (1995) also examined cultural beliefs among blacks. They conducted focus groups with individuals representing a broad range of ages and socioeconomic categories. Their results indicate that many blacks considered rest to be more important than exercise. Because many blacks, historically, had jobs that required physical labor, they felt there was no reason to exercise and that rest was more important after a hard day of work than physical activity. Women preferred group-based exercise and exercising with friends rather than with family members.

Another qualitative assessment of black women found that policy and environmental factors could be inducements to increase their activity levels. For example, providing bonuses, work relief (for example, hours or days off), vouchers to attend an exercise facility, and lower insurance rates were all suggested as incentives that would motivate black women to increase their physical activity (Carter-Nolan, Adams-Campbell, & Williams, 1996).

Several studies have investigated cultural and ethnic differences as determinants of physical activity among youths. One study (Greendorfer & Ewing, 1981) reported that the location of facilities (for example, parks and schools), opportunities to participate in games or sports, and strong values about sports (for example, the importance to the child or the child's father that he or she be good in sports) had more influence on black children than on white children. One national survey (Wilson Sporting Goods Company, 1988) revealed that black and white girls were equally as likely to be involved in sports and that their reasons for participating in and quitting sports were the same. Ethnic differences, however, were identified. Black girls participated more often through their schools than did white girls (65 percent versus 50 percent), and white girls participated more often through private organizations (21 percent versus 7 percent). Black girls were more likely than their white counterparts to feel that "boys make fun of girls who play sports" (25 percent versus 1 percent) and more often had parents who felt that sports participation was more important for boys than for girls (30 percent versus 11 percent).

Age and gender influence perceptions of physical activity barriers and facilitators. For instance, focus group data gathered from black middle school girls in Los Angeles and Houston indicate that appearance concerns (styling hair, applying makeup, and grooming after physical activity) and perceptions of gender bias by male physical education teachers are primary barriers to their involvement in physical activity during the school day (Leslie et al., 1999; Taylor, Yancey, et al., 1999).

In summary, ethnic differences related to determinants of physical activity have been reported. However, the findings have not shown a clear and consistent pattern related to ethnic and cultural influences. More research is needed to learn about physical activity for black males of various ages and to identify cultural factors. Cultural influences should be investigated independent of socioeconomic status, environmental conditions, and setting. One perspective is that other relevant determinants of physical activity may diminish the influence of ethnic and cultural differences. Another perspective (for example, Melnyk & Weinstein, 1994) is that an increasing awareness is needed of the role that cultural diversity plays in people's attitudes and behaviors toward health. For example, as Melnyk and Weinstein suggest, instead of poor motivation perhaps the lack of access to exercise facilities, the preference for social versus individual exercise regimens, and culturally based attitudes (Airhihenbuwa et al., 1995) are reasons for low levels of physical activity among black women. Because increased stress levels are commonly experienced by blacks in comparison to whites, culturally grounded stress management strategies may also play a role. In a community sample of 429 black women recruited to a nutrition and exercise pilot study, Jordan (1999) found that weight-related stress management behaviors of either turning to food or getting exercise were the single best predictors of weight status (severely overweight, moderately overweight, or normal weight). Black women who used exercise for stress management were more likely to remain at a healthy weight. Systematic and well-designed studies to assess unique cultural influences on physical activity are needed in both men and women.

Physical Activity Interventions

Physical activity interventions are programs, planned strategies, or systems designed to increase physical activity levels. Such interventions, guided by research on activity determinants, can provide opportunities for adults and youths to become more active. Interventions to increase physical activity have involved single risk factor (that is, increased physical activity only) and multiple risk factor reduction programs (that is, increased activity, smoking cessation, reduced body weight, and improved nutrition). Settings for these interventions have included schools, family homes, worksites, communities, and health care facilities. Some interventions have been designed for black adults and youths.

For black adults, eight published community studies designed to promote activity were identified (Baranowski, Simons-Morton, et al., 1990; Brownson, Smith, et al., 1996; Kanders et al., 1994; Lasco et al., 1989; Kumanyika & Charleston, 1992; Lewis et al., 1993; Williams & Olano, 1999; Yancey, McCarthy, & Leslie, 1999). The most effective interventions (Brownson et al., 1996; Kumanyika & Charleston, 1992; Lasco et al., 1989) were culturally tailored, established community coalitions, and employed community residents to lead activities such as walking groups, water exercises, low-impact aerobic classes, and aerobic jazz dance programs. The settings included churches (Kumanyika & Charleston, 1992; Yancey et al., 1999) and community or recreation centers (Baranowski, Simons-Morton, et al., 1990; Lasco et al., 1989; Yancey et al., 1999).

Some programs were designed to promote activity in families, and other programs targeted weight loss in women. Some unique features of specific interventions are highlighted in the following paragraphs.

Lewis and colleagues (1993) reported the results of a physical activity intervention in public housing communities in Birmingham, Alabama. The project solicited the involvement of the community; assessed physical activity patterns, determinants, and barriers; and designed an intervention based on this information. Community residents were hired and trained to conduct the intervention, support from community leaders was solicited, and barriers to exercise were reduced. Process data revealed variable attendance for physical activity programs in the intervention communities. Organized communities that had regular resident council meetings and involved community leaders had greater participation in physical activity classes than the less organized communities. Changes in physical activity levels across the communities were highly variable, and there were no overall differences between the treatment and control communities. Additional data analyses, however, found that physical activity levels did increase in the organized communities. This project highlighted the power of social organization to solidify the beneficial effects of the intervention program.

The Community Health Assessment and Promotion Project (CHAPP) was developed in a predominately black community in Atlanta (Lasco et al., 1989) to reduce cardiovascular risk factors. The project formed a community coalition, which conducted a needs assessment, selected cardiovascular disease as the highest priority health problem, and designed a nutrition and exercise program. A wide variety of strategies were employed to reduce barriers to class participation, including providing child care and free transportation. Over 70 percent of the participants (all black women) attended ten or more sessions over a ten-week period.

Baranowski, Simons-Morton, et al. (1990) designed and implemented a center-based program to promote activity among healthy black families with children in the sixth through seventh grades. Ninety-four families were randomly assigned to either an experimental or a control group. In the experimental group, families participated in one educational session and two fitness sessions per week for fourteen weeks. Educational sessions included individual counseling, small-group education, and aerobic activity. Free transportation and baby-sitting were provided, as well as reminders to promote attendance. Following the fourteenth week of the program, the researchers conducted a postprogram assessment. In children, physical activity increased in the control group and decreased in the experimental group. For adults, no significant differences were detected in the intervention families compared to the control families. Baranowski et al. concluded that low participation rates (M = 28 percent) were the primary reason for lack of consistent program effects. Participants cited conflicts with work and school schedules (for adults and children, respectively) as their main reason for low attendance.

One prominent intervention for youths, the Know Your Body (KYB) program (Bush et al., 1989), was started in 1983 in the Washington, D.C., public elementary schools. The participants were black students in the fourth through sixth grades. The KYB program was classroom based and teacher delivered; its three primary intervention components were improving nutrition, increasing physical activity, and preventing cigarette smoking. The physical activity component promoted the adoption of a regular program of endurance activity to supplement skill and strength activities. The evaluation indicated that the intervention group was significantly more fit than the control group at year 3. No significant differences in fitness were reported for years 2, 4, and 5.

The efficacy of a school-based aerobic exercise program for lowering blood pressure in an urban sample of high-risk, ninth-grade black girls was evaluated (Ewart, Young, & Hagberg, 1998). Girls in the intervention group received a one-semester aerobics class of fitness instruction and training designed to be enjoyable and engaging for high-risk girls. Girls randomly assigned to the control group received the standard physical education curriculum. After the one-semester class, students in aerobic exercise physical education increased their cardiorespiratory fitness and decreased their resting systolic blood pressure compared to the standard physical education control group. After completing the aerobics class, 81 percent of the girls expressed a desire to participate in a supervised exercise maintenance program for at least one additional semester.

The literature on promoting physical activity in blacks is neither extensive nor well developed. Nonetheless, more success has been reported in promoting physical activity in high-risk blacks (for example, youths with elevated blood pressure and overweight women) (Ewart et al., 1998; Lasco et al., 1989) than in promoting activity among blacks with no immediate health challenges. The most successful interventions for adults involved walking programs and aerobic programs for weight loss in black women. Studies with smaller samples and more intensive interventions have found more success than other programs. More research is needed to determine optimal strategies for involving black families and black males in health behavior change programs. Future studies should employ strategies that have been shown to be effective, such as involving the community in all aspects of program design, implementation, and evaluation. Projects funded through the On the Move! initiative in California provide excellent examples of community involvement that can be used as a template for future studies (for example, Williams & Olano, 1999). Safety in neighborhoods, activity preferences, peer norms, family values and expectations, and physical status of the participants (for example, weight, fitness levels, and chronic conditions) should be considered in designing effective programs to promote physical activity.

Future Directions

Key messages from the surgeon general's report on physical activity and health (DHHS, 1996) are that physical activity need not be strenuous to achieve health benefits and that emphasizing the amount of physical activity rather than the intensity provides more options for people to incorporate activity into their daily lives. Three recent developments are consistent with these key messages. These developments are promoting lifestyle activity, encouraging avoidance of sedentary behaviors (especially television viewing), and promoting environmental and policy approaches.

Increasing Lifestyle Activity

The lifestyle approach requires a person to accumulate, at a minimum, thirty minutes of at least moderate intensity physical activity daily in bouts as short as ten minutes and in ways adapted to that person's lifestyle. Lifestyle activities might include walking during lunchtime, lawn work, gardening, dancing, bicycling to work, pushing a stroller, or washing and waxing a vehicle and also might include more traditional forms of exercise such as jogging, going to a health club, or playing on a sports team. The lifestyle approach is being promoted because it provides more flexibility than more structured approaches (such as attending group exercise classes at prespecified times) and therefore enables improved adherence. The lifestyle approach also offers the potential for greater long-term adherence because it is not necessarily dependent on specific physical activity structures or settings. Moreover, the lifestyle approach has been shown to improve physical activity, cardiorespiratory fitness, and blood pressure for at least two years (Dunn et al., 1999). The key is for individuals to incorporate physical activity into their day in a way that works for them and is compatible with their other lifestyle habits.

Avoiding Sedentary Behaviors, Especially Television Viewing

Experimental school-based efforts with black students have succeeded in discouraging some television use, with improvements seen in body composition and fat intake but no changes found in physical activity levels (Gortmaker et al., 1999). Epstein et al. (1995) and Dietz and Gortmaker (1985) have demonstrated that obesity risk in children can be decreased by discouraging sedentary behaviors, particularly television viewing. Time spent in television viewing may displace time participating in physical activities; however, this expectation has not been documented empirically (Robinson, 1999). In addition to decreasing sedentary behaviors, encouraging physical activity while viewing television can be investigated.

Even though reductions in television viewing resulting in more physical activity have not been demonstrated, television viewing typically involves prolonged exposure to commercials promoting high-fat foods. The foods usually advertised on television are notoriously calorie rich and nutrient poor (Gamble & Cotugna, 1999). Also, national surveys (Andersen, Crespo, Bartlett, Cheskin, & Pratt, 1998; Gordon-Larsen, McMurray, & Popkin, 1999) have reported that black children view more hours of television than do children of other ethnic groups. Furthermore, in low-income ethnic minority communities, targeted commercial marketing, specifically food advertising, has been documented (Hinkle, 1997). There-fore, limiting the number of hours of television viewing is a major concern for the black community.

Promoting Environmental and Policy Approaches

To increase physical activity, environmental and policy strategies are being de-signed and promoted to change the physical and sociopolitical environments. Examples of these approaches include establishing mall-walking programs, con-structing and maintaining walking and bicycle trails, and encouraging building construction that fosters activity and organizational policies and incentives that promote physical activity during the workday (Brownson et al., 2000). Some em-pirical evidence (Brownson, et al., 2000) has demonstrated that the availability of more places to walk is associated with increased levels of walking by community residents. For the most part, however, consistent relationships among environ-mental modifications, policy changes, availability, and accessibility on the one hand and increases in physical activity on the other hand have not been docu-mented. The viability and utility of these new developments for the black com-munity should be carefully studied.

Recommendations

We offer recommendations in two categories: doing more physical activity and doing better research.

Do More Physical Activity

Health benefits can be gained by increases in activity levels, and these benefits are proportional to the amount of participation in activity. Therefore every increase in activity adds some benefit (DHHS, 1996). Emphasizing the amount of activity rather than the intensity provides more choices for including activity in daily routines. Physical activity patterns may vary from day to day to accommodate personal preferences and lifestyles. Dancing, bicycling, basketball, brisk walking, stair walking, volleyball, aerobics, lawn mowing, raking leaves, weight training, and swimming can be accommodated in a physically active lifestyle. Individuals who are engaging in some activity, even though not regularly, can gradually and incrementally increase their activity levels over an extended period of time. Indi-viduals who dislike vigorous activity or have been discouraged by structured ex-ercise programs can begin with moderate intensity physical activity accumulated over the entire day. Sedentary individuals can choose activities that easily incor-porate into their daily routines and then can gradually increase the amount of ac-tivity as they strive to achieve a physically active lifestyle.

Achieve Better Theoretical and Applied Research

Effective strategies and methods to promote physical activity can be identified from scientific research. More theory-based research, a better understanding of theoretical mediators, stronger research designs, better evaluation strategies, and reliable and valid measures of physical activity are needed to improve research in the area of physical activity (Baranowski, Anderson, & Carmack, 1998; Taylor, Baranowski, & Rohm Young, 1998). Unfortunately, only 1 percent of U.S. health-related expenditures are for health promotion research and interventions (CDC, 1992a) and an even smaller percentage is targeted to the black community. The magnitude of the potential benefit to society if a greater investment in research on physical activity were made is considerable. Most likely, better research will result from increased research. The observed synergistic health benefit of combining increased physical activity with more healthful eating offers a particularly important research opportunity (see, for example, Stefanick et al., 1998; Haskell et al., 1994; Klem, Wing, McGuire, Seagle, & Hill, 1997).

For the black community and many other communities of color, culturally relevant social incentives and reinforcers are needed. Several researchers have addressed culture (for example, Pasick, D'Onofrio, & Otero-Sabogal, 1996) and the dimensions of cultural sensitivity (for example, Resnicow, Baranowski, Ahluwalia, & Braithwaite, 1999) in relation to behavioral change strategies. Culturally relevant physical activity interventions are essential for success. The question of how best to develop these interventions in the context of a research establishment that has more often exploited than included blacks (for example, Allen, 1994; Swanson & Ward, 1995) presents a considerable challenge. Cultural adaptation is more frequently treated as a practical strategy for implementing interventions with otherwise unicultural theoretical orientations (for example, by using community locations as the intervention setting, employing black outreach staff, and choosing music or foods embraced by blacks) than as a domain of variables to be assessed within an accommodating theoretical model (Kumanyika, Morssink, & Agurs, 1992; Resnicow et al., 1999). True cultural tailoring—that is, developing or restructuring a program within the cultural framework of the target population with full involvement and participation of the target population, including leadership in senior positions—is a much rarer phenomenon (Kumanyika & Agurs-Collins, 1998; Cassady, Jang, Tanjasiri, & Morrison, 1999; Yancey, 1999).

Theoretical models that include cultural dimensions and leadership at many levels and in a variety of sectors must be fostered and mobilized to convey a sense of urgency about reversing the deleterious effects of the epidemic of sedentary behaviors among blacks (Kumanyika, 1999). For example, black leadership in the Los Angeles County municipal government (spearheaded by the Department of Health Services) is pilot testing the inclusion of ten-minute physical activity breaks in business meetings. The Richmond City Hall in Virginia features a weekly, thirty-minute lunchtime physical activity session in its main lobby as one site of a citywide physical activity promotion program named Rock! Richmond!

(Yancey, 1999). If interventions are to be effective, their planners should not view the black community as monolithic. Many different segments exist within the black community, and all of them should be encouraged to be physically active. Men, women, boys, girls, the aged, individuals with disabilities, individuals with chronic diseases, nursing home residents, students from nursery school to graduate school, and inveterately sedentary individuals all deserve opportunities to increase their physical activity levels. Effective approaches to these and other subgroups in the black community may differ.

Sisters Together: Move More, Eat Better programs (DHHS, 1999) and On the Move!, California's physical activity initiatives (Cassady et al., 1999), are examples of communities taking on the responsibility to promote physical activity. The Sisters Together program was designed to encourage black women aged eighteen to thirty-five to maintain a healthy weight by becoming more physically active and eating healthier foods. The planning of a Sisters Together program in a community includes gaining support from others, working with the media, planning activities, and measuring success (DHHS, 1999). The On the Move! initiatives were multilevel interventions in eight low-income and multi-ethnic communities, designed to encourage physically active lifestyles. Each local On the Move! program sponsored a range of activities that was consistent with the needs and interests of the community. The lessons for community leaders who intend to implement similar programs to promote physical activity are (1) create an environment that supports physical activity, (2) work with the media, (3) conduct community events, and (4) develop local partnerships to deliver the message about physical activity (Kumanyika, 1999).

Assessing personal priorities; advocating for policy and environmental changes; and encouraging neighbors, family members, and coworkers to be physically active are aspects of taking responsibility. Individuals, neighborhoods, social organizations, faith-based institutions, and community agencies all have a role to play in promoting physical activity. From the individual perspective, the application of behavioral principles can help initiate and maintain physical activity. These principles suggest beginning a physical activity routine at a comfortable level, progressing slowly and gradually to more advanced levels, setting short-term and long-term goals, and establishing a system of rewards for meeting goals. Additional principles are using environmental cues to encourage physical activity; making a formal commitment with a spouse, friend, or physician to be physically active; and identifying an activity partner or buddy (American College of Sports Medicine, 1991). Employing these and other strategies can help sustain a physically active lifestyle.

The ultimate objective is to raise expectations and change social norms. Individual motivations, community activism, and environmental and policy changes can contribute to a societal and cultural shift toward a more physically active society. With this shift, work, school, social, and community settings will become more compatible with and perhaps even encourage beneficial levels of physical activity in the black community.

Conclusion

Physical inactivity is an increasingly serious national and international problem. Promoting increased levels of physical activity can improve the physical, emotional, and psychological well-being of all members of the black community. The challenge is to make physical activity as routine a part of our lives as eating and sleeping. To meet this challenge, we must develop social norms and encourage choices that support and sustain active living. The potential benefits, particularly for the black community, are substantial and well documented.

Appendix A: Web Site Resources for Children and Parents

A number of organizations have Web sites that provide information on health and fitness for children and parents and ideas for promoting and sustaining activity in youths.

American Academy of Pediatrics
Web site: www.aap.org

This site contains the Parent Resource Guide, which is a listing of descriptions of booklets, books, and videos available for parents and children.

American College of Sports Medicine
Web site: www.acsm.org/sportsmed

The site of the American College of Sports Medicine offers advice on a number of physical activity topics.

American Council on Exercise
Web site: www.acefitness.org

This site features Fit Facts, including family exercise and good food diary examples, and information on Energy Burn, a program that uses classroom activity and a video to encourage kids to be more physically active.

Fitness Partner Connection Jumpsite
Web site: http://primusweb.com/fitnesspartner

The Fitness Partner site provides resources and support for cultivating healthy lifestyles and contains links to other fitness and nutrition Web sites for children.

International Food Information Council (IFIC)
Web site: http://ificinfo.health.org

IFIC provides information on exercise and nutrition to journalists, health professionals, educators, and consumers. This site includes the newsletter *Food Insight,* which offers information on children and fitness.

KidsHealth
Web site: http://KidsHealth.org

Tips on nutrition and exercise are offered as part of this site's information on children's health.

Melpomene Institute for Women's Health Research
Web site: www.melpomene.org

This site specializes in health issues affecting physically active women and features body image topics geared toward girls.

The Physician and Sports Medicine
Web site: www.physsportsmed.com

A personal health section on this Web site offers patient-oriented articles on exercise, nutrition, and injury prevention.

Weight-Control Information Network (WIN)
Web site: www.niddk.nih.gov/NutritionDocs.html

The WIN site has pamphlets and fact sheets on physical activity. "Helping Your Overweight Child," for example, is a pamphlet with tips for incorporating physical activity into a family's daily life.

Appendix B: Program Resources for Youths

Among the programs that have been developed to motivate and structure physical activity for youths and for which written materials are available are the following two.

Presidential Sports Award (for ages six or older)
(407) 363-6170 (to order brochures and log sheets)

The Presidential Sports Award program was developed by the President's Council on Physical Fitness and Sports. Its purpose is to motivate all Americans to become more physically active throughout life, and it emphasizes regular exercise rather than outstanding performance. The program is administered by the Amateur Athletic Union (AAU).

President's Challenge (for ages six to seventeen)
(800) 258-8146 (to order brochures and log sheets)

The President's Challenge program is administered by school physical education staff. Students aged six to seventeen are eligible for any one of four physical fitness awards for various levels of personal achievement.

Appendix C: Organizational Resources

The following physical activity information resource list was compiled by the U.S. Department of Health and Human Services and the Centers for Disease Control and Prevention. The national organizations listed here can provide information on how to promote safe and enjoyable physical activity among children, adolescents, and adults.

American Alliance for Health, Physical Education, Recreation, and Dance
1900 Association Drive
Reston, VA 20191-1599
(800) 213-7193

American Cancer Society
1599 Clifton Road NE
Atlanta, GA 30329-4251
(800) 227-2345

American College of Sports Medicine
P.O. Box 1440
Indianapolis, IN 46206-1440
(317) 637-9200

American Heart Association
7272 Greenville Avenue
Dallas, TX 75231-4596
(800) 242-8721

American School Health Association
P.O. Box 708
Kent, OH 44240-0708
(330) 678-1601

Division of Adolescent and School Health Resource Room
National Center for Chronic Disease Prevention and Health Promotion
Centers for Disease Control and Prevention
4770 Buford Highway NE, MS K-32
Atlanta, GA 30341-3724
(888) CDC-4NRG (232-4674)

National Association of Governors' Councils on Physical Fitness and Sports
201 South Capitol Avenue, Suite 560
Indianapolis, IN 46225
(317) 237-5630

National Association for Sports and Physical Education
1900 Association Drive
Reston, VA 20191-1599
(800) 213-7193, ext. 410

National Heart, Lung, and Blood Institute Information Center
P.O. Box 30105
Bethesda, MD 20824-0105
(301) 251-1222

National Recreation and Parks Association
2775 South Quincy Street, Suite 300
Arlington, VA 22206-2204
(800) 649-3042, (703) 578-5558

President's Council on Physical Fitness and Sports
701 Pennsylvania Avenue NW, Suite 250
Washington, DC 2004
(202) 272-3421

In addition, information on how to promote safe and enjoyable physical activity among young people is available from such organizations as these on the state and local levels:

Affiliates of national voluntary health organizations (for example, the American Heart Association)

State and local governments

Governor's councils on physical fitness and sports

State associations for health, physical education, recreation, and dance

Organizations that serve young people (for example, the Young Women's Christian Association)

References

Ainsworth, B. E., Berry, C. B., Schnyder, V. N., & Vickers, S. R. (1992). Leisure time physical activity and aerobic fitness in African American young adults. *Journal of Adolescent Health, 13,* 606–611.

Ainsworth, B. E., Keenan, M. L., Strogatz, D. S., Garrett, J. M., & James, S. A. (1991). Physical activity and hypertension in black adults: The Pitt County study. *American Journal of Public Health, 81,* 1477–1479.

Ainsworth, B. E., & Macera, C. A. (1998). Physical inactivity. In R. C. Brownson, P. I. Remington, & J. R. Davis (Eds.), *Chronic disease epidemiology and control* (2nd ed., pp. 191–193). Washington, DC: American Public Health Association.

Airhihenbuwa, C. O., Kumanyika, S. K., Agurs, T., & Lowe, A. (1995). Perceptions and beliefs about exercise, rest, and health among African Americans. *American Journal of Health Promotion, 9,* 426–429.

Allen, M. (1994). The dilemma for women of color in clinical trials. *Journal of the American Medical Women's Association, 49,* 105–109.

American College of Sports Medicine. (1991). *Guidelines for exercise testing and prescription* (4th ed.). Malvern, PA: Lea & Febiger.

American College of Sports Medicine. (1993). Physical activity, physical fitness, and hypertension. *Medicine and Science in Sports and Exercise, 25,* i–x.

American Heart Association. (1997). *Heart and stroke statistical update, 1997.* Dallas, TX: Author.

Andersen, R. E., Crespo, C. J., Bartlett, S. J., Cheskin, L. J., & Pratt, M. (1998). Relationship of physical activity and television watching with body weight and level of fatness among children: Results from the Third National Health and Nutrition Examination Survey. *Journal of the American Medical Association, 279,* 938–942.

Baranowski, T., Anderson, C., & Carmack, C. (1998). Mediating variable framework in physical activity interventions: How are we doing? How might we do better? *American Journal of Preventive Medicine, 15,* 266–297.

Baranowski, T., Simons-Morton, B., Hooks, P., Henske, J., Tierman, K., Dunn, J. K., Burkhalter, H., Harper, J., & Palmer, J. (1990). A center-based program for exercise change among black American families. *Health Education Quarterly, 17,* 179–196.

Blair, S. N., Kohl, H. W., III, Paffenbarger, R. S., Jr., Clark, D. G., Cooper, K. H., & Gibbons, L. W. (1989). Physical fitness and all-cause mortality: A prospective study of healthy men and women. *Journal of the American Medical Association, 262,* 2395–2401.

Brownson, R. C., Houseman, R. A., Brown, D. R., Jackson-Thompson, J., King, A. C., Malone, B. R., & Sallis, J. F. (2000). Promoting physical activity in rural communities: Walking trail access, use, and effects. *American Journal of Preventive Medicine, 18,* 235–241.

Brownson, R. C., Smith, C. A., Pratt, M., Mack, N. E., Jackson-Thompson, J., Dean, C. G., Dabney, S., & Wilkerson, J. C. (1996). Preventing cardiovascular disease through community-based risk reduction: The Bootheel Heart Health Project. *American Journal of Public Health, 86,* 206–213.

Bush, P. J., Zuckerman, A. E., Taggart, V. S., Theiss, P. K., Peleg, E. O., & Smith, S. A. (1989). Cardiovascular risk factor prevention in black school children: The "Know Your Body" evaluation project. *Health Education Quarterly, 16,* 215–227.

Carpenter, C. L., Ross, R. K., Paganini-Hill, A., & Bernstein, L. (1999). Lifetime exercise activity and breast cancer risk among post-menopausal women. *British Journal of Cancer, 80,* 1852–1858.

Carter-Nolan, P. L., Adams-Campbell, L. L., & Williams, J. (1996). Recruitment strategies for black women at risk for non-insulin-dependent diabetes mellitus into exercise protocols: A qualitative assessment. *Journal of the National Medical Association, 88,* 558–562.

Caspersen, C. J. (1989). Physical activity epidemiology: Concepts, methods, and applications to exercise. *Exercise and Sport Sciences Reviews, 17,* 423–473.

Cassady D., Jang, V., Tanjasiri, S., & Morrison, C. (1999). California gets "On the Move!" *Journal of Health Education, 30,* S6–S12.

Centers for Disease Control and Prevention. (1992a). Effectiveness in disease and injury prevention: Estimated national spending on prevention: United States, 1988. *Morbidity and Mortality Weekly Report, 41,* 529–531.

Centers for Disease Control and Prevention. (1992b). Vigorous physical activity among high school students. *Morbidity and Mortality Weekly Report, 41,* 33–35.

Centers for Disease Control and Prevention. (1997). Guidelines for school and community programs to promote lifelong physical activity among young people. *Morbidity and Mortality Weekly Report, 46*(RR-6), 1–36.

Centers for Disease Control and Prevention & American College of Sports Medicine. (1993). Summary statement: Workshop on physical activity and public health. *Sports Medicine Bulletin, 28,* 7.

Dietz, W. H., Jr., & Gortmaker, S. L. (1985). Do we fatten our children at the television set? Obesity and television viewing in children and adolescents. *Pediatrics, 75,* 807–812.

Dishman, R. K. (1996, March). *Helping people succeed when exercise programs fail.* Paper presented at the meeting of the New England Chapter of the American College of Sports Medicine, Amherst, MA.

Dunn, A. L., Marcus, B. H., Kampert, J. B., Garcia, M. E., Kohl, H. W., & Blair, S. N. (1999). Comparison of lifestyle and structured interventions to increase physical activity and cardiorespiratory fitness: A randomized trial. *Journal of the American Medical Association, 281,* 327–334.

Epstein, L. H., Valoski, A. M., Vara, L. S., McCurley, J., Wisniewski, L., Kalarchian, M. A., Klein, K. R., & Shrager, L. R. (1995). Effects of decreasing sedentary behavior and increasing activity on weight change in obese children. *Health Psychology, 14,* 109–115.

Ewart, C. K., Young, D. R., & Hagberg, J. M. (1998). School-based exercise lowers blood pressure in higher-risk adolescent girls. *American Journal of Public Health, 88,* 949–951.

Fitzgerald, J. T., Singleton, S. P., Neale, A. V., Prasad, A. S., & Hess, J. W. (1994). Activity levels, fitness status, exercise knowledge, and exercise beliefs among healthy, older African American and white women. *Journal of Aging and Health, 6,* 296–303.

Flegal, K. M., Carroll, M. D., Kuczmarski, R. J., & Johnson, C. L. (1998). Overweight and obesity in the United States: Prevalence and trends, 1960–1994. *International Journal of Obesity, 22,* 39–47.

Folsom, A. R., Cook, T. C., Sprafka, J. M., Burke, G. L., Norsted, S. W., & Jacobs, D. R. (1991). Differences in leisure-time physical activity levels between blacks and whites in population based samples: The Minnesota Heart Study. *Journal of Behavioral Medicine, 14,* 1–9.

Gamble, M., & Cotugna, N. (1999). A quarter century of food advertising targeted at children. *American Journal of Health Behavior, 23,* 261–267.

Gillum, R. F. (1987). Overweight and obesity in black women: A review of published data from the National Center for Health Statistics. *Journal of the National Medical Association, 79,* 865–891.

Gordon-Larsen, P., McMurray, R. G., & Popkin, B. M. (1999). Adolescent physical activity and inactivity vary by ethnicity: The National Longitudinal Study of Adolescent Health. *Journal of Pediatrics, 135,* 301–306.

Gortmaker, S. L., Cheung, L.W.Y., Peterson, K. E., Chomitz, G., Cradle, J. H., Dart, H., Fox, M. K., Bullock, R. B., Sobol, A. M., Colditz, G., Field, A. E., & Laird, N. (1999). Impact of a school-based interdisciplinary intervention on diet and physical activity among urban primary school children: Eat well and keep moving. *Archives of Pediatric and Adolescent Medicine, 153,* 975–983.

Greendorfer, S. L., & Ewing, M. E. (1981). Race and gender differences in children's socialization into sport. *Research Quarterly for Exercise and Sport, 52,* 301–310.

Hahn, R. A., Teutsch, S. M., Rothenberg, R. B., & Marks, J. S. (1990). Excess deaths from nine chronic diseases in the United States, 1986. *Journal of the American Medical Association, 264*, 2654–2659.

Haskell, W. L., Alderman, E. L., Fair, J. M., Maron, D. J., Mackey, S. F., Superko, H. R., Williams, P. T., Johnstone, I. M., Champaign, M. A., Krauss, R. M., & Farquhar, J. W. (1994). The effects of intensive multiple risk factor reduction on coronary atherosclerosis and clinical cardiac events in men and women with coronary artery disease: The Stanford Coronary Risk Intervention Project (SCRIP). *Circulation, 89*, 975–990.

Heath, G. W., Pratt, M., Warren, C. W., & Kann, L. (1994). Physical activity patterns in American high school students. Results from the 1990 Youth Risk Behavior Survey. *Archives of Pediatric and Adolescent Medicine, 148*, 1131–1136.

Hinkle, A. J. (1997). Community-based nutrition interventions: Reaching adolescents from low-income communities. *Annals of the New York Academy of Sciences, 817*, 83–93.

Johnson, C. A., Corrigan, S. A., Dubbert, P. A., & Gramling, S. E. (1990). Perceived barriers to exercise and weight control practices in community women. *Women and Health, 16*, 177–191.

Jones, M., & Nies, M. A. (1996). The relationship of perceived benefits and barriers to reported exercise in older African American women. *Public Health Nursing, 13*, 151–158.

Jordan, A. (1999). *The relative effects of sociocultural factors on levels of obesity among African American women.* Unpublished doctoral dissertation, Virginia Commonwealth University, Richmond.

Kanders, B. S., Ullman-Joy, P., Foreyt, J. P., Heymsfield, S. B., Heber, D., Elashoff, R. M., Ashley, J. M., Reeves, R. S., & Blackburn, G. L. (1994). The Black American Lifestyle Intervention (BALI): The design of a weight loss program for working-class African American women. *Journal of the American Dietetic Association, 94*, 310–312.

King, A. C., Blair, S. N., Bild, D. E., Dishman, R. K., Dubbert, P. M., Marcus, B. H., Oldridge, N. B., Paffanberger, R. S., Jr., Powell, K. E., & Yeager, K. K. (1992). Determinants of physical activity and interventions in adults. *Medicine Science and Sports Exercise, 24*(6, Suppl.), S221–S236.

Klem, M. L., Wing, R. R., McGuire, M. T., Seagle, H. M., & Hill, J. O. (1997). A descriptive study of individuals successful at long-term maintenance of substantial weight loss. *American Journal of Clinical Nutrition, 66*, 239–246.

Kumanyika, S. K. (1999). Physically active individuals in sedentary communities. *Journal of Health Education, 30*, S4–S5.

Kumanyika, S. K., & Agurs-Collins, T. (1998). Culturally appropriate lifestyle interventions in minority populations: Response to Gregg and Narayan. *Diabetes Care, 21*, 876–877.

Kumanyika, S. K., & Charleston, J. B. (1992). Lose weight and win: A church-based weight loss program for blood pressure control among black women. *Patient Education and Counseling, 19*, 19–32.

Kumanyika, S. K., Morssink, C., & Agurs, T. (1992). Models for dietary and weight change among African American women, identifying cultural components. *Ethnicity and Disease, 2*, 166–169.

Lasco, R. A., Curry, R. H., Dickson, V. J., Powers, J., Menes, S., & Merritt, R. K. (1989). Participation rates, weight loss, and blood pressure changes among obese women in a nutrition-exercise program. *Public Health Reports, 104*, 640–646.

Leslie, J., Yancey, A. K., McCarthy, W. J., Albert, S., Wert, C., Miles, O., & James, J. (1999). Development and implementation of a school-based nutrition and fitness promotion program for ethnically diverse middle school girls. *Journal of the American Dietetic Association, 99*, 967–970.

Lewis, C. E., Raczynski, J. M., Heath, G. W., Levinson, R., Hilyer, J. C., & Cutter, G. R. (1993). Promoting physical activity in low-income African American communities: The PARR project. *Ethnicity and Disease, 3*, 106–118.

Liu, K., Ballew, C., Jacobs, D. R., Jr., Sidney, S., Savage, P. J., Dyer, A., Hughes, G., & Glanton, M. M. (1989). Ethnic differences in blood pressure, pulse rate, and related characteristics in young adults: The CARDIA Study. *Hypertension, 14,* 218–226.

Manson, J. E., & Spelsberg, A. (1994). Primary prevention of non-insulin-dependent diabetes mellitus. *American Journal of Preventive Medicine, 10,* 172–184.

McGinnis, J. M., & Foege, W. H. (1993). Actual causes of death in the United States. *Journal of the American Medical Association, 270,* 2207–2212.

Melnyk, M. G., & Weinstein, E. (1994). Preventing obesity in black women by targeting adolescents: A literature review. *Journal of the American Dietetic Association, 94,* 536–540.

National Institutes of Health. (1998). *Clinical guidelines on the identification, evaluation, and treatment of overweight and obesity in adults.* Washington, DC: U.S. Government Printing Office.

Pasick, R. J., D'Onofrio, C. N., & Otero-Sabogal, R. (1996). Similarities and differences across cultures: Questions to inform a third generation for health promotion research. *Health Education Quarterly, 23,* S142–S161.

Pate, R. R., Long, B. J., & Heath, G. (1994). Descriptive epidemiology of physical activity in adolescents. *Pediatric Exercise Science, 6,* 434–447.

Pate, R. R., Pratt, M., Blair, S. N., Haskell, W. L., Macera, C. A., Bouchard, C., Buchner, D., Ettinger, W., Heath, G. W., King, A. C., Kriska, A., Leon, A. S., Marcus, B. H., Morris, J., Paffenbarger, R. S., Jr., Patrick, K., Pollock, M. L., Rippe, J. M., Sallis, J., & Wilmore, J. H. (1995). Physical activity and public health. *Journal of the American Medical Association, 273,* 402–407.

Popkin, B. M., & Doak, C. M. (1998). The obesity epidemic is a worldwide phenomenon. *Nutrition Reviews, 56*(4, Pt. 1), 106–114.

Resnicow, K., Baranowski, T., Ahluwalia, J. S., & Braithwaite, R. L. (1999). Cultural sensitivity in public health: Defined and demystified. *Ethnicity and Disease, 9,* 10–21.

Robinson, T. N. (1999). Reducing children's television viewing to prevent obesity. *Journal of the American Medical Association, 282,* 1561–1567.

Rohm Young, D., & King, A. C. (1995). Exercise adherence: Determinants of physical activity and applications of health behavior change theories. *Medicine, Exercise, Nutrition, and Health, 4,* 335–348.

Rowland, M., & Roberts, G. (1982). *Blood pressure levels and hypertension in persons aged 74 years: United States, 1976–1980.* (DHHS Publication No. PHS 82-1250). Hyattsville, MD: Public Health Service.

Sallis, J. F., Prochaska, J. J., & Taylor, W. C. (2000). A review of correlates of physical activity of children and adolescents. *Medicine and Science in Sports and Exercise, 32,* 963–975.

Slattery, M. L., Edwards, S. L., Boucher, K. M., Anderson, K., & Caan, B. J. (1999). Lifestyle and colon cancer: An assessment of factors associated with risk. *American Journal of Epidemiology, 150,* 869–877.

Stefanick, M. L., Mackey, S., Sheehan, M., Ellsworth, N., Haskell, W. L., & Wood, P. D. (1998). Effects of diet and exercise in men and postmenopausal women with low levels of HDL cholesterol and high levels of LDL cholesterol. *New England Journal of Medicine, 339,* 12–20.

Swanson, G., & Ward, A. (1995). Recruiting minorities into clinical trials: Toward a participant-friendly system. *Journal of the National Cancer Institute, 87,* 1747–1759.

Taylor, W. C., Baranowski, T., & Rohm Young, D. (1998). Physical activity interventions in low-income, ethnic minority, and populations with disability. *American Journal of Preventive Medicine, 15,* 334–343.

Taylor, W. C., Baranowski, T., & Sallis, J. F. (1994). Family determinants of physical activity: A social cognitive model. In R. K. Dishman (Ed.), *Advances in exercise adherence* (pp. 319–342). Champaign, IL: Human Kinetics.

Taylor, W. C., Beech, B., & Cummings, S. S. (1997). Increasing physical activity levels in youth: A public health challenge. In D. K. Wilson, J. R. Rodrique, and W. C. Taylor

(Eds.), *Health-promoting and health-compromising behaviors among minority adolescents* (pp. 107–128). Washington, DC: American Psychological Association.

Taylor, W. C., & Sallis, J. F. (1997). Determinants of physical activity in children. *World Review of Nutrition and Dietetics, 82,* 159–167.

Taylor, W. C., Yancey, A. K, Leslie, J., Murray, N. K., Cummings, S. S., Sharkey, S. A., Wert, C., James, J., Miles, O., & McCarthy, W. J. (1999). Physical activity among African American and Latino middle school girls: Consistent beliefs, expectations, and experiences across two sites. *Women and Health, 30*(2), 67–82.

Thune, I., Brenn, T., Lund, E., & Gaard, M. (1997). Physical activity and the risk of breast cancer. *New England Journal of Medicine, 336,* 1269–1275.

Thune, I., & Lund, E. (1996). Physical activity and risk of colorectal cancer in men and women. *British Journal of Cancer, 73,* 1134–1140.

U.S. Department of Agriculture. (1995). *Dietary guidelines for Americans* (4th ed.). Washington, DC: U.S. Government Printing Office.

U.S. Department of Health and Human Services. (1996). *Physical activity and health: A report of the surgeon general.* (SIN 017-023-00196-5) Atlanta, GA: U.S. Department of Health and Human Services, National Center for Chronic Disease Prevention and Health Promotion.

U.S. Department of Health and Human Services. (1999). *Sisters Together, Move More, Eat Better program guide* (NIH Publication No. 99-3329). Bethesda, MD: Author.

Washburn, R. A., Kline, G., Lackland, D. T., & Wheeler, F. C. (1992). Leisure time physical activity: Are there black/white differences? *Preventive Medicine, 21,* 127–135.

Williams, L. C., & Olano, V. R. (1999). Mobilizing and maintaining a coalition to promote physical activity among African Americans in southeast Stockton, California. *Journal of Health Education, 30*(2, Suppl.), S31–S36.

Wilson Sporting Goods Company in cooperation with the Women's Sports Foundation. (1988). *The Wilson report: Moms, dads, daughters, and sports.* River Grove, IL: Wilson Sporting Goods Co.

Wing, R. R., Kuller, L. H., Bunker, C., Matthews, K., Caggiula, A., Miehlan, E., & Kelsey, S. (1989). Obesity, obesity-related behaviors and coronary heart disease risk factors in black and white pre-menopausal women. *International Journal of Obesity, 13,* 511–519.

World Cancer Research Fund & American Institute for Cancer Research. (1997). *Food, nutrition and the prevention of cancer: A global perspective.* Washington, DC: American Institute of Cancer Research.

Yancey, A. (1999). Facilitating health promotion in communities of color. *Cancer Research Therapy and Control, 8,* 113–122.

Yancey, A., McCarthy, W., & Leslie, L. (1999). Recruiting African American women to community based health promotion research. *American Journal of Health Promotion, 12,* 335–338.

PART FIVE

ETHICAL, POLITICAL, AND ECOLOGICAL ISSUES

CHAPTER TWENTY-TWO

THE QUEST FOR ENVIRONMENTAL JUSTICE

Robert D. Bullard, Rueben C. Warren, Glenn S. Johnson

Despite significant improvements in health and environmental protection over the past several decades, millions of African Americans continue to live in unsafe and unhealthy physical environments. Many people in economically impoverished communities are exposed to greater health hazards where they live, work, and recreate than are their more affluent counterparts (Bullard, 1994a; Bryant & Mohai, 1992). When the African American race identifier and low-income status are combined, a *layering effect* occurs that results in a further worsening of health status (Warren, 1990, pp. 169–180). Public health officials and the media are contacted almost daily by people representing a community or neighborhood fighting the siting of an unsafe landfill, chemical plant, or other polluting industry. The most common complaint is adverse health affects or conditions. If we are to develop healthy African American communities, this scenario must change.

This chapter reviews the historical foundation of social context for health among African Americans and the environmental justice movement in the United States. It also briefly reviews African American health status, highlighting health conditions with possible environmental risk factors. A critique and analysis of government policies and industry practices that challenge and at times endanger the health and safety of African Americans in their neighborhoods, workplaces, and playgrounds is presented. Finally, this chapter also examines the role of grassroots groups, community-based organizations, and black institutions in dismantling the legacy of environmental racism and their efforts to ensure health improvements.

Since the first black landing in the United States in 1619, there has been a continual effort for justice in North America for people of African descent

(Bennett, 1975, p. 6). The effort has been most notable in regard to health, defining health broadly and holistically as a "synergic relationship between the physical, social, psychological, and spiritual elements that create the well-being of individuals and groups in their physical and social environments" (Warren, 1998, p. 219). This definition does not consider the absence of disease as the primary factor in health. It expands the World Health Organization's description by highlighting four important variables: relationships, the group, spirituality, and the physical and social environment (Warren, 1999, p.1). This broadened definition of health is particularly useful in addressing environmental health and justice considerations. As early as 1799, Benjamin Rush (1991, p. vi), often called the father of American psychiatry and also a signer of the Declaration of Independence, challenged the beliefs that African Americans were born inferior. Sullivan (1964), another influential thinker in psychiatry, expressed similar concerns about racism and health roles. Almost two centuries after Rush, in 1985, Secretary of the U.S. Department of Health and Human Services Margaret Heckler wrote in the *Report of the Secretary's Task Force on Black and Minority Health* that "there was a continual disparity in the burden of death and illness experienced by blacks and other minority Americans as compared with our Nation as a whole. That disparity began more than a generation ago and although our health charts do itemize steady gains in the health of minority Americans, the stubborn disparity remained . . . an affront to both our ideals and to the ongoing genius of American medicine (DHHS, 1985, p. ix).

More recently, President William J. Clinton's Commission on Race determined that health was an area in which many of the most glaring disparities between African Americans and their non-Hispanic white counterparts could be found. As a result, the Department of Health and Human Services launched a Racial and Ethnic Health Disparities Initiative focusing on six areas: infant mortality, diabetes, cardiovascular disease, cancer screening and management, HIV/AIDS, and child and adult immunization.

There are strong associations between environmental toxicants and five of these areas. For example (Johnson, 1999):

- Adverse reproductive outcomes affecting infant mortality have been found, such as central nervous system damage associated with mercury, increased premature births associated with increased blood lead levels, and decreased birthweight and gestational age associated with maternal exposure to PCBs during pregnancy.
- Environmental toxicants have been found to exacerbate diabetic and hypertensive nephropathy.
- Exposure to lead has been associated with hypertension.
- Populations living near hazardous waste sites have been found to have increased risks of cancer.
- Research under way at the Agency for Toxic Substances and Disease Registry is investigating the effect of environmental pollutants on insulin resistance in Hispanic communities.

Clearly, the continuing health disparities between African Americans and the nation as a whole cannot be fully addressed without considering environmental protection and environmental justice.

The Historical Backdrop

As recently as three decades ago the concept of environmental justice had little meaning on the radar screens of governmental, environmental, civil rights, public health, and social justice groups (Bullard, 1994b). However, it should not be forgotten that during this same period of time, in 1968, Martin Luther King Jr. was in Memphis, Tennessee, on an environmental, social, and economic justice mission for the striking black garbage workers. The strikers were demanding equal pay and better work conditions. Dr. King was assassinated before he could complete his mission.

Another landmark garbage dispute took place a decade later in Houston, Texas, when African American homeowners began a bitter fight to prevent the creation of a sanitary landfill in their suburban middle-income neighborhood (Bullard, 1983). Residents formed the Northeast Community Action Group (NECAG), and their attorney, Linda McKeever Bullard, filed a class action lawsuit to block the facility from being built. The 1979 lawsuit, *Bean v. Southwestern Waste Management, Inc.,* was the first of its kind to challenge the siting of a waste facility under civil rights law. The landmark Houston case occurred three years before the environmental justice movement gained national attention in rural, and mostly African American, Warren County, North Carolina. The environmental justice movement has measurably advanced since that humble beginning in Warren County, where a PCB landfill ignited protests and over five hundred arrests. The Warren County protests were the impetus for a U.S. General Accounting Office (GAO) (1983) study on the siting of hazardous waste landfills that documented that three-quarters of the off-site, commercial hazardous waste landfills in Region 4 (comprising eight states in the South) were located in predominantly African American communities even though African Americans made up only 20 percent of the region's population. More important, the protesters put *environmental racism* on the map. Currently, the state of North Carolina is spending over $25 million to clean up and detoxify the Warren County PCB landfill.

The protests also led the Commission for Racial Justice (1987) to publish *Toxic Waste and Race in the United States,* the first national study to correlate waste facility sites and demographic characteristics. The study documented that race was the most potent variable in predicting where waste facilities were located—more powerful than poverty, land values, and home ownership. In 1990, *Dumping in Dixie: Race, Class, and Environmental Quality* chronicled the convergence of two social movements—the movement for social justice and the environmental movement—into the environmental justice movement (Bullard, 1994a). This book highlighted African American environmental activism in the South, the same region where the modern civil rights movement began. What started out as local and often isolated community-based struggles against toxic substances and facility sitings has expanded into a multi-issue, multi-ethnic, and multiregional movement.

The First National People of Color Environmental Leadership Summit was held in Washington, D.C., in 1991. We view this summit as the most important single event in the environmental justice movement's history. The summit broadened the movement's focus from a narrow anti-toxics view to a focus on issues of public health, worker safety, land use, transportation, housing, resource allocation, and community empowerment (C. Lee, 1992). This meeting also demonstrated that it is possible to build a multiracial grassroots movement around environmental and economic justice (Alston, 1992).

Over 650 grassroots and national leaders from around the world attended the four-day summit. Delegates came from all fifty states, and people also attended from Puerto Rico, Chile, Mexico, and as far away as the Marshall Islands. People attended the summit to share their action strategies, to redefine the environmental movement, and to develop common plans for addressing environmental problems affecting people of color in the United States and around the world.

On September 27, 1991, summit delegates adopted seventeen *principles of environmental justice*. These principles were developed as a guide for organizing, networking, and relating to governmental and nongovernmental organizations (NGOs). By June 1992, Spanish and Portuguese translations of the principles were being used and circulated by NGOs and environmental justice groups at the United Nations Conference on Environment and Development (the Earth Summit) in Rio de Janeiro.

The publication of the *People of Color Environmental Groups Directory* in 1992 and 1994 further documented that environmental justice organizations are found in the United States from coast to coast, in Puerto Rico, in Mexico, and in Canada. Grassroots groups have come to embrace a wide range of issues, including public health, children's health, pollution prevention, housing, brownfields (contaminated land), community reinvestment, transportation, land use, and worker safety.

The Environmental Justice Paradigm

Despite significant improvements in environmental protection over the past several decades, millions of people who live in the United States continue to live in unsafe and unhealthy physical environments (Institute of Medicine, 1999). As we stated earlier, many economically impoverished communities and their inhabitants are exposed to greater health hazards in their homes, on the jobs, and in their neighborhoods than their more affluent counterparts are (Bullard 1994a, 1994b; U.S. Environmental Protection Agency [EPA], 1992; Bryant & Mohai, 1992; Bryant, 1995; Calloway & Decker, 1997; Collin & Collin, 1998).

Across the country, grassroots community resistance has emerged in response to practices, policies, and conditions that residents have judged to be unjust, unfair, and illegal. Among these are (1) unequal enforcement of environmental, civil rights, or public health laws; (2) differential exposure of some populations to harmful chemicals, pesticides, and other toxins in the home, school, neighborhood, and workplace; (3) faulty assumptions in calculating, assessing, and managing risks; (4) discriminatory zoning and land use practices; and (5) exclusionary practices that limit some individuals and groups from participation in decision making (C. Lee, 1992; Bullard, 1993a, 1993b, 1993c).

Environmental justice is defined as the fair treatment and meaningful involvement of all people regardless of race, color, national origin, or income with respect to the development, implementation, and enforcement of environmental laws, regulations, and policies. Fair treatment means that no group of people, including racial, ethnic, and socioeconomic groups, should bear a disproportionate share of the negative environmental consequences resulting from industrial, municipal, and commercial operations or the execution of federal, state, local, and tribal programs and policies (EPA, 1998).

During its thirty-year history, the EPA has not always recognized that many government and industry practices (intentionally or unintentionally) have had a more adverse impact on low-income people and people of color than on others. Grassroots community resistance emerged and grew in response to practices, policies, and conditions that community residents judged to be unjust, unfair, and illegal. The EPA is mandated to enforce the nation's environmental laws and protect all Americans—not just individuals or groups who can afford lawyers, lobbyists, and experts. Environmental protection is a right, not a privilege reserved for the few who can "vote with their feet" and escape or can otherwise fend off environmental health threats to themselves.

A growing body of evidence reveals that people of color and low-income persons have borne greater environmental and health risks in their neighborhoods, workplaces, and playgrounds than have members of the society at large (Johnson, Williams, & Harris, 1992; National Institute for Environmental Health Sciences [NIEHS], 1995; Institute of Medicine, 1999). The environmental justice paradigm offers an alternative. It embraces a holistic approach to address issues including developing and monitoring environmental health policies and regulations; developing risk reduction strategies for multiple, cumulative, and synergistic risks; ensuring public health; enhancing public participation in environmental decision making; promoting community empowerment; building an infrastructure to achieve environmental justice and sustainable communities; ensuring interagency cooperation and coordination; developing innovative public-private partnerships; enhancing community-based pollution prevention strategies; ensuring community-based sustainable economic development; and developing geographically oriented communitywide programming.

The environmental justice framework rests on developing tools and strategies to eliminate unfair, unjust, and inequitable conditions and decisions (Bullard,

1996). The framework attempts to challenge underlying assumptions that may contribute to differential exposure and unequal protection. It raises the *ethical* and *political* questions of who gets what, when, why, and how much. The environmental justice framework (1) adopts a public health model of health promotion, protection, and disease prevention (that is, elimination of the threat before harm occurs) as the preferred strategy; (2) shifts the burden of proof to polluters and dischargers who do harm, who discriminate, or who do not give equal protection to people of color, low-income persons, and other protected classes; (3) allows the use of disparate impact and statistical weight or an *effect* test, as opposed to *intent,* to infer discrimination; and (4) redresses disproportionate impacts through targeted action and resources. In general, this latter strategy targets resources to places where environmental and health problems are greatest (as determined by some ranking scheme that is not limited to risk assessment).

Impetus for Change

The impetus behind the environmental justice movement did not come from within the government, academia, or the mostly white and middle-class nationally based environmental and conservation groups. The impetus for change came from people of color grassroots activists and their bottom-up leadership approach. Grassroots groups organized themselves, educated themselves, and empowered themselves to make fundamental changes in the way environmental protection is performed in their communities.

Government has been slow to raise the questions of who gets help and who does not, who can afford help and who cannot, why some contaminated communities get studied and others get left off the research agenda, why industry poisons some communities and not others, why some contaminated communities get cleaned up and others do not, why some populations are protected and others are not, and why unjust, unfair, and illegal policies and practices are allowed to go unpunished.

The federal government did take some important initial steps in the early 1990s. In 1990, the Agency for Toxic Substances and Disease Registry (ATSDR) held a historic conference in Atlanta, Georgia. This ATSDR National Minority Health Conference focused on contamination (Johnson, Williams, & Harris 1992). In 1992, after meeting with community leaders, academicians, and civil rights leaders, the EPA (under the leadership of William Reilly) admitted there was a problem and established the Office of Environmental Equity. Under the Clinton administration, the name was changed to the Office of Environmental Justice.

In 1992, the EPA published *Environmental Equity: Reducing Risks for All Communities,* one of the first comprehensive documents to examine the whole question of risk, environmental hazards, and equity. Both this report and the Office of Environmental Equity were initiated only after prodding from people of color environmental justice leaders, activists, and a few academicians.

The EPA also established a twenty-five-member National Environmental Justice Advisory Council (NEJAC), under the Federal Advisory Committee Act. The NEJAC comprises stakeholders representing grassroots community groups; environmental groups; nongovernmental organizations; state, local, and tribal governments; academia; and industry. It has set up six subcommittees for its environmental justice work: Health and Research; Waste and Facility Siting; Enforcement; Public Participation and Accountability; Native American and Indigenous Issues; and International Issues.

In February 1994, seven federal agencies, including the Agency for Toxic Substances and Disease Registry, the National Institute for Environmental Health Sciences (NIEHS), the EPA, the National Institute of Occupational Safety and Health (NIOSH), the National Institutes of Health (NIH), the Department of Energy (DOE), and the Centers for Disease Control and Prevention (CDC) sponsored the national health symposium "Health and Research Needs to Ensure Environmental Justice." The conference planning committee was unique in that it included grassroots organization leaders, residents of affected communities, and federal agency representatives. The goal of the conference was to bring diverse stakeholders and those most affected by environmental hazards to the decision-making table (NIEHS, 1995). The health symposium recommended that the appropriate agencies (1) conduct meaningful health research in support of people of color and low-income communities; (2) promote disease prevention and pollution prevention strategies; (3) promote interagency coordination to ensure environmental justice; (4) provide effective outreach, education, and communications; and (5) design legislative and legal remedies.

In response to growing public concern and mounting scientific evidence, President Clinton on February 11, 1994 (the second day of the symposium), issued Executive Order 12898, "Federal Actions to Address Environmental Justice in Minority Populations and Low-Income Populations." This order attempts to address environmental injustice in existing federal laws and regulations. Executive Order 12898 reinforces the thirty-five-year-old Civil Rights Act of 1964, Title VI, which prohibits discriminatory practices in programs receiving federal funds. The order also refocuses attention on the National Environmental Policy Act (NEPA), a twenty-five-year-old law that set policy goals for the protection, maintenance, and enhancement of the environment. The goal of the NEPA is to ensure for all Americans a safe, healthful, productive, and aesthetically and culturally pleasing environment. NEPA requires federal agencies to prepare a detailed statement on the environmental effects of proposed federal actions that significantly affect the quality of human health (Council on Environmental Quality, 1997).

The Executive Order also recommends improved methodologies for collection of data on low-income and minority populations who may be disproportionately at risk, and for assessing and mitigating the impact and health effects from multiple and cumulative exposure, and the impact on subsistence fisherman and wildlife consumers. It also encourages participation of the affected populations in the various phases of assessing impacts, including scoping, data gathering, analyzing, identifying alternatives, examining mitigation methods, and monitoring.

The Executive Order mentions "subsistence" fishermen and wildlife consumers. Everybody does not buy his or her fish at the supermarket. There are many people who fish for protein, subsidizing their budgets and their diets by fishing from rivers, streams, and lakes, many of which are now polluted. These subpopulations may be underprotected when basic assumptions are made using a dominant risk paradigm.

Numerous studies reveal that African Americans and other people of color have borne greater health and environmental risk burdens than the society at large (Mann, 1991; Goldman, 1992; Goldman & Fitton, 1994; Institute of Medicine, 1999; Cooney, 1999). A recent study from the Institute of Medicine (1999) concluded that government, public health officials, and the medical and scientific communities need to place a higher value on the problems and concerns of "environmental justice" communities, environmental justice being "a concept that addresses in a cross-cutting and integrative manner the physical and social health issues related to the distribution of environmental benefits and burdens among the populations, particularly in degraded and hazardous physical environments occupied by minority or disadvantaged populations" (Institute of Medicine, 1999, p. xx). The study also confirmed what most affected communities have known for decades: people of color and low-income communities (1) are exposed to higher levels of pollution than the rest of the nation and (2) experience certain diseases in greater numbers than the more affluent, non-Hispanic white communities.

Elevated public health risks have been found in some populations even when social class is held constant. For example, race has been found to be independent of class as a predictor of the distribution of air pollution; contaminated fish consumption; the location of municipal landfills and incinerators, abandoned toxic waste dumps, and Superfund sites; and lead poisoning in children (West, Fly, Larkin, & Marans, 1990; Bryant & Mohai, 1992; Commission for Racial Justice, 1987; Goldman & Fitton, 1994; Lavelle & Coyle, 1992; Agency for Toxic Substances and Disease Registry, 1988; Pirkle et al., 1994; Stretesky & Hogan, 1998).

Communities Under Siege

Many of the nation's environmental policies distribute costs in a regressive pattern, providing disproportionate benefits for non-Hispanic whites and individuals who fall at the upper end of the education and income scale. A 1992 study, for example, uncovered glaring inequities in the way the federal EPA enforces its laws, stating: "there is a racial divide in the way the U.S. government cleans up toxic waste sites and punishes polluters. White communities see faster action, better results and stiffer penalties than communities where blacks, Hispanics and other minorities live. This unequal protection often occurs whether the community is wealthy or poor" (Lavelle & Coyle, 1992, pp. S1–S2). This study reinforced what many grassroots activists have known for decades—all communities are not treated the same. Communities located on the "wrong side of the tracks" are at greater risk from exposure to lead, pesticides (in the home and workplace), air pollution, toxic releases, water pollution, solid and hazardous waste, raw sewage, and industrial pollution (Goldman & Fitton, 1994).

Whether by design or benign neglect, African American communities ranging from the urban ghettos to rural "poverty pockets" face some of the worst environmental and health problems in the nation. Here are three instances.

Identifying Lead Poisoning in California

Childhood lead poisoning is a major threat to African American children. Lead poisoning is also preventable. Data from the Third National Health and Nutrition Examination Survey (NHANES III) (Pirkle et al., 1994) revealed that 1.7 million children (8.9 percent of children aged one to five) are lead poisoned (defined as having blood lead levels equal to or above 10 µg/dl). The NHANES III data found African American children to be lead poisoned at more than twice the rate of non-Hispanic white children at every income level. Over 28.4 percent of all low-income African American children were lead poisoned compared to 9.8 percent of low-income non-Hispanic white children. From 1976 to 1991, decreases in blood lead levels for African American and Mexican American children lagged far behind those of non-Hispanic white children.

In California a coalition of environmental, social justice, and civil libertarian groups joined forces to challenge the way the state carried out its lead screening of poor children. In *Matthews* v. *Coye,* the Natural Resources Defense Council, the National Association for the Advancement of Colored People Legal Defense and Education Fund (NAACP LDF), the American Civil Liberties Union, and the Legal Aid Society of Alameda County, California, argued that the state of California had failed to conduct federally mandated testing for lead in some 557,000 poor children who received Medicaid, winning an out-of-court settlement worth $15 million to $20 million for a program to test blood lead levels (B. L. Lee, 1992). This historic agreement triggered similar lawsuits and actions in several other states that had failed to live up to the mandate.

Closing a Smelter in Dallas

The children in a West Dallas, primarily African American neighborhood in Texas were poisoned for years by a nearby smelter that dated back to the 1930s. All the lead smelters in the city were located in either African American or Latino neighborhoods (Bullard, 1994a). The sixty-three-acre lead smelter site of West Dallas Murphy Metals (later renamed the RSR Corporation) was located next door to an elementary school and across the street from the West Dallas Boys Club and a 3,500-unit public housing project. The housing project is located just fifty feet from the sprawling lead smelter property line and in the direct path of the prevailing southerly winds. During the peak period of operation in the mid-1960s, the plant employed more than four hundred persons (few of whom lived in the West Dallas neighborhood). It pumped more than 269 tons of lead particles each year into the West Dallas air. Lead particles were blown by prevailing winds through the doors and windows of nearby residents and onto the West Dallas streets, ballparks, and children's playgrounds.

Dallas passed a stringent lead ordinance in 1968. However, lax enforcement rendered the ordinance worthless. Dallas officials were informed as early as 1972 that lead was being found in the bloodstreams of children who lived in two mostly African American and Latino neighborhoods: West Dallas and East Oak Cliff (Dallas Alliance Environmental Task Force, 1983). Another smelter, the Dixie Metals smelter, operated in the East Oak Cliff neighborhood. Living near the smelters was associated with a 36 percent increase in blood lead level. The city was urged to restrict the emission of lead into the atmosphere and to undertake a large screening program to determine the extent of the public health problem. However, it failed to take immediate action to protect the mostly African American and poor residents who lived near the smelters.

In 1980, the EPA, informed about possible health risks associated with the Dallas lead smelters, commissioned another lead screening study. This study confirmed what was already known a decade earlier: children living near the smelters were likely to have greater lead concentrations than children who did not live nearby. Lead concentrations in the soil near the RSR smelter in West Dallas, for example, averaged nine times those in the control area, and the average near the Dixie Metals smelter in East Oak Cliff was thirteen times the norm. The lead levels in the soil were so high that the West Dallas Boys Club was forced to suspend outdoor activities.

After nearly four decades of complaining to city officials, in 1981 local residents organized themselves into the West Dallas Neighborhood Committee on Lead Contamination. Staff from the Common Ground Community Economic Development Corporation, a grassroots self-help organization, assisted the committee in getting the case into the public domain, testifying at hearings, and producing reports and provided general technical assistance (Bullard, 1994a).

The city took action only after a series of articles about the lead levels made the headlines in the local Dallas newspapers (Nauss, 1983). The *Dallas Morning News* broke the headline-grabbing story of the "potentially dangerous" lead levels discovered by EPA researchers in 1981. The articles triggered widespread concern, public outrage, several class action lawsuits, and legal action by the Texas attorney general.

Although the EPA was armed with a wealth of scientific data on the West Dallas lead problem, the agency chose to play politics with the people by scrapping a voluntary plan offered by RSR to clean up the "hot spots" in the neighborhood. John Hernandez, an EPA deputy administrator, blocked the clean-up and called for yet another round of tests to be designed by the CDC with the EPA and the Dallas Health Department. The results of the new study were released in

February 1983. This study again established the smelter as the source of elevated lead levels in West Dallas children (EPA, 1983). Residents saw the response by government as insensitive, unjust, and racist. Hernandez's delay of clean-up actions in West Dallas was called tantamount to "waiting for a body count" (Lash, Gillman, & Sheridan, 1984).

Public pressure then forced the Dallas City Council to appoint a task force to study the lead problem in 1983. The Dallas Alliance Environmental Task Force (1983) concluded that Dallas "has missed many opportunities to serve and protect the community at large and two neighborhoods in particular in relation to the lead problem we now address" (p. 3).

After years of delay the West Dallas plaintiffs negotiated an out-of-court settlement worth over $45 million. The lawsuit was settled in June 1983, with RSR agreeing to a soil clean-up in West Dallas, a blood-testing program for the children and pregnant women, and installation of new antipollution equipment. The settlement, however, did not require the smelter to close. The settlement was made on behalf of 370 children—almost all of whom were poor and African American residents of the West Dallas public housing project—and 40 property owners. It was one of the largest community lead contamination settlements ever awarded in the United States.

The pollution equipment for the smelter was never installed. In May 1984, the Dallas Board of Adjustments, a city agency responsible for monitoring land use violations, requested the city attorney to order the smelter permanently closed for violating the city's zoning code. Four months later, the Dallas Board of Adjustments ordered the West Dallas smelter permanently closed.

This lead smelter operated in the mostly African American West Dallas neighborhood for fifty years without having the necessary use permits. After repeated health citations, fines, and citizen complaints against the smelter, one has to question the city's lax enforcement of health and land use regulations in its African American and Latino neighborhoods. The smelter is now closed. Although an initial clean-up was carried out in 1984, the lead problem did not go away. On December 31, 1991, EPA crews began a "comprehensive" cleanup of the West Dallas neighborhood. It was estimated that the crews would remove between 30,000 to 40,000 cubic yards of lead-contaminated soil from several West Dallas sites, including school property and about 140 private homes. The clean-up cost over $4 million.

Still, West Dallas residents wonder why they had to wait twenty years for the government to act. Why were the people in this community deserted by the city, state, and federal government? It was not because the officials did not have sufficient scientific evidence or documentation of the health problem. Having all the facts has never been sufficient when people of color are the victims. The West Dallas example typifies environmental racism. Residents of the East Oak Cliff neighborhood had to wait even longer than the residents of West Dallas. The Dixie Metals smelter was allowed to continue operating under a phase-down agreement. A coalition of African American and Latino residents were eventually successful in closing the Dixie Metals smelter under a settlement agreement in 1990, six years after the RSR lead smelter in West Dallas closed.

Relocation from Mount Dioxin

Margaret Williams, a seventy-three-year-old retired Pensacola, Florida, school-teacher, led a five-year campaign to get her community relocated once the environmental and health hazards posed by the nation's third largest Superfund site became known. The site of the Escambia Wood Treating Company was dubbed "Mount Dioxin" because of the sixty-foot-high mound of contaminated soil dug up from the neighborhood. The L-shaped mound held 255,000 cubic yards of soil contaminated with dioxin, one of the most dangerous compounds ever made. Williams led Citizens Against Toxic Exposure (CATE), a neighborhood organization formed to win relocation, into battle with the EPA officials, who first proposed to move only the 66 households most affected by the site (EPA, 1996). After prodding from CATE, the EPA then added 35 more households, for a total relocation cost of $7.54 million.

The original government plan had called for some 257 households, including an apartment complex, to be left out. Citizens Against Toxic Exposure refused to accept any relocation plan unless everyone was moved. The partial relocation was tantamount to partial justice. CATE took its campaign to the EPA's National Environmental Justice Advisory Council and succeeded in getting the NEJAC Waste and Facility Siting Subcommittee to hold a Superfund Relocation Round-table in Pensacola. At this meeting CATE's total neighborhood relocation plan won the backing of more than one hundred grassroots organizations. The EPA nominated the Escambia Wood Treating Superfund site as the country's first pilot program to help the agency develop a nationally consistent relocation policy that would consider not only toxic levels but also welfare issues such as property values, quality of life, and health and safety.

On October 3, 1996, EPA officials agreed to move all 358 households from the site at an estimated cost of $18 million. EPA officials deemed the mass relocation to be "cost efficient" after city planners decided to redevelop the area for light industry rather than clean the site to residential standards (Escobedo, 1996). This decision marked the first time that an African American community had been relocated under the EPA's Superfund program, and it was hailed as a landmark victory for environmental justice.

The Right to Breathe Clean Air

Air pollution problems have been with us for some time now. Before the federal government stepped in, state and local governments handled most issues related to air pollution. Because these state and local governments did such a poor job, however, the federal government established national clean air standards. Congress enacted the Clean Air Act (CAA) in 1970 and mandated the EPA to carry out this law (which has been amended twice, in 1977 and 1990). The CAA was a response to states' unwillingness to protect air quality. Indeed, many states used their lackadaisical enforcement of environmental laws as lures for business and economic development (Reitze, 1991).

National Argonne Laboratory researchers discovered in 1992 that 437 of the 3,109 U.S. counties and independent cities failed to meet at least one of the EPA ambient air quality standards. African Americans and Latinos are more likely to live in areas with reduced air quality than are non-Hispanic whites. Specifically, 57 percent of whites, 65 percent of African Americans, and 80 percent of Hispanics live in the 437 counties and independent cities with substandard air quality. Nationwide, 33 percent of non-Hispanic whites, 50 percent of African Americans, and 60 percent of Hispanics live in the 136 counties in which two or more air pollutants exceed standards. Similar patterns have been found for the 29 counties designated as nonattainment areas for three or more pollutants. Again, 12 percent of non-Hispanic whites, 20 percent of African Americans, and 31 percent of Hispanics lived in the worst nonattainment areas (Wernette & Nieves, 1992).

The Atlanta metropolitan region is a nonattainment area for ozone, one of the six criteria pollutants listed under the National Ambient Air Quality Standards (NAAQS). There is a price to be paid for nonattainment. Costs include potential loss of future federal assistance (in other words, transportation dollars are often tied to states' conforming with requirements of the Clean Air Act) and public health concerns (rising asthma and other respiratory illnesses). In the Atlanta nonattainment area, motor vehicles account for primary source for both volatile organic compounds (VOCs) and nitrogen oxides (NOx) (Research Atlanta, Inc., 1997).

The public health community has insufficient information to determine the exact magnitude of air pollution-related health problems. However, it is known that persons suffering from asthma are particularly sensitive to the effects of carbon monoxide, sulfur dioxides, particulate matter, ozone, and NOx (Mann, 1991). Ground-level ozone may exacerbate health problems such as asthma, nasal congestion, throat irritation, respiratory tract inflammation, reduced resistance to infection, changes in cell function, loss of lung elasticity, chest pains, lung scarring, formation of lesions in the lungs, and premature aging of lung tissues (Ozkaynk et al., 1996; American Lung Association, 1995).

Asthma is an emerging epidemic in the United States. The annual age-adjusted death rate from asthma increased by 40 percent between 1982 and 1991, from 1.34 to 1.88 per 100,000 people (CDC, 1995a). During the period from 1980 to 1993, the highest rates were consistently reported among blacks aged fifteen to twenty-four years old (CDC, 1996). Poverty and minority status are important risk factors for asthma mortality.

Children are at special risk from ozone pollution (Pribitkin, 1994). Children also carry a considerable share of the asthma burden. It is the most common chronic disease of childhood in the United States. Asthma affects almost five million children under eighteen years of age. It is the fourth leading cause of disability among these children (CDC, 1995b). Although the annual age-adjusted hospital discharge rate for asthma among children under fifteen years old decreased slightly from 184 to 179 per 100,000 between 1982 and 1992, that decrease was slower than the decrease in other childhood diseases (National Center for Health Statistics, 1995, Tables 83, 84, 86, 87), resulting in a 70 percent increase in the proportion of hospital admissions related to asthma during the 1980s. Inner-city children have the highest rates for asthma prevalence, hospitalization, and mortality (CDC, 1995a). Bad air is making a lot of children sick (Soto, 1999). A 1999 study from the Clean Air Task Force, a coalition of environmental and consumer groups, linked asthma and respiratory problems and smog (Abt Associates & Clean Air Task Force, 1999). High smog levels are associated with rising hospital admissions and emergency room visits for respiratory reasons in cities across the nation (see Table 22.1).

The Atlanta, Georgia, metropolitan region is a nonattainment area for ozone, one of the six criteria pollutants listed in the National Ambient Air Quality Standards (NAAQS). A 1994 CDC-sponsored study showed that pediatric emergency department visits at Atlanta's Grady Memorial Hospital increased by one-third following peak ozone levels. The study also found that the asthma rate among African American children was 26 percent higher than the asthma rate among non-Hispanic white children (White, Etzel, Wilcox, & Lloyd, 1994).

TABLE 22.1. OZONE-RELATED ADVERSE HEALTH EFFECTS BY CITY, APRIL–OCTOBER 1997.

Metropolitan Area	Respiratory Hospital Admissions	Respiratory Emergency Room Visits	Asthma Attacks
Atlanta	580	1,740	100,000
Baltimore	630	1,890	86,000
Chicago	1,500	4,500	200,000
Cincinnati	390	1,170	57,000
Cleveland	760	2,280	89,000
Detroit	930	2,790	100,000
Hartford	660	1,980	75,000
Miami/Ft. Lauderdale	1,200	3,600	110,000
Minneapolis/St. Paul	479	1,410	66,000
New York	4,100	12,300	520,000
Philadelphia	1,600	4,800	200,000
Pittsburgh	730	2,190	79,000
St. Louis	610	1,830	100,000
Tampa/St. Petersburg	780	2,340	68,000
Washington, D.C.	800	2,400	130,000

Source: Abt Associates & Clean Air Task Force, 1999.

Because children with asthma in Atlanta may not have visited the emergency department for their care, the true prevalence of asthma in the community is likely to be higher. Atlanta had sixty-nine days of unhealthy air during the summer of 1999 (Soto, 1999).

A 1996 report from the CDC shows hospitalization and death rates from asthma increasing for persons twenty-five and younger. The greatest increases occurred among African Americans. African Americans are two to six times more likely than non-Hispanic whites to die from asthma (CDC, 1992). The hospitalization rate for African Americans with asthma is three to four times the rate for non-Hispanic whites (White et al., 1994; Crain et al., 1994).

Conclusion

The environmental justice movement emerged in response to environmental inequities, threats to public health, unequal protection, differential enforcement, and disparate treatment received by the poor and people of color. The movement redefined environmental protection as a basic right. It also emphasized pollution prevention, waste minimization, and cleaner production techniques as strategies to achieve environmental justice for all people in the United States without regard to race, ethnicity, color, national origin, or income.

Both race and class factors place African American communities at special risk. Although public health, environmental and civil rights laws have been established for more than three decades, all communities have not received the same benefits from their application, implementation, and enforcement. Having an industrial facility in one's community does not automatically translate into jobs for nearby residents. Many industrial plants are located at the fence line with African American communities. Some are so close that local residents could walk to work. More often than not, however, African American residents are stuck with the pollution and poverty, and other people commute in for the industrial jobs.

The environmental justice movement has established clear goals of eliminating unequal enforcement of environmental, civil rights, and public health laws. Grassroots and national leaders are calling for an end to the elevated exposure of African Americans and other people of color to harmful chemicals, pesticides, and other toxins in the home, school, neighborhood, and workplace. They are also calling on scientists, researchers, and policy analysts to reexamine their assumptions in calculating, assessing, and managing risks in communities that are overburdened with environmental health threats.

Finally, environmental justice leaders are demanding that no community or nation, rich or poor, urban or suburban, regardless of race and ethnic background, should be allowed to become a "sacrifice zone" or dumping ground. They are also pressing local, state, and federal governments to live up to their mandate to protect the environment and the health of all citizens.

References

Abt Associates & Clean Air Task Force. (1999). *Out of breath: Health effects from ozone in the eastern United States.* Washington, DC: Abt Associates, Inc.

Agency for Toxic Substances and Disease Registry. (1988). *The nature and extent of lead poisoning in children in the United States: A report to Congress.* Atlanta, GA: Centers for Disease Control and Prevention, Agency for Toxic Substances and Disease Registry.

Alston, D. (1992). Transforming a movement: People of color unite at summit against environmental racism. *Sojourner, 21*(1), 30–31.

American Lung Association. (1995). *Out of breath: Populations at-risk to alternative ozone levels.* Washington, DC: Author.

Bennett, L. (1975). *The shaping of black America.* Chicago: Johnson.

Bryant, B. (1995). *Environmental justice: Issues, policies, and solutions.* Washington, DC: Island Press.

Bryant, B., & Mohai, P. (Eds.). (1992). *Race and the incidence of environmental hazards.* Boulder, CO: Westview Press.

Bullard, R. D. (1983). Solid waste sites and the black Houston community. *Sociological Inquiry, 53,* 273–288.

Bullard, R. D. (1993a). *Confronting environmental racism: Voices from the grassroots.* Boston: South End Press.

Bullard, R. D. (1993b). Environmental racism and land use. *Land Use Forum 2*(1), 6–11.

Bullard, R. D. (1993c). Race and environmental justice in the United States. *Yale Journal of International Law, 18*(1), 319–335.

Bullard, R. D. (1994a). *Dumping in Dixie: Race, class, and environmental quality.* Boulder, CO: Westview Press.

Bullard, R. D. (1994b). Grassroots flowering: The environmental justice movement comes of age. *Amicus Journal, 16,* 32–37.

Bullard, R. D. (1996). *Unequal protection: Environmental justice and communities of color.* San Francisco: Sierra Club Books.

Calloway, C. A., & Decker, J. A. (1997, January). Environmental justice in the United States: A primer. *Michigan Bar Journal, 76,* 62–68.

Centers for Disease Control and Prevention. (1992). Asthma: United States, 1980–1990. *Morbidity and Mortality Weekly Report, 39,* 733–735.

Centers for Disease Control and Prevention. (1995a). Asthma: United States, 1982–1992. *Morbidity and Mortality Weekly Report, 43,* 952–955.

Centers for Disease Control and Prevention. (1995b). Disabilities among children aged less than or equal to 17 years: United States, 1991–1992. *Morbidity and Mortality Weekly Report, 44,* 609–613.

Centers for Disease Control and Prevention. (1996). Asthma mortality and hospitalization among children and young adults: United States, 1980–1993. *Morbidity and Mortality Weekly Report, 45,* 350–353.

Collin, R. W., & Collin, R. M. (1998). The role of communities in environmental decisions: Communities speaking for themselves. *Journal of Environmental Law and Litigation, 13,* 37–89.

Commission for Racial Justice. (1987). *Toxic wastes and race in the United States.* New York: United Church of Christ.

Cooney, C. M. (1999). Still searching for environmental justice. *Environmental Science and Technology, 33,* 200–205.

Council on Environmental Quality. (1997). *Environmental justice: Guidance under the National Environmental Policy Act.* Washington, DC: Author.

Crain, F., Weiss, K., Bijur, J., Hersh, M., Westbrook, L., & Stein, R. (1994). An estimate of the prevalence of asthma and wheezing among inner-city children. *Pediatrics, 94,* 356–362.

Dallas Alliance Environmental Task Force. (1983). Final Report. Dallas, TX: Dallas Alliance.

Escobedo, D. (1996, October 4). EPA gives in, will move all at toxic site. *Pensacola News Journal,* p. A1.

Goldman, B. (1992). *The truth about where you live: An atlas for action on toxins and mortality.* New York: Random House.

Goldman, B., & Fitton, L. J. (1994). *Toxic wastes and race revisited.* Washington, DC: Center for Policy Alternatives, NAACP, & United Church of Christ.

Institute of Medicine. (1999). *Toward environmental justice: Research, education, and health policy needs.* Washington, DC: National Academy Press, p. 2.

Johnson, B. L. (1999). *Impact of hazardous waste on human health.* Boca Raton, FL: CRC Press.

Johnson, B. L., Williams, R. C., & Harris, C. M. (1992). *Proceedings of the 1990 National Minority Health Conference: Focus on environmental contamination.* Princeton, NJ: Scientific Publishing.

Lash, J., Gillman, K., & Sheridan, D. (1984). *A season of spoils: The Reagan administration's attack on the environment.* New York: Pantheon Books.

Lavelle, M., & Coyle, M. (1992, September). Unequal protection. *National Law Journal,* pp. S1–S2.

Lee, B. L. (1992, February). *Environmental litigation on behalf of poor, minority children: Matthews v. Coye: A case study.* Paper presented at the annual meeting of the American Association for the Advancement of Science, Chicago.

Lee, C. (1992). *Proceedings: The First National People of Color Environmental Leadership Summit.* New York: United Church of Christ, Commission for Racial Justice.

Mann, E. (1991). *L.A.'s lethal air: New strategies for policy, organizing, and action.* Los Angeles: Labor/Community Strategy Center.

National Center for Health Statistics. (1995). *Health, United States, 1995* (DHHS Publication No. PHS 95-1232). Hyattsville, MD: Author.

National Institute for Environmental Health Sciences. (1995). *Proceedings of the Health and Research Needs to Ensure Environmental Justice Symposium.* Research Triangle Park, NC: Author.

Nauss, D. W. (1983, July 17). The people vs. the lead smelter. *Dallas Times Herald,* pp. 18–26.

Ozkaynk, H., Spengler, J. D., Spengler, M. O., Uue, J., Zhou, H., Gilbert, K., & Ramstrom, S. (1996). Ambient ozone exposure and emergency hospital admissions and emergency room visits for respiratory problems in thirteen U.S. cities. In American Lung Association, *Breathless: Air pollution and hospital admissions/emergency room visits in 13 cities.* Washington, DC: American Lung Association.

Pirkle, J. L., Brody, D. J., Gunter, E. W., Kramer, R. A., Paschal, D. C., Glegal, K. M., & Matte, T. D. (1994). The decline in blood lead levels in the United States: The National Health and Nutrition Examination Survey (NHANES III). *Journal of the American Medical Association, 272,* 284–291.

Pribitkin, A. E. (1994). The need for revision of ozone standards: Why has the EPA failed to respond? *Temple Environmental Law and Technology Journal, 13,* 104.

Reitze, A. W., Jr. (1991). A century of air pollution control law: What worked; what failed; what might work. *Environmental Law, 21,* 1549.

Research Atlanta, Inc. (1997). *The costs of nonattainment: Atlanta's ozone imbroglio.* Atlanta: Georgia State University.

Rush, B. (1991). Observations . . . Transactions of the American Philosophical Society, 1799. In A. Thomas & S. Sillen (Eds.), *Racism and Psychiatry* (p. B1). New York: Carol, 289–297.

Soto, L. (1999, October 6). Take it from kids: Bad air hurts. *Atlanta Journal and Constitution,* p. B1.

Stretesky, P., & Hogan, M. J. (1998). Environmental justice: An analysis of Superfund sites in Florida. *Social Problems, 45,* 268–287.

Sullivan, H. (1964). *The fusion of psychology and social science.* New York: Norton.

U.S. Department of Health and Human Services. Task Force on Black and Minority Health. (1985). *Report of the Secretary's Task Force on Black and Minority Health* (Vol. 1, Executive Summary). Washington, DC: U.S. Government Printing Office.

U.S. Environmental Protection Agency. (1983). *Report of the Dallas Area Lead Assessment Study.* Dallas: Author.

U.S. Environmental Protection Agency. (1992). *Environmental equity: Reducing risks for all communities.* Washington, DC: Author.

U.S. Environmental Protection Agency. (1996, August). Escambia Wood Treating Company interim action: Addendum to April 1996 Superfund Proposed Plan Fact Sheet. Atlanta, GA: Author.

U.S. Environmental Protection Agency. (1998). *Guidance for incorporating environmental justice in EPA's NEPA compliance analysis.* Washington, DC: Author.

U.S. General Accounting Office. (1983). *Siting of hazardous waste landfills and their correlation with racial and economic status of surrounding communities.* Washington, DC: U.S. Government Printing office.

Warren, R. (1990). Oral health for the poor and underserved. *Journal of Health Care for the Poor and Underserved, 1,* 169–180.

Warren, R. (1998). Toward new models. In V. De La Cancela, J. Chin, & Y. Jenkins (Eds.), *Community health psychology: Empowerment for diverse communities* (pp. 219–221). New York: Routledge.

Warren, R. (1999). *Oral health for all: Policy for available, accessible and acceptable care.* Washington, DC: Center for Policy Alternatives.

Wernette, D. R., & Nieves, L. A. (1992). Breathing polluted air. *EPA Journal, 18,* 16–17.

West, P., Fly, J. M., Larkin, F., & Marans, P. (1990). Minority anglers and toxic fish consumption: Evidence of the state-wide survey of Michigan. In B. Bryant & P. Mohai (Eds.), *Race and the incidence of environmental hazards* (pp. 100–113). Boulder, CO: Westview Press.

White, M. C., Etzel, R. A., Wilcox, W. D., & Lloyd, C. (1994). Exacerbations of childhood asthma and ozone pollution in Atlanta. *Environmental Research, 65,* 56.

CHAPTER TWENTY-THREE

RESEARCH AND ETHICS

A Legacy of Distrust

Giselle Corbie-Smith, Kimberly R. Jacob Arriola

When medical research and research ethics are viewed through the prism of race and ethnicity, conflicting values are revealed. Often the weight placed on various ethical principles is determined by the cultural context of the individual. For example, most of the empirical literature dealing with the process of informed consent in clinical and research settings uses the western model of autonomy as its underpinning. As assessments of benefits and harm are culturally mediated, it might be more useful to explore certain ethical principles, specifically those of autonomy and beneficence, using culturally specific criteria as elicited from or defined by the patient.

For African Americans and other ethnic groups in the United States, the community or family is often a more central construct than the individual. Often the social and interpersonal responsibilities of being part of a community or family are just as important (if not more important) as the individual's personal freedom in making decisions, particularly decisions related to health care. It is within this social context that ethical issues related to medical research involving communities of color need to be considered. The history of racism in medicine, the distrust of the medical community, and the complexities of informed consent in communities of color and the vulnerable communities in which African Americans are represented, sometimes disproportionately, are among the layers of important issues raised in examining research ethics in the black community. This chapter discusses these issues and also outlines the historical context of research participation in the African American community, with an emphasis on the U.S. Public Health Service study of untreated syphilis at Tuskegee, which has become a lasting metaphor for the difficulty of trust in a racist environment.

Medical and Scientific Racism

Medical racism, stemming from a desire to protect the self-interest of those who hold the greatest power, has been defined as the misuse of an individual or group of individuals in the context of medical research or practice (Jones, 1997). The targets of medical racism are typically those who do not fit within the dominant group. In the United States these individuals are often ethnic and racial minorities, female, homosexual, disabled, or of low socioeconomic status. Although medical racism is not confined to any of these groups, the most prominent and well-known instances have affected black Americans.

Scientific racism may be defined as the use of scientific research methods to uphold racist beliefs, either intentionally or unintentionally. For example, during the eighteenth century, Thomas Malthus, a British professor of political economy, argued that poverty was a necessary condition because it made available cheap labor (Chase, 1977). Craniometry, the "science" of measuring human skulls, was a development of the nineteenth century. One of its uses was to "prove" blacks' inferiority. Intelligence testing has been put to a similar use in the twentieth century (Gould, 1981). What these movements have in common is a strong influence from the sociopolitical climate of the times, either an explicit or implicit motive to demonstrate white superiority and black inferiority, and widely publicized cases of ethical misconduct (for example, Cyril Burt's fabrication of IQ data and Samuel George Morton's fudging and finagling of data on skull measurement) (Gould, 1981; Kamin, 1974).

Although instances of intentional scientific misconduct are relatively rare, the subtle introduction of bias in scientific research is common (Altman & Hernon, 1997). Research is influenced by the investigator's attitudes, beliefs, and values as well as by the social, cultural, and political context in which the research occurs (Longino, 1994). Values associated with each of these contexts have the potential to influence research practices, research questions, the description of the data, and specific and global assumptions about the topic. Because racism and discrimination are deeply entrenched in American society, they have undoubtedly influenced the various contexts within which scientific research has been conducted.

Given the social and political history of the United States, investigators should be cautious in interpreting apparent racial differences in diseases and manifestations of illness. Because race is a socially defined construct, investigators should be mindful that racial differences not be exclusively interpreted as genetic (Cooper & David, 1986). Scientists' willingness to use supposed genetic and biological differences as an explanation for susceptibility to disease has led to stereotyping or stigmatizing of groups. Therefore, when examining differences in morbidity and mortality, for example, priority should be given to exploring the possible social, cultural, economic, and environmental determinants of disease before resorting to biological differences between groups as an explanation for differences in health outcomes. Wyatt (1994) argues that the overuse of race as a grouping variable in epidemiological studies of disease prevalence has the potential to overemphasize between-group differences, to downplay other defining characteristics, and to cause misinterpretation when race is confounded with some other factor (for example, economic status).

The U.S. Public Health Service Study at Tuskegee

The tendency of African Americans to avoid participating in medical research has been linked to the history of racism in that research (Gamble, 1997; Thomas & Quinn, 1991; Brandt, 1978; Caplan, Edgar, & King, 1992; Edgar, 1992; King, 1992; Corbie-Smith, 1999). The most powerful example of this racism is the Tuskegee Syphilis Study. As Jones (1993) tells us: "For many blacks, the Tuskegee Study became a symbol of their mistreatment by the medical establishment, a metaphor for deceit, conspiracy, malpractice, and neglect, if not outright racial genocide. . . . . [N]o scientific experiment inflicted more damage to the collective psyche of black Americans than the Tuskegee Study" (p. 220) (see also Jones, 1992).

The U.S. Public Health Service study at Tuskegee, an observational study of over four hundred sharecroppers with untreated syphilis, began in 1932 in Macon County, Alabama. The study was to document the course of the disease in blacks and racial differences in the clinical manifestations of syphilis. Despite the availability of treatment, initially arsenic and bismuth, then penicillin in the 1940s, the men were not told they had syphilis, not given counseling on avoiding spread of the disease, and not given treatment throughout the forty-year course of the study. At the conclusion of the trial over one hundred of the men had succumbed to syphilis or related complications. The U.S. Public Health Service study at Tuskegee, the longest nontherapeutic experiment on humans in the history of medicine, ended in 1972 when a front-page newspaper article detailed ethical concerns about the study (Jones, 1993).

Over a quarter of a century after the study was ended, references to Tuskegee still appear in the lay press and media, keeping this study a humbling reminder of the powerful influence of society and racism on medicine. Television, radio, and print media are full of discussion about this troubling mark in medical history. On May 16, 1997, the continuing unrest around this study precipitated a formal apology from the president of the United States on behalf of the U.S. government.

Several authors have argued that knowledge of the Tuskegee Syphilis Study is an important deterrent to African Americans' participation in health promotion and research (Cox, 1998; Des Jarlais & Stepherson, 1991; Green, Maisiak, Wang, Britt, & Ebeling, 1997; Guinan, 1993; Wolinsky, 1997; Thomas & Quinn, 1991). However, mistrust of the medical establishment has been supported by more than the Tuskegee study. The use of Mexican American women for the study of contraceptives, inadequate and differential access to health care for numerous groups, and military experiments with Agent Orange are among the more recent examples that are given as justifications for mistrust (Corbie-Smith, Thomas, Williams, & Moody-Ayres, 1999; Levine, 1986). In fact, mistrust of the medical community can be justified by a long history of exploitation in the name of research that dates back to the time of slavery and continues to the present day (Dula, 1994; Gamble, 1993, 1997). Given a history that runs from experimentation performed on slaves to public health efforts gone awry in sickle cell screening and involuntary sterilization, conspiracy theories cannot be simply written off as paranoia or hypersensitivity.

Distrust of the medical establishment has profound implications for the prevention and treatment of disease. For example, HIV/AIDS is a disease that was initially discovered in the United States among homosexual white males but very quickly spread to communities of color. In the less than twenty years since HIV/AIDS was first discovered, the burden of it has overwhelmingly fallen on communities of color. Although blacks make up only 13 percent of the U.S. population, they make up 46 percent of all AIDS cases (National Center for Health Statistics, 1999). AIDS is the leading cause of death for blacks between twenty-five and forty-four years of age (Hoyert, Kochanek, & Murphy, 1999). Fortunately, HIV/AIDS can be prevented through behavior modification. However, prevention efforts geared toward African Americans are surrounded by the legacy of medical misuse and distrust.

This underlying distrust has contributed to beliefs that needle exchange programs and policies that limit the reproductive rights of HIV-positive women are also based on genocidal intentions (Dalton, 1989; Thomas & Quinn, 1991). This distrust is also likely to have fueled the conspiracy theories that claim AIDS was created in governmental laboratories for the purpose of eliminating people who are unwanted by society, African Americans in particular (Dalton, 1989; Heck & Capitanio, 1994; Thomas & Quinn, 1991).

Although this belief is not supported by scientific evidence, it is held by many community leaders and members. The issue has been vigorously debated in the popular press, as evidenced by segments devoted to it on television (for example, *Tony Brown's Journal*), in newspapers (for example, *The Los Angeles Sentinel*), and in magazines (for example, *Essence*). The deliberate creation of AIDS is generally regarded as a myth in the scientific community. Nevertheless scientists and public health officials must take this myth seriously insofar as it imposes a barrier to African Americans' health seeking behaviors. It must be viewed as a legitimate reaction to the legacy of Tuskegee and other misuses of blacks and others in the name of science before the necessary steps can be taken to dismantle the barrier it raises.

In order to address the lasting legacy of the Tuskegee Syphilis Study and other real or perceived instances of ethical misconduct in minority communities, investigators need first to arm themselves with an appreciation of the significance of these events. The Tuskegee study is a barrier at several levels to minority populations' participation in clinical trials. This study highlights the powerful subtext of trust in the doctor-patient relationship and gives us an opportunity to examine closely the relationship between investigators and minority participants in the context of clinical research.

Research Participation and African Americans

The ongoing effects of the Tuskegee Syphilis Study are demonstrated most strikingly by unsuccessful attempts at improving representation of minority patients in clinical trials. In the wake of the medical experiments carried out on Jewish and other populations in Nazi-occupied Europe and, later, on African Americans in the Tuskegee Syphilis Study, biomedical research has emphasized the protection of the individual patient (Chavkin, 1994). This concern for the protection of human subjects was formally codified in the Nuremberg Code in 1949, which was the beginning of a cascade of regulations emphasizing the protection of human subjects. Some of the most prominent events in this process have been the 1964 Declaration of Helsinki (World Medical Association, 1964), the establishment and strengthening of the institutional review board (IRB), the exclusion of women of childbearing potential from the early phases of drug trials (NIH, 1979), and the publication of the Belmont Report by the National Commission for the Protection of Human Subjects of Biomedical and Behavioral Research (1978). Many of the regulations that were designed during this period to protect vulnerable populations such as minority populations from potential abuse led in fact to excluding them from research.

More recently, however, the scientific community began questioning the exclusion of certain groups. First, the bioethical principle of justice requires that the burdens and benefits associated with participating in research be distributed within a society. If excluded groups are to benefit from the fruits of research, they will have to be included among those who bear the burden of research as subjects. Otherwise, the ability to generalize and apply research findings from a homogeneous study sample to racially and ethnically diverse populations is limited. These and other concerns led to the creation of the National Institutes of Health (NIH) Office of Research on Women's Health and the NIH Office of Research on Minority Health and culminated in the passage of the NIH Revitalization Act by Congress in 1993 (NIH, 1993). This act both mandates the inclusion of women and minorities as subjects in clinical research and makes it incumbent upon investigators to understand and respond to the attitudes and beliefs of potential research participants.

In response to the NIH recommendations, researchers have begun actively recruiting minority populations. However, recruitment efforts are often unsuccessful. As discussed earlier, public knowledge of the historical relationship between federally funded research and minority patients has contributed to a sense of distrust of the medical profession in general and of medical research in particular. As Mark Smith, a physician from the Henry J. Kaiser Family Foundation, pointed out in 1990 during testimony before the National Commission on AIDS, the Tuskegee Syphilis Study "provides validation for common suspicions about the ethical even-handedness in medical research . . . when it comes to black people" (Jones, 1993, p. 236).

Thus the absence of trust has emerged as a stumbling block in efforts to include African Americans in clinical research. Beyond the evidence of Tuskegee, HIV infection, Agent Orange exposure, and CIA distribution of crack cocaine in black communities are used as contemporary evidence that biomedical abuse continues in minority communities (Corbie-Smith et al., 1999). Some authors have suggested that trust developed between a primary care provider and a patient is the only kind of trust that will be able to overcome fear of exploitation in research (El-Sadr & Capps, 1992) and that lack of trust in the researcher is the primary barrier to African American participation in clinical trials (Mouton, Harris, Rovi, Solorzano, & Johnson, 1997).

Despite a historical context that has led to mistrust of the medical and research community, African American patients are still willing to give suggestions on how to increase their involvement in research. When asked during focus group interviews how participation in research might be improved, participants expressed the desire for more honest and respectful interaction from physicians and other research personnel and stated the importance of providing complete information about the risks and benefits of the research. Although money and other incentives are often considered powerful motivators, focus group members emphasized their need to be sure that as research participants they had full knowledge about what they were being asked to do and were given sufficient time to consider their options. Information concerning the details of research participation should come from several sources, and participants should be given time to filter the information through their own social networks. Finally, in order to increase the involvement of African Americans, many focus group members believed that more must be done to improve the understanding of why research is important and how science is conducted and to raise awareness about the purpose of research and opportunities to participate, not only among potential participants but also among the community as a whole. They felt these efforts would dispel myths and misconceptions about research involving human subjects, resulting in a greater willingness to consider research participation (Corbie-Smith et al., 1999).

Investigators would do well to solicit and incorporate the suggestions of African American community members and potential participants in designing research protocols and recruitment strategies. The model of community consent and a collaborative relationship with the population under investigation is not new, and its use in the United States (Freeman, 1993; Kaluzny et al., 1993; Gorelick et al., 1996) and in international communities (Barry, 1988) has been described. However, finding ways to effectively implement community approval, as a complement to individual consent, may be particularly important in those African American and other ethnic minority populations where the collective community may be valued as highly as the individual. This inclusive approach not only might lead to fewer failed efforts but also could help forge strong community partnerships that would transcend the devastating effects of societal mistrust.

Informed Consent and Communities of Color

Ensuring that participants enrolling in clinical research studies are fully informed before they agree to participate has been and continues to be a tremendous challenge. The difficulty of informed consent is magnified when cultural differences exist between the study team and the participant (Corbie-Smith, 1999). Currently, the process of informed consent hinges on a consent document in which the risks are disclosed. This method may be a major hindrance to obtaining fully informed consent in patients of varying socioeconomic backgrounds (Taylor, Bezjak, & Fraser, 1998; Williams et al., 1995). For patients with lower levels of English fluency or limited formal education, the language of written documents often outstrips the ability of these groups to comprehend the information being conveyed (Davis, Holcombe, Berkel, Prammanik, & Divers, 1998). In addition to literacy issues, cultural and linguistic barriers may complicate comprehension of written materials (Smith, 1993). Despite overall increased educational attainment, lower literacy levels remain an important problem for African Americans. For some urban hospitals it is estimated that almost 80 percent of individuals seeking care in those hospitals are either marginally or functionally illiterate (Williams et al., 1995). In light of these high numbers of functionally or marginally illiterate patients seeking care in public hospitals, it is important to ask whether patients are able to access the information they are offered about their care.

Informed Consent in a Clinical Setting

The need for informed consent also arises in the broader context of the doctor-patient or investigator-participant interaction. In this context it is again important to acknowledge the history of abuse of certain subgroups in the United States. For African Americans, the history of involuntary or poorly informed participation in experimentation from the time of slavery to the present has created mistrust and the perception of unethical behavior in the medical profession. It is important for health care providers to familiarize themselves with this history because patients often are aware of examples of perceived exploitation by the medical community, events possibly distorted or modified through repeated retellings. It is important to be cognizant of this backdrop for many patients in underserved communities. To try to dismiss these concerns as unfounded or unimportant does little to improve the rapport between doctor and patient. Because trust developed between the primary care provider and the patient may be the only way this general mistrust can be overcome, taking patients' concerns about trust seriously is critical.

Yet another factor, however, is that in a trusting clinical relationship, there is always the possibility that interpersonal trust may override a truly informed and carefully deliberate decision. For many patients in underserved populations, finally finding a health care provider who will see them on a consistent basis and with whom they feel trust may hinder their ability to weigh carefully the risks and benefits of a particular procedure. This patient may feel the need to please his or her physician, thereby falling into a paternalistic model of health care decision making. In short, trust is essential, yet it can impinge on one's ability to provide informed consent.

Influencing all these factors in obtaining adequate informed consent in vulnerable populations is the environment in which these patients seek care. Often they receive their health care in teaching hospitals where financial resources are severely limited, where time constraints are constant, and where a significant amount of the care is provided by medical trainees. Medical students and residents are often inexperienced and do not feel comfortable with their ability to convey the information necessary to obtain adequate informed consent. In addition, because a team of trainees is usually caring for the patient, there may be several people involved in the consent process, each of whom may believe that another has adequately disclosed to the patient the risks and benefits of a particular medical treatment. Moreover, patients who use emergency departments as their primary source of care are typically under pressure to make decisions rapidly, they are often separated from their family and friends, and they lack a long-term trusting relationship with their caregivers. These factors also impair their ability to understand what information is supplied to them and to give informed consent.

Recently the possibility of waiving consent for emergent or emergency room research has been raised (Biros et al., 1995; Brody, Katz, & Dula, 1997). We would advocate extreme caution in taking this step with populations, such as the African American community, that are particularly sensitive to the implications of being involved in research without their consent. Although the researchers advocating these changes in informed consent have described explicit and ethically sound guidelines for waiver of informed consent for specific protocols, we would strongly suggest that IRBs reviewing these protocols take into consideration not only the scientific integrity of the proposed research but also the history of medical experimentation among the intended research subjects.

Informed Consent for Vulnerable Populations

The issue of informed consent takes on an added level of complexity in research involving populations of uncertain decision-making capacity such as children and adolescents, and also individuals whose power of free choice is limited or nonexistent, such as those who are undereducated or incarcerated. Children and adolescents, the poor and the undereducated, and the incarcerated are considered vulnerable populations because their capacity to provide consent is limited, making them particularly susceptible to exploitation by the scientific research enterprise. (Other segments of society are equally vulnerable—the mentally disabled and the institutionalized elderly, for example—but are not discussed here for the sake of brevity.) The following sections discuss important issues relevant to conducting research with individuals in each of these three groups as well as current regulations and guidelines that have been developed to protect these individuals.

Minors. Minors, individuals less than eighteen years of age, are legally considered to have limited capacity to provide informed consent. They may be immature in their affect, behavior, and cognition. Additionally, authority figures such as parents and teachers have a power advantage over them, and these authority figures are influential in determining a child's or adolescent's participation in research (Sieber, 1992). In light of these issues, ethicists have debated whether clinical research should be conducted on children at all (for example, see Ramsey, 1976; McCormick, 1974). The primary issues are who is most able to reasonably decide whether minors can participate in research and how minors can be involved in research for the sake of social benefit when they themselves have not consented to participate (Melton & Stanley, 1996). In order to clarify this ethical debate, the National Commission for the Protection of Human Subjects of Biomedical and Behavioral Research (1977), the U.S. Department of Health and Human Services ("Additional Protections for Children Involved as Subjects in Research," 1983), and the Society for Adolescent Medicine (1995) have established recommendations to guide research involving children and adolescents.

These recommendations stipulate that research on children be preceded by research on animals and adults when possible, that the privacy of the children and their parents be protected, and that the assent of children, when possible, and the permission of their parents be solicited. There are additional recommendations for children in special situations (for example, neglected or abused children) that entail the waiving of parental or guardian permission requirements when other mechanisms of protection can be substituted.

The recommendations supporting research involving adolescents include the following: (1) research must be done to enhance adolescents' health and well-being; (2) an understanding of adolescent social, psychological, and cognitive development must guide the protection of adolescents in the research enterprise; (3) parents must play an important role in protecting the adolescent to the extent possible; (4) the potential risks and benefits of participating in research must be evaluated; (5) members of the target population should be included in the development and conduct of the research; (6) the principles of beneficence, respect, and justice must provide a useful framework for determining adolescent involvement in research; and (7) IRBs should have guidelines to assist their interpretation of federal regulations as they apply to adolescent research. These sets of recommendations have been useful in protecting children and adolescents from harm as well as encouraging their participation in much needed research. The health of African American children and adolescents has been positively influenced by children no longer being "therapeutic orphans," the term used by Levine (1986) to describe the consequences of the general reluctance to conduct research on drug safety and efficacy in children.

Poor and Undereducated Populations. In the United States, African Americans are disproportionately represented among those who live in poverty. In 1998, for example, 26.1 percent of all African Americans lived in poverty, a figure unchanged from the previous year (U.S. Census Bureau, 1999b). In that same year the median income among blacks was $25,351 (U.S. Census Bureau, 1999a), a level that mirrors the educational attainment of this group. In 1997, approximately 25 percent of black adults aged twenty-five and older had not completed high school (U.S. Census Bureau, 1998). Because of lower socioeconomic status, these individuals have a disproportionate lack of health insurance compared to more affluent populations and are more likely to report poor mental and physical health. The combination of unmet subsistence needs and the offer of monetary remuneration or compensation along with increased access to medical care may serve to coerce poor and undereducated people to participate in medical research. Undue emphasis on compensation for research participation may infringe on these individuals' ability to weigh the risks and benefits carefully and to make decisions voluntarily about research involvement for themselves or their children.

Levine (1986) and Sieber (1992) have highlighted these ethical dilemmas in this population. Sieber argues that to conduct ethically sound community-based intervention research within this population requires (1) working in collaboration with members of the community's existing social structure (the "gatekeepers") to achieve their buy-in to the intervention; (2) understanding and respecting the community culture; (3) involving members of the community in the process of developing the study; (4) using the participants' basic assumptions, as opposed to the researchers', as a foundation for all communication; (5) building trust within the community; and (6) focusing on disease prevention, coalition building, and empowerment.

Incarcerated Populations. People of color, and African Americans in particular, are overrepresented among inmates in the U.S. correctional system. For many of these inmates, their power outside the facility is limited by their comparatively low economic and educational status, and their power inside the facility is stripped away by the U.S. penal system. Correctional institutions purposefully use implicit and explicit messages of isolation, intimidation, and restraint to produce conformity. In addition, some inmates may hope that exhibiting "good behavior" will reduce their sentences (Levine, 1986). Thus the values and cultural norms of the penal system are inherently in conflict with the environment necessary for ethically sound research. If coercion implicitly influences inmates' consent processes, then fundamental ethical conflicts arise.

There is widespread agreement that inmates need to provide consent before agreeing to participate in research. However, if this consent is provided under the influence of coercion, it becomes invalid (Levine, 1986). Goldiamond (National Commission for the Protection of Human Subjects of Biomedical and Behavioral Research, 1978) argued that institutions can be coercive in at least two ways.

First, they can set up conditions for participation that carry critical consequences (for example, linking eligibility for early parole to research participation). However, for the second form of coercion, the institution need not deliver the critical consequence; instead, it benefits from a consequence that should occur naturally. For example, among sick inmates the promise of recovery should not be linked to research participation because this is an unconditional right to which they are entitled. Moreover, just as in the case of those who are poor or undereducated, incentives that are overly rewarding may be effectively coercive and therefore violate fundamental ethical principles. Thus monetary compensation for participation in research should be comparable to compensation for other jobs in the prison or jail facility.

As a result of these and other issues related to this population, the National Commission for the Protection of Human Subjects of Biomedical and Behavioral Research (1976) established guidelines for conducting research with inmates. These guidelines include the following recommendations: IRBs that review protocols to be conducted with inmates must include a prisoner or prisoner advocate and should consider factors such as the risk-benefit ratio, the procedures for obtaining informed consent, the safeguards to protect individual rights, the procedures for selecting participants, and the provisions for compensation should injury occur.

Conclusion

Attention to the ethical issues involved in carrying out clinical research should be expected of all investigators, and especially of those engaging African American communities in such research. To conduct culturally appropriate research, investigators need an appreciation of the history of medical and scientific racism, past and current instances of ethical misconduct, and the underpinnings of mistrust in the African American community. To actively engage communities of color, investigators need to be willing to invite community participation at the inception of the study and to continue community partnerships long after the scientific goals of the research project have been met. Long-term partnerships between investigators and African American communities are needed to address continued racial and ethnic disparities in health and health care.

References

Additional protections for children involved as subjects in research. Fed. Reg. 48, 9814–9820 (1983).

Altman, E., & Hernon, P. (1997). *Research misconduct: Issues, implications, and strategies.* Greenwich, CT: Ablex.

Barry, M. (1988). Ethical considerations of human investigation in developing countries: The AIDS dilemma. *New England Journal of Medicine, 319,* 1083–1085.

Biros, M., Lewis, J., Olson, C. M., Runge, J., Cummins, R., & Fost, N. (1995). Informed consent in emergency research: Consensus statement from the Coalition Conference of Acute Resuscitation and Critical Care Researchers [Special communication]. *Journal of the American Medical Association, 273,* 1283–1287.

Brandt, A. (1978). Racism and research: The case of the Tuskegee Syphilis Study. *Hastings Center Report, 8*(6), 21–29.

Brody, B., Katz, J., & Dula, A. (1997). In case of emergency: No need for consent. *Journal of the American Medical Association, 27,* 7–12.

Caplan, A., Edgar, H., & King, P. (1992). Twenty years later: The legacy of the Tuskegee Syphilis Study. *Hastings Center Report, 22,* 29–38.

Chase, A. (1977). *The legacy of Malthus: The social costs of the new scientific racism.* New York: Knopf.

Chavkin, W. (1994). Women and clinical research. *Journal of the American Medical Women's Association, 49*(4), 99–100.

Cooper, R., & David, R. (1986). The biological concept of race and its application to public health and epidemiology. *Journal of Health Politics, Policy, and Law, 11,* 97–116.

Corbie-Smith, G. (1999). The continuing legacy of the Tuskegee Syphilis Study: Considerations for clinical investigation. *American Journal of the Medical Sciences, 317,* 5–8.

Corbie-Smith, G., Thomas, S., Williams, M., & Moody-Ayres, S. (1999). Attitudes and beliefs of African Americans toward participation in medical research. *Journal of General Internal Medicine, 14,* 537–546.

Cox, J. (1998). Paternalism, informed consent and Tuskegee [Editorial and comments]. *International Journal of Radiation Oncology, Biology, and Physics, 40,* 1–2.

Dalton, H. L. (1989). AIDS in blackface. *Daedalus (118),* 205–227.

Davis, T., Holcombe, R., Berkel, H., Prammanik, S., & Divers, S. (1998). Informed consent for clinical trials: A comparative study of standard versus simplified forms. *Journal of the National Cancer Institute, 90,* 668–674.

Des Jarlais, D. C., & Stepherson, B. (1991). History, ethics, and politics in AIDS prevention research. *American Journal of Public Health, 81,* 1393–1394.

Dula, A. (1994). African American suspicion of the healthcare system is justified: What do we do about it? *Cambridge Quarterly of Healthcare Ethics, 3,* 347–357.

Edgar, H. (1992). Outside the community. *Hastings Center Report, 22*(6), 32–35.

El-Sadr, W., & Capps, L. (1992). The challenge of minority recruitment in clinical trials for AIDS. *Journal of the American Medical Association, 267,* 954–957.

Freeman, H. P. (1993). The impact of clinical trial protocols on patient care systems in a large city hospital: Access for the socially disadvantaged. *Cancer, 72,* 2834–2838.

Gamble, V. N. (1993). A legacy of distrust: African Americans and medical research. *American Journal of Preventive Medicine, 9*(6, Suppl.), 35–38.

Gamble, V. N. (1997). Under the shadow of Tuskegee: African Americans and healthcare. *American Journal of Public Health, 87,* 1773–1778.

Gorelick, P. B., Richardson, D., Hudson, E., Perry, C., Robinson, D., Brown, N., & Harris, Y. (1996). Establishing a community network for recruitment of African Americans into a clinical trial: The African-American Antiplatelet Stroke Prevention Study (AAASPS) experience [Editorial]. *Journal of the National Medical Association, 88,* 701–704.

Gould, S. J. (1981). *The mismeasure of man.* New York: Norton.

Green, B. L., Maisiak, R., Wang, M. Q., Britt, M. F., & Ebeling, N. (1997). Participation in health education, health promotion, and health research by African Americans: Effects of the Tuskegee syphilis experiment. *Journal of Health Education, 28,* 196–201.

Guinan, M. (1993). Black communities' belief in "AIDS as genocide": A barrier to overcome for HIV prevention. *Annals of Epidemiology, 3,* 193–195.

Heck, G. M., & Capitanio, J. P. (1994). Conspiracies, contagion, and compassion: Trust and public reactions to AIDS. *AIDS Education and Prevention, 6,* 365–375.

Hoyert, D. L., Kochanek, K. D., & Murphy, S. L. (1999). Deaths: Final data for 1997. *National Vital Statistics Reports* (Vol. 47, No. 19). Hyattsville, MD: National Center for Health Statistics.

Jones, J. H. (1992). The Tuskegee legacy: AIDS and the black community. *Hastings Center Report, 22*, 38–40.

Jones, J. H. (1993). *Bad blood: The Tuskegee syphilis experiment.* New York: Macmillan.

Jones, J. M. (1997). *Prejudice and racism* (2nd ed.). Hillsdale, NJ: Erlbaum.

Kaluzny, A., Brawley, O., Garson-Angert, D., Shaw, J., Godley, P., Warnecke, R., & Ford, L. (1993). Assuring access to state-of-the-art care for U.S. minority populations: The first 2 years of the minority-based community clinical oncology program. *Journal of the National Cancer Institute, 85*, 1945–1950.

Kamin, L. J. (1974). *The science and politics of IQ.* Hillsdale, NJ: Erlbaum.

King, P. (1992). The dangers of difference. *Hastings Center Report, 22*(6), 35–38.

Levine, R. J. (1986). *Ethics and regulation of clinical research* (2nd ed.). Baltimore, MD: Urban & Schwarzenberg.

Longino, H. (1994). Gender and racial bias in scientific research. In K. Shrader-Frechette (Ed.), *Ethics of scientific research* (pp. 139–151). Lanham, MD: Rowman & Littlefield.

McCormick, R. A. (1974). Proxy consent in the experimentation situation. *Perspectives in Biology and Medicine, 18*, 2–20.

Melton, G. B., & Stanley, B. H. (1996). Research involving special populations. In B. H. Stanley, J. E. Sieber, & G. B. Melton (Eds.), *Research ethics: A psychological approach* (pp. 177–202). Lincoln: University of Nebraska Press.

Mouton, C. P., Harris, S., Rovi, S., Solorzano, P., & Johnson, M. S. (1997). Barriers to black women's participation in clinical trials. *Journal of the National Medical Association, 89*, 721–727.

National Center for Health Statistics. (1999). *Health, United States, 1999, with health and aging chartbook* (DHHS Publication No. PHS 99-1232). Hyattsville, MD: Author.

National Commission for the Protection of Human Subjects of Biomedical and Behavioral Research. (1976). *Research involving prisoners: Report and recommendations* (DHEW Publication No. OS 76-132). Washington, DC: U.S. Government Printing Office.

National Commission for the Protection of Human Subjects of Biomedical and Behavioral Research. (1977). *Research involving children: Report and recommendations* (DHEW Publication No. OS 77-0005). Washington, DC: U.S. Government Printing Office.

National Commission for the Protection of Human Subjects of Biomedical and Behavioral Research (1978). *The Belmont Report: Ethical principles and guidelines for the protection of human subjects of research.* (DHEW Publication No. OS 78-0012). Washington, DC: U.S. Government Printing Office.

National Institutes of Health. (1979). *The Belmont Report: Ethical principles and guidelines for the protection of human subjects of research* (DHEW Publication No. OS 78-0013 and No. OS 78-0014). Washington, DC: Author.

National Institutes of Health. (1993). *NIH Revitalization Act* (Subsection A, Pt. 1). Washington, DC: Author.

Nuremberg Code. (1949). In *Trials of war criminals before the Nuremberg Military Tribunals under Control Council Law No. 10: Vol. 2. Nuremberg, October 1946–April 1949* (pp. 181-182). Washington, DC: U.S. Government Printing Office.

Ramsey, P. (1976). The enforcement of morals: Nontherapeutic research on children. *Hastings Center Report, 6*(4), 21–30.

Sieber, J. E. (1992). *Planning ethically responsible research: A guide for students and internal review boards.* Thousand Oaks, CA: Sage.

Smith, R. (1993). Deception in research, and racial discrimination in medicine [Editorial and comments]. *British Medical Journal, 306*, 668–669.

Society for Adolescent Medicine. (1995). Guidelines for adolescent research. *Journal of Adolescent Health, 17,* 264–269.

Taylor, K., Bezjak, A., & Fraser, H. (1998). Informed consent for clinical trials: Is simpler better? *Journal of the National Cancer Institute, 90,* 644–645.

Thomas, S. B., & Quinn, S. C. (1991). The Tuskegee Syphilis Study, 1932–1972: Implications for HIV education and AIDS risk education programs in the black community. *American Journal of Public Health, 81,* 1498–1505.

U.S. Census Bureau. (1998). *Educational attainment of persons 25 years old and over, by sex, region, and race: March 1997* [On-line]. Available: www.census.gov/population/socdemo/race/black/ tabs97/tab07.txt

U.S. Census Bureau. (1999a). *Money income in the United States* (USDC Publication No. P60-206). Washington, DC: U.S. Government Printing Office.

U.S. Census Bureau. (1999b). *Poverty in the United States* (USDC Publication No. P60-207). Washington, DC: U.S. Government Printing Office.

Williams, M. V., Parker, R. M., Baker, D. W., Parikh, N. S., Pitkin, K., Coates, W. C., & Nurss, J. R. (1995). Inadequate functional health literacy among patients at two public hospitals. *Journal of the American Medical Association, 274,* 1677–1682.

Wolinsky, H. (1997). Steps still being taken to undo damage of "America's Nuremberg." *Annals of Internal Medicine, 127,* I43–I45

World Medical Association. (1964). *World Medical Association Declaration of Helsinki: Recommendations guiding medical doctors in biomedical research involving human subjects* (1975 revision of original 1964 version). Cambridge, MA: MIT Press, 328–329.

Wyatt, G. E. (1994). The sociocultural relevance of sex research: Challenges for the 1990s and beyond. *American Psychologist, 49,* 748–754.

CHAPTER TWENTY-FOUR

HEALTH POLICY CHALLENGES

Bailus Walker Jr.

The compelling challenge of bettering the health status of the black community elevates into sharper focus the importance of policy development, application, and analysis. This challenge is also making it necessary to transcend traditional notions of public health while applying more rigorously integrated molecular, social, behavioral, clinical, and measurement sciences in policy formulation and policy impact assessment.

As the variations in health status between racial groups continue to provoke public discussions, doctoral dissertations, and other scholarly papers, it is increasingly clear that health care policy formulation must consider the interrelated areas of organization, funding, and delivery of health services in the United States and in other countries as well. It must also speak to primary, secondary, and tertiary care; the dynamic changes in health services delivery systems; the relationship between health services and social services; the patterns of productivity and utilization of health services; forms of participation; and satisfaction with services provided.

Further, health policy interventions should alter or control environmental and occupational risk factors for disease and reduce behavioral risks such as smoking and excesses and imbalances in food consumption. The line here is almost impossible to draw rigorously in practical policy terms because the boundaries between what is medical and what is social, what is biological and what is environmental is beginning to blur as we learn more about the complexity of contemporary problems of morbidity and mortality in the black community.

In summary the health issues confronting the black community in the twenty-first century call for a policy perspective that draws on the intellectual tradition that places health care in the broader context of environmental and physical, cultural, and political and socioeconomic determinants of health. There are many benefits to understanding the multiple dimensions of health for an entire population. Although it would be useful to address all these issues, the purpose here is to examine a sample of the health policy themes that have dominated the evolving health services landscape since the first edition of *Health Issues in the Black Community* in 1992 and that are relevant to the health concerns of black Americans.

Before addressing the main topic of this chapter, it seems useful to emphasize that policies are made regularly at all levels of the health care system. Clearly identifiable today are three levels at which health policy is made. *Public policy* includes federal, state, and local initiatives that affect the entire population or certain segments of it. This multivalent policy environment is rooted in our federal system, with the separation of powers across the branches of the federal government and the existence of fifty sovereign states. Another level at which health policy is made is the *health care system* itself. Private and public sector components of the health care system make policy decisions about staffing, scope and quality of services, purchasing, and relationships with other health and nonhealth enterprises. A third level of policymaking is the *practice*, or *clinical*, level. Clinicians and other health care providers make numerous decisions that set policy affecting patient care.

To observers who do not appreciate the intricate history of health policy in the United States, this diversity and complexity of policies can seem frustrating for health care providers and consumers. But we cannot ignore the fact that polyinterventions—many different policies imposed by a number of institutions functioning in the same setting—may be beneficial as well. The system permits some degree of flexibility and prevents the likelihood that one institution or individual could unilaterally impose policies with broad-scale negative impacts.

In the following sections, health policy initiatives of governments are more closely examined.

Health Policy Developments

Health policy developments in the 1990s were fueled, to some extent, by the revolution in the organization and financing of health care that was evident in the 1980s. It is difficult to fully assess these changes. Some aspects are clear; others are still in the process of evolution. Certainly, advances in the biomedical sciences and in technological innovations have altered approaches to the delivery of health care and added to the cost of care. Society has generally valued innovation in health services, and has supported public policies that encourage the development of new medical technology. At the same time, technology is vilified as one of the dominant factors responsible for the continuing escalation of medical costs. It is also apparent that the critical issue may not be medical technology per se but the combination of economic, professional, and social incentives that elevates the importance of cost decisions about patient care. These considerations coupled with a broad constellation of market forces significantly affected the price paid for health care. Thus, in the decades of the 1980s and 1990s, costs became an important—indeed the central—policy issue.

In response to these interlocking concerns, including concern about the multivalent policy environment, President Clinton, on November 26, 1993, transmitted to Congress the administration's health care reform proposal. It was designed to guarantee comprehensive and secure health care coverage. The plan (U.S. House of Representatives, 1993) of more than 1,200 pages would have redesigned almost every component of the health care industry, from the number of doctors that hospitals would train each year to the finest details of the insurance policy everyone in America would be required to buy. Indeed, under the president's proposal every eligible individual would have been guaranteed coverage under a health plan including comprehensive benefits defined in law. The proposal provoked considerable debate in the Congress, stimulated editorials in leading newspapers, and was the principal topic in many forums of public discussion. At social gatherings in Washington, one often heard the plan described as "too big," "too complex," and "ham-handed." The proposal was not enacted into law; the various reasons for its failure have been widely recited, and they will not be repeated here.

The Market Approach

The 1994 failure of health care reform on the federal level led to favorable consideration of the market rather than the government as an approach to address the increasing cost of health services. The period from 1994 to 1996 can be characterized as the triumph of the market because enrollment in managed care plans surged; for-profit hospitals and health care plans expanded at a much greater rate than their not-for-profit competitors, which served among others the black community. At the same time, federal, state, and local policymakers promoted managed care as the most productive approach to controlling Medicare and Medicaid costs.

Indeed, the potential advantages of managed care were widely advertised, especially those of health maintenance organizations, with their capitation payments to physicians and hospitals. By embracing managed competition, many policymakers endorsed market principles, implicitly sanctioning a shake-up in the organization of health care. Managed care as a national health policy imposes enormous pressure for change on institutions that provide health care. As hospitals—long a resource in the health, civic, and economic environment of the black community—merge, consolidate, or close, the communities they serve are negatively affected, not only by a reduction in vital services but also by a loss of jobs. Compensating for these losses, especially for unskilled workers, has been difficult. Black physicians and other health care practitioners feel the constraints of market pressures as well. Finding a managed care plan to hire them became a vexed issue. Black physicians resented the loss of control that came with market consolidations. Choices, such as where to hospitalize their patients and when to discharge them, were dictated by accountants located at some distance from the site where patients' problems were clinically managed. The turbulent triumph of the marketplace had other influences as well. Some forty-nine states (all except Alaska) have steered roughly one-half of the nation's forty million Medicaid recipients into managed care plans and into similar arrangements. This trend was part of a central social policy innovation of the 1990s, as governments turned to the private sector to deliver major health and social programs.

Prior to the 1990s, public policy prohibited states from requiring Medicaid beneficiaries to enroll in managed care. To make managed care mandatory, states had to seek waivers from this Medicaid policy. In 1997, that policy was changed. The Balanced Budget Act of 1997 allowed states to make managed care mandatory without a waiver (Schoenman, 1999). In exchange for this new flexibility in adopting managed care, states must meet requirements for enrollment procedures and choice of plans. At a minimum, they must establish standards for access and procedures for monitoring the quality and appropriateness of care. The evidence of the success of this program is mixed. Low reimbursement rates and poor provider participation have made beneficiaries—many of whom are black—overly reliant on emergency departments and clinics that see mostly Medicaid patients.

Tennessee was one of the first states to revamp its Medicaid by shifting virtually all Medicaid beneficiaries statewide into capitated managed care arrangements. A 1994 review of the Tennessee program, known as TennCare, revealed that rapid expansion into managed care created confusion for patients, providers, and health plans. These problems were exacerbated by weaknesses in the state's oversight infrastructure. The speed with which TennCare was implemented, the limited involvement of stakeholders in program design and implementation, and the state's limited experience with managed care (both in Medicaid and the commercial market) were important factors contributing to the program's tumultuous first year. Five years later, a follow-up study found that the financial status of participating plans had deteriorated, raising questions about the long-term viability of TennCare and its impact on the health status of Tennessee's black community (Gold, Fazer, & Schoen, 1995; Aizer & Gold, 1999).

No less important is the Ohio experience with managed care Medicaid. In the spring of 1995, Ohio implemented a policy that required most people who receive Medicaid benefits to join a private health maintenance organization. Patients had a choice of six health plans. By early 1999, all but one of those plans had disappeared from the program, leaving thirty thousand people in the state no alternative but to get out of managed care. In Cincinnati, one of the plans that dropped out of the government insurance program for the poor essentially abandoned more than nine thousand people, including a substantial number of blacks. This defection in the winter of 1999 was part of a series of obstacles that has challenged—and finally defeated—Ohio, with its large black population, as it attempted to implement a policy of integrating poor patients into managed care (Goldstein, 1999).

In California, where the managed care system was viewed as a model not so long ago, the system is fraying, annual premiums are increasing almost geometrically, and nearly a third of the state's more than three hundred medical networks (medical groups that act as intermediaries between individual physicians and health maintenance organizations) have closed or entered bankruptcy proceedings. These networks have been described as bureaucracies that took money out of the system without improving it. Evaluations of the policies in Tennessee, Ohio, California, and other states of expanding Medicaid managed care illuminate the complexity of enrolling the medically disadvantaged in managed care (Rundle, 1999). This complexity arises primarily because the medically disadvantaged are a heterogeneous group: some are eligible for Medicaid because their income and assets are only somewhat above the normal Temporary Aid to Needy Families (TANF) threshold. Others, however, are eligible because they incur high medical costs and spend their assets down to eligible levels. Some states are attempting to address this complexity by creating managed care that extends across Medicare and Medicaid. The evaluations of the outcomes of these policy initiatives are still evolving.

Managed Care and the Uninsured

Numerous explanations have been proffered as the root causes of the "failure" of managed care. From an employers' perspective, Bob Galvin (1999), physician-director of health care for General Electric, suggests that a weakness of managed care is that two stakeholders—physicians and patients—have not been engaged. He goes on to point out that health maintenance organizations (HMOs) have delivered only half of what employers wanted from managed care: "HMOs have exploited the overcapacity in the system but have not fully developed their networks into organized systems of high quality care" (p. 166). Commenting further on the behavior of managed care plans, Galvin laments the fact that a court directive—from the U.S. Court of Appeals for the Ninth Circuit—was needed to ensure that HMOs provided basic customer services. The issue in this case was the apparent lack of response by HMOs to Medicare members' appeals, which prompted the court to require plans to respond to appeals within five days in legible, understandable language.

Steve Schroeder (1996) of the Robert Wood Johnson Foundation attributes some of managed care's problems to past market failures. The most obvious failure is that many millions of Americans lack health insurance. In late 1999, 44.3 million Americans (16.3 percent of the U.S. population) were without health insurance coverage. Despite a strong economy and sustained economic growth with historically low levels of unemployment, the number of Americans without health insurance continues to grow. Many of these individuals are low- and moderate-income workers. The cost of health insurance is rising as well. Rising health care costs can have a direct effect on the number of uninsured. Higher costs can raise substantial questions of equity. For instance, Congress has wrestled with the fairness of a Medicare program that does not include prescription medication coverage. In 1998, the number of people covered through Medicaid declined by more than one million, a side effect of federal policy that is moving people off welfare.

This most recent portrait of the uninsured includes over 44 million uninsured—over 18 percent of the total nonelderly population. Over half of the uninsured Americans have low incomes, making less than 20 percent of the federal poverty level ($32,000 for a family of four in 1998). Approximately 15.7 million women, eighteen to sixty-four years of age, were without health insurance in 1998—a more than 10 percent increase within this decade (The Henry J. Kaiser Family Foundation, 2000). These data also reflect the impact of welfare policy on women whose government assistance is curtailed and who are moved into low-end jobs without fringe benefits such as health care coverage. Thus the unresolved problem of how to address the health care needs of the uninsured is among the critical challenges on the current agendas of managed care proponents and of policymakers. Health insurance is important for black Americans because it removes one of the most critical barriers to access to the health care system. For instance, Schoen, Lyons, Rowland, Davis, and Puleo (1997) surveyed two thousand low-income adults in five states. Twenty-two percent of the uninsured interviewed did not get needed care in 1996, the year before the survey, which is three times the rate of failure to get care reported by those who are privately insured.

There is general agreement that having a regular provider or source of primary care enhances access to preventive services and to timely care that can reduce the number of hospitalizations. It can be plausibly argued that without health insurance coverage, many blacks are not benefiting from state-of-the-art screening, diagnostic procedures, and treatments. The counterargument, of course, is that access is not the only issue with broad policy implications. Equal treatment is also a problem for blacks in many parts of the country. Even with full insurance, black patients are less likely to receive coronary bypasses or bone marrow transplants. A study by Schulman et al. (1999) found that the race of the patient affects decisions about whether to refer patients for cardiac catheterization. The findings were most striking for black women. More recent research has added kidney transplantation to the growing list of medical procedures that are less available to black Americans. Moreover, evidence from a large-scale study indicates that blacks suffering from kidney failure are nearly as likely as whites to want a transplant. These findings undercut the notion, often put forth as an explanation for such racial disparities, that blacks are less likely than white patients to choose aggressive care. In what can be characterized as a terrible indictment of medical care systems, black patients in the study were also less likely than whites to report that their primary nephrologist provided all the medical information they desired. Thus black patients were more likely than white patients to report that they had received worse medical care than other patients. The results of this study may well reflect the failure of policy implementation at several levels. The consequences of racial disparities in care are particularly acute in kidney disease, where prevalence is much higher in blacks than in whites.

These data raise a serious question about whether the vision of the original formulators of Medicaid policy to provide low-income people with mainstream medical care has been blurred by time and ideology, resulting in tiers of health care. Each tier varies in expanse of services and in quality of care—a construction that exacerbates health disparities between blacks and whites. The tier for many poor blacks continues to be the so-called health care safety net: urban public hospitals, community health centers, some inner-city teaching hospitals, and local health departments. Thus the growing number of the uninsured, including the rise in persons who are employed but lack health insurance, has etched in sharp relief a particular concern of the black community: the financial viability of the safety net institutions. Teaching hospitals, for example, like other hospitals, have taken steps to respond to federal policies that have cut government payments and to the demands of managed care for lower hospital fees and shorter stays. Yet they still shoulder the extra obligations that teaching hospitals have long assumed: training new physicians including minority physicians, conducting medical research, and providing charity, that is, uncompensated, care. Teaching hospitals have also developed community outreach programs to address health conditions in black neighborhoods. These functions have traditionally been indirectly underwritten at least in part by the private sector. Assessments of difficulties facing teaching hospitals identify increases in managed care and the growth of more competitive markets as among the forces that have made it difficult for academic medical centers to use patient revenue to subsidize education and research functions and to subsidize care for the uninsured. Some managed care arrangements have disrupted the flow of patients to teaching hospitals, jeopardizing the patient base required to carry out clinical research and education. These pressures are especially severe in New York City, which has the nation's largest concentration of teaching hospitals.

Community health centers (CHCs), to take another example, have also been a significant health resource in the black community since they were established in the 1960s as a part of President Johnson's War on Poverty. They deliver services to poor and medically underserved patients through a network that includes migrant health centers, homeless health centers, and other community-based centers. An analysis of CHCs issued by the Commonwealth Fund (Davis, Collins, & Hall, 1999) revealed that although the centers can contract with and participate in managed care plans, the discounted payments offered by plans can lead to substantial losses in Medicaid revenues. This reduction in Medicaid funding is exacerbated by the fact that safety net providers are losing market share. Even as the population of uninsured patients continues to grow, financial constraints could well curtail the ability of CHCs to meet the primary health care needs of the uninsured. Far more than is commonly realized, CHCs provide cost-effective care while also improving access to care, reducing emergency room use, and increasing preventive services. Encouragingly, female health center patients are more likely to obtain mammograms and Pap smears than are patients in other health service facilities.

Ensuring the financial viability of CHCs should be an important objective of federal and state health policies designed to maintain the health care safety net for high-risk populations. Broadly speaking, these policies should speak to two issues in ways specific to CHCs: paying for care for the uninsured and safeguarding essential providers in an era of market-based managed care. To be fair, in the closing days of its 1999 session, Congress attempted to shore up these key parts of the black community's health care infrastructure by restoring more than $12 billion that was cut from Medicare in 1997. This allocation was part of an overall appropriation of $229 billion for mandatory programs such as Medicaid. The adequacy of this investment, when measured by the need, will be the subject of much debate well into 2001 and beyond.

The Incremental Approach

Another theme that has dominated the health policy sphere since the 1994 failure of national health reform is the current incremental approach to health policymaking. This approach has often been criticized as an undesirable strategy. For instance, the House of Representatives Committee on Education and Labor writes: "Those who argue that incremental reforms would solve most of the problem, and that we cannot afford universal coverage, are simply wrong" (U.S. House of Representatives, 1994, p. 567).

But incrementalism appears to be attractive to some policymakers. Indeed, some students of health policy seem committed to the approach. Incrementalism views public policy making as the continuation of past government activities with augmenting modifications. Several examples are illustrative. In 1996, Congress passed the Health Insurance Portability Act (HIPA). Its policy objective is to increase the number of persons who have and maintain access to health insurance. The Health Insurance Portability Act is designed to increase access by making it more difficult for insurers to segment an insurance risk pool and deny or revoke access to specific individuals or groups on the basis of health status. By setting minimum federal standards for certain aspects of private health insurance held by over 160 million Americans, HIPA established important new federal responsibility. The policy set minimum standards of protection to improve access to health insurance for people obtaining coverage through employment as well as for those purchasing it as individuals. For example, HIPA limits the time for which preexisting conditions may be excluded from coverage. Since the enactment of HIPA, the Congress has enacted additional federal health insurance requirements, including minimum standards affecting benefits for mental health care, maternal and newborn care, and reconstruction after mastectomy.

For instance, Congress enacted the Mental Health Parity Act in 1996. It took effect in January 1998. This act was a response to the growing discrepancy between insurance benefits for mental health services and medical care. For instance, in 1996 a number of employer-sponsored mental health plans had imposed limits on the number of covered outpatient visits or inpatient days. Medical plans generally had no such limits. The Mental Health Parity Act does not require employers to offer mental health coverage, but it does require that dollar limits on mental health coverage must be equal to dollar limits on medical benefits if that coverage is offered. Under the provisions of the act, employers and insurers also have the option of dropping mental health benefits altogether. It should be noted that many states have passed their own mental health parity laws in the past several years; by 1998, nineteen states had adopted some form of parity mandate that imposed further requirements on employers. The overarching goal of parity policy is to achieve more equitable, nondiscriminatory provision of health services for individuals with mental illness. It is still not clear whether the Mental Health Parity Act is significantly increasing access to mental health care or otherwise improving mental health insurance benefits.

Continuing the incremental approach to health policymaking, Congress created the State Children's Health Insurance Program (SCHIP) in 1997, with the goal of significantly reducing the number of uninsured low-income children. Under SCHIP, a state enacting a low-income children's health insurance program has the choice of (1) expanding Medicaid and thus building upon an existing program; (2) establishing a separate, stand-alone program that can include cost sharing and that allows the state to adopt a benefit package that meets one of several employer-based benchmarks; or (3) combining these two approaches. The State Children's Health Insurance Program appropriates about $40 billion over ten years. By October 1999, however, states had used less than 25 percent of the money made available up to that time. This slow progress in enrolling children prompted President Clinton to direct federal officials to visit U.S. schools and register low-income children in a state health insurance program. The president also proposed to train Americorp and Vista volunteers, who deal directly with low-income families, to enroll children in Medicaid (Pear, 1999).

With 11.3 million children uninsured, expanding coverage for this group was a laudable policy objective. However, evidence abounds that low-income adults are also at high risk of being uninsured, due in large part to fluctuations in public health care programs and in the private insurance market. Blacks without a link to the workforce, for example, and also many who are linked may not have access to affordable insurance. In a related policy shift, the Personal Responsibility and Work Opportunity Reconciliation Act, commonly known as welfare reform, severed the link between Medicaid and cash assistance, enhancing the opportunity to restructure Medicaid as a health insurance program rather than a welfare program.

As the first generation of managed care was coming to end and as polls began showing that the public believed it important for government to address the increasing numbers of the uninsured, other incremental health policy initiatives began to emerge. The Republican leadership in the House of Representatives unveiled a bill that would create a variety of tax breaks designed to make coverage more affordable to individuals and small businesses. Intellectual reinforcement was given these proposals by a number of analyses that illuminated the large subsidies (in the form of tax deductions or exclusions) available to affluent Americans with employer-provided insurance. Most working families without that coverage get little or no help to pay for insurance or for the direct costs of health care. In advocating the expansion of access to health care through tax reform, Butler and Kendall (1999) posit that it is neither feasible nor probably desirable to design a federal policy that seeks to address every aspect and issue associated with a health care coverage system for the uninsured. One problem is that the federal government by itself does not control all the financial mechanisms and resources for expanding coverage through tax credits. Butler and Kendall conclude that policymakers thus should see a federal tax credit as one element of a national, not federal, strategy to expand choice and coverage. This assertion is debatable.

The 2000 election at the federal and state level may well determine what health policies will be pursued after January 2001. Early evidence suggests that patients' bill of rights and payment for prescription drugs will be high on the domestic agenda along with coverage for the uninsured. It is reasonable to anticipate that the debate will have some of the same themes heard in the preelection health policy discussions. Before it adjourned, the House of Representatives passed a comprehensive patients' rights bill. Most of the provisions involved fairly standard consumer protections: managed care providers would be required to make full disclosure of costs and benefits, to have enough doctors and other resources to provide promised services, and to refrain from gagging doctors, that is, asking them to avoid mentioning costly courses of treatment. If enacted into law, such policies could go a long way toward easing public concerns about managed care.

In one of the most important steps by the federal government to help disabled people since the passage of the Americans with Disabilities Act in 1990, Congress and the administration in the fall of 1999 agreed on a bill expanding Medicaid and Medicare to give the increasing population of disabled people more access to health care. Under the provisions of the bill, which sailed through the House in October 1999, states could provide Medicaid to workers who are not actually disabled but have physical or mental impairments that make them "reasonably expected" to become severely disabled in the absence of treatment. This could be a significant benefit to black Americans who have been infected with HIV, the virus that causes AIDS, but have yet to develop symptoms of the disease. Medicaid would help them get protease inhibitors and other powerful pharmaceuticals so they can fight off AIDS and continue to be employed.

Conclusion: The Future

It is far too soon to tell if the sum vector of these incremental proposals and policies will ultimately bring to full fruition universal coverage, without which every black American remains at risk of losing his or her health insurance. Universal coverage means what it says. Unless health care for every black American is covered, some black Americans will fall through the cracks. And until everyone is covered, no one can be secure in the knowledge that he or she will not be in a group to which incremental reforms did not quite reach.

The options through which the U.S. could achieve universal coverage and the methods to pay for it are limited. Universal coverage could be achieved through a government program such as the single-payer approach advocated by the American Public Health Association and many others. Alternatively, universal coverage could be achieved through the private sector by building on the current employer-sponsored system, which now covers about two-thirds of the U.S. population. Under this approach, all employers would have to insure their employees, and those who were not employed or were self-employed would have to be insured through some other means.

Thus, generally speaking, there are three possible ways to achieve universal coverage: through employer mandates, individual mandates, or taxes. Using a combination of these three methods has also been suggested as a viable approach. But for black Americans, the focus on future health reforms that would achieve universal coverage must go beyond money. Future policies should pay attention to the organization of health services and to broad preventive measures to reduce illness and injury and improve healthy functioning. For the black community, health policies in the future should be formulated and legitimatized in ways that result in impact. *Policy impact* is not the same as *policy output*. To assess policy impact we must know more than the level of government activity (for example, the dollars spent or the number of consumers served) that we use to assess policy output. Impact must be measured by actual changes in the practices and in the conditions that are targeted by the government activity. For example, future health policy must confront more forcefully than in the past the potential for rationing of treatment based on race or national origin, health status, or anticipated need for health services. Bolder policy initiatives will be needed to ensure constant monitoring and surveillance of the content of medical care. The health care system needs a more effective mechanism for keeping tabs on health care errors made by physicians, nurses, pharmacists, and other members of the health care team with the goal of correction and prevention. The policy impact needed in all these instances is a tangible, not a symbolic, effect.

Observant students of community-oriented primary care and of public health have long worried about the waste caused by the misplaced incentives in the health care system, including higher reimbursement rates for diagnosis and treatment than for health promotion and disease prevention services. To halt this waste, future policies must encourage long-term investments in prevention. Including a broad spectrum of preventive services in a universally available, comprehensive benefit package will encourage everyone to use these services that prevent costly illnesses or detect them early, at stages when they can be treated relatively easily and at lower cost. Early testing and diagnosis of treatable illnesses can improve the quality of life for black Americans and in many cases yield substantial monetary savings. For example, a nonfatal case of colorectal cancer—a disease for which blacks are at high risk—incurs medical costs of $30,000 to $40,000. A fatal case can cost approximately $110,000. Effective screening for this disease alone has the potential to realize savings in excess of $5 billion in health care costs nationally (U.S. House of Representatives, 1993). Of course, such long-term savings through prevention can be achieved only through short-term investments associated with providing early screening and detection of disease and subsequent prevention of progression.

Another issue that future health policy initiatives must address is the public health infrastructure. A failure to take the public health system seriously enough in the past has left the health care system burdened by preventable disease and ill equipped to deal with the reemerging problem of infectious disease. Today it is clearer than ever that a sound public health system provides the infrastructure on which improvements in the health care system can be built. It solves collectively those problems that no one consumer can solve—from the control of ambient air pollutants that may provoke asthmatic stress to the regulation of the safety of food, water, and housing. It provides the safety net under the inevitable gaps that will occur in any health reform plan, whether such gaps affect the homeless or other residents of underserved inner cities. When all the necessary elements come together, public health can make significant reductions in morbidity and mortality. A case in point is the successful eradication of smallpox, an undertaking that was predicated on a public health system of shared goals, warning system, safety net services, research, and personnel. Similarly, the poliomyelitis immunization initiative was dependent on a defined public health infrastructure. In the same manner, public health services have reduced the incidence of milk-borne disease and other diseases that could disrupt not just the health care system but the economy of a community.

The opportunity exists for a policy to be effected that guarantees funding to ensure that public health activities are constant and certain. Funding by any other mechanism is inherently less reliable than a guaranteed funding approach and could place the health security of the American public at serious risk.

It bears repeating that each time Congress has struggled with questions on how best to ensure health security for all Americans, it has had to come to grips with an essential reality. Comprehensive health care reform is difficult to craft, disruptive to the established and entrenched interests, and complicated to structure and explain because of the interwoven parts that must be balanced. It is costly to finance and perturbing to those individuals who believe that they are well insured now but are afraid that reforms will leave them less protected. Moreover, the diversity that makes the health care system uncoordinated and expensive also makes it difficult to find common ground. Overcoming these barriers is a challenge posed to each American. And it is a challenge posed to all Americans.

References

Aizer, A., & Gold, M. (1999). Managed care and low-income populations: Four years' experience with TennCare. Menlo Park, CA: Kaiser Family Foundation.

Butler, S., & Kendall, D. B. (1999). Expanding access and choice for healthcare consumers through tax reform. *Health Affairs, 18,* 45–57.

Davis, K., Collins, K. S., & Hall, A. (1999). *Community health centers in a changing U.S. healthcare system* [Policy brief]. New York: Commonwealth Fund.

Galvin, R. (1999). An employer's view of the U.S. healthcare market. *Health Affairs, 18,* 166–169.

Gold, M., Fazer, H., & Schoen, C. (1995). Managed care and low income populations: A case study of managed care in Tennessee. Menlo Park, CA: Kaiser Family Foundation.

Goldstein, A. (1999, October 4). Million more lacked health coverage in 1998, U.S. study finds. *Washington Post,* p. 1.

The Henry J. Kaiser Family Foundation. (2000, April). *The uninsured: Kaiser public opinion update.* Menlo Park, CA: Author.

Pear, R. (1999, October 26). President urges governments to reach uninsured children. *New York Times,* p. 12.

Rundle, R. L. (1999, November 15). California doctors face piles of unpaid claims as care systems fray. *Wall Street Journal,* p. 1.

Schoen, C., Lyons, B., Rowland, D., Davis, K., & Puleo, E. (1997). Insurance matters for low income adults: Results from a five-state survey. *Health Affairs, 16,* 163–171.

Schoenman, J. A. (1999). Impact of BBA on Medicare HMO payments for rural areas. *Health Affairs, 18,* 244–250.

Schroeder, S. (1996). *The triumph of the market* (Annual report of the Robert Wood Johnson Foundation). Princeton, NJ: Robert Wood Johnson Foundation.

Schulman, K. A., Berlin, J. A., Harless, W., Kerner, J. F., Sistrunk, S., Gersh, B. J., Dube, R., Taleghani, C. K., Burke, J. E., Williams, S., Eisenberg, J. M., and Escarce, J. J. (1999). The effect of race and sex on physicians' recommendation for cardiac catheterization. *New England Journal of Medicine, 340,* 618–624.

U.S. House of Representatives. 103rd Congress. 1st Session. (1993). Comprehensive health security. (HR Doc 103–174). Washington, DC: U.S. Government Printing Office.

U.S. House of Representatives. 103rd Congress. 2nd Session. (1994). Health Security Act: Report of the Committee on Education and Labor on HR 3600 together with minority and supplemental views. Washington, DC: U.S. Government Printing Office.

CHAPTER TWENTY-FIVE

CULTURAL SENSITIVITY
IN PUBLIC HEALTH

Ken Resnicow, Ronald L. Braithwaite

That health promotion and health care must be practiced with cultural sensitivity is one of the most widely accepted principles of public health. It is virtually self-evident, at least in a general sense, that health promotion programs should be tailored to the social and cultural characteristics of the target population. However, what such tailoring entails, how to achieve it, and its impact on psychosocial and behavioral outcomes has not been adequately described or empirically examined. Much of the cultural sensitivity literature has emanated from nursing and social work ("AAN Expert Panel Report," 1992; Caudell, 1996; Facione, 1993; Henderson, Sampselle, Mayes, & Oakley, 1992; London, 1991; Sawyer et al., 1995; Schiele, 1996; Schlesinger & Devore, 1995; Swendson & Windsor, 1996), whereas the relevant public health literature has been limited mostly to HIV and substance use prevention (Airhihenbuwa, DiClemente, Wingood, & Lowe, 1992; Baldwin et al., 1996; Bayer, 1994; Catalano, Hawkins, et al., 1993; Orlandi, 1986; Singer, 1991; Stephens, Braithwaite, & Taylor, 1998). In this chapter we address the issue of cultural sensitivity as it relates to developing health promotion programs for African American populations. We begin by

Development of this chapter was supported with funding from U.S. Center for Substance Abuse Prevention Grant 8602, National Cancer Institute Grant CA-69668, National Heart, Lung, and Blood Institute Grant HL-64959, and National Heart, Lung, and Blood Institute Grant HL-62659 to Ken Resnicow. Parts of this chapter appeared previously in K. Resnicow, R. Braithwaite, J. Ahluwalia, & T. Baranowski (1999), "Cultural Sensitivity in Public Health: Defined and Demystified," *Ethnicity and Disease, 9,* 10–21, and K. Resnicow, R. Soler, R. Braithwaite, J. Ahluwalia, & J. Butler (2000), "Cultural Sensitivity in Substance Use Prevention," *Journal of Community Psychology, 28,* 271–290.

providing definitions and a conceptual framework for understanding cultural sensitivity and a discussion of the rationale for tailoring health promotion programs. We provide specific examples of ways health promotion programs can be tailored for racial and ethnic populations, and we conclude by highlighting priority areas for future research. Much of our research has focused on African Americans and, to a lesser extent, Hispanic populations. Therefore most of the examples provided here relate to these two groups. Nonetheless, the principles discussed should be applicable to other subpopulations defined by race and ethnicity or by sociodemographic characteristics.

Defining the Terms

The lack of theoretical clarity and empirical research about cultural sensitivity is due in part to the inconsistent if not confusing terminology that surrounds the construct. Cultural sensitivity is discussed under many names: for example, cultural competence, cultural relevance, cultural diversity, cultural pluralism, cultural tailoring, and cultural targeting. In addition, one may be culturally syntonic, culturally appropriate, culturally consistent, multicultural, culturally legitimate, or ethnically sensitive (Airhihenbuwa et al., 1992; "AAN Expert Panel Report," 1992; Bayer, 1994; Henderson et al., 1992; Isaacs & Benjamin, 1991; Marin et al., 1995; Schlesinger & Devore, 1995; Singer, 1991). Although definitions and distinctions for these terms have been offered (Amuleru-Marshall, 1993; "AAN Expert Panel Report," 1992; Bayer, 1994; Bazron, Dennis, & Isaacs, 1989; Isaacs & Benjamin, 1991; Morris, 1993; Sue, Mak, & Sue, 1998; Sue & Sue, 1999; Sussman, Parker, et al., 1995), the terminology as yet has no accepted standards. In response to this need, the following definitions are proposed (Dole, 1995; Pasick, D'Onofrio, & Otero-Sabogal, 1996; Yee, Fairchild, Weizmann, & Wyatt, 1993):

- *Cultural sensitivity.* The incorporation of the ethnic and cultural characteristics, experiences, norms, values, behavioral patterns, and beliefs of a target population and the acknowledgment of the relevant historical, environmental, and social forces in the design, delivery, and evaluation of targeted health promotion materials and programs.
- *Cultural competence.* The capacity of an individual to exercise interpersonal cultural sensitivity (Marin et al., 1995). (Thus a practitioner may exhibit cultural competence, whereas intervention programs, materials, and messages may exhibit cultural sensitivity.)
- *Multicultural.* Incorporating and appreciating perspectives of multiple racial and ethnic groups without assumptions of superiority or inferiority. (Culturally competent individuals and culturally sensitive interventions are implicitly multicultural.) Cultural pluralism is a synonym for multiculturalism.

- *Cultural tailoring.* The process of creating culturally sensitive interventions, often involving the adaptation of existing programs, materials, and messages for racial and ethnic subpopulations (Pasick et al., 1996).
- *Culturally based.* Using culture, ethnicity, history, and core values as media to motivate behavioral change. (Messages and programs, for example, may be culturally based.) (Singer [1991, p. 276] uses a similar term, *culturally innovative*, to define programs that use culture therapeutically.)
- *Ethnic identity.* The extent to which individuals identify with and gravitate to their racial or ethnic group. Ethnic identity includes such elements as taking pride in one's race or ethnicity, feeling affinity for the group culture (as expressed, for example, in food, media, and language), sharing specific group attitudes toward the majority culture, involving oneself with group members, having experiences with racism and attitudes toward racism, sharing attitudes toward intermarriage, and placing importance on preserving one's culture and aiding others of like background (Resnicow & Ross, 1997; Thompson, 1992). For immigrant groups, ethnic identity includes aspects of acculturation, that is, adoption of values and practices of the host country (Dana, 1996; Neff & Hoppe, 1992; Sue et al., 1998; Sue & Sue, 1999).

Cultural Sensitivity Further Defined

It is useful to think of cultural sensitivity as functioning in two primary dimensions (Resnicow, Braithwaite, Ahluwalia, & Baranowski, 1999): *surface structure* and *deep structure*. In regard to surface structure, cultural sensitivity involves matching intervention materials and messages to observable social and behavioral characteristics of a target population. For audiovisual materials, achieving a culturally sensitive surface structure may involve using people, places, language, music, foods, brand names, locations, and clothing familiar to and preferred by the target audience. It may include identifying the channels (for example, media) and settings (for example, churches or schools) that are most appropriate for the delivery of messages and programs. It also entails understanding various characteristics of the behavior in question, for example, the product brands that are used or the context in which a health behavior occurs. In sum, a surface structure is culturally sensitive to the extent to which interventions *fit* within the culture, experience, and behavioral patterns of the audience. In other words, appropriateness of surface structure sensitivity is analogous to face validity of psychological measures: it is a necessary but insufficient prerequisite for construct validity. Like face validity, culturally sensitive surface structure is generally achieved through expert and community review as well as the involvement of the target population in the intervention development process (Resnicow, Braithwaite, et al., 1999). Cultural competence, or interpersonal sensitivity, is essential at the surface level also. It involves using ethnically matched staff to recruit participants as well as to design, deliver, and evaluate programs (Sawyer et al., 1995).

The second dimension in which intervention sensitivity must function, deep structure, is the level at which the programs and messages reflect the ways cultural, social, psychological, environmental, and historical factors influence health behaviors differently across racial and ethnic populations (Airhihenbuwa et al., 1992; Marin et al., 1995; Morris, 1993; Pasick et al., 1996; Sabogal, Otero-Sabogal, Pasick, Jenkins, & Perez-Stable, 1996). This includes understanding how members of the target population perceive the cause, course, and treatment of illnesses as well as their perceptions regarding the determinants of specific health behaviors. In turn, this understanding involves an appreciation of how religion, family, society, economics, and the government, both in perception and in fact, influence the target behavior. Among many African Americans for example, there is a belief that the U.S. government may be covertly encouraging the spread of HIV/AIDS, guns, and drugs in their communities (Cochran & Mays, 1993; Gasch, Poulson, Fullilove, & Fullilove, 1991). Including messages that acknowledge these beliefs (though not necessarily either accepting or refuting them) will likely enhance program acceptance and effectiveness.

Core cultural values for African Americans include communalism, religion and spiritualism, expressiveness, respect for verbal communication skills, connection to ancestors and history, commitment to family, and intuition and experience (as opposed to empiricism) (Akbar, 1984; Butler, 1992; Cochran & Mays, 1993; Goddard, 1993b; Harris, 1992; Heath, 1989; Morgan, 1991; Nobles, Goddard, Cavil, & George, 1993). African American culture is also characterized by a unique sense of time, a unique rhythm, and a unique communication style (Butler, 1992; Hecht, Collier, & Ribeau, 1993; Nobles et al., 1993). The use of oral communication (that is, direct personal communication rather than communication through the audiovisual channels) as well as stories, religious and spiritual themes, and historical references to convey messages should be considered when developing health promotion programs for African Americans.

Whereas an appropriate surface structure generally increases the receptivity, comprehension, or acceptance of messages (Simons-Morton, Donohew, & Crump, 1997), an appropriate deep structure conveys *salience*. Surface structure establishes feasibility, whereas deep structure determines program impact.

Group Differences: The Rationale for Cultural Sensitivity

The rationale for targeted and tailored health promotion programs derives essentially from observations of three areas of difference among racial and ethnic groups: (1) differences in disease prevalence rates, (2) differences in the prevalence of the behavioral risk factors, and (3) differences in the predictors of health behaviors. Whereas the first two factors provide the rationale for *targeted* health promotion and disease prevention programs (that is, programs delivered to specific subpopulations), it is the latter factor that is the basis for *tailored* programs and messages (those adapted for subpopulations). Stated differently, factors one and two relate more to surface structure cultural sensitivity, whereas the latter factor has significant deep structure implications.

Differences in Disease and Behavioral Risk Factor Prevalence

As of 1996, life expectancy for African American males was sixty-six years, compared to seventy-four years for white males. The difference is slightly less for African American women (seventy-four years compared to eighty years for white women) but still alarmingly discrepant (Pamuk, Makuc, Heck, & Lochner, 1998). With regard to specific causes of death, African Americans have higher rates of heart disease, stroke, most cancers, pneumonia, influenza, chronic liver disease, diabetes, HIV, unintentional injuries, and homicide (Baquet, Horm, Gibbs, & Greenwald, 1991; Hahn, Teutsch, Franks, Chang, & Lloyd, 1998; Pamuk et al., 1998). They also exhibit higher rates of hypertension (males and females) and obesity (females only) (Centers for Disease Control and Prevention [CDC], 1994; Hahn, Teutsch, et al., 1998; Pamuk et al., 1998; Winkleby, Kraemer, Ahn, & Varady, 1998; Winkleby, Robinson, Sundquist, & Kraemer, 1999), and they are less physically active (CDC, 1994; Crespo, Keteyian, Heath, & Sempos, 1996; Winkleby, Kraemer, et al., 1998).

The Unique Case of Substance Use. Conversely, perhaps with the exception of marijuana (U.S. Department of Health and Human Services [DHHS], 1998a; Kann et al., 1998), African American youths exhibit lower rates of use for all legal and illicit substances than whites do (DHHS, 1998a; Oetting & Beauvais, 1990; University of Michigan, 1997; Vega, Zimmerman, Warheit, Apospori, & Gil, 1993; Wallace & Bachman, 1993; Wills & Cleary, 1997). This difference does not appear to be solely the result of underreporting or differential validity of self-reports (Oetting & Beauvais, 1990; Wallace & Bachman, 1993; Wills & Cleary, 1997).

Not only do rates differ but patterns of use also vary by racial and ethnic group. For example, African Americans are far more likely than other groups to smoke menthol cigarettes (Hymowitz et al., 1995; Royce, Hymowitz, Corbett, Hartwell, & Orlandi, 1993). African Americans are less likely than whites to be heavy smokers (Hahn, Folsom, Sprafka, & Norsted, 1990; Hymowitz et al., 1995; Novotny, Warner, Kendrick, & Remington, 1988; Royce et al., 1993) but are less likely to smoke light or low-tar cigarettes (Hahn, Folsom, et al., 1990; Hymowitz et al., 1995). There may also be racial or ethnic differences in how nicotine is processed. Compared to whites, African Americans exhibit equal or higher serum levels of nicotine metabolites despite smoking fewer cigarettes per day, and they appear to clear nicotine more slowly (Perez-Stable, Herrera, Jacob, & Benowitz, 1998).

Interestingly, whereas during adolescence African Americans exhibit lower alcohol, tobacco, and other drug use rates, by adulthood rates equal or even exceed those of whites (DHHS, 1998a, 1998b; Pamuk et al., 1998). Although the reasons for this paradox are not entirely understood, it is in part due to later initiation and lower quit rates (Fiore et al., 1990; Headen, Bauman, Deane, & Koch, 1991; Novotny et al., 1988; Royce et al., 1993; DHHS, 1998b).

Socioeconomic Versus Ethnic and Genetic Explanations. Because African Americans tend to have lower socioeconomic status (SES) than whites, and numerous health indicators are related to SES variables (Lantz et al., 1998), it is important when examining between-group difference in health indices to account for SES differences (Diez-Roux, Nieto, Tyroler, Crum, & Szklo, 1995; Gorey & Vena, 1994; Williams, 1990). Failure to do so may lead to inappropriate attribution of differences to ethnic, racial, or genetic factors rather than to socioeconomic disparities, which in turn may perpetuate views of racial inferiority as well as misdirect health care research and service dollars (Williams, 1995). As they are among whites, total mortality and cancer rates as well as some chronic disease risk factors are inversely related to income and education among African Americans (Patterson & Block, 1988; Smith, Neaton, Wentworth, Stamler, & Stamler, 1996; Smith, Wentworth, Neaton, Stamler, & Stamler, 1996), and the magnitude of the association also appears similar in African Americans and whites, at least with regard to all-cause mortality rates (Lantz et al., 1998), cancer rates (Gorey & Vena, 1994), and smoking prevalence (Wagenknecht et al., 1990). Black-white differences in the risk for several cancers (Baquet et al., 1991; Gorey & Vena, 1994) and smoking rates (Wagenknecht et al., 1990) diminish or even reverse after controlling for SES, further suggesting that racial and ethnic differences may be related more to SES than to ethnic, cultural, or biological factors.

However, differences in adult death rates and infant mortality rates as well as in other health indicators such as obesity, body image preferences, high blood pressure, sedentariness, smoking quit rates, diabetes markers, poor diet, and health knowledge remain higher in African Americans than in whites even after adjustment for education or income or both (Becker, Yanek, Koffman, & Bronner, 1999; CDC, 1994; Hahn et al., 1998; Harrell & Gore, 1998; Krieger, Rowley, Herman, Avery, & Phillips, 1993; Neaton, Kuller, Wentworth, & Borhani, 1984; Pappas, Queen, Hadden, & Fisher, 1993; Resnicow, Wang, et al., in press; Shea et al., 1991; Sprafka, Folsom, Burke, & Edlavitch, 1988; Wagenknecht et al., 1990; Winkleby, Kraemer, et al., 1998; Winkleby, Robinson, et al., 1999). Conversely, African American adolescents appear less likely than whites to smoke cigarettes, independent of SES (Winkleby, Robinson, et al., 1999), and African American adults have higher dietary carotenoid intake even after adjusting for education and income (Nebeling, Forman, Graubard, & Snyder, 1997). Thus some ethnic differences in health indicators appear to be independent of sociodemographic factors.

One explanation for these inconsistent results is that there are often an insufficient number of middle and upper socioeconomic level African American participants in epidemiological studies. Thus conclusions about the effects of SES on health indicators across ethnic groups are often based on small samples and unstable parameter estimates (Harrell & Gore, 1998; Herd, 1990; Lillie-Blanton, MacKenzie, & Anthony, 1991; Resnicow, Wang, et al., in press; Winkleby, Kraemer, et al., 1998). Another explanation is that socioeconomic factors function differently among African Americans and whites. For example, African Americans reap a lower increase in income per year of education, and they have lower net worth at all income levels than whites do (Krieger et al., 1993; Williams, 1995). It is also possible that ethnicity, genetics, and socioeconomic factors may each influence the same health indicator independently.

Differences in the Predictors of Health Behavior

Differences in disease and risk factor prevalence rates provide the rationale for targeted interventions. However these differences provide little guidance for tailoring interventions. Effective adaptation of interventions to subpopulations derives from understanding how the correlates and predictors of health behaviors differ across racial and ethnic populations. For example, there are ethnic differences in the relative effects of peers and parents on substance use behavior. Numerous studies have found that peers exert a stronger influence on cigarette and other drug use among whites and Hispanics than among African Americans (Gottfredson & Koper, 1996; Headen et al., 1991; Koepke, Flay, & Johnson, 1990; Landrine, Richardson, Klonoff, & Flay, 1994; Sussman, Dent, Flay, Hansen, & Johnson, 1987; Dusenbury et al., 1992; Ringwalt & Palmer, 1990). Conversely, parents appear to have a greater impact on alcohol, tobacco, and other drug (ATOD) use among African American than among white youths (Catalano, Morrison, et al., 1992; Clark, Scarisbrick-Hauser, Gautam, & Wirk, 1999; Koepke et al., 1990; Ringwalt & Palmer, 1990; Robinson, Klesges, Zbikowski, & Glaser, 1997). Smoking among African American youths is inversely associated with parental disapproval, whereas no such association is evident among whites (Gritz et al., 1998). One explanation for this stronger impact of parents can be found in a survey of 256 white and 51 African American parents (Clark et al., 1999) that found African American parents were far more likely than white parents to believe they could influence their children's smoking behavior (See Table 25.1). They were more likely to establish clear rules and expectations regarding smoking in the household and, in another study, were more likely than whites to prohibit smoking in their cars (Royce et al., 1993). African American parents are also more likely than whites to set and reinforce rules with their children about other drug use, to be proactive family managers, to punish unacceptable behavior, and to exert influence over whom their children choose as friends; each of these behaviors may help explain the lower substance use rates among African American adolescents (Catalano, Morrison, et al., 1992; Koepke et al., 1990).

Alcohol, tobacco, and other drug use may serve different functions across racial and ethnic groups. For example, African Americans may be more likely to use drugs to "anesthetize" the emotional effects of racism, poverty, oppression, and lack of opportunity (Amuleru-Marshall, 1993; Dawkins, 1988; Goddard,

TABLE 25.1. ETHNIC DIFFERENCES IN PARENTAL
ATTITUDES TOWARD YOUTH SMOKING.

Attitude	Percentage of Parents Who Agree	
	White (%)	Black (%)
All kids will try tobacco, it's part of growing up	54	33
Punishing children for trying tobacco is not likely to keep them from trying it again	72	22
If parents forbid teens to use tobacco, teens will only want to use it more	50	12
Schools can be more effective than parents in teaching children about the dangers of smoking	32	9

Source: Data from Clark et al., 1999.

1993a; Harvey, 1985; Schiele, 1996; DHHS, 1990a). However, in one study, depression was a significant predictor of smoking initiation in white adolescents but not in African Americans or Hispanics (Gritz et al., 1998). And although African American youths' greater involvement in religion is sometimes cited as a reason for their lower substance use rates, in one study religiosity was protective against drug use in whites but not African Americans (Amey, Albrecht, & Miller, 1996).

Substance use behaviors cluster with other health and social risk behaviors differently among African Americans, whites, and Hispanics. For example, cigarette use in whites is correlated with smokeless tobacco use, but there is no such association in African Americans or Hispanics (Escobedo, Reddy, & DuRant, 1997). Similarly, deviance and risk taking and their association with substance use and sexual behavior appear to manifest differently across racial and ethnic groups (Bettes, Dusenbury, Kerner, James-Ortiz, & Botvin, 1990; DiIorio, Dudley, & Soet, 1998; Headen et al., 1991; Koepke et al., 1990; Landrine et al., 1994; Sussman, Dent, et al., 1987).

Another example of ethnic differences appears in the ideal body image and the meaning of being overweight for African Americans and whites. Compared to whites, African American women and men appear to prefer fuller body types. African American women report a higher ideal body weight and are more likely to be satisfied with their weight, even when they are statistically overweight, than are white women (Desmond, Price, Hallinan, & Smith, 1989; Kumanyika, Wilson, & Guilford-Davenport, 1993; Parnell et al., 1996; Stevens, Kumanyika, & Keil, 1994). How these cultural differences developed is a matter of debate (Kumanyika, Morssink, & Agurs, 1992); however, it appears that in the African American community, being "large" conveys a different social image than it does among whites. When designing weight control interventions for African Americans, it therefore may be useful to deemphasize thinness as an outcome and focus instead on spiritual, physical, or psychological benefits, such as gaining personal control; improving physical functioning; or being better able to fulfill social roles such as parent or church member.

Ethnic differences also exist in the predictors of sexual behaviors and social relationships. For example, in one study, self-efficacy was significantly associated with condom use among white but not black college females (Soet, DiIorio, & Dudley, 1998). Another study found that black women felt a greater sense of control over their relationships than white women did (Soet, Dudley, & DiIorio, 1999). African American males initiate sex earlier and report more partners, yet they are also more likely to use condoms (DiIorio et al., 1998). Racial and ethnic differences in the prevalence of socioeconomic and environmental risk factors associated with health behavior are also evident. For African Americans these include higher school drop-out rates and a greater likelihood of low socioeconomic status and of chaotic family life (Catalano, Hawkins, et al., 1993; Headen et al., 1991; Schinke, Moncher, Palleja, Zayas, & Schilling, 1988; DHHS, 1990b). More specifically, compared to whites, African Americans experience a greater number of negative stressful events; moreover, they experience different types of stressors and employ different types of coping strategies in response to stress (Airhihenbuwa & Cole, 1988; Fitzpatrick & Boldizar, 1993; Garrison, Schoenbach, Schluchter, Kaplan, & Berton, 1987). They also derive social support, a buffer against stress, from different sources (Thomas, Bethlehem, & Holmes, 1992). African American adolescents are more likely than their white counterparts to be the victim of or witness to violence, to experience the death of a parent or sibling, to be involved in the criminal justice system, and to have parents whose income has recently decreased (Fitzpatrick & Boldizar, 1993; Garrison et al., 1987). African American youths also rate the impact of stressful events differently than do white adolescents (Newcomb, Huba, & Bentler, 1986). Another important source of stress for African Americans is racism (Amuleru-Marshall, 1993; Cochran & Mays, 1993; Goddard, 1993a), which can increase feelings of anger, hostility, alienation, and helplessness, all of which have been associated with negative health outcomes (Barefoot, Dahlstrom, & Williams, 1983; Scherwitz et al., 1992). This higher level of risk appears inconsistent with the lower rates of ATOD use among African Americans. One explanation for this apparent paradox is that the predictors of substance use, both the risk and the protective factors, function differently across racial and ethnic subgroups.

Practice Implications

Understanding ethnic and cultural differences in the predictors and determinants of health behavior is an essential element in developing culturally sensitive health promotion interventions. Program planners could use these findings to shape their interventions in several ways. For example, ATOD interventions for African American youths may be more effective when they engage parents and other adult models, whereas interventions for European American youths should perhaps focus more on altering perceptions of peer use and peer approval.

Although some of the differences cited previously, such as the relative influence of peers versus the influence of parents as well as the relative impacts of culturally bound stressors, can serve as a starting point for program developers, it is important to examine these etiological pathways in each population that will be served to determine their relevance and how they might be incorporated into intervention messages and services. Factors such as socioeconomic status, urbanicity, geographic differences, secular trends, and numerous other factors can alter the ways these phenomena affect health behaviors in specific populations. As will be discussed later, formative research with the local target population is a prerequisite for the development of sensitive interventions.

In defining these populations, program developers must also consider the issue of *within*-group heterogeneity. Failure to appreciate the heterogeneity not only between ethnic groups but within each group can lead to what has been called "ethnic glossing" (Longshore, 1997; Trimble, 1990–1991) and ultimately to insensitive and ineffective interventions. To achieve cultural sensitivity, at the level of surface or deep structure, it is essential to understand the variations within the target population (Pasick et al., 1996; Sabogal et al., 1996). For example, among African American youths living in low-income public housing complexes (a seemingly homogeneous population), there will be considerable variability with regard to important predictors of behavior such as parental attitudes and behaviors, religiosity, educational attainment, and political beliefs. Although it may not be feasible or desirable to develop interventions targeted to each of these parameters, interventions can nonetheless incorporate multiple perspectives that appeal to a broad spectrum of the target population. In effect, through audience segmentation, even materials designed for a single racial and ethnic group can be multicultural (Simons-Morton et al., 1997). A related phenomenon is the fluidity of racial and ethnic group membership. Racial and ethnic populations may be defined by external parameters established by researchers rather than by any indigenous cultural ethos. For example, defining African Americans by church membership will yield a different cultural subgroup than defining them by income status (Sasao, 1998).

An important dimension for which heterogeneity should be assumed is racial and ethnic identity. Such identity varies considerably within any superficially homogeneous racial and ethnical population (Cross, 1991; Cross, Parham, & Helms, 1991). For some individuals, race or ethnicity is central to their self-concept, whereas for others it plays a less prominent role. Among African Americans, for example, ethnic identity can comprise various permutations of problack-antiblack and prowhite-antiwhite beliefs (Cross, 1991; Parham & Helms, 1985b; Resnicow & Ross, 1997).

Ethnic identity has been associated with substance use in African Americans. For example, antiwhite attitudes have been associated with increased substance use in adolescents (Resnicow, Soler, Braithwaite, Selassie, & Smith, 1999), whereas problack attitudes have been associated with stronger antidrug attitudes (Gary & Berry, 1985; Resnicow, Soler, et al., 1999). In adults, involvement in black networks and increased awareness of sociopolitical issues pertaining to blacks are associated with decreased alcohol use (Herd & Grube, 1996). For several cultural groups, ethnic identity has been related to numerous other psychological characteristics and health behaviors in adults and youths (Baldwin, 1984; Belgrave et al., 1994; Brook, Whiteman, Balka, Win, & Gursen, 1998; Helms, 1990; Herd & Grube, 1996; Klonoff & Landrine, 1997; Munford, 1994; Oyserman, Gant, & Ager, 1995; Parham & Helms, 1985a, 1985b; Phinney & Chavira, 1992; Scribner, Hohn, & Dwyer, 1995; Vega et al., 1993).

The heterogeneity of ethnic identity has significant implications for developing culture-based interventions. In recent years, many health and social programs for African American youths have been based on African-centered principles. Participants are immersed in African culture and tradition to enhance cultural esteem and inoculate them against harmful behaviors (Damond, Breuer, & Pharr, 1993; Foster et al., 1993; Greene, Smith, & Peters, 1995; Nobles et al., 1993; Randolph & Banks, 1993; Schiele, 1996; Ward, 1995). Substance use and violence prevention programs, for example, have incorporated such culture-based elements as the study of African history, Kwanzaa, the Nguzo Saba, and African traditions such as unity circles and rites of passage ceremonies. Culture-based interventions have also been used with Hispanic, Native American, and Asian American populations (Baldwin et al., 1996; Lalonde, Rabinowitz, Shefsky, & Washienko, 1997; Marin et al., 1995; Ramirez, Gallion, Espinoza, McAlister, & Chalela, 1997; Shintani, Beckham, O'Connor, Hughes, & Sato, 1994; Singer, 1991). One application of culture-based messages involves using communal and family preservation as a motivation for behavior change. For example, messages such as "do it for the sake of your community" or "do it because your people need you to be strong" may offer salient reasons for health behavior change to African Americans with strong ethnic identities (Resnicow, Braithwaite, et al., 1999; Resnicow, Vaughan, Futterman, Weston, & Harlem Health Connection Study Group, 1997). Similarly, messages might address how tobacco or alcohol manufacturers target African Americans or how smoking and drugs are modern forms of slavery. Given the variability in ethnic identity, however, Afrocentric and other culture-based programs and messages, although on one hand potentially salient, must be carefully pretested. Segments of the population that do not place a high priority on, for example, ethnic identity, Afrocentrism, or community survival may find them irrelevant, inflammatory, or offensive.

Nevertheless, some contend that any program for African American youths should be based on Afrocentric (as opposed to Eurocentric) principles (Akbar, 1984; Asante, 1988). This assumption is based on the premise that historically African Americans have been stripped of their cultural heritage, and that (re)discovering and celebrating their African roots will enhance their cultural esteem (and therefore their self-concept) and facilitate positive behaviors. Also, some contend that it is not only a pragmatic but also a moral imperative to formulate programs from an African perspective, consistent with the psychobiology of African people (Akbar, 1984; Asante, 1988).

Developing Culturally Sensitive Interventions

The process of developing culturally sensitive health promotion programs should begin with an analysis of disease rates and behavioral risk factors and, more important, the unique behavioral predictors in the target population. Although much of this information can be culled from the scientific literature, this process will likely require collection of new data, particularly to elucidate the predictors of behavior. Data for this analysis can be obtained through both quantitative surveys and qualitative techniques. Qualitative data collection may include exploratory or formative focus group as well as pretesting techniques based on principles of social marketing and health communication (Andreasen, 1995; Maibach & Parrott, 1995; Resnicow, Braithwaite, et al., 1999; Simons-Morton et al., 1997). Quantitative methods may include surveys and secondary analysis of existing data sets or archival information.

Focus groups are a potentially valuable means for developing culturally sensitive intervention messages. At the formative level of program development, members of the target population are convened to explore thoughts, feelings, experiences, associations, language, assumptions, and environmental enabling and constraining factors regarding specific behaviors; for example, focus group members might be asked about frequency and context of physical activity. Specific guidelines for conducting focus groups can be found elsewhere (see, for example, Basch, 1987; Krueger, 1988). Exploratory focus groups also provide an opportunity to examine the possible role of culturally based messages in a program. Although potentially costly, it may be valuable when developing interventions for minority groups to conduct a few focus groups with European Americans. Though some might view this as ethnocentric (by establishing white values and practices as the norm) or as simply a waste of resources, contrasting responses from racial and ethnic subpopulations to those of the majority culture can help program developers crystallize the extent of tailoring required.

Focus groups may elucidate the language connected with a particular topic. For example, focus groups we conducted with African American smokers in Harlem revealed the term loosies, which refers to single cigarettes purchased at newspaper stands, generally for $.25. Incorporating such terminology can increase the surface structure sensitivity of an intervention. It may also be useful to explore with the focus group how the target population perceives the prevalence, expression, and determinants of the target health behavior to differ in their community relative to the European American community. For example, in exploratory groups for a smoking cessation program for low-income African Americans, participants reported that for many African Americans smoking served as a stress reduction technique, whereas "white folk," they felt, "can just take a vacation" (Resnicow, Vaughan, et al., 1997).

One focus group strategy for delineating cultural differences is what we have called ethnic mapping (Resnicow, Braithwaite, et al.,1999). It entails asking participants to rate aspects of the target behavior along the continuum shown in Figure 25.1. First, several *anchors* are presented, items for which responses have been generally consistent across African American populations. For example, the anchors might be rap music and Kwanzaa (generally rated mostly black things), skiing and caviar (generally rated mostly white things), and Christmas and television (generally rated equally black and white things). Once participants become comfortable with the classification schema, they are asked to use the same categories to classify elements of the target behavior. In a recent series of four focus groups conducted during the development of an intervention to increase fruit and vegetable consumption among African American adults, participants were asked to rate approximately twenty-five foods using this schema (Resnicow, Braithwaite, et al., 1999; Resnicow, Coleman-Wallace, et al., 2000). If more than 50 percent of the participants rated an item in one of the three categories, it was considered a consensus. As shown in Table 25.2, results of the ethnic mapping indicated that foods such as asparagus, tomato juice, pumpkin pie, and artichokes should probably not be emphasized in the proposed program or, if these foods were to be included, that they should be presented as foods that many participants would not previously have eaten or did not typically consume. Table 25.3 presents the ethnic mapping results for various forms of physical activity (along with specific responses) from four focus groups of adults from Atlanta-area black churches. In this analysis, the percentages of respondents choosing each option are shown. This process provided information that was not available from quantitative data sources. The ethnic mapping technique may also be useful for examining other health behaviors, such as smoking (to determine brand prefer-

FIGURE 25.1. ETHNIC MAPPING CONTINUUM.

Mostly a Black Thing	Equally a Black and White Thing	Mostly a White Thing

TABLE 25.2. RESULTS OF ETHNIC MAPPING BY FOUR FOCUS GROUPS OF FRUIT AND VEGETABLE INTAKE.

Mostly Black	Equally Black and White	Mostly White
Turnip greens	Apples	Artichokes
Collards	Pears	Asparagus
Sweet potato pie	Bananas	Beets
Watermelon	Peaches	Bean salad
	Grapes	Tomato juice
	Pineapple	Pumpkin pie
	Oranges	Apricots
	Raisins	

Note: (N = 33).

TABLE 25.3. RESULTS OF ETHNIC MAPPING BY FOUR FOCUS GROUPS OF PHYSICAL ACTIVITY.

	Mostly Black (%)	Equally Black and White (%)	Mostly White (%)
Black and White			
Jogging	0	82.7	17.2
Aerobics at home (using video)	0	72.4	27.6
Jazz or ballroom dancing	10.3	62.1	27.6
Walking at work	21.0	79.0	0
Walking for exercise	3.4	75.9	20.7
Bicycling indoor	0	79.3	20.7
Bicycling outdoor	0	55.2	44.8
Gardening	3.4	58.6	38.0
Housework at home	27.6	58.6	13.8
Bowling	3.4	93.1	3.4
Tennis	0	72.4	27.6
YMCAs and community health facilities	5.0	70.0	25.0
Swimming at pool	3.4	86.2	10.3
Weight lifting or power lifting	0	86.2	13.8
Body building	20.0	80.0	0
Rollerblading	3.4	55.2	41.4
Football	17.2	86.2	0
Mostly White			
Aerobics at health club	0	50.0	50.0
Square dancing	0	6.9	93.1
Hiking	0	3.4	96.6
Raquetball or squash	0	17.2	82.8
Private health club (not including YMCAs)	0	0	100.0
Swimming at beach or lake	0	40.0	60.0
Soccer	0	34.5	65.5
Baseball and softball	0	41.4	58.6
Ice skating	0	6.9	93.1
Mostly Black			
Basketball	65.0	30.0	5.0
Housework for your job	84.2	15.8	0
Jumping rope or double dutch	72.4	27.6	0

Note: (N = 29).

ences, quitting techniques, and perceptions about smokers) and HIV-related and substance use behaviors.

Focus groups can also be used for pretesting. In this process, members of the target audience are exposed to program materials and messages to obtain feedback about format and content at both the surface and deep structure levels. Pretesting should be distinguished from pilot testing. The former typically involves exposing potential participants, under controlled conditions, to subelements of an intervention such as specific messages, artwork, or intervention themes to determine their appropriateness and potential salience. Pilot testing usually entails delivering the actual intervention, under real-world circumstances, to a small number of participants to determine the feasibility of the intervention delivery process. During pretesting, participants are typically asked to rate materials on dimensions such as comprehension, interest, and attractiveness. It may also be useful to inquire specifically about the cultural sensitivity of the materials and messages. This is often done with questions such as, How appropriate are these materials for people like yourself? or, How appropriate are these materials for people with your background?

Occasionally, racial and ethnic populations may prefer audiovisual materials that represent or are designed for multiple racial and ethnic groups as opposed to more narrowly targeted materials. In some cases audiences may perceive targeted interventions as singling out or casting an unfavorable light on their community. This reaction may be more likely to surface when addressing behaviors or illnesses associated with a social stigma, such as HIV and substance use, or issues connected with a belief that the government contributes to the problem, such as guns, drugs, and HIV. Additionally, a low-income group may show a preference for images that portray individuals from their same racial or ethnic group but from a higher socioeconomic bracket. Similarly, it cannot always be assumed that racial and ethnic groups will prefer or will be more responsive to same-group practitioners (Parham & Helms, 1981). Examples of the ways formative research have been used to develop culturally sensitive health promotion programs can be found elsewhere (see, for example, Harrington & Donohew, 1997; Ramirez et al., 1997).

Key Research Questions

We have contended that culturally sensitive health promotion programs are necessitated by differences in disease rates, risk factor distribution, and especially, behavioral predictors. Controlled research demonstrating how these factors can be incorporated into prevention interventions and what impact, if any, they have on outcomes is lacking however. Although the ethical and philosophical arguments for cultural sensitivity may not require scientific evidence, there are nonetheless several key empirical questions regarding feasibility and effectiveness that merit investigation.

With regard to developing a culturally sensitive surface structure, some of the assumptions appear a priori valid. For example, it is largely self-evident that interventions should be written in the language of their intended audience or at an appropriate reading level. However, other surface structure issues such as whether materials should portray role models exclusively from the target audience or role models of mixed racial and ethnic backgrounds or whether images should reflect the socioeconomic background of the audience or a higher income bracket require empirical examination. Some bilingual populations may prefer interventions in English whereas others may prefer a mix of languages (Lalonde et al., 1997; Ramirez et al., 1997). Program developers may need to explore these issues each time they plan to introduce an intervention into a racial or ethnic subpopulation.

Little is known about just how much differently racial and ethnic groups may respond to health promotion interventions or about how much tailoring is needed (Dent et al., 1996). If, for example, the predictors of substance use are in fact different across groups, then it would be expected that response to interventions would also vary. In one study, African American youths rated a multicultural drug prevention video intervention more highly than whites did, and there was some indication that the program had a greater impact on the behavioral intentions of African Americans (Freimuth, Plotnick, Ryan, & Schiller, 1997). Similarly, numerous studies have shown that adolescents' perceptions of the prevalence and acceptability of substance use among their peers is one of the strongest predictors of their own substance use, and interventions that focus on altering these perceptions may be more effective than programs that target refusal skills (Donaldson, Graham, Piccinin, & Hansen, 1995; Donaldson, Graham, & Hansen, 1994; Hansen & Graham, 1991). Because peer influences appear less predictive of substance use in African Americans, it follows that normative education and peer resistance programs may be less effective for this population. There has been little research testing this hypothesis however. In fact most substance use prevention programs that are based on skills training have generally worked as well, if not better, among minority students (Botvin, Baker, Dusenbury, Botvin, & Diaz, 1995; Botvin & Dusenbury, 1992; Botvin, Batson, Witts-Vitale, Bess, & Dusenbury, 1989; Ellickson & Bell, 1990; Graham, Johnson, Hansen, Flay, & Gee, 1990). To date there is little evidence documenting that substance use prevention programs, including those that involve peer resistance skills training, are more or less effective among minority youths.

A key phenomenon that remains underresearched is the substantially lower substance use rates that have been documented among African American (and Asian) youths. These lower rates suggest an opportunity to use African American culture as an exemplar for African American youths, rather than approaching the problem as a deficit in that culture. The possible protective role of parental monitoring, family bonding, spirituality, and other positive attributes of African American family life and culture that may buffer African American youths from ATOD use has not been adequately explored (Gary & Littlefield, 1998; Goddard, 1993b; Pinkett, 1993). Other avenues to explore include how exposure to problem drug use and to the crime and violence associated with the sale and use of drugs in the home and the community may discourage use among minority youths. Additional research is needed to understand ethnic differences in alcohol, tobacco, and other drug use and, eventually, how the protective factors identified can be incorporated into prevention programs for both minority and majority youths.

As little as is known about surface structure sensitivity, even less is known about the efficacy of culturally sensitive deep structure messages. Controlled trials comparing the efficacy of culturally sensitive and standard (non-culturally

sensitive) materials are needed. To a great extent it is not known whether culturally sensitive programs are in fact more effective (Dent et al., 1996). Continuing
with the example of substance use prevention programs, in one study the effects
of a culturally tailored substance use prevention intervention were not superior to
a generic intervention among a sample of African American and Latino youths
at one-year follow-up (Botvin, Schinke, Epstein, & Diaz, 1994), although effects
for the tailored intervention appeared to be superior at the two-year follow-up
(Botvin, Schinke, Epstein, Diaz, & Botvin, 1995). To obtain results with a high
degree of internal validity when investigating the efficacy of culturally sensitive
materials, it is important to compare materials that are similar in as many dimensions as possible. For example, it may be possible to hold constant the key
scientific content and health education messages of an intervention and also the
length of any video or print material and vary only the method of conveying
that content. In one such study, Ahluwalia, Richter, Mayo, and Resnicow
(1999) found little difference in six-month smoking cessation rates among African
American smokers randomized to receive a culturally sensitive cessation video
and a standard video developed for European Americans. Another example of
this investigative approach can be found in Sussman, Parker, et al. (1995).

Similarly, despite the inherent appeal of using culture to enhance self-esteem
and motivate positive behavior change, little is known about the feasibility (acceptance) or efficacy (salience) of culture-based interventions. Many programs
have incorporated culture-based themes, but they have rarely been isolated ex-
perimentally, so the unique impact of the culture-based components is not well
understood (Davis, Lambert, Cunningham-Sabo, & Skipper, 1995; Freimuth et
al., 1997; Harrington & Donohew, 1997; Lalonde et al., 1997; Long, 1993; Maypole & Anderson, 1987; Nobles et al., 1993; Ramirez et al., 1997). It should be
noted that some might contend that the assumed need for controlled research
documenting the efficacy of such interventions is an ethnocentric (and perhaps
unnecessary) assumption, that their value is intuitively known and inherent.
Nonetheless, given the diversity of ethnic identity among African Americans, it is
possible that programs that use culture-based messages may be not only ineffective, but somewhat paradoxically, even culturally insensitive for some African
American populations (Cross, 1991). Afrocentric interventions may, for example,
be more acceptable and salient than other interventions among African American teens and less acceptable among older African Americans. Controlled studies comparing culture-based and standard interventions are needed.

Additional research issues include determining how surface and deep structure messages may function differently across racial or ethnic subpopulations and
sociodemographic subpopulations, which populations are more or less responsive
to culture-based messages, and which elements of ethnicity and culture are independent of socioeconomics. Research is also needed to delineate core cultural
values across racial and ethnic populations, the extent to which individuals sub-
scribe to these values, and how these values can be incorporated into disease prevention and health promotion programs.

Conclusion

The rationale for culturally sensitive health programs is driven by epidemiologic, sociologic, philosophic, and pragmatic factors. Although in some ways the need for and benefits of tailoring health programs for specific ethnic, racial, and sociodemographic populations may appear to be self-evident, numerous empirical questions regarding the process and impact of tailoring remain unanswered. The framework provided in this chapter may be helpful to researchers and practitioners interested in further defining what cultural sensitivity is and how to achieve it.

References

AAN Expert Panel Report: Culturally competent health care. (1992). *Nursing Outlook, 40,* 277–283.

Ahluwalia, J. S., Richter, K. P., Mayo, M. S., & Resnicow, K. (1999). *Quit for life: A randomized trail of culturally sensitive materials for smoking cessation in African Americans.* Journal of Global Information Management, 14, (Supplement 2), 6.

Airhihenbuwa, C., & Cole, G. (1988). Results of a pilot study of the relationships of psychosocial measures among black adolescent students. *The Western Journal of Black Studies, 12,* 204–209.

Airhihenbuwa, C. O., DiClemente, R. J., Wingood, G. M., & Lowe, A. (1992). HIV/AIDS education and prevention among African Americans: A focus on culture. *Journal of AIDS Education and Prevention, 4,* 267–276.

Akbar, N. (1984). Afrocentric social sciences for human liberation. *Journal of Black Studies, 14,* 395–414.

Amey, C. H., Albrecht, S. L., & Miller, M. K. (1996). Racial differences in adolescent drug use: The impact of religion. *Substance Use and Misuse, 31,* 1311–1332.

Amuleru-Marshall, O. (1993). *Political and economic implications of alcohol and other drugs in the African American community* (DHHS Publication No. SMA 93-2015). Rockville, MD: Substance Abuse and Mental Health Services Administration.

Andreasen, A. (1995). *Marketing social change: Changing behavior to promote health, social development, and the environment* (1st ed.). San Francisco: Jossey-Bass.

Asante, M. (1988). *Afrocentricity.* Trenton, NJ: Africa World Press.

Baldwin, J. A. (1984). African self-consciousness and the mental health of African Americans. *Journal of Black Studies, 15,* 177–194.

Baldwin, J. A., Rolf, J. E., Johnson, J., Bowers, J., Benally, C., & Trotter, R. T. (1996). Developing culturally sensitive HIV/AIDS and substance abuse prevention curricula for Native American youth. *Journal of School Health, 66,* 322–327.

Baquet, C., Horm, J., Gibbs, T., & Greenwald, P. (1991). Socioeconomic factors and cancer incidence among blacks and whites. *Journal of the National Cancer Institute, 83,* 551–556.

Barefoot, J., Dahlstrom, W., & Williams, R., Jr. (1983). Hostility, CHD incidence, and total mortality: A 25-year follow-up study of 255 physicians. *Psychosomatic Medicine, 45,* 59–63.

Basch, C. (1987). Focus group interview: An underutilized research technique for improving theory and practice in health education. *Health Education Quarterly, 14,* 411–448.

Bayer, R. (1994). AIDS prevention and cultural sensitivity: Are they compatible? *American Journal of Public Health, 84,* 895–898.

Bazron, B. J., Dennis, K. W., & Isaacs, M. R. (1989). *Toward a culturally competent system of care* (Vol. 1). Washington, DC: Georgetown University Child Development Center.

Becker, D. M., Yanek, L. R., Koffman, D. M., & Bronner, Y. C. (1999). Body image preferences among urban African Americans and whites from low income communities. *Ethnicity and Disease, 9*, 377–386.

Belgrave, F. Z., Cherry, V. R., Cunningham, D., Walwyn, S., Letkala-Rennert, K., & Phillips, F. (1994). The influence of Africentric values, self-esteem, and black identity on drug attitudes among African American fifth graders: A preliminary study. *Journal of Black Psychology, 20*, 143–156.

Bettes, B. A., Dusenbury, L., Kerner, J., James-Ortiz, S., & Botvin, G. J. (1990). Ethnicity and psychosocial factors in alcohol and tobacco use in adolescence. *Child Development, 61*, 557–565.

Botvin, G. J., Baker, E., Dusenbury, L., Botvin, E., & Diaz, T. (1995). Long-term follow-up results of a randomized drug use prevention trial in a white middle-class population. *Journal of the American Medical Association, 273*, 1106–1112.

Botvin, G. J., Batson, H. W., Witts-Vitale, S., Bess, V., & Dusenbury, L. (1989). A psychosocial approach to smoking prevention for urban black youth. *Public Health Reports, 104*, 573–582.

Botvin, G. J., & Dusenbury, L. (1992). Smoking prevention among urban minority youth: Assessing effects on outcome and mediating variables. *Health Psychology, 11*, 290–299.

Botvin, G. J., Schinke, S. P., Epstein, J. A., & Diaz, T. (1994). Effectiveness of culturally focused and generic skills training approaches to alcohol and drug abuse prevention among minority youths. *Psychology of Addictive Behaviors, 8*, 116–127.

Botvin, G. J., Schinke, S. P., Epstein, J. A., Diaz, T., & Botvin, E. M. (1995). Effectiveness of culturally focused and generic skills training approaches to alcohol and drug abuse prevention among minority adolescents: Two-year follow-up results. *Psychology of Addictive Behaviors, 9*, 183–194.

Brook, J. S., Whiteman, M., Balka, E. B., Win, P. T., & Gursen, M. D. (1998). Drug use among Puerto Ricans: Ethnic identity as a protective factor. *Hispanic Journal of Behavioral Sciences, 20*, 241–254.

Butler, J. (1992). Of kindred minds: The ties that bind. In M. Orlandi, R. Weston, & L. Epstein (Eds.), *Cultural competence for evaluators: A guide for alcohol and other drug abuse prevention practitioners working with ethnic communities* (DHHS publication no. 92-1884, pp. 23–54). Rockville, MD: Alcohol, Drug Abuse, and Mental Health Administration, Office for Substance Abuse Prevention.

Catalano, R. F., Hawkins, J. D., Krenz, C., Gillmore, M., Morrison, D., Wells, E. A., & Abbott, R. (1993). Using research to guide culturally appropriate drug abuse prevention. *Journal of Consulting and Clinical Psychology, 61*, 804–811.

Catalano, R. F., Morrison, D. M., Wells, E. A., Gillmore, M. R., Iritani, B., & Hawkins, J. D. (1992). Ethnic differences in family factors related to early drug initiation. *Journal of Studies on Alcohol, 53*, 208–217.

Caudell, K. A. (1996). Incorporating cultural sensitivity into educational programs is an important consideration for nurses. *ONS News, 11*(5), 5.

Centers for Disease Control and Prevention. (1994). Prevalence of selected risk factors for chronic disease by education level in racial/ethnic populations. *Morbidity and Mortality Weekly Report, 43*, 894–899.

Clark, P. I., Scarisbrick-Hauser, A., Gautam, S. P., & Wirk, S. J. (1999). Anti-tobacco socialization in homes of African American and white parents, and smoking and nonsmoking parents. *Journal of Adolescent Health, 24*, 329–339.

Cochran, S., & Mays, V. (1993). Applying social psychological models to predicting HIV-related sexual risk behaviors among African Americans. *Journal of Black Psychology, 19*, 142–154.

Crespo, C. J., Keteyian, S. J., Heath, G. W., & Sempos, C. T. (1996). Leisure-time physical activity among U.S. adults. *Archives of Internal Medicine, 156,* 93–97.

Cross, W. (1991). *Shades of black diversity in African American identity.* Philadelphia: Temple University Press.

Cross, W., Parham, T., & Helms, J. (1991). The stages of black identity development: Nigrescence models. In R. Jones (Ed.), *Black psychology* (3rd ed., pp. 319–338). Hampton, VA: Cobb & Henry.

Damond, M. E., Breuer, N. L., & Pharr, A. E. (1993). The evaluation of setting and a culturally specific HIV/AIDS curriculum: HIV/AIDS knowledge and behavioral intent of African American adolescents. *Journal of Black Psychology, 19,* 169–189.

Dana, R. H. (1996). Assessment of acculturation in Hispanic populations. *Hispanic Journal of Behavioral Sciences, 18,* 317–328.

Davis, S. M., Lambert, L. C., Cunningham-Sabo, L., & Skipper, B. J. (1995). Tobacco use: Baseline results from Pathways to Health, a school-based project for Southwestern American Indian youth. *Preventive Medicine, 24,* 454–460.

Dawkins, M. (1988). Alcoholism prevention and black youth. *The Journal of Drug Issues, 18,* 15–20.

Dent, C. W., Sussman, S., Ellickson, P., Brown, P., and others (1996). Is current drug abuse prevention programming generalizable across ethnic groups? *American Behavioral Scientist, 39,* 911–918.

Desmond, S., Price, J., Hallinan, C., & Smith, D. (1989). Black and white adolescents' perceptions of their weight. *Journal of School Health, 59,* 353–358.

Diez-Roux, A. V., Nieto, F. J., Tyroler, H. A., Crum, L. D., & Szklo, M. (1995). Social inequalities and atherosclerosis. The Atherosclerosis Risk in Communities study. *American Journal of Epidemiology, 141,* 960–972.

DiIorio, C., Dudley, W. N., & Soet, J. (1998). Predictors of HIV risk among college students: A CHAID analysis. *Journal of Applied Biobehavioral Research, 3,* 119–134.

Dole, A. (1995). Why not drop race as a term? *Journal of the American Psychological Association, 50,* 40.

Donaldson, S., Graham, J., Piccinin, A., & Hansen, W. (1995). Resistance-skills training and onset of alcohol use: Evidence for beneficial and potentially harmful effects in public schools and in private Catholic schools. *Health Psychology, 14,* 291–300.

Donaldson, S. I., Graham, J. W., & Hansen, W. B. (1994). Testing the generalizability of intervening mechanism theories: Understanding the effects of adolescent drug use prevention interventions. *Journal of Behavioral Medicine, 17,* 195–216.

Dusenbury, L., Kerner, J. F., Baker, E., Botvin, G., James-Ortiz, S., & Zauber, A. (1992). Predictors of smoking prevalence among New York Latino youth. *American Journal of Public Health, 82,* 55–58.

Ellickson, P., & Bell, R. (1990). Drug prevention in junior high: A multi-site longitudinal test. *Science, 247,* 1299–1305.

Escobedo, L. G., Reddy, M., & DuRant, R. H. (1997). Relationship between cigarette smoking and health risk and problem behaviors among U.S. adolescents. *Archives of Pediatric and Adolescent Medicine, 151,* 66–71.

Facione, N. C. (1993). The Triandis model for the study of health and illness behavior: A social behavior theory with sensitivity to diversity. *Advances in Nursing Science, 15,* 49–58.

Fiore, M. C., Novotny, T. E., Pierce, J. P., Giovino, G. A., Hatziandreu, E. J., Newcomb, P. A., Surawicz, T. S., & Davis, R. M. (1990). Methods used to quit smoking in the United States: Do cessation programs help? *Journal of the American Medical Association, 263,* 2760–2765.

Fitzpatrick, K., & Boldizar, J. (1993). The prevalence and consequences of exposure to violence among African-American youth. *Journal of the American Academy of Child and Adolescent Psychiatry, 32,* 424–430.

Foster, P. M., Phillips, F., Belgrave, F. Z., Randolph, S. M., and others (1993). An Africentric model for AIDS education, prevention, and psychological services within the African American community. *Journal of Black Psychology, 19,* 123–141.

Freimuth, V. S., Plotnick, C. A., Ryan, C. E., & Schiller, S. (1997). Right turns only: An evaluation of a video-based, multicultural drug education series for seventh graders. *Health Education and Behavior, 24,* 555–567.

Garrison, C., Schoenbach, V., Schluchter, I., Kaplan, M., & Berton, H. (1987). Life events in early adolescence. *Journal of the American Academy of Child and Adolescent Psychiatry, 26,* 865–872.

Gary, L., & Berry, G. (1985). Predicting attitudes toward substance use in a black community: Implications for prevention. *Community Mental Health Journal, 21,* 42–51.

Gary, L., & Littlefield, M. (1998). The protective factor model: Strengths-oriented prevention for African American families. In F. Brisbane (Ed.), *Cultural competence for health care professionals working with African-American communities: Theory and practice* (CSAP Cultural Competence Series No. 7, DHHS Publication No. 98-3228, pp. 81–105). Rockville, MD: Center for Substance Abuse Prevention.

Gasch, H., Poulson, D. M., Fullilove, R. E., & Fullilove, M. T. (1991). Shaping AIDS education and prevention programs for African Americans amidst community decline. *Journal of Negro Education, 60,* 85–96.

Goddard, L. (1993a). *Background and scope of the alcohol and other drug problem* (DHHS Publication No. SMA 93-2015). Rockville, MD: Substance Abuse and Mental Health Services Administration.

Goddard, L. (1993b). *Natural resistors in AOD abuse prevention* (DHHS Publication No. SMA 93-2015). Rockville, MD: Substance Abuse and Mental Health Services Administration.

Gorey, K. M., & Vena, J. E. (1994). Cancer differentials among U.S. blacks and whites: Quantitative estimates of socioeconomic-related risks. *Journal of the National Medical Association, 86,* 209–215.

Gottfredson, D. C., & Koper, C. S. (1996). Race and sex differences in the prediction of drug use. *Journal of Consulting and Clinical Psychology, 64,* 305–313.

Graham, J. W., Johnson, C. A., Hansen, W. B., Flay, B. R., & Gee, M. (1990). Drug use prevention programs, gender, and ethnicity: Evaluation of three seventh-grade Project SMART cohorts. *Preventive Medicine, 19,* 305–313.

Greene, L., Smith, M., & Peters, S. (1995). "I Have a Future" comprehensive adolescent health promotion: Cultural considerations in program implementation and design. *Journal of Health Care for the Poor and Underserved, 6,* 267–281.

Gritz, E. R., Prokhorov, A. V., Hudmon, K. S., Chamberlain, R. M., Taylor, W. C., DiClemente, C. C., Johnston, D. A., Hu, S., Jones, L. A., Jones, M. M., Rosenblum, C. K., Ayars, C. L., & Amos, C. I. (1998). Cigarette smoking in a multiethnic population of youth: Methods and baseline findings. *Preventive Medicine, 27,* 365–384.

Hahn, L. P., Folsom, A. R., Sprafka, J. M., & Norsted, S. W. (1990). Cigarette smoking and cessation behaviors among urban blacks and whites. *Public Health Reports, 105,* 290–295.

Hahn, R. A., Teutsch, S. M., Franks, A. L., Chang, M. H., & Lloyd, E. E. (1998). The prevalence of risk factors among women in the United States by race and age, 1992–1994: Opportunities for primary and secondary prevention. *Journal of the American Medical Women's Association, 53,* 96–104, 107.

Hansen, W., & Graham, J. (1991). Preventing alcohol, marijuana, and cigarette use among adolescents: Peer pressure resistance training versus establishing conservative norms. *Preventive Medicine, 20,* 414–430.

Harrell, J. S., & Gore, S. V. (1998). Cardiovascular risk factors and socioeconomic status in African American and Caucasian women. *Research in Nursing and Health, 21,* 285–295.

Harrington, N. G., & Donohew, L. (1997). Jump start: A targeted substance abuse prevention program. *Health Education and Behavior, 24,* 568–586.

Harris, N. (1992). A philosophical basis for an Afrocentric orientation. *Western Journal of Black Studies, 6,* 154–159.

Harvey, W. (1985, Winter). Alcohol abuse and the black community: A contemporary analysis. *Journal of Drug Issues,* pp. 81–90.

Headen, S., Bauman, K., Deane, G., & Koch, G. (1991). Are the correlates of cigarette smoking initiation different for black and white adolescents? *American Journal of Public Health, 81,* 854–858.

Heath, S. (1989). Oral and literate traditions among black Americans living in poverty. *American Psychologist, 44,* 363–373.

Hecht, M. L., Collier, M. J., & Ribeau, S. A. (1993). *African American communication: Ethnic identity and cultural interpretation.* Thousand Oaks, CA: Sage.

Helms, J. E. (1990). *Black and white racial identity: Theory, research, and practice.* Westport: CT: Greenwood Press.

Henderson, D. J., Sampselle, C., Mayes, F., & Oakley, D. (1992). Toward culturally sensitive research in a multicultural society. *Health Care for Women International, 13,* 339–350.

Herd, D. (1990). Subgroup differences in drinking patterns among black and white men: Results from a national survey. *Journal of Studies on Alcohol, 51,* 221–232.

Herd, D., & Grube, J. (1996). Black identity and drinking in the U.S.: A national study. *Addiction, 91,* 845–857.

Hymowitz, N., Corle, D., Royce, J., Hartwell, T., Corbett, K., Orlandi, M., & Piland, N. (1995). Smokers' baseline characteristics in the COMMIT trial. *Preventive Medicine, 24,* 503–508.

Isaacs, M. R., & Benjamin, M. P. (1991). *Toward a culturally competent system of care* (Vol. 2). Washington, DC: Georgetown University Child Development Center.

Kann, L., Kinchen, S. A., Williams, B. I., Ross, J. G., Lowry, R., Hill, C. V., Grunbaum, J. A., Blumson, P. S., Collins, J. L., & Kolbe, L. J. (1998). Youth risk behavior surveillance: United States, 1997 (CDC Surveillance Summaries). *Morbidity and Mortality Weekly Report, 47,* 1–89.

Klonoff, E. A., & Landrine, H. (1997). Distrust of whites, acculturation, and AIDS knowledge among African Americans. *Journal of Black Psychology, 23,* 50–57.

Koepke, D., Flay, B., & Johnson, C. (1990). Health behaviors in minority families: The case of cigarette smoking. *Family and Community Health, 13,* 35–43.

Krieger, N., Rowley, D., Herman, A., Avery, B., & Phillips, M. (1993). Racism, sexism, and social class: Implications for studies of health, disease, and well-being. *American Journal of Preventive Medicine, 9,* 82–122.

Krueger, R. A. (1988). *Focus groups: A practical guide for applied research.* Thousand Oaks, CA: Sage.

Kumanyika, S. K., Morssink, C., & Agurs, T. (1992). Models for dietary and weight change in African-American women: Identifying cultural components. *Ethnicity and Disease, 2,* 166–175.

Kumanyika, S. K., Wilson, J., & Guilford-Davenport, M. (1993). Weight-related attitudes and behaviors of black women. *Journal of the American Dietetic Association, 93,* 416–422.

Lalonde, B., Rabinowitz, P., Shefsky, M. L., & Washienko, K. (1997). *La Esperanza del Valle:* Alcohol prevention novellas for Hispanic youth and their families. *Health Education and Behavior, 24,* 587–602.

Landrine, H., Richardson, J., Klonoff, E., & Flay, B. (1994). Cultural diversity in the predictors of adolescent cigarette smoking: The relative influence of peers. *Journal of Behavioral Medicine, 17,* 331–346.

Lantz, P. M., House, J. S., Lepkowski, J. M., Williams, D. R., Mero, R. P., & Chen, J. (1998). Socioeconomic factors, health behaviors, and mortality: Results from a nationally representative prospective study of U.S. adults. *Journal of the American Medical Association, 279,* 1703–1708.

Lillie-Blanton, M., MacKenzie, E., & Anthony, J. C. (1991). Black-white differences in alcohol use by women: Baltimore survey findings. *Public Health Reports, 106,* 124–133.

London, F. (1991). How-to's for greater cultural sensitivity. *Advancing Clinical Care, 6*(6), 42.

Long, L. (1993). *An Afrocentric intervention strategy* (DHHS Publication No. SMA 93-2015). Rockville, MD: Substance Abuse and Mental Health Services Administration.

Longshore, D. (1997). Treatment motivation among Mexican American drug-using arrestees. *Hispanic Journal of Behavioral Sciences, 19,* 214–229.

Maibach, E., & Parrott, R. (1995). *Designing health messages: Approaches from communication theory and public health practice.* Thousand Oaks, CA: Sage.

Marin, G., Burhansstipanov, L., Connell, C. M., Gielen, A. C., Helitzer-Allen, D., Lorig, K., Morisky, D. E., Tenney, M., & Thomas, S. (1995). A research agenda for health education among underserved populations. *Health Education Quarterly, 22,* 346–363.

Maypole, D. E., & Anderson, R. B. (1987). Culture-specific substance abuse prevention for blacks. *Community Mental Health Journal, 23,* 135–139.

Morgan, G. (1991). Afrocentricity in social science. *Western Journal of Black Studies, 15,* 197–206.

Morris, M. (1993). *The complex nature of prevention in the African American community: The problem of conceptualization* (DHHS Publication No. SMA 93-2015). Rockville, MD: Substance Abuse and Mental Health Services Administration.

Munford, M. B. (1994). Relationship of gender, self-esteem, social class, and racial identity to depression in blacks. *Journal of Black Psychology, 20,* 157–174.

National Center for Health Statistics. (1998). *Health, United States, 1998 with socioeconomic status and health chartbook* (DHHS Publication No. PHS 98-1232). Hyattsville, MD: Author.

Neaton, J. D., Kuller, L. H., Wentworth, D., & Borhani, N. O. (1984). Total and cardiovascular mortality in relation to cigarette smoking, serum cholesterol concentration, and diastolic blood pressure among black and white males followed up for five years. *American Heart Journal, 108*(3, Pt. 2), 759–769.

Nebeling, L. C., Forman, M. R., Graubard, B. I., & Snyder, R. A. (1997). The impact of lifestyle characteristics on carotenoid intake in the United States: The 1987 National Health Interview Survey. *American Journal of Public Health, 87,* 268–271.

Neff, J., & Hoppe, S. (1992). Acculturation and drinking patterns among U.S. Anglos, blacks, and Mexican Americans. *Alcohol and Alcoholism, 27,* 293–308.

Newcomb, M., Huba, G., & Bentler, P. (1986). Desirability of various life change events among adolescents: Effects of exposure, sex, age, and ethnicity. *Journal of Research in Personality, 20,* 207–227.

Nobles, W., Goddard, L., Cavil, W., & George, P. (1993). *An African-centered model of prevention for African-American youth at high risk* (DHHS Publication No. SMA 93-2015). Hyattsville, MD: U.S. Department of Health and Human Services, Center for Substance Abuse Prevention.

Novotny, T. E., Warner, K. E., Kendrick, J. S., & Remington, P. L. (1988). Smoking by blacks and whites: Socioeconomic and demographic differences. *American Journal of Public Health, 78,* 1187–1189.

Oetting, E. R., & Beauvais, F. (1990). Adolescent drug use: Findings of national and local surveys. *Journal of Consulting and Clinical Psychology, 58,* 385–394.

Orlandi, M. (1986). Community-based substance abuse prevention: A multicultural perspective. *Journal of School Health, 56,* 394–401.

Oyserman, D., Gant, L., & Ager, J. (1995). A socially contextualized model of African American identity: Possible selves and school persistence. *Journal of Personality and Social Psychology, 69,* 1216–1232.

Pamuk, E., Makuc, D., Heck, K., & Lochner, K. (1998). *Health, United States 1998: Socioeconomic status and health chartbook.* Hyattsville, MD: National Center for Health Statistics, DHHS publication no. 98-1232.

Pappas, G., Queen, S., Hadden, W., & Fisher, G. (1993). The increasing disparity in mortality between socioeconomic groups in the United States, 1960 and 1986. *New England Journal of Medicine, 329,* 103–109. (See also the notice of an error in this article in *New England Journal of Medicine, 329,* 1139)

Parham, T., & Helms, J. (1981). The influence of black students' racial identity attitudes on preferences for counselor's race. *Journal of Counseling Psychology, 28,* 250–257.

Parham, T., & Helms, J. (1985a). Attitudes of racial identity and self-esteem of black students: An exploratory investigation. *Journal of College Student Personnel, 26,* 143–147.

Parham, T., & Helms, J. (1985b). Relation of racial identity attitudes to self-actualization and affective states of black students. *Journal of Counseling Psychology, 32,* 431–440.

Parnell, K., Sargent, R., Thompson, S. H., Duhe, S. F., Valois, R. F., & Kemper, R. C. (1996). Black and white adolescent females' perceptions of ideal body size. *Journal of School Health, 66,* 112–118.

Pasick, R., D'Onofrio, C., & Otero-Sabogal, R. (1996). Similarities and differences across cultures: Questions to inform a third generation for health promotion research. *Health Education Quarterly, 23*(Suppl.), S142–S161.

Patterson, B., & Block, G. (1988). Food choices and the cancer guidelines. *American Journal of Public Health, 78,* 282–286.

Perez-Stable, E. J., Herrera, B., Jacob, P., III, & Benowitz, N. L. (1998). Nicotine metabolism and intake in black and white smokers. *Journal of the American Medical Association, 280,* 152–156.

Phinney, J. S., & Chavira, V. (1992). Ethnic identity and self-esteem: An exploratory longitudinal study. *Journal of Adolescence, 15,* 271–281.

Pinkett, J. (1993). *Spirituality in the African American community* (DHHS Publication No. SMA 93-2015). Rockville, MD: Substance Abuse and Mental Health Services Administration.

Ramirez, A. G., Gallion, K. J., Espinoza, R., McAlister, A., & Chalela, P. (1997). Developing a media- and school-based program for substance abuse prevention among Hispanic youth: A case study of Mirame: Look at me. *Health Education and Behavior, 24,* 603–612.

Randolph, S. M., & Banks, H. D. (1993). Making a way out of no way: The promise of Africentric approaches to HIV prevention. *Journal of Black Psychology, 19,* 204–214.

Resnicow, K., Braithwaite, R., Ahluwalia, J., & Baranowski, T. (1999). Cultural sensitivity in public health: Defined and demystified. *Ethnicity and Disease, 9,* 10–21.

Resnicow, K., Coleman-Wallace, D., Jackson, A., DiGirolamo, A., Odom, E., Wang, T., Dudley, W., Davis, M., & Baranowski, T. (2000). Dietary change through black churches: Baseline results and program description of the Eat for Life Trial. *Journal of Cancer Education, 15,* 156–163.

Resnicow, K., & Ross, D. (1997). Development of a racial identity questionnaire for African American adults. *Journal of Black Studies, 23,* 239–254.

Resnicow, K., Soler, R., Braithwaite, R., Selassie, M., & Smith, M. (1999). Development and validation of a racial identity scale for African American adolescents: The Survey of Black Life. *Journal of Black Psychology, 25,* 171–188.

Resnicow, K., Vaughan, R., Futterman, R., Weston, R., & Harlem Health Connection Study Group. (1997). A self-help smoking cessation program for inner-city African Americans: Results from the Harlem Health Connection Project. *Health Education and Behavior, 24,* 201–217.

Resnicow, K., Wang, T., Dudley, W. N., Wallace, D., Jackson, A., Ahluwalia, J. S., Baranowski, T., & Braithwaite, R. L. (in press). Risk factor distribution among sociodemographically diverse African American adults. *Journal of Urban Health.*

Ringwalt, C., & Palmer, J. (1990). Differences between white and black youth who drink heavily. *Addictive Behaviors, 15,* 455–460.

Robinson, L. A., Klesges, R. C., Zbikowski, S. M., & Glaser, R. (1997). Predictors of risk for different stages of adolescent smoking in a biracial sample. *Journal of Consulting and Clinical Psychology, 65,* 653–662.

Royce, J. M., Hymowitz, N., Corbett, K., Hartwell, T. D., & Orlandi, M. A. (1993). Smoking cessation factors among African Americans and whites [COMMIT Research Group]. *American Journal of Public Health, 83,* 220–226.

Sabogal, F., Otero-Sabogal, R., Pasick, R., Jenkins, C., & Perez-Stable, E. (1996). Printed health education materials for diverse communities: Suggestions learned from the field. *Health Education Quarterly, 23*(Suppl.), S123–S141.

Sasao, T. (1998). The cultural context of epidemiologic research. In F. Brisbane (Ed.), *Cultural competence for health care professionals working with African-American communities: Theory and practice* (CSAP Cultural Competence Series No. 7, DHHS Publication No. 98-3228, pp. 183–212). Rockville, MD: Center for Substance Abuse Prevention.

Sawyer, L., Regev, H., Proctor, S., Nelson, M., Messias, D., Barnes, D., & Meleis, A. I. (1995). Matching versus cultural competence in research: Methodological considerations. *Research in Nursing and Health, 18,* 557–567.

Scherwitz, L., Perkins, L., Chesney, M., Hughes, G., Sidney, S., & Manolio, T. (1992). Hostility and health behaviors in young adults: The CARDIA Study (Coronary Artery Risk Development in Young Adults Study). *American Journal of Epidemiology, 136,* 136–145.

Schiele, J. H. (1996). Afrocentricity: An emerging paradigm in social work practice. *Social Work, 41,* 284–294.

Schinke, S., Moncher, M., Palleja, J., Zayas, L., & Schilling, R. (1988). Hispanic youth, substance abuse, and stress: Implications for prevention research. *International Journal of the Addictions, 23,* 809–826.

Schlesinger, E. G., & Devore, W. (1995). Ethnic sensitive social work practice: The state of the art. *Journal of Sociology and Social Welfare, 22,* 29–58.

Scribner, R., Hohn, A., & Dwyer, J. (1995). Blood pressure and self-concept among African-American adolescents. *Journal of the National Medical Association, 87,* 417–422.

Shea, S., Stein, A., Basch, C., Lantigua, R., Maylahn, C., Strogatz, D., & Novick, L. (1991). Independent associations of educational attainment and ethnicity with behavioral risk factors for cardiovascular disease. *American Journal of Epidemiology, 134,* 567–582.

Shintani, T., Beckham, S., O'Connor, H., Hughes, C., & Sato, A. (1994). The Waianae Diet Program: A culturally sensitive, community-based obesity and clinical intervention program for the Native Hawaiian population. *Hawaii Medical Journal, 53*(5), 136–141, 147.

Simons-Morton, B. G., Donohew, L., & Crump, A. D. (1997). Health communication in the prevention of alcohol, tobacco, and drug use. *Health Education and Behavior, 24,* 544–554.

Singer, M. (1991). Confronting the AIDS epidemic among IV drug users: Does ethnic culture matter? *AIDS Education and Prevention, 3,* 258–283.

Smith, G. D., Neaton, J. D., Wentworth, D., Stamler, R., & Stamler, J. (1996). Socioeconomic differentials in mortality risk among men screened for the Multiple Risk Factor Intervention Trial: 1. White men. *American Journal of Public Health, 86,* 486–496.

Smith, G. D., Wentworth, D., Neaton, J. D., Stamler, R., & Stamler, J. (1996). Socioeconomic differentials in mortality risk among men screened for the Multiple Risk Factor Intervention Trial: 2. Black men. *American Journal of Public Health, 86,* 497–504.

Soet, J. E., DiIorio, C., & Dudley, W. N. (1998). Women's self-reported condom use: Intra- and interpersonal factors. *Women and Health, 27,* 19–32.

Soet, J. E., Dudley, W. N., & DiIorio, C. (1999). The effects of ethnicity and perceived power on women's sexual behavior. *Psychology of Women Quarterly, 23,* 707–723.

Sprafka, J. M., Folsom, A. R., Burke, G. L., & Edlavitch, S. A. (1988). Prevalence of cardiovascular disease risk factors in blacks and whites: The Minnesota Heart Survey. *American Journal of Public Health, 78,* 1546–1549.

Stephens, T., Braithwaite, R., & Taylor, S. (1998). Model for using hip-hop music for small group HIV/AIDS prevention counseling with African American adolescents and young adults. *Patient Education and Counseling, 35,* 127–137.

Stevens, J., Kumanyika, S. K., & Keil, J. (1994). Attitudes toward body size and dieting: Differences between elderly black and white women. *American Journal of Public Health, 84,* 1322–1325.

Sue, D., Mak, W. S., & Sue, D. W. (1998). Ethnic identity. In L. C. Lee & N.W.S. Zane (Eds.), *Handbook of Asian American psychology* (pp. 289–323). Thousand Oaks, CA: Sage.

Sue, D. W., & Sue, D. (1999). *Counseling the culturally different: Theory and practice* (3rd ed.). New York: Wiley.

Sussman, S., Dent, C., Flay, B., Hansen, W., & Johnson, C. (1987). Psychosocial predictors of cigarette smoking onset by white, black, Hispanic, and Asian adolescents in Southern California. *Morbidity and Mortality Weekly Report, 36*(4, Suppl.), 11S–16S.

Sussman, S., Parker, V. C., Lopes, C., Crippens, D. L., Elder, P., & Scholl, D. (1995). Empirical development of brief smoking prevention videotapes which target African-American adolescents. *International Journal of the Addictions, 30,* 1141–1164.

Swendson, C., & Windsor, C. (1996). Rethinking cultural sensitivity. *Nursing Inquiry, 3,* 3–10, 11–12.

Thomas, M., Bethlehem, L., & Holmes, B. (1992). Determinants of satisfaction for blacks and whites. *Sociological Quarterly, 33,* 459–472.

Thompson, V. S. (1992). A multifaceted approach to the conceptualization of African American identification. *Journal of Black Studies, 23,* 75–85.

Trimble, J. (1990–1991). Ethnic specification, validation prospects, and the future of drug use research. *International Journal of the Addictions, 25,* 149–170.

University of Michigan. (1997). *Monitoring the Future study: 1997 results.* [On-line]. Available: www.icpsr.umich.edu/cgi/ab.prl?file=247

U.S. Department of Health and Human Services. (1990a). *Alcohol and other drug use among Hispanic youth* (DHHS Publication No. ADM 90-1726). Rockville, MD: Alcohol Drug Abuse, and Mental Health Administration, Office for Substance Abuse Prevention.

U.S. Department of Health and Human Services. (1990b). *Ecology of alcohol and other drug use: Helping black high-risk youth* (OSAP Prevention Monograph No. 7, DHHS Publication No. ADM 90-1672). Rockville, MD: Alcohol Drug Abuse, and Mental Health Administration, Office for Substance Abuse Prevention.

U.S. Department of Health and Human Services. (1998a). *Prevalence of substance use among racial and ethnic subgroups in the United States, 1991–1993* (DHHS Publication No. SMA 98-3202). Rockville, MD: Substance Abuse and Mental Health Services Administration, Office of Applied Studies.

U.S. Department of Health and Human Services. (1998b). *Tobacco use among U.S. racial/ethnic minority groups: A report of the surgeon general.* Atlanta, GA: National Center for Chronic Disease Prevention and Health Promotion, Office on Smoking and Health.

Vega, W. A., Zimmerman, R. S., Warheit, G. J., Apospori, E., & Gil, A. G. (1993). Risk factors for early adolescent drug use in four ethnic and racial groups. *American Journal of Public Health, 83,* 185–189.

Wagenknecht, L. E., Perkins, L. L., Cutter, G. R., Sidney, S., Burke, G. L., Manolio, T. A., Jacobs, D. R., Jr., Liu, K. A., Friedman, G. D., Hughes, G. H., & Hulley, S. B. (1990). Cigarette smoking behavior is strongly related to educational status: The CARDIA Study. *Preventive Medicine, 19,* 158–169.

Wallace, J. M., Jr., & Bachman, J. G. (1993). Validity of self-reports in student-based studies on minority populations: Issues and concerns. In *Drug abuse among minority youth* (NIDA Research Monograph No. 130, pp. 167–200). Bethesda, MD: National Institutes of Health, National Institute on Drug Abuse.

Ward, J. V. (1995). Cultivating a morality of care in African American adolescents: A culture-based model of violence prevention. *Harvard Educational Review, 65,* 175–188.

Williams, D. R. (1990). Socioeconomic differentials in health: A review and redirection. *Social Psychology Quarterly, 53,* 81–99.

Williams, D. R. (1995). U.S. socioeconomic and racial differences in health: Patterns and explanations. *Annual Review of Sociology, 21,* 349–386.

Wills, T. A., & Cleary, S. D. (1997). The validity of self-reports of smoking: Analyses by race/ethnicity in a school sample of urban adolescents. *American Journal of Public Health, 87,* 56–61.

Winkleby, M. A., Kraemer, H. C., Ahn, D. K., & Varady, A. N. (1998). Ethnic and socio-economic differences in cardiovascular disease risk factors: Findings for women from the Third National Health and Nutrition Examination Survey, 1988–1994 [see the comments]. *Journal of the American Medical Association, 280,* 356–362.

Winkleby, M. A., Robinson, T. N., Sundquist, J., & Kraemer, H. C. (1999). Ethnic variation in cardiovascular disease risk factors among children and young adults: Findings from the Third National Health and Nutrition Examination Survey, 1988–1994. *Journal of the American Medical Association, 281,* 1006–1013.

Yee, A., Fairchild, H., Weizmann, F., & Wyatt, G. (1993). Addressing psychology's problem with race. *American Psychologist, 48,* 1132–1140.

CHAPTER TWENTY-SIX

CLOSING THE GAP

Eliminating Health Disparities

Stephen B. Thomas, Sandra Crouse Quinn

The purpose of this chapter is to provide the reader with a social and historical context for understanding how best to improve the health status of African Americans. To accomplish our task we must go back to the future. In other words, we believe solutions to the problem of poor health status among African Americans already exist and can be harvested from black history. It is not only a history of pain and suffering but also a history of self-reliance and creativity. For black people in the twenty-first century, health promotion and disease prevention can become a mass movement, on the scale of the civil rights movement of the 1960s. Mobilization of black people in such a mass movement can generate multiracial coalitions that can drive the political will essential to addressing the full range of health issues described in this book, from organ and tissue donation to environmental justice.

The disparity in health status between black and white Americans was not new when it was so well documented in the 1985 *Report of the Secretary's Task Force on Black and Minority Health* (U.S. Department of Health and Human Services [DHHS], 1985). The task force identified the six leading causes of preventable excess deaths for minority populations: cancer, cardiovascular disease, diabetes, infant mortality, chemical dependency, and homicide/unintentional injury. It employed the term *excess death* to describe the difference between the number of deaths for each age group in racial minority populations and the numbers of deaths that would be expected in those same age groups in the white majority population; by this standard, blacks experienced a 42 percent excess mortality rate when compared to whites. In 1985, these findings led to the creation of the Office of Minority Health in the U.S. Department of Health and Human Services (DHHS).

On June 14, 1997, President Clinton announced an unprecedented national campaign titled One America in the Twenty-First Century: The President's Initiative on Race. This initiative was described as a critical element in the president's effort to prepare our country to live united as one nation (DHHS, 1998). The president called together the members of his cabinet and requested that each of them respond to the challenge of living as one nation within the context of their agencies. The secretary of Health and Human Services, Donna Shalala, responded to the president's call with a broad community-based campaign focused on the health status of racial and ethnic minority populations.

In 1998, the president committed the nation to an ambitious goal to be achieved by the year 2010: eliminate the disparities experienced by racial and ethnic minority populations in six areas of health status while continuing the progress made in improving the overall health of the American people. The priority areas for elimination of health disparities are (1) infant mortality, (2) cancer screening and management, (3) cardiovascular diseases, (4) diabetes, (5) HIV/AIDS, and (6) adult and child immunization. DHHS secretary Shalala spearheaded the Closing the Gap campaign, with leadership from David Satcher, former surgeon general of the United States (Goodwin, 2000; DHHS, 1998).

Eliminating Racial and Ethnic Health Disparities

It is noteworthy that the goals embodied in the Closing the Gap campaign have been made an integral component of Healthy People 2010, the nation's health objectives for the twenty-first century. This unprecedented effort will require a major national commitment to identifying and addressing the underlying causes of higher levels of disease and disability in the African American community. The ultimate aim is to uncover social, cultural, and environmental factors beyond the factors found in the biomedical model and address a broad range of issues. This approach includes, but is not limited to, breaking the cycle of poverty, increasing access to quality health care, eliminating environmental hazards in homes and neighborhoods, and implementing effective prevention programs tailored to specific community needs. Engaging the African American community as partners in health promotion and disease prevention in this campaign requires an appreciation for cultural identity in the context of an increasingly diverse American society.

The Burdens of Race and History

For more than two hundred years the United States has been the most culturally diverse country in the world. That diversity continues with the influx of individuals from more and more cultures from the around the globe. Racial and ethnic minorities are the fastest-growing segments of the U.S. population, composing almost 20 percent of the total population in 1990 and increasing to 25 percent by the turn of the century. Nonwhite children, those younger than nineteen years of age, are expected to account for one-third of all children in the year 2000 (Yax, 1999). Culture also affects how chronic and disabling conditions are defined and treated. For example, white Americans typically emphasize physical survival and functional capacity and therefore tend to battle against chronic conditions and disabilities that they see inflicted on them. In contrast, many Asian cultures emphasize living in harmony with nature; thus a chronic condition is seen as part of the normal cycle of life. A person's culturally based health beliefs and practices determine what problems he or she will recognize as needing traditional Western medical care and whether he or she will follow through with prescribed treatment, change lifestyle behaviors, or reduce exposure to environmental factors associated with the illness. An additional factor for African Americans is that because of historical inequalities and racism in the health care system, many African Americans may delay seeking care. Beliefs about health and illness also influence community responses to health communication messages designed to promote health and prevent disease. Moreover, language differences and cultural differences can hinder communication between public health professionals and members of ethnic and racial minority populations (Joseph-Di Caprio, Garwick, Kohrman, & Blum, 1999).

Cultural Identity Defined

The classic definition of culture, written in 1871 by Edward Burnett Tylor, states that "culture . . . is that complex whole which includes knowledge, beliefs, art, morals, law, customs, and any other capabilities and habits acquired by man as a member of society" (quoted in Saraf, 1997, p. 874). In 1952, Kroeber and Kluckhohn cited 164 definitions of culture, ranging from "learned behavior" to "ideas in the mind" (quoted in Saraf, 1997, p. 874). Culture depends upon the ability, possessed by humans alone, of *symboling*, which consists of "assigning to things and events certain meanings that cannot be grasped with the senses alone." Language is a good example of symboling (Saraf, 1997, p. 847).

To understand cultural identity in the context of public health, we must focus on those worldviews shared by the people we seek to serve. It is from this perspective that the meanings of words used to describe diseases and the adaptive behaviors needed to prevent premature illness and death must be explored. We must be cognizant that people live their lives as simultaneous members of and participants in a multiplicity of social contexts. Thus cultural identity may be shaped in part by the location where an individual spent his or her youth— a rural, urban or suburban setting. But cultural identity is complex. It is also necessary to take into consideration an individual's language, age, gender, cohort, family configuration, race, ethnicity, religion, nationality, socioeconomic status, occupation, education, sexual orientation, political ideology, migration status, and stage of acculturation into the society in which he or she currently lives (Falicov, 1995).

The science of epidemiology enables public health professionals to systematically assess the health status of populations. However, when illness and death data are used without an appreciation for social context, unintended consequences can result. For example, it is not uncommon to use surveillance data to describe populations as "noncompliant," "intravenous drug users," "homeless," "high risk," and "hard to reach." Although such categorization enables public health professionals to focus scarce resources where the need is greatest, it also stigmatizes the very people in greatest need of assistance by implying that they are somehow responsible for their diseases. Ethnic and racial minority populations have historically suffered the burden of stigma directly related to the ways public health data is presented to policymakers and the general public.

Because culture influences the way communities view and take action on disease conditions that can be treated and prevented, public health professionals seeking to close the health status gap will increasingly need to understand the cultural context in which disease prevention and health promotion strategies are delivered. In particular, we must overcome the persistent legacy of abuses from the past, from slavery to the syphilis study at Tuskegee.

Anatomy of the President's Apology for the Tuskegee Syphilis Study

Back in the 1940s, when Nazi doctors went on trial for unethical experiments on humans, the world heard the term *research crime* for the first time. Most Americans thought such abuses could never happen here. However, on a hot summer day in July 1972, the front-page story in newspapers across the nation described an experiment sponsored by the U.S. government. In Macon County, Alabama, a sample of black men was left untreated for syphilis. Over four decades, even as some of these men died, the government went to great lengths to ensure that men in the Tuskegee Syphilis Study were denied treatment, even after penicillin became the standard of care in the mid 1940s.

A quarter century after that public revelation, on May 16, 1997, in the East Room of the White House, President Bill Clinton issued a formal apology for the longest nontherapeutic experiment on human beings in the history of medicine and public health. The study, conducted under the auspices of the U.S. Public Health Service (PHS), was originally projected to last six months but spanned forty years, from 1932 to 1972. The purpose of the study was to determine the effect of untreated syphilis in black men. The men were never told that they had the sexually transmitted disease. Instead, government doctors told the men they had "bad blood," a term that was commonly used to describe a wide range of unspecified maladies. The 600 black men in the study (399 with syphilis and a control group of 201 who did not have the disease) were the sons and grandsons of slaves. Most had never been seen by a doctor. When announcements were made in churches and in the cotton fields about a way to receive free medical care, the men showed up in droves. Little did they know the high price they would pay over the next four decades as they were poked and prodded by an endless array of government medical personnel. Even as some men went blind and insane from advanced (tertiary) syphilis, the government doctors withheld treatment, remaining committed to observing their subjects through to the study's predetermined "end point," autopsy. To ensure that the families would agree to this final procedure, the government offered them burial insurance, at most fifty dollars, to cover the cost of a casket and grave.

The research project was finally stopped after Peter Buxtun, a former venereal disease investigator with the PHS, shared the truth about the study's unethical methods with a reporter from the Associated Press. On July 25, 1972, news accounts sparked a public outcry that ultimately brought the notorious experiment to an end. Congressional hearings led to federal legislation that strengthened the guidelines for protection of human subjects in research. Fred Gray, a civil rights attorney, filed a $1.8 billion class action lawsuit on behalf of the men that resulted in a $10 million out-of-court settlement for the victims, their families, and their heirs (Thomas & Quinn, 1997; Jones, 1993; Thomas & Quinn, 1991; Clinton, 1997; Thomas & Quinn, 2000). Almost twenty-five years later, however, there remains among many African Americans a legacy of deep mistrust that hampers efforts to promote health and prevent disease.

During the ceremony in the East Room of the White House, the president directed his words to Carter Howard, Frederick Moss, Charlie Pollard, Herman Shaw, Fred Simmons, Sam Doner, Ernest Hendon, and George Key (the study's sole survivors)—all of whom are over ninety years old and the first five of whom were present for the occasion—saying:

> [They] are a living link to a time not so very long ago that many Americans would prefer not to remember but we dare not forget. It was a time when our nation failed to live up to its ideals, when our nation broke the trust . . . that is the very foundation of our democracy. The United States government did something that was wrong, deeply, profoundly, morally wrong. To the survivors, to the wives and family members, the children and the grandchildren, I say what you know: No power on Earth can give you back the lives lost, the pain suffered, the years of internal torment and anguish. What was done cannot be undone. But we can end the silence. We can stop turning our heads away. We can look at you in the eye and finally say on behalf of the American people, what the United States government did was shameful, and I am sorry [Clinton, 1997].

Clinton and the other persons present experienced the power of forgiveness from men who suffered at the hands of doctors in the PHS. In that emotional statement, the president apologized on behalf of the American people, something his five predecessors had not done. He placed responsibility for the abuse on the medical research establishment when he stated, "The people who ran the study at Tuskegee diminished the stature of man by abandoning the most basic ethical precepts. They forgot their pledge to heal and repair." The government, Clinton announced, was providing a $200,000 grant to help establish a center for bioethics in research and health care at Tuskegee University as part of a lasting "memorial" to the study's victims. Shaw, aged ninety-four, expressed gratitude to Clinton "for doing your best to right this wrong tragedy and to resolve that Americans should never again allow such an event to occur." The legacy of Tuskegee goes well beyond the syphilis study; it is a defining part of the history of racism and discrimination in the United States.

On May 15, 1999, the authors of this chapter went to Macon County, Alabama, to participate in the anniversary of the president's apology. Parts of Macon County look the same as they did in 1932. The route to Tuskegee Square pushes past shaky mobile homes and a decrepit motel, between eroded embankments of red clay that look like gashes in flesh. We shook the hands of three of the eight men still alive from the 623 who unwittingly took part in the Tuskegee Study. The leather-soft hands of Mr. Charles Pollard, 93 at the time; Mr. Herman Shaw, who was 95; and Mr. Fred Simmons, who was 103, were strong as a vise. These men have lived long enough to see a definitive chapter in the history of race and medicine in America. The president of the United States apologized to them on behalf of the government that wronged them. Today, however, the survivors of the Tuskegee Syphilis Study remain economically poor, living in the same town and attending the same churches where they were recruited into the study back in 1932.

For many black people the legacy of Tuskegee generates anger that hangs in the air like smoke. People are not laboratory animals. No one should be allowed to suffer when a proven treatment is available, as penicillin was available for the treatment of syphilis by the early 1940s. Using people in medical research without their informed consent is ethically unconscionable. It is particularly so when one engages in a subterfuge to do so and when the people are as vulnerable as the men in the Tuskegee Study were because of their poverty and lack of access to any other medical care. For far too many African Americans, the legacy of Tuskegee is a shadow over biomedical research, medicine, and public health practice. This shadow can be used as a reason not to take full advantage of early treatment for preventable diseases and not to participate in clinical research. Additionally, the underrepresentation of blacks as blood donors, their reluctance to sign organ donor cards, their fear of being tested for AIDS, and their hesitancy to have their children immunized threatens the health and well-being of us all. Trust, once given unconditionally, now must be earned. How can black people now trust what their doctor tells them, what public health agencies tell them, when they know the men in the Tuskegee study had syphilis and were not treated?

Yet for others the presidential apology is the thorn on the rose. Remarkably, the Tuskegee study still has its defenders; some of them are African Americans (White, 1999; Benedek, 1999; White, 2000). Some say it was a valid and well-intentioned effort to learn more about a disease that was rampant among black men in Macon County. They say the men were not harmed and probably were helped by taking part in the study. The government doctors who ran the study were viewed as progressive compared to local physicians at the time. The Rosenwald Fund that financed the initial syphilis control work was dedicated to increasing the number of "Negro" health professionals in the South. It is indeed ironic that over the forty years of the Tuskegee study the men had regular visits from government doctors. Today, Tuskegee, Alabama, has no twenty-four-hour health care facility. The men in the Tuskegee study trusted their doctors; today, syphilis is an epidemic in parts of the South where many black people do not trust the treatment (Gamble & Fletcher, 1996; Thomas & Thomas, 1999; Thomas et al., 1999).

The nation and the African American community heard "I'm sorry" from a president who was not even alive in 1932 when the Tuskegee study began. Over the years the Tuskegee study has undergone a transformation from science to conspiracy to metaphor. It is an American tragedy made of a volatile confluence of race, science, and medicine. It is part of the collective memory of many African Americans, fueling their suspicion and fear of medical and public health research. The legacy of Tuskegee is still being deeply woven into the tapestry of life and living in America. An indelible pattern is evolving as each of us responds to the contingencies and values the Tuskegee study exposed. This legacy connects us to all people who suffer under oppression, from the Africans on the middle passage, to the Native American tribes forced to extinction, to the victims of the Holocaust, to the survivors of apartheid. The president's apology is an expression of our humanity, a balm on our sores of resentment and retaliation.

An apology from the president will not heal all the wounds, but it is an essential gesture in the healing process and a cue for the rest of us to move toward atonement and racial reconciliation. The president's apology may be the crucial first step in addressing the fear and mistrust that shapes the behavior and attitudes of many African Americans not only toward participating in medical research but also toward receiving the health care that they need and deserve.

It is important that we learn from mistakes of the past. However, we must also harvest black history to acknowledge the leaders and replicate the successful public health programs developed by and for African Americans. Booker T. Washington and his National Negro Health Week are a good place in the past from which to chart a future course for health of the black community.

Back to the Future: Lessons from the National Negro Health Movement, 1915 to 1951

Booker T. Washington, founder of the Tuskegee Institute, viewed the poor health status of black Americans as an obstacle to economic progress, and in 1914, he issued a call for "the Negro people . . . to join in a movement which shall be known as Health Improvement Week" (Patterson, 1939, p. 13). Health Improvement Week evolved into the National Negro Health Week, which lasted for thirty-five years. This section presents an overview of the structure and activities of the National Negro Health Week and suggests implications for public health in the black community today.

Although the 1985 secretary's task force report was heralded as the first comprehensive assessment of minority health, in the early part of the twentieth century the health status gap between whites and blacks was already clearly chronicled in local and state health data. In 1906, W.E.B. Du Bois edited *The Health and Physique of the Negro American*, a volume that documented that disparity. In 1914, Booker T. Washington reported that "at the last session of the Tuskegee Negro Conference, some startling facts were brought out concerning the health of the colored people of the U.S. . . . [Forty-five] percent of all deaths among Negroes were preventable; there are 450,000 Negroes seriously ill all the time; the annual cost of this illness is 75 million dollars; that sickness and death cost Negroes annually 100 million dollars" (Patterson, 1939, p. 13). These data fueled the energies of an emerging public health leadership in the black medical and lay communities that launched a thirty-five-year national movement to improve the health of black Americans. The history of this effort and its most public manifestation, the National Negro Health Week (NNHW), has long gone unnoticed in medical and public health literature.

NNHW Origins

In the early twentieth century, much of the black population lived in poverty and was concentrated in the rural South. Formal health care was often nonexistent, sanitation was poor, nutrition was inadequate, and housing substandard. The great black migration to urban areas in the North began as a search for greater economic opportunity. However, the poverty that accompanied these African Americans to the Northern cities combined with poor housing conditions and lack of access to health care contributed to the continuation of a disproportionate burden of illness and death from chronic and infectious diseases. Death rates in 1915 were 20.2 per 1,000 for blacks as compared to 12.9 for whites. The infant mortality rate for blacks was 180.6 per 1,000 live births compared to 98.6 for white babies (U.S. Public Health Service [PHS], 1950). Summarizing this disparity, Louis Dublin of the Metropolitan Life Insurance Company stated, "it is only fair to say that the Negro is by the usual measures of mortality at a point where the white race was only thirty years ago" (Dublin, 1928, p. 200, 216).

Blacks were also poorly represented in the health professions. According to Dublin (1928), there was only 1 black physician per 3,000 blacks compared to 1 physician for every 670 whites. The ratios for black dentists and nurses were comparable. However, emerging in the early part of the century was a spark of leadership in black medical and nursing associations and a strong lay public health movement predominantly spearheaded by educated black women. In 1905, under the leadership of Monroe Work, the Men's Sunday Club in Savannah, Georgia, with a focus on improving community health, was one of numerous lay efforts to address the black community's health needs. In 1906, the Atlanta Conference for the Study of the Negro Problem called for "the formation of local health leagues among colored people for the dissemination of better knowledge of sanitation and preventive medicine" (Du Bois, 1906, p. 110). Concerned about tuberculosis and syphilis, black health professionals, hospitals, churches, and civic organizations cooperated in a variety of efforts to improve the health status of black Americans.

Mounting interest in the improvement of black health status spawned two events that constitute the origins of National Negro Health Week. First, a communitywide sanitation campaign, conducted by the Negro Organization Society of Virginia in 1913, caught the attention of Booker T. Washington, who believed that "the future of the race depends upon the conservation of its health" (PHS, 1950, p. 2). The Virginia campaign helped to stimulate the 1914 Worker's Day at the Annual Tuskegee Negro Conference, during which exhibits and programs focused on the theme "fifty years of Negro health improvement in preparation for efficiency." Charts prepared by Monroe Work at Tuskegee Institute projected a reduction in death rates from 24 per 1,000 for blacks in 1913 to 12 per 1,000 in 1963. Posters featured the economic losses from disease and premature death and recommended that "length of life increases wherever sanitary science and preventive medicine are applied" (Brown, 1937, p. 554).

These two events underscored Washington's understanding of the role of health in the economic development of the black community. He stated, "Without health, and until we reduce the high death rate, it will be impossible for us to have permanent success in business, in property getting, in acquiring education, or to show other evidences of progress" (Jackson, 1924, p. 236). Washington viewed economic success, built on racial solidarity and group unity, as a key to acceptance into the mainstream of American society. It was from this vantage point that he launched the national Health Improvement Week in 1915: "Because of these facts I have thought it advisable to ask the Negro people of the whole country to join in a movement which shall be known as 'Health Improvement Week' beginning April 11 to April 17, inclusive, 1915. By means of these organizations and agencies [churches, civic organizations, business, barbershops, and so on], all the colored people can be reached and influenced. They can be taught what to do to aid in improving their health conditions. Thus the amount of sickness among us can be lessened and the number of deaths annually greatly decreased" (Patterson, 1939, p. 13). Washington and the National Negro Business League (an organization founded by Washington with the backing of industrialist Andrew Carnegie) initially promoted this week that ultimately became known as National Negro Health Week. Robert R. Moton, principal of the Tuskegee Institute following Washington's death, stated that although the National Negro Health Week "originated within the race itself," it was meant to be a cooperative effort between whites and blacks (Brown, 1937, p. 553). Washington, in a 1915 address to the first public health conference for black Marylanders in Baltimore, stated, "white people and black people throughout this State can cooperate in encouraging the Negro wherever he lives to have a clean, sanitary, healthy community" (Brown, 1937, p. 555). This theme was echoed years later during a National Negro Health Week radio broadcast by R. A. Vonderlehr (1939), a white PHS officer, when he stated, "Quite obviously the color line cannot be drawn where the prevention of disease is concerned" (p. 1).

An oversight committee at Tuskegee Institute managed the NNHW. There were two primary objectives: "(1) to provide practical suggestions for the local health week committees that conducted the week's events and (2) to stimulate the people as a whole to cooperative endeavor in clean-up, educational, and specific hygienic and clinical services for general sanitary improvement of the community and for health betterment of the individual, family, and home" (Brown, 1937, p. 555). Ultimately, a week in early April, running from Sunday to Sunday, became the regular time of the week's observance, as a memorial to Booker T. Washington whose birthday was April 5.

NNHW Community Mobilization

In the early years the annual *Health Week Bulletin,* published by the Tuskegee Institute, presented (1) the objective for the specific year's observance, (2) suggestions for each day's activities, (3) a list of organizations that could be potential collaborators, and (4) a plan of organization for local communities. The strategy for community mobilization recommended the following steps: (1) win the support of all public-spirited agencies; (2) if there is an official health department, consult the executive officer of that department and ask him to convene a meeting; (3) invite representatives from churches, schools, health agencies, medical and nursing associations, civic groups such as the Rotary and Kiwanis, fraternal orders, women's clubs, business leaders, the chamber of commerce, and all other interested groups; and (4) organize a health week central committee, choose officers, and appoint necessary subcommittees (PHS, 1926, p. 4).

This community mobilization approach was not unlike strategies advocated for contemporary efforts to develop community partnerships for public health programs. It was suggested that the central committee conduct a needs assessment survey of the community to determine the most significant health problems. The central committee then used its findings to prioritize issues to be addressed during the week. Although the Tuskegee oversight committee recommended an organizational structure for the week's activities that included a central committee and separate committees for each day, it also recognized that individual communities would ultimately determine their own organizational structure. Calling for community mobilization in a way that was sensitive to the needs of individual communities allowed the involvement of a broad array of organizations and institutions, both white and black.

Structure and Breadth of NNHW Activities

The Tuskegee oversight committee published and distributed a set of goals and activities for each day of the week. Sunday was termed Mobilization Day and featured a heavy focus on sermons about health during church services and popular mass meetings. Though the mass meetings had as one goal to announce the schedule for the remainder of the week, specific topics were also suggested by the oversight committee. In one year for example, one speaker was to focus on the human and economic cost of tuberculosis, venereal diseases, and other prevalent health conditions, and another speaker was to emphasize the effectiveness of prevention in the reduction of morbidity and mortality from these diseases. Finally, a third speaker was to stress the "value of buoyant health" (PHS, 1926). The organizers stressed the need for good speakers and good music. Sunday was chosen to start the week because the church could then play its pivotal role in mobilizing community involvement.

The focus of Monday, Home Hygiene Day, was on the "establishment of a sanitary home" (PHS, 1926, p. 4). Lectures, pamphlets, and demonstrations, both for adults and children, were the suggested educational methods. Tuesday, Community Sanitation Day, used the same educational methods to focus activities on ensuring safe water, food, and milk supplies; proper waste disposal; clean streets; safe wells; and destruction of swamp breeding grounds for insects. Collaboration with the local health department was suggested in order to carry out these activities. As Special Campaign Day, Wednesday concentrated on the specific health problem identified in the community needs assessment conducted by the health week central committee. Activities suggested included a noonday conference focusing on the specific problem with the goal of developing and immediately implementing a plan of action. For example, "if a community decided to make a renewed attack on tuberculosis, it may conclude at the noon-day conference that an additional public health nurse is necessary. With the support of the business men and others, it may be possible, before the day closes, to raise funds with which this nurse may be employed" (PHS, 1926, p. 7). Adult Health Day on Thursday emphasized annual health examinations for adults through health education programs of men's and women's organizations and clinics operated by the local medical society. Maternal and infant health clinics were also a focus for adult health day. Friday, School Health Day, offered health education programs and school-based health services. Clinics established in schools conducted screenings and provided vaccinations. Health education programs employed health essays, songs, games, and plays to focus on good health habits, and parental involvement was heavily emphasized. School clean-up activities were organized. Emphasizing health as a primary aim of education was a theme.

Designated General Cleanup Day, Saturday focused on cooperative, large-scale clean-up activities and inspection of community health campaign results. Collecting data and taking pictures for reports and newspaper stories was a key activity. As Reports and Follow-up Day, Sunday had as its focal point, community gatherings through the church and large civic meetings. The week was scheduled to end on a Sunday for the same reason it began on a Sunday, to take advantage of the role of the church as a major convener of community groups. The week culminated in a review of all activities and achievements intermingled with food, music, and inspirational speeches.

Involvement of the U.S. Public Health Service

From its inception in 1915, the Tuskegee oversight committee organized the week's activities with the support of other organizations (Brown, 1937). In a 1921 letter to Surgeon General H. S. Cumming, Moton requested assistance from the PHS in promoting National Negro Health Week and implementation of a year-round program. In response, Roscoe Brown (a dentist who had become a PHS lecturer and consultant on health education) attended that year's Annual Tuskegee Negro Conference. In 1921, the PHS assumed publication of the *NNHW Bulletin,* as the week's bulletin was now called, and beginning in 1927, produced the health week poster. Also in 1921, the U.S. surgeon general convened the first annual NNHW conference in Washington, D.C. The purpose of that meeting, which included representatives of all cooperating agencies, was the planning and evaluation of campaign activities. The conference also featured exhibits of health week reports and of the poster contest entries and a public meeting on health issues.

NNHW Strategies

Clearly, one of the most impressive aspects of the week was the scope of the activities and the breadth of the target audiences reached through a truly comprehensive effort to improve community health. The strategies used constitute an effective health communication campaign conducted through a variety of channels to reach large audiences. From church, school, clinic, and community settings, a multitude of blacks from childhood through adult years were mobilized. The use of radio broadcasts, newspapers, posters, and brochures was extensive. For example, in 1933, sixty-one radio broadcasts were reported, and in 1937, the *National Negro Health News* applauded newspapers for their extensive coverage of the week. This coverage included editorials, announcements, photographs, schedules, special news articles, and in some areas, special editions during health week (PHS, 1933b, 1937). Interpersonal communication through mass meetings, health education sessions, and individual contacts with public health professionals reinforced the annual theme and messages during the week. Themes chosen for the annual observance illustrated an appreciation for the multiple levels of intervention necessary to improve black health status. Among them were, in 1929, "a complete health examination for everybody"; in 1932, "help yourself and your community to better health"; in 1935, "the family and home as the unit of community health"; in 1936, "the child and the school as factors in community health"; and in 1939, "the citizen's responsibility for community health" (Brown, 1937; Vonderlehr, 1939).

Each year, the PHS created a set of standardized materials that were supplemented with local materials from public health departments and voluntary organizations. Standard materials included (1) the *National Negro Health Week News*, published quarterly after 1933; (2) the NNHW poster; (3) the NNHW school leaflet; (4) the NNHW radio broadcast; and (5) the NNHW sermon. The materials featured that year's theme and were available to NNHW committees at no cost.

For example, for the twentieth anniversary of National Negro Health Week, the official poster featured a photograph of Booker T. Washington with the theme inscribed: "Let Us Honor Him with the Fruits of Our Endeavors" (PHS, 1933b). Illustrated leaflets were prepared for students to stimulate their participation in the health week poster contest for the upcoming year's observance (PHS, 1933b). School leaflets illustrated to engage children's interest featured a health education message.

Radio broadcasts, prepared for use by local stations, often featured an interview with a PHS official such as the surgeon general. Representatives from other sponsoring groups such as the National Association of Colored Graduate Nurses also participated in broadcasts (PHS, 1945). Topics included the history of the week, the health status of blacks, and a call for more effective health practices. Local broadcasts featuring individuals involved in a specific community's observance expanded beyond a discussion of the history and health status of blacks to announce local activities. These local broadcasts also reflected the breadth of involvement at the community level. John Turner, a physician in Philadelphia, observed during his April 8, 1944, broadcast interview on station WPEN that "during the week from April 9 to 16, practically every Negro agency for uplift in Philadelphia was or will be the center of activity featuring some phase of program relating to National Negro Health Week. Some of these agencies are our two hospitals—Douglass and Mercy—YWCA and YMCA, Health Centers, churches, beautician and barber headquarters" (PHS, 1944, p. 9).

In recognition of the key role of the black church, the official sermon was published and distributed to communities for their use. As a 1933 *National Negro Health News* editorial stated, "The church can render a most helpful service in the Health Week Anniversary by making occasional announcements and by starting the Health Week proper with a good message to the church assemblies of the day" (PHS, 1933b, p. 9). Local central committees often had a subcommittee for church involvement that would issue a call for involvement of local pastors. Building upon the week's theme, the official sermon combined health education with scripture and gave religious support to the week's activities.

The modern concern with cultural sensitivity in public health programs was certainly a critical issue during NNHW. In 1923, Roscoe Brown described an exhibit created for the 1922 health week activities, stating that "the 'Keeping Fit' exhibit for colored boys and young men is an adaptation of the original exhibit with no less content of the ideals of physical fitness but with subjects of the colored population to make the challenge and appeal more personal" (p. 13). Announcements for each year's observance included photographs of activities conducted at the local level in the previous year's observance.

NNHW Program Evaluation Methods

The NNHW provided a model for process and impact evaluation across multiple communities and organizations. The PHS distributed standardized reporting forms for activities that asked about the following broad categories: (1) objectives; (2) community and home clean-up activities; (3) educational activities, including numbers of lectures, exhibits, and sermons, numbers in attendance, and the number of educational brochures distributed; (4) attendance at practical—clinic visits, and community health events; (5) local prizes awarded; (6) other accomplishments; (7) field service, which included the number of organizations participating, community exhibits, and associated lectures and conferences; and (8) media coverage (articles, photos, and so forth). Though the final report on activities was dependent on reporting by local or state NNHW committees, the 1933 statistical report provides evidence of the breadth of activities. In twenty-five participating states, there were 2,941 lectures attended by 269,572 people; 3,872 outhouses improved or constructed; and 477 health clinics conducted (PHS, 1933c). In recognition of community efforts for the week, the awards committee gave certificates of merit, trophies, and medals for various levels of effort.

Implications for Health Promotion in the Black Community Today

Ultimately, National Negro Health Week evolved into a comprehensive year-round program, the National Negro Health Movement, that integrated community development, health education, professional training, and health policy initiatives—all designed to improve black health status. The movement came under the auspices of the Office of Negro Health Work in the U.S. Public Health Service, and when the move toward integration led to the dismantling of the office in 1951, the National Negro Health Movement came to an end. Although the week and the movement were not without their critics during their time, their thirty-five-year history represents the longest sustained health promotion and disease prevention campaign for black Americans in public health history. A historical look at the week provides some valuable lessons for public health professionals seeking to reduce the excess morbidity and mortality experienced by the African American community today.

Too often today as we work in the arena of categorical funding for programs, the broader scope of issues that affect the health of a community are neglected.

The NNHW broadly defined its scope as ranging from environmental and sanitation issues and individual behavior to efforts to increase the numbers of black health professionals and promote access to care. This range is not inconsistent with the recommendations of the *Report of the Secretary's Task Force on Black and Minority Health* (DHHS, 1985), which emphasized health education, research on individual risk factors, and training of black health professionals. The broad scope of the NNHW also reflects closely the breadth of issues uncovered today when community members are full participants in defining their own health agendas.

Addressing the disparity in health status is an awesome task that is too frequently undertaken by local health departments and a few community organizations. The NNHW was sustained by and flourished because of the broad-based participation of a multitude of organizations from schools, churches, businesses, and work sites to local health departments, professional associations, the media, and civic groups. Although the week originated at Tuskegee Institute, support from the PHS was critical to sustaining the effort over time. Nevertheless, along with the standardized materials and framework for the week's observance, local communities also had the freedom to modify their activities to suit their needs. This combination of governmental support, collaboration among a multitude of organizations, and freedom to develop a campaign appropriate to individual communities suggests a model for community-based public health campaigns today.

Today, efforts to acquire funding for health promotion programs are dependent upon identifying the needs and deficits of the black community. Although it is critical to identify needs, focusing solely on those needs can have a demoralizing effect when communities are made to feel that only outside assistance can address their concerns. Furthermore, a focus on needs and deficits, particularly as we have seen today in the portrayal of violence in the black community by the mass media, can result in people's not focusing on the needs but seeing whole communities as deficient or bankrupt. Through its use of internal resources and indigenous organizations, the NNHW provides a model for building on the strengths of black communities. Drawing on racial pride and the hopes of the black community for progress provided a positive tone and goal for the week. At the same time, even though racial pride was clearly a motivating factor, it was not emphasized to the exclusion of collaborative efforts with white organizations. If today's public health campaigns can draw on racial pride and strengths and assets in the black community and also work in interracial coalitions, we will enhance our likelihood of success. (See Braithwaite, Taylor, and Austin, *Building Health Coalitions in the Black Community*, 2000, for a more comprehensive discussion of the viability of health coalitions in the black community.)

The National Negro Health Week provides a valuable lesson in cultural sensitivity for those seeking to work successfully with the African American community. Although cultural sensitivity frequently begins and ends with materials development for health education programs, the NNHW's reliance on credible black institutions and local community leaders demonstrates how sensitivity includes community empowerment. Public health professionals can play a supportive role to those in the black community with the necessary credibility to reach the populations in greatest need. (Resnicow and Braithwaite, in Chapter Twenty-Five in this volume offer a more theory-grounded discussion of cultural sensitivity in health promotion programming.)

The complexities of race and health today mirror similar concerns from the period of the NNHW. Though the week's observance was a prime example of the creation of services and health promotion campaigns embedded in the black community, leaders of the black community simultaneously demanded universal access to care during the days of segregation. This same duality is very much evident today, as calls for culturally sensitive and community-based programs must be blended with a continuing demand for full access to health care. Furthermore, the activism of those who were involved in the week suggests the advocacy necessary to ensure that as managed care becomes the predominant system of health insurance in this country, the populations that are most vulnerable and therefore most costly to care for are fully incorporated into that system.

Today, many poor black communities have suffered from the flight of those middle-class blacks no longer restricted by segregation. However, the middle-class black activists responsible for planning and implementing the NNHW in many communities saw their fate tied to that of those blacks less educated and poorer, and the lesson of the NNHW suggests that middle-class blacks must use their resources and skills to work with communities still struggling with poverty and inequality.

Where Do We Go from Here?

Even though National Negro Health Week ended over forty years ago, its significance is still honored today. In April 1994, the Ohio Commission on Minority Health called for celebration of the seventy-ninth anniversary of National Negro Health Week during Ohio's annual Minority Health Month. In identifying National Negro Health Week as "the forerunner to Minority Health Month," the commission stated, "To the best of our knowledge, Negro Health Week was the beginning of the minority health movement in the U.S." (Ohio Commission on Minority Health, 1994, back cover).

Just as Booker T. Washington believed that the health of black America was tied to African Americans' economic progress and social acceptance into the broader society, we believe that the health status of black people is still indelibly bound to the role African Americans play in the nation today and their role in our country's future. Advances in medical science have not removed the possibility that a large segment of black America will continue to suffer from preventable death even while standing in the shadow of a medical wonder world. Over fifty years ago, *National Negro Health News* stated: "It is a time for remembering the health of the race and how essential it is to our racial progress. There is no better time to think of this than now, when we shall need every racial resource to make the progress we should make in these days" (PHS, 1943b, p. 6). On October 31, 2000, the United States Congress directed the National Institutes of Health to establish a center to study health disparities among the nation's minority populations. "Equal access to health care is not a privilege, it is a fundamental right," said Representative John Lewis, D-GA ("Congress approves . . . ," 2000). Thus, at the dawn of a new century the African Americans have appealed to moral responsibility and congressional mandate to improve the health status of blacks and other minority populations.

We call upon public health professionals to examine black history for guidance and to join with the African American community now in an interracial coalition to promote health and prevent disease among African Americans. When we accept the moral imperative to improve the health status of poorly served, underserved, and never served segments of our society, we truly demonstrate the principles of public health as social justice. From this perspective the National Negro Health Movement represents a significant contribution from African Americans to the history of public health—a contribution worthy of replication today.

References

Benedek, T., & Erlen, J. (1999). The scientific environment of the Tuskegee Study of Syphilis, 1920–1960. *Perspectives in Biology and Medicine, 43*(1), 1–30.

Braithwaite, R. L., Taylor, S. E., and Austin, J. N. (2000). *Building health coalitions in the black community*. Thousand Oaks, CA: Sage.

Brown, R. (1923). The work of the U.S. Public Health Service with Negroes. *Opportunity 1,* 12–13.

Brown, R. (1937). The National Negro Health Week movement. *Journal of Negro Education, 6,* 553–564.

Clinton, W. (1997). *Remarks by the president in apology for study done in Tuskegee*. Washington, DC: The White House, Office of the Press Secretary.

Congress approves center to study health disparities. (2000, October 31). *Associated Press Wire Service.*

Du Bois, W.E.B. (1906). *The health and physique of the Negro American*. Atlanta, GA.: Atlanta University Press.

Dublin, L. (1928). The health of the Negro. *Opportunity, 2,* 198–200, 216.

Falicov, C. (1995). Training to think culturally: A multidimensional comparative framework. *Family Process, 34,* 375–381.

Gamble, V., & Fletcher, J. (1996). *Final report of the Tuskegee Syphilis Legacy Committee*. Atlanta, GA: Centers for Disease Control and Prevention.

Goodwin, N. (2000). The presidential initiative to eliminate racial and ethnic disparities in health: An interview with the surgeon general of the United States, David Satcher. *Health Promotion Practice, 1*(1), 29–31.

Jackson, A. (1924). The need for health education among Negroes. *Opportunity, 2,* 235–237.

Jones, J. H. (1993). *Bad blood: The Tuskegee syphilis experiment*. (2nd ed.). New York: Free Press.

Joseph-Di Caprio, J., Garwick, A., Kohrman, C., & Blum, R. (1999). Culture and the care of children with chronic conditions: Their physicians' views. *Archives of Pediatrics and Adolescent Medicine, 153,* 1030–1035.

Ohio Commission on Minority Health. (1994). *April 1994 calendar of events: Minority Health Month.* Columbus, OH: Author.

Patterson, F. (1939, April–June). [Statement concerning National Negro Health Week.] *National Negro Health News, 7,* 13.

Saraf, J. (Ed.). (1997). *Concept and components of culture.* (15th ed., vol. 16). Chicago: Encyclopaedia Britannica, 874–893.

Thomas, J., Clark, M., Robinson, J., Monnett, M., Kilmarx, P., & Peterman, T. (1999). The social ecology of syphilis. *Social Science and Medicine, 48*(8), 1081–1094.

Thomas, J., & Thomas, K. (1999). Things ain't what they ought to be: Social forces underlying racial disparities in rates of sexually transmitted diseases in a rural North Carolina county. *Social Science and Medicine, 49*(8), 1075–1084.

Thomas, S., & Quinn, S. (1991). The Tuskegee Syphilis Study, 1932–1972: Implications for HIV education and AIDS risk education programs in the black community. *American Journal of Public Health, 81,* 1498–1505.

Thomas, S., & Quinn, S. (1997). Presidential apology for the study at Tuskegee. *1998 Medical and Health Annual.* Chicago: Encylopaedia Britannica.

Thomas, S., & Quinn, S. (2000). Light on the shadow of the syphilis study at Tuskegee. *Health Promotion Practice, 1*(3), 234–237.

U.S. Department of Health and Human Services. (1998). *Health Care RX: Access for all: The president's initiative on race.* Rockville, MD: Health Resources and Services Administration.

U.S. Department of Health and Human Services. Task Force on Black and Minority Health. (1985). *Report of the Secretary's Task Force on Black and Minority Health* (Vol. 1, Executive Summary). Washington, DC: U.S. Government Printing Office.

U.S. Public Health Service. (1926). *National Negro Health Week announcement, April 4 to 10, 1926: The Twelfth Annual Observance* [Brochure]. Washington, DC: U.S. Government Printing Office.

U.S. Public Health Service. (1933a). [Editorial.] *National Negro Health News, 1,* 9.

U.S. Public Health Service. (1933b). The 1934 health week. *National Negro Health News, 1,* 7.

U.S. Public Health Service. (1933c). Statistical report. *National Negro Health News, 1,* 2–3.

U.S. Public Health Service. (1937). Cooperation of newspapers in the health week publicity. *National Negro Health News, 5,* 19.

U.S. Public Health Service. (1943a). Application: National Negro Health Week poster contest. *National Negro Health News, 11,* 23.

U.S. Public Health Service. (1943b). Health and race progress. *National Negro Health News, 11,* 6.

U.S. Public Health Service. (1944). National Negro Health Week: A radio broadcast. *National Negro Health News, 12,* 9–10.

U.S. Public Health Service. (1945). 1945 National Negro Health Week recorded radio broadcast. *National Negro Health News, 13,* 1–2.

U.S. Public Health Service. (1950). The National Negro Health Movement. *National Negro Health News, 18,* 1–6.

Vonderlehr R. (1939). The citizen's responsibility for community health. *National Negro Health News, 7,* 1–3.

White, R. (1999). Grand dragon or windmill: Why I opposed the presidential apology for the Tuskegee study. *Journal of the National Medical Association, 89*(11), 719–720.

White, R. (2000). Unraveling the Tuskegee study of untreated syphilis. *Archives of Internal Medicine, 160,* 585–598.

Yax, L. K. (1999). *National Estimates: Annual population estimates by sex, race, and hispanic origin, selected years from 1990 to 1998.* Washington, DC: U.S. Bureau of the Census, Population Division.

AFTERWORD

John E. Maupin Jr.

The authors assembled for this edition of *Health Issues in the Black Community* provide an awesome mosaic of the health challenges facing the African American population. This collective work by some of America's most respected scholars and experts on health issues that confront communities of color examines the problems and experiences of blacks in the health care system. While not intended as an exhaustive glossary of all the diseases and health conditions that disproportionately affect black America, this edition more than adequately explores the breadth and depth of a wide variety of contemporary health issues and concerns.

Using epidemiological data, various chapters examine specific health problems while others focus on the health issues of specific subpopulations in the black community. In addition, this book critically examines the environmental and behavioral forces that have an impact on the condition of an individual's health—and shape the health status and practices of a community. The data presented herein further underscore the fact that gender, age, and environment all create differential health experiences.

This edition also focuses on the context and nature of barriers to care as well as effective intervention strategies. More important, however, both individually and collectively the authors also present an excellent discourse on the dynamic interplay between the physical, social, psychological, and spiritual elements that create the well-being of individuals and groups in their various environments.

The variety of subjects covered and the authors' style differences in presenting them help highlight the complexity of the challenges that affect communities of color. The data presented in this book reaffirm one conclusion: America has been, and remains, a country divided by inequities in health care. The supposition that health care reflects the general condition and quality of life within a given population or subpopulation is reiterated throughout the book. Each author provides evidence that health care reflects the matrix of social, economic, and political influences that divide American society.

Furthermore, the multidisciplinary approaches presented in this book effectively convey the magnitude of the problem and the urgency. While we contemplate the approaches and strategies put forth by the authors, we must also recognize the new threats impinging on the quality of life for all Americans. In the midst of the aforementioned complexities, science is discovering more strains of bacterial and viral infections with increased resistance to the medicines with which to combat them. In addition to addressing this concern, we must also contend with diseases brought to our shores by increased global travel and commerce.

The World Health Organization defines health as "a state of complete physical, mental, and social well-being and not merely the absence of disease or infirmity." Reading this book and focusing on the word "complete" in this definition makes one question whether it is possible to ever achieve a healthy life given the nonsupportive environment in which most blacks live. The problem of race-based health status disparity is of course not new. Such disparities have remained a consistent reality.

Fortunately, each chapter of this book also conveys a sense of hope grounded in the presentation of a variety of culturally-sensitive intervention strategies designed to ameliorate health status inequities, foster healthier lifestyles, and encourage good health practices. I, too, have a sense of hope based on commitments from private foundations to fund scholarly efforts that attempt to explain why inequities in health status continue to exist. I am encouraged by the growing number of biomedical scientists committed to investigating the disproportionately high levels of disease and disability. And last, but not least, I am encouraged by the increased level of federal sensitivity, understanding, and—more important—funding specifically targeted toward making a difference. "Healthy People 2010" signals a new level of commitment by the federal government to address this disgraceful state of affairs.

The second chapter, written by Alwyn T. Cohall and Hope E. Bannister, "The Health Status of Children and Adolescents," discusses a holistic approach to health status inequities that examines and modifies the social context of African American children and adolescents. The authors also provide a useful model in designing a more comprehensive, systematic effort of sustained intensity and duration. This approach appropriately emphasizes the following areas: building social capital; improving access to care; training health care professionals; improving screening, management referral, and coordination of care; reducing environmental hazards; and improving life options. Cohall and Bannister also stated that failure to aggressively "counter the pathogens of poverty, lack of health insurance, and cultural insensitivity is no less a disgrace than withholding treatment for syphilis. While the cure for health disparities is not as simple as a shot of penicillin, there are concrete, tangible efforts that can be made today."

We are also aptly reminded in the last chapter of the book that time is of the essence. As quoted from the *National Negro Health News* published fifty years ago, "It is a time for remembering the health of the race and how essential it is to our racial progress. There is no better time to think of this than now when we shall need every racial resource to make the progress we should make in these days" (U.S. Public Health Service, 1943, p. 6). Reducing health disparities will not only require individual responsibility but a broad approach that includes the four estates of society: clergy, academia, government, and media. Therefore, assuring health is the responsibility and obligation of everyone.

Reference

U.S. Public Health Service. (1943). Health and race progress. *National Negro Health News, 11*, 6.

Nashville, Tennessee　　　　　　　　　John E. Maupin Jr.
April 2001　　　　　　　　　　　　　President, Meharry Medical College

NAME INDEX

SUBJECT INDEX

A

"AAN Expert Panel Report," 516, 517, 533

Abortion, 23, 254, 255

Abstinence-based interventions, 318–322, 336

Abt Associates, 484, 486

Abuse. *See* Child abuse; Domestic violence

Academic performance and achievement, 29, 412; and asthma, 291, 294–295; cigarette smokers and, 356; and stigma of inferiority, 112

Access to care disparity, overview of, 3

Accident mortality rates: age adjusted, *8, 9*; for children and adolescents, *16, 17, 18*, 19, 37; for men, 62, 70

Accidental and intentional injuries: mortality rates for, by cause, 19; preventing, 34–35

Acculturation, 109; defined, 518

Acquired immune deficiency syndrome (AIDS). *See* HIV/AIDS

Action stage, defined, 357

Active lifestyle approach, 456, 457, 459

"Additional Protections for Children Involved as Subjects in Research," 497, 499

Adherence and compliance: in asthma treatment, 287, 288; in diabetes treatment, 237–238; in dietary change interventions, 438; in physical activity interventions, 454, 456; in tuberculosis treatment, 275–276

Adolescents. *See* Children and adolescents

Adult Health Day, 553

Adult-supervised recreational activities, 35

Adventist Health Study, 434

Advisory Committee on Diet, Nutrition, and Cancer Prevention, 441

Advocating practices, *138–141*, 145

Aerobic programs, success of, 455

African American Action Team, 368–369

African American Health Issues Forum, 75

African American Male Initiative, 75

African history, study of, incorporating, 526

African proverb, 412

African tribes, modern-day, churches as, 142

African-American Breast-Cancer Alliance, 222

Afrocentric principles, basing programs on, 337, 338, 368, 381, 526

Agency for Health Care Policy and Research (AHCPR), 371

Agency for Healthcare Research and Quality, 64, 78

Agency for Toxic Substances and Disease Registry (ATSDR), 472, 476, 477, 478, 486

Agent Orange experiments, 492, 494

Aggravated assault, 25, 154

Aggressive behavior, and lead poisoning, 22

Aging, understanding, life-course approach to, 81–92

Agricultural Research Service, 447

Aid to Families with Dependent Children (AFDC), 33, 432. *See also* Welfare reform

AIDS Project, 147

Air pollution: and asthma, 21, 285, 292, 299, 482–485; distribution of, 478; in urban areas, *484*

Alan Guttmacher Institute, 14, 23, 38, 333, 339